S0-AYV-112

Phil Stoddart

    With kind regards

and good wishes for the

future

           J. Mustarde

16/12/71

PLASTIC SURGERY
IN INFANCY AND CHILDHOOD

PLASTIC SURGERY
IN INFANCY AND CHILDHOOD

EDITOR

JOHN CLARK MUSTARDÉ

B.Sc., M.B., Ch.B. (Distinct.), D.O.M.S., F.R.C.S. (Eng.), F.R.C.S. (Glas.)

Consultant Plastic Surgeon to West of Scotland Plastic
Surgery Unit, Canniesburn Hospital, Glasgow; Ballochmyle Hospital, Ayrshire; Royal Hospital for Sick Children, Yorkhill, Glasgow; Seafield Sick Children's
Hospital, Ayrshire

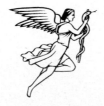

E. & S. LIVINGSTONE
EDINBURGH AND LONDON
1971

© Longman Group Limited, 1971

All rights reserved. No part of this publication may be
reproduced, stored in a retrieval system, or transmitted
in any form or by any means, electronic, mechanical,
photocopying, recording or otherwise, without the prior
permission of the publishers (E. & S. Livingstone, Teviot
Place, Edinburgh)

ISBN 0 443 00724 1

Printed in Great Britain

PREFACE

The past ten to fifteen years have seen considerable changes in the scope and function of the plastic surgeon. On the one hand, much that was formerly regarded as basic plastic surgery practice is now, as a result of enlightened post-graduate training, performed as a routine by surgeons in other disciplines, and the application of skin grafts or the usage of local flaps is no longer the prerogative of the plastic surgeon. Offsetting this, however, there has been a growing involvement of the plastic surgeon in problems hitherto considered to be outwith his normal field. The recent rapid development of neurosurgery-plastic surgery techniques for correction of gross cranio-facial deformities, the greater involvement of the plastic surgeon in urological problems affecting the urethra and bladder, and the increasing acceptance of responsibility for the whole spectrum of surgery of the hand are but three examples of this widening of the plastic surgery horizon.

Although advances have been made in almost every aspect of plastic surgery it is probable that it is in the treatment of congenital defects that the greatest strides forward have been made, both with regard to the increased scope of the plastic surgeon within the field itself, and, perhaps more important, with regard to the intensity of effort being applied to the development of more satisfactory techniques. Inevitably the literature concerned with this aspect of plastic surgery has been growing rapidly, and with the constant increase in the number of new journals in which communications concerning these problems may be published the surgeon who is called on to deal with this type of work is faced with a considerable problem if he is to keep up-to-date with current thought and practice.

As the majority of congenital deformities are treated in childhood the expanding field of plastic surgery particular to children has inevitably become almost a sub-specialty, and it has been apparent for some time that there was a need for the production of a publication which would gather together in the convenient vehicle of a single volume as much of modern thought and experience on the subject as seems of practical value. Such a book should by definition be confined to plastic surgery as it applies to children, with all the considerable differences in growth potential and healing that children possess, and it should not merely be a repetition of procedures to be found in any standard work on plastic surgery in general. Where surgical management and operative treatment are the same as in adults, this should be briefly stated and no further elaboration made: it should draw comparisons between the two regimes where necessary, but, whilst stating in detail what should be done for child patients, must ruthlessly eschew any tendency to become merely another text-book on plastic surgery with a bias towards the treatment of children.

Despite the fact that the scope of this book is limited to plastic surgery in infancy and childhood, this field of surgery is in itself already too wide for any one individual to be able to write authoritatively on all of its aspects. By inviting the views of twenty-seven different contributors, all of whom are recognised as undoubted experts in the particular subjects concerning which they have written, it is hoped that, whilst this inevitably gives rise to considerable variations in style and quality of writing, the reader will find the best of current thought on every aspect of the field.

The use of addenda to certain chapters, whilst perhaps an innovation, has enabled what is believed to be relevant material from sources other than the main contributor to be included: in only one instance was this practice objected to and the addendum to that particular chapter was omitted. Although the context of each chapter was fairly well-defined at the outset, it became obvious in time that a number of the contributions would inevitably overlap. Where the overlap was merely repetitious an attempt has been made to set a balance in the editing—without, it is hoped, giving offence to any whose work has been thus mutilated—but where the overlap seemed to be of value, in that it put forward a different point of view, it has been retained.

In a single volume it is not possible to include numerous alternative operations, nor was this ever intended, and the contributors were each invited to produce a practical, working blue-print rather than an exhaustive study of their separate subjects. Sufficient references have been included, however, to allow the reader to carry out a more detailed study if he so desires. For some a favourite technique may have been omitted, or a technique advocated with which they do not agree: this must be inevitable if the size of the work is restricted to a single volume and this last consideration was regarded as a basic essential, from the point of view of convenience as well as cost, when the project was originally planned.

The inclusion of certain subjects, such as ectopia vesicae and spina bifida may be regarded as stretching the boundary of plastic surgery in children beyond the usual limits. It is hoped, however, that the book will prove of value, not only to plastic surgeons, but to paediatric surgeons, oral surgeons and general surgeons, and indeed to all who may be called on to carry out this type of work on children. To this end the list of contributors includes several eminent paediatric and oral surgeons who have helped to produce a broader, more widely acceptable viewpoint, and to them, as to each of the plastic surgeons who have helped to make the publication of this book possible, I extend my sincere thanks. I should like to acknowledge the very considerable debt I owe to Mrs Hilda Dennison for the long hours of work entailed in preparing the index.

1971   J. C. M.

LIST OF CONTRIBUTORS

J. E. ADAMSON

M.D., F.A.C.S.
Chief, Division of Plastic Surgery, Norfolk General Hospital, Norfolk, Virginia; Consultant in Plastic Surgery, United States Naval Hospitals, Bethesda, Maryland and Portsmouth, Virginia.

A. J. BARSKY

D.D.S., M.D.
Professor of Plastic Surgery, Albert Einstein College of Medicine, New York; Visiting Surgeon, Chief of Plastic Surgery, Albert Einstein Affiliated Hospitals, New York; Attending Surgeon, Chief of Plastic Surgery, Beth Israel Hospital, New York.

W. R. BURSTON

Ph.D., D.Orth.R.C.S., L.D.S.
Consultant Orthodontist, Paediatric and Plastic Surgery Units, the United Liverpool Hospitals and Liverpool Regional Hospital Board; Honorary Lecturer in Child Health, University of Liverpool.

JOHN MARQUIS CONVERSE

M.D.
Lawrence D. Bell Professor of Plastic Surgery, Institute of Reconstructive Plastic Surgery, New York University Medical Centre; Chief of Department of Plastic Surgery and Ophthalmology, Manhattan Eye, Ear and Throat Hospital.

W. M. DENNISON

M.D., F.R.C.S. (Ed.), F.R.C.S. (Glasg.), F.A.A.P. (Hon).
Barclay Lecturer in Surgery of Infancy and Childhood, University of Glasgow; Senior Surgeon and Chairman of the Division of Surgery, Royal Hospital for Sick Children and Surgical Paediatric Unit, Stobhill Hospital, Glasgow; Paediatric Surgeon, Royal Maternity Hospital, Glasgow.

A. J. EVANS

F.R.C.S.
Consultant Plastic Surgeon, Plastic Surgery and Burns Centre, Queen Mary's Hospital, Roehampton, London and the S.W. Metropolitan Regional Hospital Board.

P. FOGH-ANDERSEN

M.D.
Plastic Surgeon, Queen Louise's Children's Hospital and Deaconess Hospital, Copenhagen.

G. FRANCESCONI

L.D.
Director of the Department of Plastic Surgery, Hospital of Lucca; Consultant in Plastic Surgery, Dermatological Clinic, University of Pisa; Lecturer in Plastic Surgery, University of Milan.

T. GIBSON

F.R.C.S. (Ed.), F.R.C.S. (Glasg.).

Regional Director, West of Scotland Plastic Surgery Unit, Canniesburn Hospital, Glasgow; Visiting Professor, Bio-Engineering Unit, University of Strathclyde; Consultant Plastic Surgeon, Western Infirmary, Glasgow; Senior Lecturer in Tissue Transplantation, Glasgow University.

C. E. HORTON

M.D., F.A.C.S.

President of the Educational Foundation of the American Society of Plastic and Reconstructive Surgeons, Inc.; Consultant to U.S. Naval Hospitals, Bethesda, Maryland and Portsmouth, Virginia; Consultant, U.S. Public Health Hospital, Norfolk, Virginia.

I. T. JACKSON

F.R.C.S. (Glasg.), F.R.C.S. (Ed.).

Consultant Plastic Surgeon, West of Scotland Plastic Surgery Unit, Canniesburn Hospital, Glasgow.

W. K. LINDSAY

M.D., B.Sc., F.R.C.S. (C), F.A.C.S., M.S.

Associate Professor, Department of Surgery, University of Toronto; Chairman, Inter-Hospital Coordinating Committee for Plastic Surgery, Department of Surgery, University of Toronto; Chief, Division of Plastic Surgery, The Hospital for Sick Children, Toronto.

D. N. MATTHEWS

O.B.E., M.D., M.Ch., F.R.C.S.

Surgeon in Charge of Plastic Surgery, University College Hospital, London; Plastic Surgeon, Hospital for Sick Children and Royal Masonic Hospital; Civilian Consultant in Plastic Surgery to the Royal Navy.

R. A. MLADICK

M.D.

Attending Surgeon and Director of Head and Neck Tumor Clinic, Norfolk General Hospital, Norfolk, Virginia; Consultant, Hampton V.A. Hospital, Portsmouth Naval Hospital and U.S. Public Health Hospital, Norfolk, Virginia.

J. C. MUSTARDÉ

B.Sc., D.O.M.S., F.R.C.S. (Eng.), F.R.C.S. (Glasg.).

Consultant Plastic Surgeon, West of Scotland Plastic Surgery Unit, Canniesburn Hospital, Glasgow, Ballochmyle Hospital and Seafield Sick Children's Hospital, Ayrshire, and Royal Hospital for Sick Children, Yorkhill, Glasgow.

H. H. NIXON

M.A., F.R.C.S.

Consultant Paediatric Surgeon, Hospital for Sick Children and St. Mary's Children's Hospital, London.

H. L. OBWEGESER
M.D., D.M.D.

Professor and Chief of Oral and Maxillofacial Surgery and Chief of Oral Diagnosis, Zahnärztliches Institut, University of Zurich.

I. P. TANGUY
M.D.

Professor of Plastic Surgery, Catholic University of Rio de Janeiro; Chief of Plastic Surgery Department, Santa Casa de Misericordia General Hospital.

J. RANSOHOFF
M.D.

Consultant, Department of Neurosurgery, New York Uuiversity Medical Center.

T. D. REES
M.D., F.A.C.S.

Associate Professor of Clinical Surgery (Plastic), New York University School of Medicine.

P. P. RICKHAM
M.D., M.S., F.R.C.S., D.C.H.

Senior Consultant Paediatric Surgeon, Alder Hey Children's Hospital, Liverpool; Director of Paediatric Surgical Studies, University of Liverpool.

BLAIR O. ROGERS
B.A., M.D.

Attending Surgeon, Department of Plastic Surgery, Manhattan Eye, Ear and Throat Hospital, New York City; Assistant Professor of Clinical Surgery, Institute of Reconstructive Plastic Surgery, New York University School of Medicine; Consultant in Plastic Surgery to the United Nations Medical Staff, New York City.

N. L. ROWE
F.D.S.R.C.S. (Eng., Ed. and Glasg.), L.R.C.P., M.R.C.S., L.M.S.S.A.

Consultant in Oral Surgery, the Westminster Hospital, Queen Mary's Hospital, Roehampton and the Institute of Dental Surgery, London; Civilian Consultant to the Royal Navy and the British Army.

P. TESSIER
M.D.

Surgeon in Charge, Plastic Surgery Department, Hospital Foch Suresnes, Paris.

D. I. WILLIAMS
M.D., M.Ch. (Camb.), F.R.C.S.

Genito-Urinary Surgeon, The Hospital for Sick Children and St. Peter's Hospital, London.

G. B. WINTER

B.S., B.D.S., F.D.S.R.C.S., D.C.H.
Professor of Children's Dentistry of the University of London; Honorary Consultant Dental Surgeon, Eastman Dental Hospital and Queen Elizabeth Hospital for Children, London.

D. WOOD-SMITH

F.R.C.S.E.
Consultant, Institute of Reconstructive Plastic Surgery, New York University Medical Center.

CONTENTS

Section 1
HEAD AND NECK

CHAPTER   PAGE

I   HARE LIP AND CLEFT PALATE   D. N. Matthews   1

II   THE EARLY ORTHODONTIC TREATMENT OF CLEFT LIP AND PALATE IN INFANTS   W. R. Burston   37

III   DEFORMITIES OF THE JAWS   H. L. Obwegeser   46

IV   VERTICAL AND OBLIQUE FACIAL CLEFTS (ORBITO-FACIAL FISSURES)   P. Tessier   94

V   LIPS, TONGUE AND FLOOR OF MOUTH   W. K. Lindsay   102

VI   TUMOURS OF THE JAW IN CHILDHOOD   N. L. Rowe and G. B. Winter   130

VII   TRAUMATIC LESIONS OF THE JAWS AND TEETH   N. L. Rowe and G. B. Winter   154

VIII   OSTEITIS OF THE MAXILLA   W. M. Dennison   176

IX   FACIAL INJURIES IN CHILDREN   J. M. Converse   178
          Addendum: THE FORESHORTENED NOSE   J. C. Mustardé   202

X   THE ORBITAL REGION   J. C. Mustardé   207

XI   HYPERTELORISM   P. Tessier   238
          Addendum 1: ONE-STAGE CRANIOFACIAL OSTEOTOMY IN HYPERTELORISM WITH PARAMEDIAN RESECTION AND PRESERVATION OF THE OLFACTORY NERVES   J. M. Converse and J. Ransohoff   248
          Addendum 2: CORRECTION OF MINOR DEGREES OF HYPERTELORISM   J. C. Mustardé   251

XII   CRANIO-FACIAL DYSOSTOSIS (DISEASES OF CROUZON AND APERT)   P. Tessier   254

XIII   THE NOSE   A. J. Barsky   261
          Addendum: BIFID NOSE: HEMI-ABSENCE OF NOSE   G. Francesconi   268

XIV   CORRECTIVE AND RECONSTRUCTIVE SURGERY IN DEFORMITIES OF THE AURICLE IN CHILDREN   J. M. Converse and D. Wood-Smith   274
          Addendum: CORRECTION OF PROMINENT EARS USING BURIED MATTRESS SUTURES   J. C. Mustardé   306

XV   CONGENITAL FACIAL PARALYSIS (PALSY): UNILATERAL AND BILATERAL   Blair O. Rogers   314

CHAPTER   PAGE

XVI   SPECIAL PROBLEMS OF FACIAL PARALYSIS IN CHILDHOOD: THE USE OF THE STERNOCLEIDOMASTOID MUSCLE C. E. Horton, J. E. Adamson and R. A. Mladick   322

XVII   FACIAL HEMIATROPHY IN CHILDHOOD T. D. Rees   326

XVIII   FACIAL HEMIATROPHY (THE USE OF AUTOGENOUS MATERIALS) I. Pitanguy   332

XIX   ACQUIRED FACIAL HEMI-HYPERTROPHY (HEMI-GIGANTISM) J. C. Mustardé   337

XX   CONGENITAL SCALP DEFECTS. R. A. Mladick, C. E. Horton, and J. E. Adamson   345

XXI   CRANIUM BIFIDUM P. P. Rickham   348

XXII   HYDROCEPHALUS IN CHILDHOOD P. P. Rickham   352

XXIII   THE NECK W. K. Lindsay   360

SECTION 2
TRUNK

XXIV   SPINA BIFIDA W. M. Dennison   381

XXV   THE SURGICAL TREATMENT OF SPINA BIFIDA J. C. Mustardé   386

XXVI   HYPOSPADIAS C. E. Horton   396

XXVII   EPISPADIAS AND EXSTROPHY D. I. Williams   427

XXVIII VAGINAL AGENESIS P. Fogh-Andersen   437

XXIX   HERMAPHRODITISM AND PROBLEMS OF SEXUAL DEFINITION R. A. Mladick, C. E. Horton and J. E. Adamson   443

XXX   SACROCOCCYGEAL TERATOMA, DERMAL SINUS AND POSTANAL PITS H. H. Nixon   447

XXXI   PLASTIC SURGERY OF THE INFANTILE AND ADOLESCENT BREAST C. E. Horton, J. E. Adamson and R. A. Mladick   452

SECTION 3
LIMBS

XXXII   THE UPPER EXTREMITY A. J. Barsky   463

XXIII   THE LOWER EXTREMITY A. J. Barsky   509

CHAPTER PAGE

SECTION 4
GENERAL

XXXIV PIGMENTED NAEVI T. Gibson 514

XXXV HAEMANGIOMA T. Gibson 519

XXXVI LYMPHANGIOMA W. M. Dennison 526

XXXVII THE TREATMENT OF BURNS IN INFANCY AND CHILDHOOD
A. J. Evans 531

XXXVIII KELOIDS AND HYPERTROPHIC SCARS I. T. Jackson 561

XXXIX SCLERODERMA J. E. Adamson, C. E. Horton and R. A.
Mladick 566

XL UNRECOGNISED TRAUMA IN INFANTS AND CHILDREN W. M.
Dennison 572

INDEX 575

SECTION 1

HEAD AND NECK

CHAPTER I

HARE LIP AND CLEFT PALATE

INCIDENCE AND AETIOLOGY

The bald statement that the average incidence in the newborn of a deformity of lip or palate, or both, is one in one thousand live births gives no conception of the amount of work involved in treating patients suffering from this deformity. All except the most trivial need to be under continuous review through childhood and adolescence into adult life, and many need several operations in institutions equipped to treat young babies and staffed with experts in several specialities.

Written and sculpted records of bygone civilisations prove the existence of this deformity for many thousands of years and in differing races which include the Chinese, the Egyptians, the Incas, the Greeks and the Romans. There is widespread belief as the result of recent statistical surveys that the incidence of both cleft lip and cleft palate is increasing, after allowing for such factors as better record-keeping and more money spent on genetic research, but the reason is unknown.

The aetiology of clefts is obscure, although many facts are known both as the result of human genetic study and from animal experiment. Clefts of lip and alveolus and backward continuation through the palate, whether unilateral or bilateral, may be due to genetic aberration producing an abnormal chromosomal pattern; their hereditary transmission is usually through a male sex-linked recessive gene. Cleft palate alone, however, reaching no further forward than the posterior margin of the premaxilla when due to genetic abnormality is believed to be caused by a female dominant aberration which is not sex-linked. Hence one sometimes encounters a striking family history in which several female siblings are affected, without malformations having occurred in previous generations.

By no means all clefts, however, of lip and palate are due to hereditary factors, and environmental mischance is believed to be capable of producing exactly the same malformations. Little is known about these environmental factors but it is widely believed that they include irregularities in vitamin intake, especially vitamin A, virus infections, the action of antimetabolites and hormonal failures. The evidence, however, is mostly based on animal experiment and this is not necessarily valid in man. Intra-uterine posture has also for long been thought capable of causing deformities including failures of lip and palate; for example it has been suggested that the retroposed tongue, in consequence of under-development of the mandible, is responsible for the cleft palate in the Pierre Robin syndrome. Occasionally in a practice over many years one meets a case in which the imprint of a digit in a malformation is unmistakeable.

Much further research needs to be done before many of the parents with whom the surgeon is confronted can be accurately advised of an increased risk, and its degree. But genetic counselling in cases of hereditary clefts can be accurate enough to be of great value when the family history of both partners is known and chromosomal studies can be made.

EMBRYOLOGY AND CLASSIFICATION

In essence the causation of clefts of lip and palate is a failure of separate mesodermal masses to meet and fuse, as the result of which the overlying epithelium is stretched until it is so attenuated that it gives way. Where small amounts of mesoderm have met and fused, bridges, called Simonart's bands, persist. This basic concept has replaced the view hitherto widely held that clefts resulted from the failure of separate facial processes to unite and is the outcome of several studies, of which the most important in recent times are those of Fogh-Andersen (1942), Tondury (1955) and Stark (1968).

Stark has elucidated the problem still further by demonstrating from a study of six human embryos that the formation of the normal lip is due to the down growth of a single mesodermal mass into the ecto-endodermal cover as a three-pronged wedge. The central prong is not only responsible for the prolabium but also for the pre-maxillary palate as far as the incisor foraminae; the lateral prongs are responsible for the formation of the remainder of the lip; for this reason Stark recommends that clefts of lip and of the alveolus should all be known as clefts of the primary palate. Clefts of the remainder of the hard palate and of the soft palate (the secondary palate) result from failure, either partial or complete, of the ingrowth and fusion of lateral shelves which normally complete the separation of the oral and nasal cavities. Stark states that these first project downwards and later turn upwards to effect fusion. He suggests that failures in the primary palate occur between the fourth and seventh weeks after conception and failures of the secondary palate between the seventh and twelfth weeks. Thus a failure of lip, alveolus and the complete palate would postulate the continuation of the effect of a genetic abnormality or the harmful effect of an environmental influence over all this length of time, whilst failures of the primary or secondary palates alone would imply its restriction to the appropriate weeks. This theory does not, however, satisfy completely in that the backward continuation of a unilateral cleft of lip and alveolus produces a different anatomical abnormality of the palate from that seen in a cleft of the secondary palate alone. This fact, however, does not in any way detract from the importance of Stark's observation that the premaxillary palate is formed from the same mesoderm which makes the lip, and is the mainspring from which recent alterations in classification have stemmed.

Hitherto clefts had been classified as: Group 1 (lip), Group 2 (palate) and Group 3 (complete); this was suggested by Davis and Ritchie in 1922. It remained unchallenged until Kernahan and Stark put forward their ideas in 1958. Thereafter the International Confederation for Plastic and Reconstructive Surgery adopted the following in 1967:

Clefts of lip, alveolus and palate

(Classification based on embryological principles)

Group 1: Clefts of anterior (primary) palate
   (*a*) Lip: right and/or left.
   (*b*) Alveolus: right and/or left.

Group 2: Clefts of anterior and posterior (primary and secondary) palate
  (*a*) Lip: right and/or left.
  (*b*) Alveolus: right and/or left.
  (*c*) Hard palate: right and/or left.
  (*d*) Soft palate: medial.

Group 3: Clefts of posterior (secondary) palate
  (*a*) Hard palate: right and/or left.
  (*b*) Soft palate: medial.

(For further subdivision the terms 'total' and 'partial' should be used.)

Rare facial clefts

(Classification based on topographical findings)
  (*a*) Median clefts of upper lip with or without hypo- or aplasia of premaxilla.
  (*b*) Vertical clefts (oro-orbital).
  (*c*) Transverse clefts (oro-auricular).
  (*d*) Clefts of lower lip, nose and other very rare clefts.

A number of suggestions have been made for pictorial recording of clefts, based on the new understanding of the embryology, of which the most thoroughly worked out are the cross-hatched diagrammatic pattern of Pfeiffer and Schuchardt and the Greek symbolism of Vilar-Sancho. Both have advantages, but the former is somewhat cumbersome and the latter relies upon a dead language. The need still remains for the evolution of a simple graphic recording chart which will have world-wide application.

CURRENT VIEWS

Social attitudes to congenital deformities have varied greatly over the years and in different civilisations. At times ignorance and superstition have conspired to confer supernatural powers amounting sometimes to witchcraft upon such sufferers, inspiring fear which resulted in infanticide. But there are records as far back as the Chin dynasty of attempts to correct the deformities of lip and palate. An immense amount of time, effort and skill have been expended upon them over the last hundred years and much technical progress has been made. This has been greatly facilitated by the amenities of the modern hospital, progress in anaesthetic and orthodontic techniques, the understanding of the physiology of shock, the discovery of antibiotics and the development of paediatrics as a specialty. With these advantages the modern surgeon can devote his whole attention, unhurried, to the meticulous correction of the deformity. Research has also widened his understanding of the nature of the deformity and has thus directed his attention more precisely to what is needed to effect a cure. There remains, however, much still to be learnt with the consequence that there are many differing views on technical matters and on the timing of surgical intervention.

It is most important, however, to remember that the surgeon cannot know whether the final result of his efforts will be good, bad or indifferent until the child is fully grown; he may thus have to wait 15 years or more. He must, therefore, profit by the experience of others; it is only too easy, by failing to do so, to repeat the mistakes of the past. Nowhere is this truer than in the surgery of the nose tip, where a satisfactory operation in childhood may eventuate with a hideous deformity in the adolescent.

There has for long been disquiet at the possibility that early surgical intervention may cause deformities which would not have occurred if surgery had been delayed; in particular there is the possibility that growth of the maxilla may be retarded. But in modern society this risk is generally accepted because the social, educational and psychological handicaps which delay precipitates are unacceptable to most patients, parents and surgeons. As compensation the surgeon has the assistance of the orthodontist and the prosthetist in his battle with the collapsed maxilla.

Appreciation of the fact that children with clefts are suffering from a deficiency of tissue and not merely a displacement of normal tissues is one of the major advances in understanding in recent times and has resulted in endeavours to make good the losses with soft tissue flaps and bone grafts. The former have been in the surgeon's armamentarium long enough to have proved their worth, whilst the latter are still on trial. Without doubt too much has been expected of a rib strut spanning the alveolar gap. It cannot be the means of promoting the development of a normal maxilla during childhood for which much else is required. Over-expectation has led to disappointment and the abandoning of all early bone grafting by some workers. This probably represents too great a swing of the pendulum, and early grafting may well be found to be of lasting value, but the verdict must be delayed. In a seven-year follow-up of 94 cases the author has found that arch alignment of the opposed ends of the grafted segments had been maintained in 60 per cent. of cases and that teeth had grown into the bone-filled space in 31·5 per cent. In severe bilateral cases in which the premaxilla had been set back the insertion of bone grafts simultaneously had prevented collapse of the premaxilla, so that the results were as good as those in milder cases in which closure had been possible without setting the premaxilla back.

The strut has so far proved of value in these respects, but it cannot of course reverse an inborn failure of maxillary growth potential, nor can it resist the tendency to lateral segmental collapse which is enhanced both by constricting stresses from the surrounding soft tissues and by the scarring resulting from closure of the secondary palate.

If early bone grafting is to be employed the graft should be inserted when the lip is closed. To add another operation subsequently for this purpose must increase scar formation and is unjustifiable; this may well account for the conclusion by Robertson and Jollys in their series (1968) that the insertion of a graft is actually harmful. It is also of course essential to avoid any damage to marginal tooth buds. They are of value to all developing arches and are of special value if a graft is used since it provides a matrix into which they can migrate. They are often set into slender alveolar projections and are easily traumatised unless meticulous care is taken.

The author's belief on present evidence is that insertion of an alveolar strut to make good a deficiency is worthwhile and is not harmful, that it is not a passport to a normal maxilla for which rapid expansion and late bone grafting in adolescence may be the answer, and that greater use should be made of orthodontic appliances throughout childhood following early grafting to resist lateral collapse.

Pre-operative orthodontics

The purpose of this recently introduced technique (which is further discussed in Chapter II) is to align the segments correctly. To succeed it should be commenced by the time the child is 2 weeks old; at this early age the parts are easily moved, but every week's delay after this gives the orthodontist several more weeks work. If started at the proper time the orthodontist's work is always complete by the time the surgeon wants to operate unless he favours immediate closure of the lip at birth. In the author's experience pre-operative orthodontics are invaluable in three specific conditions: unilateral complete clefts of lip and palate with collapse of the lesser segment; unilateral cleft of the lip including the alveolus to correct its obliquity (Fig. **1**, 1) and bilateral complete clefts with collapse of the lateral segments and moderate protrusion of the premaxilla. The lateral segments can be expanded and the premaxilla set back. Minor degrees of premaxillary protrusion need no pre-operative orthodontics and gross protrusion cannot be set back orthodontically without buckling the septum to the point of obstruction of the airway. If pre-operative orthodontics are to be undertaken it is in the author's opinion essential to fill the alveolar gap with a rib graft; without this the advantages of the orthodontic treatment are largely thrown away. Conversely if a rib graft is to be used at all it can only have a chance of conferring a beneficial long-term effect on the alveolar arch if this is correctly aligned orthodontically beforehand. An incompletely expanded lateral segment will swing inwards like a pendulum on a bone graft, and is a likely cause of the failures which have been reported. Contrary to general belief pre-operative orthodontics is not heavy on bed occupancy; this has been pointed out by Burston (1958) who did most of the pioneer work. The addition of the 15 minutes to the length of the surgical operation for lip closure which the use of a rib graft entails is of no account in practice, however much it may be thought harmful in theory; in an experience of continuous use over 10 years in a large practice no case has given anxiety, including the occasional one in which the pleura has been opened. It only needs to be closed

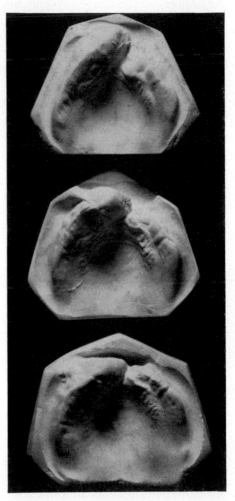

Fig. **1**, 1

Pre-operative orthodontics. Models to show the correction of alveolar deformity by the use of a splint over a period of three weeks.

with a single catgut stitch whilst the lung is expanded by the anaesthetist. If primary bone grafting is ultimately discarded it will be because of failure to influence the growing maxillary arch sufficiently; not for reasons of technical hazard.

Unilateral cleft lip

It is now widely accepted that in all but minor defects there is a deficiency of tissue great enough to produce a short lip if closure is effected by straight suture. Some kind of flap is required to increase the vertical height of the lip and to use the available tissue to best advantage to make good the deficiency. There are several types in common use and all gain length at the expense of width. The advantages and dis-advantages of each can be argued, and the truth is that there is room for the individual preference of the operator who, if he is experienced, will vary any standard procedure in detail to suit his own likes and to meet the individual features which every case presents. The basic decision is to use a flap. Flap repairs are by no means new and were reported in detail by Malgaigue in 1844 and by others too at about the same time. In the earlier part of this century they fell into disuse because many experienced surgeons, such as Kilner, felt that the use of a flap might imperil the subsequent growth of the rotated muscle. Their re-introduction largely stems from the work of Le Mesurier, who produced a variation of the flap described by Hagedorn in 1884; the results have stood the test of time and have provoked a large number of alter-natives, of which perhaps the Tennison (1952) and the Millard (1960) are the most popular today. All can be easily combined with the introduction of a rib graft using either the Stellmach or the Schuchardt flap or one of the modifications (Stellmach, 1955; Schuchardt, 1960). The author's preference is to use the Le Mesurier technique with a variation of the medial flap, similar to that published by Brauer in 1953. This has been in continuous use for fifteen years and has stood the test of time. Since 1960 it has been combined with the Stellmach flap to enclose the rib graft.

In cases in which there is no alveolar gap requiring a bone graft but where the palate is also cleft the lip repair is combined with closure of the anterior third of the palate, as advocated by Veau (1931, 1938).

Bilateral cleft lip

When complete this deformity is the most difficult of all to treat because of the protrusion of the premaxilla, which is the keystone of the maxillary arch. Its displace-ment allows the lateral segments to collapse towards each other producing a 'dog-mouth' deformity. In mild degrees of protrusion the arch can be restored by pre-operative orthodontics to distract the lateral segments and the insertion of alveolar bone grafts to maintain them in their proper alignment. In most instances, and certainly unless the operator is experienced in the technique, the two sides should be repaired separately at an interval of three weeks. Sufficient bone for both sides is cut from one rib at the first operation and half of it buried subcutaneously for use at the second procedure.

If the premaxilla is more than slightly protruding pre-operative orthodontics includes the exertion of pressure upon it to set it back (Fig. **1**, 2). The subsequent operative procedure is then the same as for the mild case. If, however, the premaxilla is grossly rotated it can only be set back surgically. This can either be done by removal of a triangular piece of septum immediately behind it at the time of primary closure as recommended by Denis Browne (1949), or it can be treated similarly months, or even years, after primary closure. Fortunately, cases severe enough to need septal resection are rare, since it is extremely important not to impinge upon the small swelling of the septum situated about a centimetre behind the premaxilla. Denis Browne maintained that this swelling was caused by a suture line at the growing edge of what he described as the pre-vomerine bone. Whether or not this is so, it is undoubtedly true that if this area is encroached upon subsequent growth of the premaxilla is much impaired. If the premaxilla is set back at primary closure bone grafts are of great value in stabilising it.

Primary closure of the lip in bilateral cases should be by straight suture to the two sides of the prolabium and only the mucosa of the two sides should meet below it. The rotation of skin flaps below it results in a long, ugly lip which is tight and indrawn. Even small prolabial segments are adequate for attachment of the lateral segments and often develop surprisingly well after operation. In many of these cases, however, the columella is virtually non-existent and draws the nose tip down in an ugly curve.

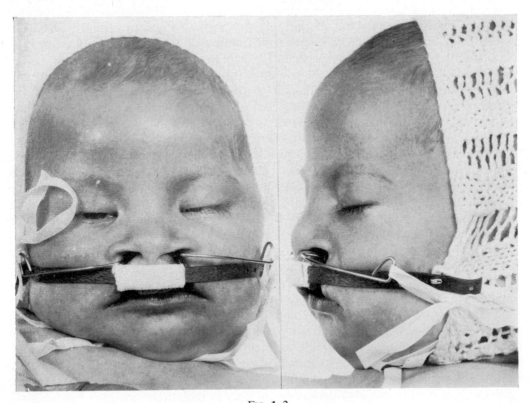

FIG. 1, 2

Pre-operative orthodontics. Showing splint and elastic attachment with which to set the premaxilla back.

This is unavoidable and is later corrected by lifting the prolabial skin to fashion the columella, which in turn may precipitate the need to remake the prolabium from the lower lip with an Abbe flap. But these are not primary procedures.

Cleft palate

The object of closure of a cleft palate is to enable the child to develop normal speech; with this will come swallowing without regurgitation. To achieve normal speech the soft palate must be sufficiently mobile to move freely and rapidly, and long enough to close the oro-nasal sphincter in conjunction with the contraction of the superior constrictor muscle. These are the essential requirements of a successful operation. There are several ways in which they may be achieved.

In the author's opinion the operation should be performed before the child reaches the age of 18 months when it will be making conscious efforts to learn to talk by repeating the words and phrases it hears. It needs the normal anatomy of the mouth to do so. To achieve a normal palate, however, is a considerable test of surgical skill and the operation takes time. It is unwarranted to put the child to this lengthy procedure before the speech apparatus is needed. It is the author's practice, therefore, to repair the palate when the child is between 12 and 15 months old, and to do so as a routine by an operation of the Veau-Wardill type, to which is added a Z-plasty to lengthen the nasal mucosa of the soft palate, backward dislocation of the greater palatine arteries after removal of the posterior wall of the bony canals, and wide dissection of the lateral palatal spaces with fracture of the hamular processes. Dissection of the lateral spaces is between the superior constrictor and tensor palate muscles medially, and the internal pterygoid muscle laterally. This dissection can safely be carried deeply without danger to the nerve supply since this enters the muscles from above, and is an essential part of the operation if a mobile soft palate is to be obtained free of tension.

Some surgeons feel it is necessary to carry out a primary push-back operation and to use an island flap or a free graft to supplement the nasal mucosa to obtain adequate length. Others, including Stark (1968), believe that the combination of a primary pharyngoplasty with closure of the cleft palate is needed. A third approach to the problem is to close only the soft palate and leave the hard for several years, using a prosthesis. This course is advocated because of the proven restricting effect of operative scarring on the expansion and development of the lateral segments particularly in the neighbourhood of the maxillary tuberosities. If followed, the closure of the maxilla must be postponed at least until completion of eruption of the secondary dentition. The wearing of a prosthesis through school life is a high price for a child to pay for a maxillary arch. Those who advocate it, however, believe that it is worthwhile and that the gap in the hard palate becomes progressively smaller so that it is easy to close if closure is needed at all. The author does not believe that any of these procedures is necessary or desirable as a primary procedure in the average cleft, although all may be of great assistance when faced with an unusually hypoplastic velum. These differences of approach not only indicate a universal desire to improve upon present results but also underline the axiom that there are very few surgical problems in which there is only one 'right' way of correcting them.

TECHNIQUE OF PRIMARY CLOSURE

Unilateral cleft lip

The design of the quadrilateral flap of Le Mesurier (1949), shown in Figure **1**, 3, the triangular flap of Tennison (1952) shown in Figure **1**, 4 or the rotation flap of Millard (1960) shown in Figure **1**, 5 can always be used in conjunction with the insertion of a rib graft using a Stellmach flap (Fig. **1**, 6) to cover it (Stellmach (1955)).

The procedure is undertaken when the child is 3 months old under general anaesthetic delivered through an intra-tracheal tube. A bony alveolar gap is closed at the same operation with a rib graft after pre-operative orthodontics. The rib graft is taken first. With the child lying on its right side and the arm drawn forwards to lift the scapula an appropriate length of the seventh rib is removed subperiosteally from below the angle of the scapula. The edges of the latissimus dorsi and serratus magnus muscles are cut with the diathermy to expose the rib and subsequently resutured. The child is then turned on its back and the lip marked out in accordance with the method selected. Marking includes the septal Stellmach flap. In wide clefts the buccal mucosa

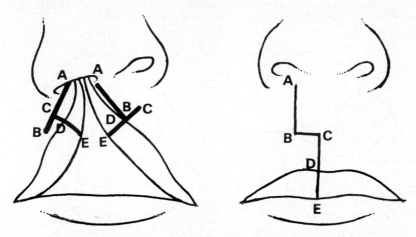

FIG. **1**, 3

Le Mesurier right-angled flap. Two points A are chosen which will form a satisfactory nostril floor.

Marking the lateral flap: D is sited on the muco-cutaneous junction at the point where the mucosa begins to narrow. C is 5 mm (3/16 in.) from D at right-angles to the muco-cutaneous junction. The line AC is drawn; in narrow clefts where there is plenty of tissue available it can be slightly convex away from the cleft to add slight pouting to the lip. The line CB is equal to CD and the point B so placed that an imaginary line from B to the muco-cutaneous junction is two-thirds the length of the line CD. This provides the elevation of the cupid's bow on completion of the operation.

Marking the medial flap: point D is marked on the muco-cutaneous junction so that the line AD is equal in length to AB on the lateral flap. A line DC is drawn at right-angles to the muco-cutaneous junction and equal in length to the line CD on the lateral flap.

A line DE is drawn across the mucosa as a straight downward continuation of the line CD. When the flaps are cut the flap ABC fits into the angle opened out on the lateral flap ABD.

The symmetry of the cupid's bow depends upon the length of the line AB and its extension from B to the muco-cutaneous junction on the lateral flap being equal to the distance on the uncleft side from the nostril floor to the apex of the cupid's bow.

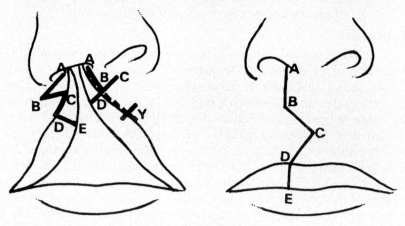

FIG. 1, 4

Tennison triangular flap. A piece of wire is cut equal to the distance from the nostril floor to the point of the cupid's bow on the uncleft side (AY) and folded into three equal lengths to mark the lateral incisions (ABCD). On the medial side only two of the three segments of the wire are used for the incision (ABCD).

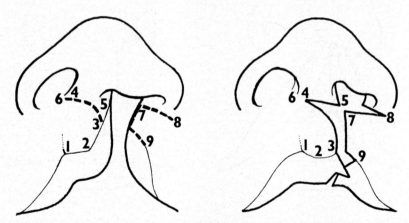

FIG. 1, 5

Millard flap. The design is based on a vertical flap to fall along the line of the philtrum, and a horizontal flap to tie in the alar base.

Rotation-advancement equation:

$$1-2=2-3 \qquad 3-5=1-6$$
$$3-4=9-7 \qquad 4-5<7-8$$

is freely incised in the buccal sulcus laterally, and the flap freed from the surface of the maxilla without damaging its periosteum or the infra-orbital nerve. The mucosa is similarly cut on the medial side across the philtral band and the mucosa of the floor of the opposite nostril freed if there is much columellar obliquity. In extreme cases the lower edge of the septal cartilage can be freed from the nasal spine by careful dissection without damaging it to assist in columellar straightening.

Another useful manoeuvre when the width of the gap is such that the ala is very

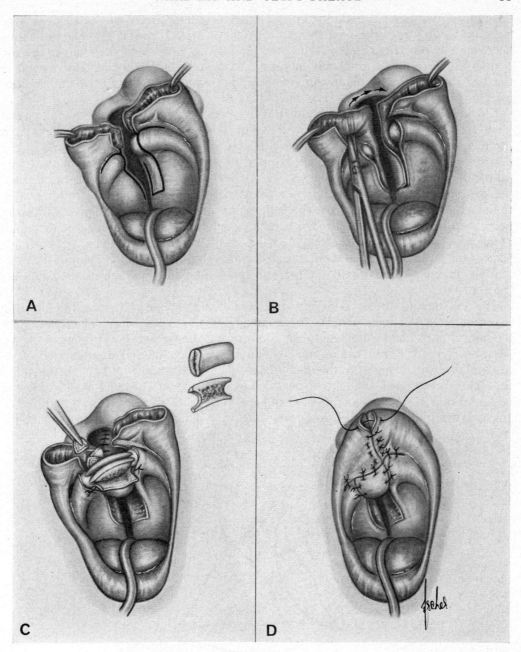

FIG. 1, 6

Stellmach flap. (A) A quadrilateral flap is taken from the side of the septum and based anteriorly. (B) It is turned so that its raw surface covers the rib graft in the alveolar gap, and the alar cartilage is freed with scissors from the skin to the nose-tip to restore normal curvature. (C) The rib is split longitudinally and inserted in two pieces. Both are notched at each end to wedge them securely against the bony margins. Surplus fragments of cartilage are used to support the alar base. (D) The buccal mucosa stitched to the anterior edge of the septal flap to complete the cover of the rib graft.

flat is to separate the alar skin from the underlying lateral crus of the alar cartilage right up to the tip of the nose by blunt dissection with scissors. The alar wall thus becomes a two-ply structure enabling the underlying mucosa-cartilage layer to slide on the skin to restore normal alar curvature. No disturbance of subsequent growth of the alar cartilage occurs from this, the essential requirement being the undisturbed attachment of the cartilage to the mucosa.

Closure commences with attachment of the medial to the lateral layers of the nasal mucosa at the level of the alveolus with two or three interrupted catgut stitches. Then the rotated Stellmach flap is sutured with two fine silk stitches to each side of the alveolar gap. These four stitches are inserted so that their knots are on the posterior mucosal surface of the flap. Its raw surface, which faces forwards, forms the bed for the bone graft. This is inserted as two pieces created by splitting the rib longways; these are securely wedged across the gap one on top of the other, their ends having been shaped by cutting small recesses with bone nibbling forceps. One of the small bone chips so created can be inserted on the contra-lateral side of the septal cartilage against the nasal spine if the septum is so deviated that it does not come into the midline by closure of the soft tissues. Spare fragments of cartilage are used to support the alar base.

The remainder of the nasal layer is then closed and the bone graft buried by suturing the free edge of the Stellmach flap to the cut edge of the buccal mucosa advanced with the lateral flap. The lip is then closed to complete the operation. Ordinarily the Le Mesurier type of flap is the author's preference but the medial flap is cut back in triangular fashion, similar to the method described by Brauer (Fig. 1, 7), if it is found that there is too much tissue to allow the lateral flap to sit correctly in place. It will be found that in wide gaps no tissue will need to be resected since it is all required to give a natural fullness to the formation of the lip. A Denis Browne bow is applied for

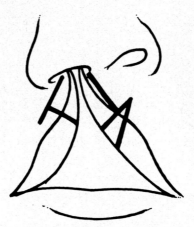

FIG. 1, 7

Modification of Le Mesurier flap. Triangular excision of skin and mucosa on the medial side as used by the author, and similar to the modification described by Brauer.

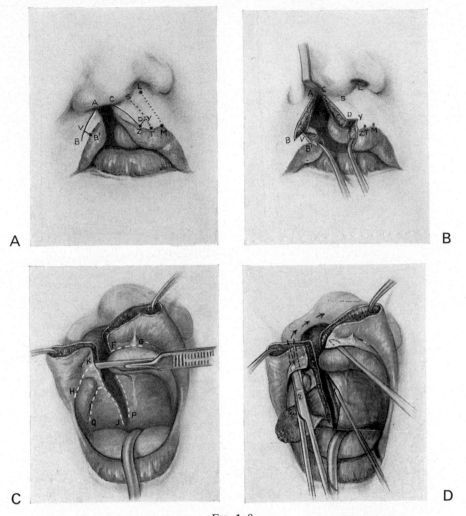

FIG. 1, 8

Unilateral cleft. Closure with Le Mesurier lip flap and Veau palate flap. (A) Lip
incisions marked. (B) Lip flaps cut so as to produce a length on the cleft side equal
to the distance LM. (C) Buccal and palatal incisions outlined. (D) Flaps cut and
scissors inserted to free nasal skin from alar cartilage for restoration of nostril
curvature.

a week to relieve the suture line of tension when the child cries, and the nostril is
packed daily with a carrot of cotton wool soaked in liquid paraffin to ensure adhesion
of the two-ply lateral alar wall to create a rounded ala.

Primary closure of the unilateral complete cleft in which there is no bony alveolar
gap requiring a graft is also undertaken at the age of three months. Lip closure is
combined with closure of the alveolar mucosa and the anterior part of the hard
palate. Nasal flaps are joined with interrupted catgut stitches tied on the nasal surface,
and these are backed with a mucoperiosteal flap from the buccal surface of the lesser

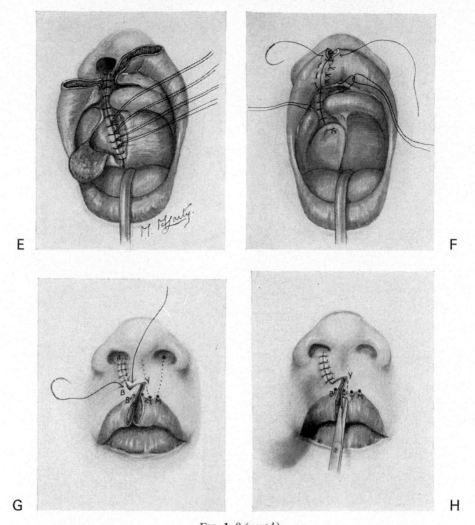

FIG. 1, 8 (*contd.*)

(E) Nasal layer closed. (F) Palatal covering flap attached and buccal covering flaps being stitched. (G) Skin incisions closed down to quadrilateral flap. (H) Excision of triangular area of skin ZTY and dependent mucosa.

segment as advocated by Veau, and further forward by labial flaps liberated by incisions in both buccal sulci (Fig **1**, 8).

Bilateral cleft lip

The lateral flaps are cut straight and designed so that their muco-cutaneous junctions meet the prolabium to form the apices of the cupid's bow; only their mucosal extensions pass beneath it to meet each other (Fig. **1**, 9). The passage of skin flaps beneath the prolabium produces too long a lip even with a small prolabium. Failure, however,

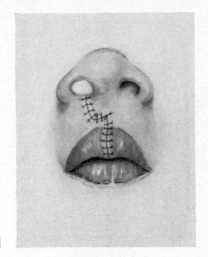

FIG. **1**, 8 (*contd.*)
(I) Operation completed.

to pass mucosal extensions beneath the prolabium often leads to a midline mucosal defect with an ugly notch.

Where the premaxilla is grossly protruded it is set back by removing septal bone immediately behind it. Its stability is restored by transfixing it with a pin which engages the septal cartilage (Fig. **1**, 10). In these rare severe cases the columella is so underdeveloped that the nose tip is inevitably drawn down and needs lengthening secondarily later.

As with unilateral clefts all bony alveolar gaps are closed with rib grafts no matter whether the premaxilla has been set back or not. It is safer, unless the operator is very experienced, to raise only one Stellmach septal flap at a time, leaving an interval of three weeks between closure of the first and second sides. It is essential to do this if the premaxilla has been set back to obviate risk of avascular necrosis. Sufficient bone is cut at the first operation for grafting both sides and the piece needed for the second operation is buried subcutaneously in the chest wound.

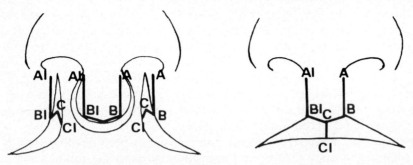

FIG. **1**, 9
Bilateral cleft. Closure with straight skin flaps to the apices of the cupid's bow and mucosal flaps below the prolabium.

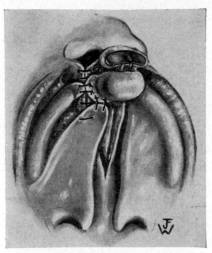

FIG. **1**, 10

Reposition of the premaxilla. Triangular wedge of bone is removed behind the premaxilla and its stability restored by transfixion with a pin.

In bilateral clefts in which there are no bony defects large enough to require bone grafts it is the author's practice to close both sides at the same time, using palatal flaps from the maxillae to cover the nasal suture lines closing the anterior part of the palate, as recommended by Veau; the post-alveolar part of the palate is of difficult access if it is not closed with the lip. There is, of course, no reason why the operation should not be performed in two stages, with a three-week interval, if the operator prefers, but the induration remaining after the first procedure can add to the difficulties of securing symmetry of the cupid's bow if this is done.

Cleft palate

Personal preference is for the two or four flap Veau-Wardill type of closure rather than the Langenbeck repair, but the standard procedure is varied in several important respects.

The operation commences with wide dissection of the lateral palatal spaces and fracture of the hamular processes to carry the superior constrictor and tensor palati muscles medially; this space is virtually bloodless (Fig. **1**, 11).

After elevation of the flaps the musculo-tendinous attachment of the soft palate to the posterior bony margin of the hard palate is completely freed. This necessitates sacrifice of the small lesser palatine sensory nerves, but this does not lead to any permanent reduction of sensitivity of the soft palate. The posterior margin of the greater palatine foramen is removed by two cuts with a 5 mm osteotome. The medial cut should be made first; if the lateral cut is made first the bony wing of the hard palate is weakened and if small can be fractured as the medial cut is made. The greater palatine artery is dislocated backwards through the resected bony channel to allow reposition of the posterior flap. Corresponding reposition of the nasal mucosal layer is achieved by a side cut into it on each side to allow triangles to open out. The cuts are staggered, the first being made just posterior to the back of the bony palate and the second about a centimetre further back. This additional length is of course gained at the expense of width and in very wide gaps with grossly underdeveloped segments of soft palate care must be taken not to make these side cuts so deep that there is excessive tension on the palate when sutured. In practice this situation hardly ever arises if the lateral palatal spaces are opened up accurately and completely; adequate relaxation is secured by this essential manoeuvre to meet the requirements of all except the most exceptionally wide gaps.

In cases in which a primary alveolar bone graft has been covered by a Stellmach flap it is essential to carry the anterior dissection through the rotated mucosa of the flap to expose the back edge of the rib graft; unless this is done an oro-nasal continuity of mucosa persists and a fistula will form.

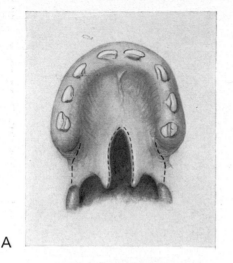
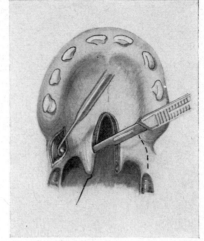

A
B

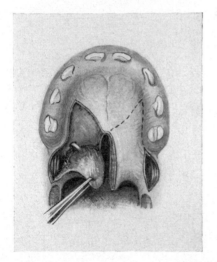
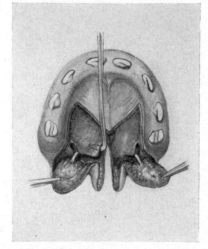

C
D

FIG. **1**, 11

Repair of cleft palate. (A) Incisions. (B) Lateral space opened and hamulus fractured.
(C) Buccal muco-periosteal flap raised containing the greater palatine artery.
(D) Nasal mucosal flaps elevated from the hard palate.

Palatal closure is in two layers both of which contain muscle as well as mucosa in
the soft palate. Interrupted catgut sutures are used and the buccal layer is reinforced
with a few fine monofilament nylon stitches. The apices of the two or four flaps are
held to the nasal layer by a figure-of-eight catgut stitch and the anterior nasal flaps
usually incorporate small flaps turned from the septum. The lateral palatal spaces
are packed for a week with ribbon gauze wrung out of a benzoin-mastic mixture*;

* Composition of Benzoin Mastic: mastic 800 g, caster oil 25 ml, benzene to 2 litres—40 per cent solution
of mastic in benzene.

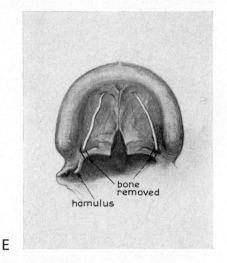

E

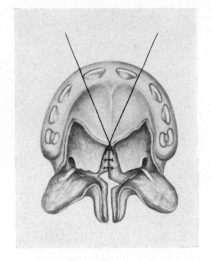

F

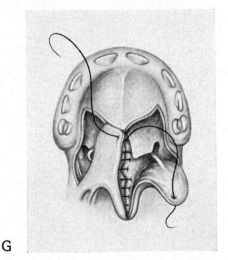

G

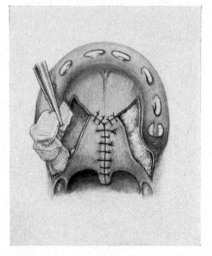

H

FIG. **1**, 11 (*contd.*)

(E) Showing bone to be removed to allow backward displacement of the greater palatine arteries. (F) Nasal mucosal flaps lengthened. (G) Nasal layer sutured and buccal flaps attached. (H) Lateral spaces packed with gauze soaked in benzoin mastic.

these act as splints to relieve the median suture line of tension and prevent food and saliva from lodging in the spaces. They can be removed without anaesthetic by the nursing staff with the child restrained by wrapping it firmly in a blanket.

A tongue stitch is inserted on completion of the operation to control the airway without the need for instrumentation, which is otherwise a possible source of damage to the suture line. Tonsillectomy is sometimes required if the size of the tonsils is such that the airway might be obstructed by them after suture of the palate; it must be undertaken in all doubtful cases, despite the well recognised advantage of leaving them to help closure of the postnasal space when they constitute no risk. Tracheostomy is occasionally needed in children with very underdeveloped mandibles, and the decision for or against performing it will be much influenced by the nursing skill available in the post anaesthetic period. If performed the opening should be made as low in the trachea as practicable, and well away from the cricoid ring to minimise the likelihood of formation of a tracheal fistula. In young children these can be very difficult to close and the site of the tracheostomy is the single most important factor in their avoidance. A plastic tracheostomy tube should be used.

Pierre Robin syndrome

This consists of the association of a cleft palate with a hypoplastic mandible. It may give rise to recurrent attacks of respiratory embarrassment in the neonate, persisting for about two months and causing permanent cerebral damage from anoxia. During an attack the tongue becomes wedged in the cleft with the result that cyanosis is rapid and progressive. It can be overcome by hooking the tongue down with a right-angled metal spatula. In many cases the infant can be nursed through these dangerous weeks without surgery by careful positioning in the cot and by the use of an incubator. But the desirability of relying on this regime depends upon the availability of skilled nurses day and night. The alternative is either to attempt to fix the tongue by suturing it to the lip or buccal sulcus, or to perform a tracheostomy; many suturing operations have been described but none is very satisfactory and tracheostomy is preferable if surgical intervention is required.

A case nursed successfully through the first few weeks of life rarely gives any subsequent anxiety except in the few hours after operation for closure of the cleft palate. The reduction of the airway by the operation and the muscular hypotonia consequent upon anaesthesia and surgery produce conditions in which an emergency can readily arise. It is often desirable to perform a tracheostomy at the end of the operation, and essential to have medical cover immediately and continuously available for intubation in case of emergency if tracheostomy has not been performed. The frequency and seriousness of postoperative obstruction justifies postponement of closure of the cleft palate in cases of Pierre Robin syndrome for longer than for ordinary cases of cleft palate if it is the wish of the surgeon or parents to minimise the chances of having to perform a tracheostomy.

SECONDARY SOFT TISSUE CORRECTIONS

The choice of time at which an operation is performed on a growing child is often of great importance, and much harm can be done in the long term by disturbance of tissues despite an apparently excellent initial result; the final outcome may well be hideous and produce much greater reconstructive problems than the original disability. In general, however, but with some exceptions, soft tissue repairs can be performed safely in time to minimise the child's embarrassment when going to school. The importance of this needs no emphasis.

The lip

Scar excisions, secondary flap procedures to equalise the length of the two sides of the lip, and adjustment of the cupid's bow can all be safely carried out as soon as the lip is judged by the surgeon to be large enough for accurate correction. It is the author's practice to perform all such operations at about the age of $3\frac{1}{2}$ years, which gives ample time for the new scars to fade before the child goes to school when 5 years old. Similarly, the columella may be lengthened at the same age in bilateral cases in which it is underdeveloped and the nose tip drawn down. Many techniques are available of which that described in 1960 by Millard (Fig. **1**, 12) and in 1952 and 1964 by Matthews (Fig. **1**, 13) will be found to give satisfactory results. In cases in

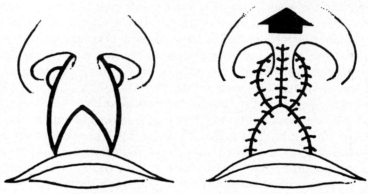

FIG. **1**, 12
Nose tip elevation. Millard flap. Using vertical labial flaps.

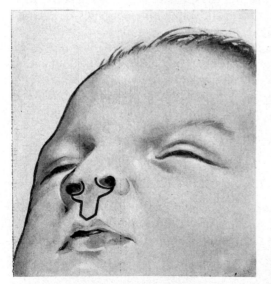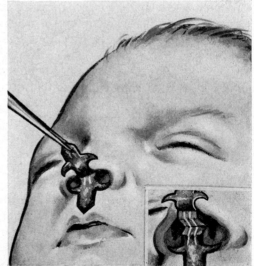

FIG. **1**, 13
Nose tip elevation. Matthews flap. Using winged flaps inset into the sides of the columella.

which tethering of the nose tip is severe, or those in which the upper lip is tight, or both, utilisation of the prolabial skin for the columella may necessitate the introduction of a flap from the lower lip as substitution for the prolabium by the technique described in 1898 by Abbe (Fig. **1**, 14). Young children withstand the combination of these procedures in one operation very well and they can be safely undertaken in 3-year-olds.

Occasionally the proximity of the lips when the Abbe flap is inset embarrasses respiration if the nasal airways are also small. This is easily overcome by fixing a short length of rubber tubing between the lips. Feeding constitutes no problem and the children enjoy having 'two mouths' through which to feed. If approached as a game all children join in and feed enthusiastically. It is wise to guard against possible tension on the flap in the immediate post-operative period, and for a few days thereafter, from crying by placing a single strong mono-filament nylon stitch as a mattress from the upper to the lower lip on each side. If tied over small bone shirt buttons they leave no marks; they are not needed for more than four days even in the most fractious child provided sedatives are intelligently used.

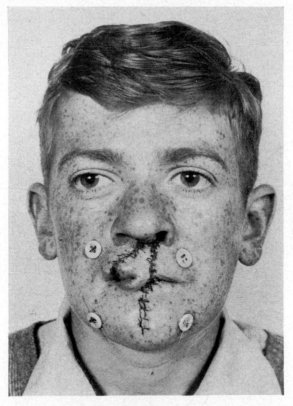

FIG. **1**, 14
Abbe flap. Two nylon stitches are tied over buttons to prevent stretching of the suture lines in the first few days after operation.

Nose tip

Deformities of the nose tip are amongst the most difficult to correct. In children under about 10 years of age it is a golden rule, which any surgeon can prove by experience and to the cost of his patients, that no operation should be undertaken which separates the alar cartilage from the underlying mucosa or which involves cutting of the cartilage even with the mucosa attached. Much subsequent difficulty and distress will be avoided if this is accepted by the inexperienced.

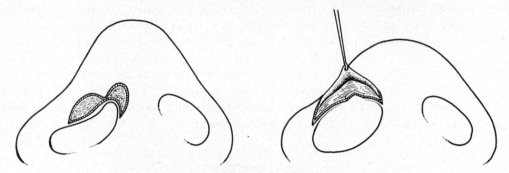

FIG. **1**, 15
Nostril inroll. Modification of the Joseph flap.

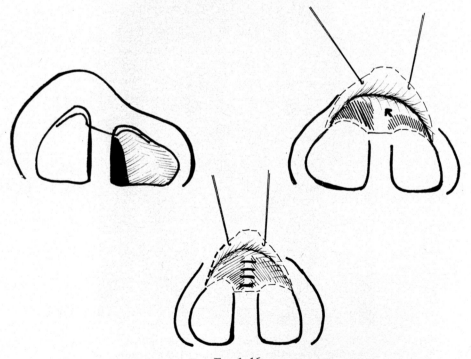

FIG. **1**, 16
Flying-bird incision. Used to approximate the alar cartilages.

In the 3½-year age group, when help is often urgently needed to improve appearance before schooling starts, small inequalities of the alar tip can be corrected by the Joseph inroll, or the author's modification of it (Fig. **1**, 15). These corrections are only of the skin and mucosa. The cartilage is not shortened. It is not therefore applicable to gross downward displacements of the tip in which the cartilage also shares. These can either be treated by suturing the two alar cartilages to each other after exposure through a 'flying-bird' incision (Fig. **1**, 16), or by lifting the alar cartilage complete with its mucosal lining as a rotation flap (Fig. **1**, 17). The choice

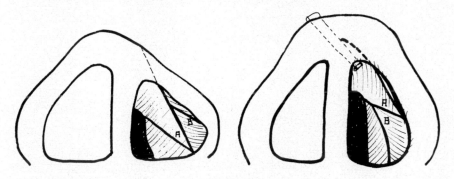

FIG. **1**, 17

Rotation flap. To elevate the alar cartilage. Flap B consists of mucosa and is used to restore the fullness of the vestibular lining.

is to some extent the surgeon's preference, although it is usually found that unilateral cases do best with rotation flaps and bilateral cases with suture through the flying-bird incision.

Any inadequacy left by either of these procedures, neither of which involve separation of the cartilage from the mucosa, should be left until the child is approaching puberty, by which time the alar cartilage will have grown to a good size. Then they should be approached through a flying-bird incision and their lateral crura completely dissected from the underlying mucosa up to their angles. Their medial crura are undisturbed. The lateral crura are then balanced symmetrically by suturing them to each other along the bridge-line, and even by turning a part of an overlarge lateral crus from one side to supplement an underdeveloped crus on the opposite side. The two balanced crura are then resutured to the mucosal lining in symmetrical positions, and the nostril margins equalised by suitable skin excisions prior to resuture. In the author's experience this is much the most effective way of restoring the nose tip in all cleft cases and is the only operation performed if the degree of deformity does not call for interference at an earlier age.

Pharyngoplasty and push-back operations

The purpose of these operations is to close an inadequate oro-nasal sphincter which is impairing speech or causing nasal regurgitation. It is no use doing this for speech impediment unless this is proved to be due to inadequacy of the sphincter. Simple tests like blowing and sucking through a straw give a very fair indication of

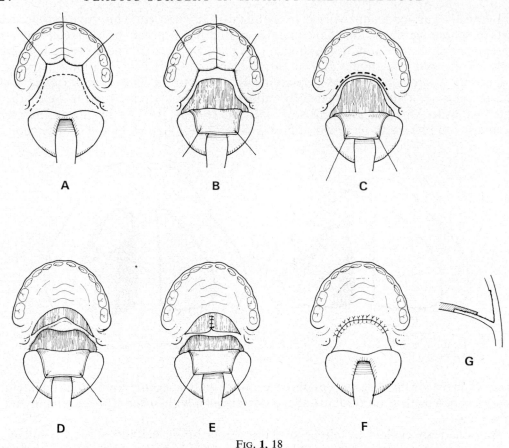

FIG. 1, 18

Rosenthal pharyngoplasty. (A) Incision on posterior pharyngeal wall. (B) Pharyngeal flap raised. (C) Incision on posterior border of soft palate. (D) Raw surface created on soft palate by undermining. (E) Raw surface of nasal layer of soft palate elongated by midline sutures. (F) Pharyngeal flap sutured in place. (G) Sectional view to show approximation of raw surfaces of nasal layer of soft palate and of pharyngeal flap.

this, and the evidence can be confirmed by an X-ray or with cine-radiography. Where the palate is short, and particularly where this is combined with excessive tension reducing movement, the best results are obtained by a flap from the posterior pharyngeal wall. This can either be based above (Sanvenero-Rosselli) or below (Rosenthal) (Fig. 1, 18); the author prefers the latter for two reasons. First the nasal layer of the soft palate, after dissection through an incision along its posterior border, can be lengthened by suture to form a backing for the front portion of the flap, and second the partial re-attachment of the flap to the posterior pharyngeal wall postoperatively pulls the palate both upwards and backwards where it should be. The author has not noticed any increased tendency to middle ear infection after using the Rosenthal flap, as has been reported, so long as care is taken to keep the incision clear of the eustachian cushions. When gross scarring is present in the adenoid bed the upward based Rosselli flap has an advantage since its anterior convexity comes from well below this area.

If pharyngoplasty is reserved for the correction of speech defects and regurgitation
due to deficiencies of the oro-nasal sphincter the question of its utilisation at 15 months
with primary closure of the palate does not arise. It is not proved to be needed until
the child is about 3 years old. At this age a skilled paediatric anaesthetist can safely
give a hypotensive anaesthetic. The meticulous accuracy of dissection and suture
which are essential if the operation is to be of value is much easier to achieve in a
bloodless field. Working at the bottom of a small hole without hypotension, it is very
difficult to obtain it in any other way. The routine hypotensive anaesthetics which the
anaesthetist provides for the author would in his opinion be justification enough for
postponing operation until this age, even if no other considerations supported this.

Pharyngoplasty can be combined with a push-back operation whenever the shortness of the palate demands this. For a push-back to be effective the muscle must be
detached from the back of the hard palate and the nasal mucosa cut transversely at

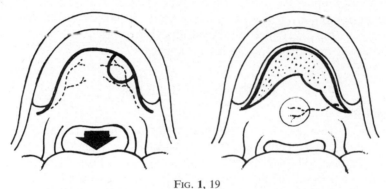

Fig. 1, 19

Millard island flap. Using an island of buccal mucosa based on the greater
palatine artery with which to make good the deficiency in the nasal mucosa
after the palate has been set back.

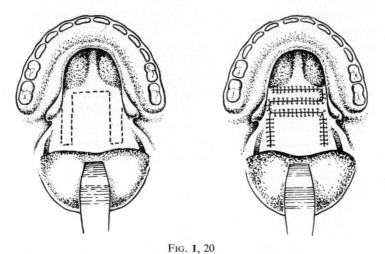

Fig. 1, 20

Hynes pharyngoplasty. Using lateral flaps including the salpingopharyngeus
muscles with which to build forward the posterior pharyngeal wall.

the same level; otherwise it not only limits reposition but increases the tendency of the soft tissues to creep forwards postoperatively. There has been much dispute as to whether it is necessary to resurface the diamond-shaped defect opened up in the nasal mucosa by the transverse incision. It is probably best to do so, although on many occasions epithelial regenesis appears to be quite adequate. A simple effective method is to tack a thin diamond-shaped skin graft in place with four loosely tied stitches at the corners. An alternative is the island flap (Millard, 1960) from the anterior palate (Fig. 1, 19) or the 'sandwich' flap using two flaps from the anterior palate, one for the nasal surface and the other for the buccal (Moore and Chong, 1967).

Oro-nasal sphincter inadequacy may sometimes be demonstrable as the cause of a speech defect or of regurgitation when the palate is seen and proved to be of adequate length and mobility. Many such cases have large lateral recesses behind the posterior pillars of the fauces and the deficiencies can then often be very satisfactorily corrected by a pharyngoplasty of the Hynes type (Fig. 1, 20). The small flaps sutured across the posterior pharyngeal wall which contain the salpingo-pharyngeus muscles may contribute to the excellence of the results, but in the author's view the main benefit is conferred by closure of the lateral spaces.

BONY CORRECTIONS

Late bone grafting

The operation is used in cases of collapse of the maxillary arch and the object is to maintain normal dental occlusion after expanding the fragments orthodontically, using fixed appliances. These consist of segmental cap splints fixed to the teeth and set in acrylic into which a Fischer expansion screw is incorporated. The procedure can be used with a mixed dentition as soon as sufficient permanent teeth have erupted in each fragment, but it is best to wait until the patient is about 18 when skeletal development of the mandible is virtually complete so that the bite can be arranged in proper occlusion for adult life. Expansion cannot be made using deciduous teeth since they are always dislodged and lost if pressure is exerted upon them.

Expansion using permanent teeth takes place along the line, or lines, of the original cleft and displaces the whole segment without rotation of the teeth or alveolus. The secret of success is to expand the fragments rapidly taking no more than three weeks to achieve the desired position. This is in complete contrast to the principle of slow movement of individual teeth over a period of months or years by conventional orthodontics. It also achieves distances of movement which are impossible to effect with conventional orthodontics, no matter how long such methods are tried.

Fears that expansion might not be restricted to the displaced fragment have not been realised; this is probably due to the steadying influence of normal occlusion with the mandible of a fragment when it reaches its correct position. The angle at which the Fischer expansion screw is placed, however, is of great importance and is determined by careful examination of study models. For example in a unilateral cleft when only lateral displacement of the lesser segment is needed the screw is set transversely (Fig. 1, 21), whilst when more movement is required at its anterior than its posterior end the screw is set obliquely, or two screws are included for selective

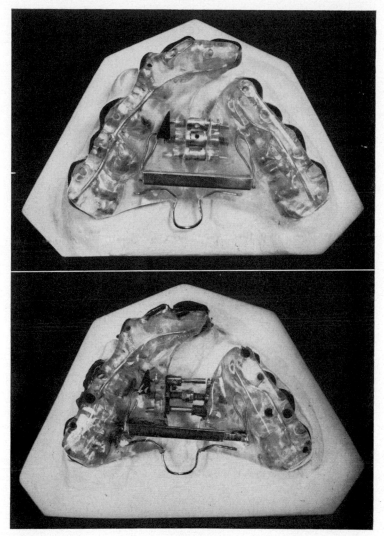

Fig. **1**, 21

Rapid expansion of unilateral cleft. Splints on models before and after expansion showing single expansion screw set transversely.

expansion. In bilateral clefts one screw is set transversely to expand the lateral segments whilst another is incorporated at right angles to it to push a collapsed maxilla forward (Fig. **1**, 22).

The screw is turned by means of a pin which engages the screw mechanism and the manoeuvre can easily be performed by the patient or a relative. It should be turned one revolution at least three times in the 24 hours. The larger type of screw permits 11 mm of expansion; if more than this is needed the acrylic in which it is embedded is cut away with a dental drill and a second unexpanded screw incorporated using rapidly setting acrylic. The palatal mucosa must be protected from damage by the

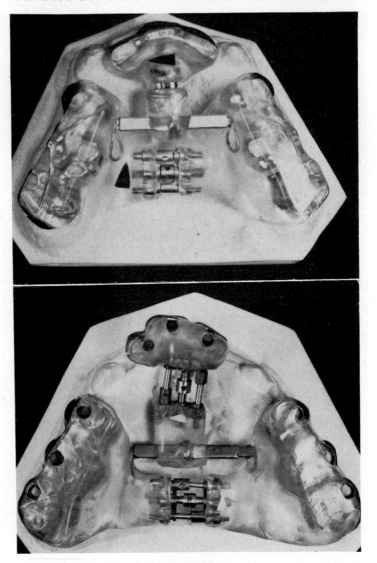

FIG. 1, 22

Rapid expansion of bilateral cleft. Splints on models showing one screw
set transversely to expand the lateral segments and another at right angles
to push the premaxilla forward.

acrylic with a strip of silver foil which is withdrawn as soon as the acrylic has set
(Fig. 1, 23).

Maximum movement occurs in the first few days as can be demonstrated radiologically. During this time the patient complains of a sense of heaviness in the
maxilla but rarely of any sensation amounting to pain. An early observation by
almost every patient is the restoration of the airway in a nostril previously blocked.
All surgeons who have attempted to restore the airway in cleft cases by other methods

will know that it is well-nigh impossible; rapid expansion is the only sure way of achieving this and may well be an even more important result of treatment than restoration of normal occlusion. In school age children, whose nasal obstruction is precipitating otitis media and deafness, there is good reason to undertake rapid expansion without delaying until they are fully grown to avoid permanent impairment of hearing. Another welcome achievement of expansion and bone grafting is improvement in appearance. Fullness is restored to the sunken maxilla and the alar

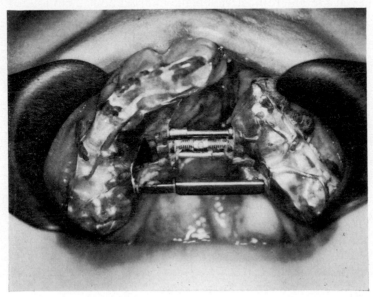

FIG. 1, 23

Rapid expansion of the unilateral cleft. Fixed expansion splints set in place on the teeth with single expansion screw.

base is supported. A lingually deviated tooth bordering the cleft may also come forward into the space created by expansion so that with the subsequent aid of conventional orthodontics it forms a useful component of the dental arch.

Expansion does not cause breakdown of the mucosa, nor does it macroscopically increase the size of existing fistulae. It causes slight separation of both buccal and nasal mucosa from the edges of the bones bordering the cleft. These small spaces are useful starting points from which to commence the surgical separation of the nasal from the buccal layer.

The operation consists of incising the mucosa in the buccal sulcus to expose the bones bordering the cleft. The nasal mucosa is then meticulously separated from the buccal layer as far back as the posterior margin of the hard palate. All pre-existing fistulae are sutured prior to the insertion of the bone graft. This is taken from the inner table of the ilium and includes its periosteum. It is shaped to fit the defect; its widest part fills the defect in the bony palate; its narrowest part fills the alveolar gap; an extension to support the alar base can usually be usefully left anteriorly. Ordinarily the periosteal surface faces downwards into the mouth, but if there has been a difficult nasal fistula to close it is best to fashion the graft so that its periosteal surface is on the nasal side, since the periosteal surface is the least vulnerable to infection (Fig. 1, 24). It is of paramount importance that the graft sits well down into the alveolar gap and is tightly wedged there. It is useless to allow the graft to ride upwards and lie in the pyriform opening of the nose. In order to increase the firmness of the fixation of the graft in the alveolar gap a small bony peg, shaped like a matchstick, can with advantage be placed above it along its medial and lateral borders. Each matchstick lies in the antero-posterior plane and is about 2 cm long. Fixation with

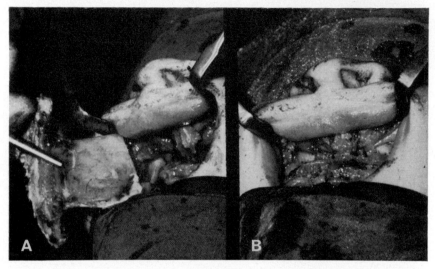

FIG. 1, 24

Insertion of bone graft. Bilateral cleft after expansion and separation of the maxillary spine to free the nose tip. (A) Shaped bone graft ready for insertion. (B) Graft *in situ* and held by small matchstick peg at each end.

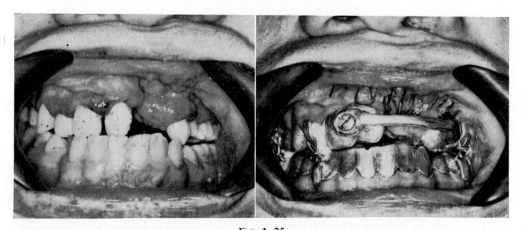

FIG. 1, 25

Lateral osteotomy in addition to rapid expansion and bone graft of cleft. Using sectional cap splints and a pre-cast locking bar, the anterior open bite of the lesser segment has been brought down by lateral osteotomy and the bony gap grafted as well as the main cleft.

the expansion apparatus is maintained for seven weeks after which it is taken off and a removable tooth bearing prosthesis substituted.

In bilateral clefts both sides are closed at the same operation using a similar graft for each side. The incision in the buccal sulcus can safely be made right round from one lateral segment to the other.

If angulation of the lesser segment is present in unilateral cases or elevation or depression of the premaxilla in bilateral cases these can be corrected by suitable osteotomies at the same time as the bone graft is inserted. This is achieved by removing the expansion apparatus on the morning of operation and substituting segmental cap splints with screw attachments for pre-cast locking bars. The segmental splints and locking bars are made from models taken prior to expansion and cut so that they can be properly aligned on the mandibular model The unilateral case is treated by lateral osteotomy below the antral floor and the bilateral case by severing the nasal spine with a dental drill to mobilise the premaxilla. In both cases gaps left by moving the bones are filled by bone grafts additional to those used to graft the main clefts (Fig. 1, 25)

Maxillary osteotomy

In some cases examination of study models reveals a maxillary arch capable of satisfactory occlusion but retroposed; a class III occlusion due to maxillary hypoplasia rather than mandibular prognathism. A similar condition can sometimes be produced by expansion and bone grafting of a small maxilla; the arch is restored but the maxilla remains retroposed. This condition, no matter whether it is after expansion and bone grafting or not, is amenable to treatment by horizontal osteotomy of the maxilla and advancement of the lower fragments. The steps of the operation are submucous division of the cartilaginous and bony septum immediately above the palatal arch, section of the lateral maxillary walls with a dental drill through mucosal incisions in the buccal sulcus as far forward as the pyriform opening, and severance of the pterygoid laminae and maxillary and palatine tuberosities with an osteotome. With the antral mucosa freed from the bone this can be easily moved forward into occlusion without damaging the air sinus, and fixed with cap splints and precast locking bars. The vascularity of the severed fragment is not imperilled by this procedure and the soft tissues of the palate are no hinderance to its free forward movement (Fig. 1, 26).

Nasal reduction

In essence this operation is similar to cosmetic rhinoplasty and like it should not be undertaken until the bony structures have reached adult proportions. This means that it should not be performed before the mid-teens; if performed on a child subsequent growth of the bones may be considerably reduced.

In all complete unilateral clefts the nose is considerably deviated away from the cleft side, the septum is curved and there is asymmetry of all bony and cartilaginous elements of the lateral nasal walls, including the turbinates. More often than not the alar cartilages also need adjustment and equalisation; a convenient approach for all this work, except resection of the base of the bony pyramids and turbinectomy, is the

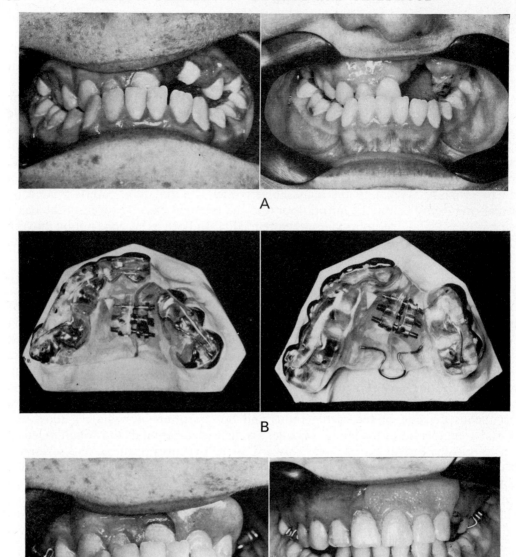

A

B

C

FIG. 1, 26

Maxillary osteotomy after rapid expansion and bone graft. (A) Before and after expansion and bone graft showing restoration of arch but persistent class III occlusion. (B) Splints on models before and after expansion.
(C) Before and after restoration of class III occlusion by maxillary osteotomy. Gap created by expansion and bone graft filled with denture.

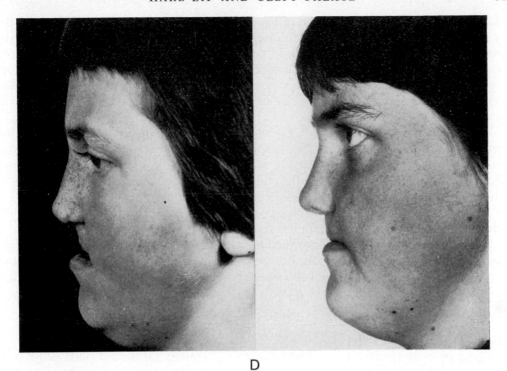

D

FIG. **1**, 26 (*contd.*)
(D) Profile pictures before and after maxillary osteotomy.

flying-bird incision. The whole bridgeline can be reached and visualised from it and the septum dealt with as well. No other incision gives such satisfactory exposure of the alar cartilages. Additional support to the tip is sometimes needed in unilateral and bilateral cases, and an angled bone graft or an acrylic implant can be accurately placed under direct vision through this incision. It can also be safely combined with a secondary soft tissue correction of the lip if this is required.

The bases of the nasal pyramids are best approached for section through separate small stab incisions in the mucosa at the lower margin of each nasal bone. The larger nasal bone in deviated noses can be reduced by removing the excess from the base of the pyramid through this incision if desired, although it is the author's preference to remove the excess along the bridgeline where the nasal bone is under direct vision.

RARE FACIAL CLEFTS

Median cleft lip

This is caused by failure of development of the median nasal processes which are responsible for the prolabium, columella and premaxilla as far back as the incisive foraminae. It is a failure of the primary palate. When complete the deformity is associated with intracranial malformations, and the child is often still-born. The commonest is failure of division into hemispheres with absence of the corpus callosum.

PS C

Failure of development of the Sylvian aqueduct may accompany this with consequent hydrocephalus. There may also be failures of development of the skull, of which the commonest is absence of the sphenoid sinus with a midline defect of the sphenoid bone through which the meninges project into the nasal roof causing obstruction. Unless the surgeon is aware of this possibility the swelling may be mistaken for hypertrophied adenoid tissue with disastrous consequences if such a misdiagnosis is acted upon.

Mental subnormality is usually associated with all severe degrees of this deformity, but lesser degrees and minor midline notching of the lip may not cause any detectable lowering of the intelligence quotient in early childhood, and special schooling is not necessary. Even in these, however, the child usually drops behind the age group as the educational requirements advance; this must be recognised and allowed for if signs of stress appear around puberty. It is easy for a school teacher, anxious for the child's advancement, to mistake this cerebral handicap for laziness.

The surgical correction of minor median clefts can usually be achieved by straight closure with a fair cosmetic result, but on the rare occasions when severe cases need surgery an Abbe flap is required to restore both lip and columella, and a prosthesis is needed as a substitute for the missing bone and incisor teeth. Happily this very serious type of cleft is a rarity.

Oro-orbital (vertical) clefts

These pass upwards towards the orbit and are often associated with gross mal-formation of both sides of the lip and of the palate. The vertical cleft skirts the alar base and traverses the cheek to end in bifurcation of the lower eyelid. The whole orbit is then likely to be small and its contents disorganised with a tiny sightless globe. The nasal wall on the affected side is always short and the alar base is drawn upwards bringing the lip with it. Repair of the eyelid and cheek are straightforward but it is extremely difficult to lengthen the nose and bring the ala down to the same level as on the opposite side. This difficulty stems from the hypoplasia of the underlying maxilla and pyriform opening. Additional soft tissue has often to be introduced into the lateral nasal wall for both lining and cover; this is best done with an inturned lining flap surfaced with a free graft. The restoration of adequate length to the nasal wall drops the lip to give it correct height. (See also Chap. IV.)

The naso-lacrymal apparatus is usually normal in this type of cleft, being in con-tinuity with the punctum on the medial portion of the split eyelid. This is in contrast to its abnormality in cases in which there is a 'third nostril' (Fig. **1**, 27). These accessory nostrils are in fact naso-lacrymal ducts opening separately through an orifice on the skin lateral to the nostril; this is easily demonstrated by the injection of dye through the punctum; it can be incorporated in the nostril without great difficulty and its orifice used to increase the diameter of the nostril if this is small, as is often the case. (See also 'lateral proboscis' p. 267.)

Transverse clefts

These run from the oral commissure towards the ear. In simplest form they consist only of macrostoma, whilst in complete cases the cheek is cleft to within 2 cm of the

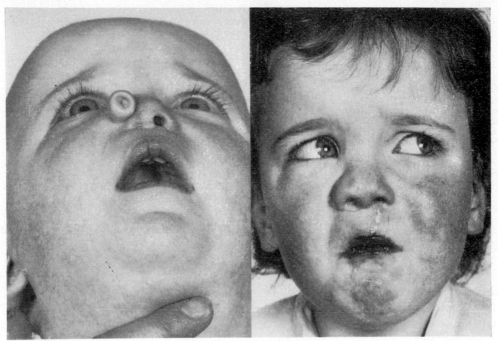

FIG. 1, 27

'Third nostril.' This segment contains the opening of the naso-lachrymal duct and is incorporated into the stenosed nostril to enlarge it. (See also 'lateral proboscis', p. 267.)

tragus. All intermediate grades occur. Occasionally the upper extremity of the cleft is the epithelium of the parotid duct which has failed to form a tube. In all severe transverse clefts there is hypoplasia of the face and ear, with underdevelopment of the mandible and malformation of the auricle, which may only be represented by a lobular tag set low down, level with the angle of the mandible (p. 269). The external auditory canal is also missing in such cases and exploration fails to find more than primitive ossicles.

Treatment of macrostoma necessitates dissection of the separated fibres of the orbicularis oris muscle and their careful suture. If reliance is placed upon closure of mucosa and skin the mouth always shows deformity during the play of facial expression and there is a tendency for the commissure to be stretched with relapse to the pre-operative state.

Closure of the more extensive clefts of the cheek is also straightforward, but the difficulty of achieving a satisfactory cosmetic result centres round the reconstruction of the ear and enlargement of the mandible. The former can either be attempted by the Tanzer technique or by the introduction of new skin supported by an acrylic inlay. The deformity of the mandible is best disguised by onlay grafts of split rib set into the buccal sulcus, whilst shortness of the ascending ramus may necessitate lengthening by a bone graft or by an acrylic joint depending upon the degree of failure.

D. N. MATTHEWS

ACKNOWLEDGMENTS

I acknowledge with thanks the permission to publish certain of the illustrations granted by the Editor of the British Journal of Plastic Surgery, Ethicon Ltd., and Professor K. Schuchardt.

REFERENCES

ABBE, R. (1898). *Med. Rec. N.Y.* **53**, 477.
BRAUER, R. O. (1953). *Plastic reconstr. Surg.* **11**, 275.
BROWNE, D. (1949). *Ann. R. Coll. Surg.* **5**, 169.
BURSTON, W. R. (1958). *Dent. Prac.* **9**, 41.
DAVIS, J. S. & RITCHIE, H. P. (1922). *J. Am. med. Ass.* **70**, 1323.
FOGH-ANDERSON, P. (1942). *Inheritance of Hare Lip and Cleft Palate.* Copenhagen: Arnold Busch.
HAGEDORN, U. (1884). *Zentbl. Chir.* **11**, 756.
HYNES, W. (1950). *Br. J. plast. Surg.* **3**, 128.
KERNAHAN, D. A. & STARK, R. B. (1958). *Plastic reconstr. Surg.* **22**, 435.
KILNER, T. P. (1937). In *Postgraduate Surgery*, Vol. 3, p. 3800, ed. Maingot, R. London: Medical Publishers.
LE MESURIER, A. B. (1949). *Plastic reconstr. Surg.* **4**, 1.
MATTHEWS, D. N. (1952). *Br. J. plast. Surg.* **5**, 77.
MATTHEWS, D. N. (1968). *Br. J. plast. Surg.* **21**, 153.
MATTHEWS, D. N. & GROSSMANN, W. (1964). In *Transactions of the Third International Congress of Plastic Surgeons*, Amsterdam: Exerpta Medica.
MILLARD, D. R. (1960). *Plastic reconstr. Surg.* **24**, 595.
MOORE, F. T. & CHONG, J. K. (1967). *Br. J. Oral Surg.* **4**, 183.
PFEIFFER, G. & SCHUCHARDT, K. (1964). In *Transactions of the Third International Congress of Plastic Surgeons*, Amsterdam: Exerpta Medica.
ROBERTSON, N. R. E. & JOLLEYS, A. (1968). *Plastic reconstr. Surg.* **42**, 414.
SCHUCHARDT, K. (1960). *Klin. Chir.* **295**, 850.
STARK, R. B. (1968). *Cleft Palate.* New York: Harper & Row.
STELLMACH, R. (1955). *Fortschr. Kieferorthop.* **16**, 247.
TANZER, R. C. (1959). *Plastic reconstr. Surg.* **23**, 1.
TENNISON, C. M. (1952). *Plastic reconstr. Surg.* **9**, 115.
TONDURY, G. (1955). *Fortschr. Kiefer- u. Gesichts-chir.* **1**, 1.
VEAU, V. (1931). *Division Palatine.* Paris: Masson.
VEAU, (1938). *Bec de Lièvre.* Paris: Masson.
VILAR-SANCHO, R. (1962). *Plastic reconstr. Surg.* **30**, 263.

CHAPTER II

THE EARLY ORTHODONTIC TREATMENT OF CLEFT LIP AND PALATE INFANTS

McNeil (1954) first introduced the concept of providing a dental plate for the neonate suffering from a cleft palate. The original intention was to reduce the width of the cleft prior to surgery by denying the tongue access to the cleft and also by stimulating growth in the palatal shelves by inducing a hyperaemia of the parts. Considerable controversy arose as to whether or not it was possible to obtain non-surgical closure in the region of the anterior palate. Undoubtedly the provision of a plate greatly facilitated feeding. McNeil extended his work to the treatment of clefts of the lip and palate and found that it was possible to mould the deformed maxillary segments into better position by providing a series of plates that 'did not quite fit'. The natural chewing and sucking action of the infant then caused the bones to conform to the plate which was then changed for a further correction plate.

The author has followed this latter aspect of McNeil's work. Attention has been drawn (Burston, 1960) to the underlying nature of the cleft deformity, especially the function of the cartilaginous interorbital nasal septum and its influence on the overlying facial bones. Further work by Latham and Burston (1964) on the role of the sutures in cleft lip and palate infants suggested that the plates fitted were influencing growth at the sutures. More recently a much more detailed analysis by Latham

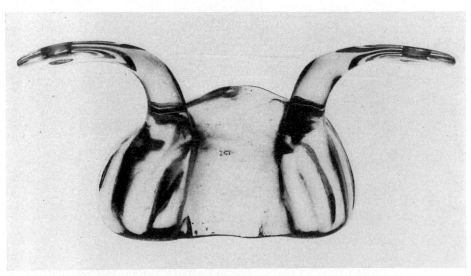

Fig. 2, 1

Plate made in clear acrylic so that the tissues can be seen with the plate *in situ*. Wings are provided to facilitate the insertion and withdrawal of the plate and holes are provided in the wings for the attachment of tape to stabilise the plate in the child's mouth.

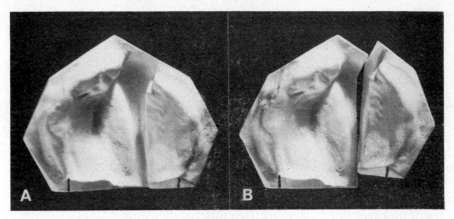

Fig. 2, 2

(A) Plaster cast taken from an impression of the child's mouth. (B) The same model divided and correction applied. When the plate is made to this corrected model it will bring pressure on the maxillary segments, thus moving these into better position.

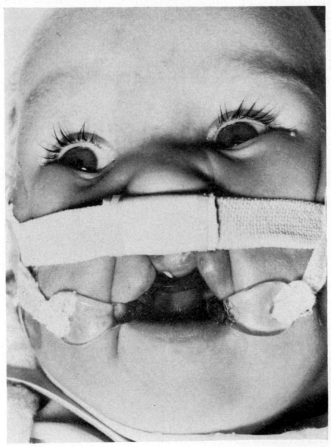

Fig. 2, 3

External elastic traction applied to control the premaxilla in the bilateral condition.

(1969) has shown that the original concept of the role of the nasal septum was an oversimplification. The original defect influences the growth of the cartilage to produce the characteristic deformity but later in foetal life the maxillary bones tend to follow their own genetic pattern of growth. However, the sutures act as planes of adjustment which can be influenced by correction plates in obtaining a much better relationship of the facial bones prior to surgery. This is true of all cases of cleft lip and palate but is best seen in the severe bilateral cases.

The object of early treatment is to assist the surgeon in producing an acceptable cosmetic result and in producing a maxillary arch of adequate shape and size. This latter factor has great importance on tongue action in speech and also renders later orthodontic treatment much more feasible. A not unimportant aspect of orthodontic treatment is the maintenance of general dental health. In the ordinary way patients seeking orthodontic treatment are a carefully selected sample of the population where parents have taken great care to ensure their children have received adequate routine dental treatment. In the writer's experience this is unhappily far from true in the cleft population so that there is a severe restriction on what may be accomplished by later orthodontic treatment. For these reasons alone it would appear desirable to obtain an optimum result as early as possible in the child's life.

As practised in the Liverpool Unit the orthodontist sees the mother and child as soon after birth as possible with the object of fitting a feeding plate (Fig. 2, 1), ideally before the infant has its first feed. The orthodontist also visits as the representative of the team to cushion the parents, particularly the mother, against the shock she will have received. The importance of the family having direct access to informed opinion and advice in the early critical weeks must be kept in mind in the overall management of the condition. It is at this time too that the decision has to be taken as to whether the child can be treated in the home or whether it is desirable to hospitalise the baby; if the latter, it is most desirable to have special accommodation staffed by nurses trained to deal with these conditions.

In the normal way the feeding plate will be replaced in a week by a correction plate (Figs. 2, 2A and B). When an individual is at rest the teeth are separated, the position of the mandible being dictated by the resting length of the muscles attached thereto. The same is true of the gum pads of the infant. The plate is so made as to hold the jaw a little more open so as to secure reflex chewing activity, which, together with the action of the tongue, produces the desired forces on the maxillary segments. The action of the plate may be reinforced by external pressure strapping (Fig, 2, 3). In the unilateral condition such pressure will be used to correct the mid-line deviation; in the bilateral cleft the pressure will correct the eversion of the premaxilla and reposition the latter structure on the septum. In both cases the plate will be moving the lateral maxillary element (or in the bilateral cases, elements) forward and, if necessary, outward.

The object is to secure a symmetrical maxillary arch lying outside the mandible. In the writer's experience the majority of cases yield satisfactorily to plate therapy (Figs. 2, 4A and B; 2, 5A and B). In these situations there would appear every good reason for including an anterior palate repair at the time of lip operation to stabilise the parts prior to final fixation at palate repair proper.

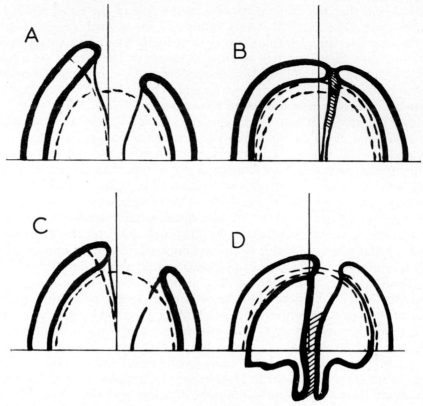

FIG. 2, 4

(A) Original position of the maxillary segments, the dotted line representing the super-imposition of the mandible on the maxillary arch. (B) The corrected arch lying outside the mandible, the shaded area representing an anterior palate repair. (C) The original position of the maxillary segments. Note in this case the mandible is well forward at birth. In this situation it may be impossible to secure apposition of the maxillary segments outside the line of the mandible and the best result that can be achieved is as in (D). In this situation the anterior repair is omitted at lip repair and later may be again deferred in the interests of avoiding contraction.

In the unilateral condition which has not lined up satisfactorily (Fig. 2, 4c and d) although it would be possible to approximate the alveolar processes in a position of symmetry, this could only be done at the expense of producing a depressed middle third of the face. In these circumstances an anterior palate repair is not carried out at the time of lip operation and attempts are made to improve the situation between this operation and the time of palate repair by further plate therapy. If at palate repair there is still an alveolar defect the soft palate and part of the hard palate is repaired, the intention being to fill the anterior fistula with a chipped rib graft when the child is approximately 3 years old. The bone graft is regarded as a space-filling procedure of a non-contractile nature. If it is postponed until 3 years the deciduous teeth will have fully erupted and therefore any minor adjustment to the occlusion may be carried out by cap splint therapy on the teeth. It will also be possible to insert a post-operative retainer to guard against any possible distortion to the arch by oedema of

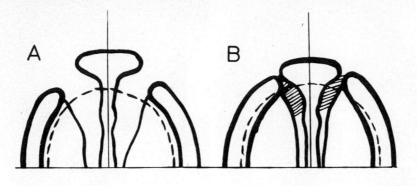

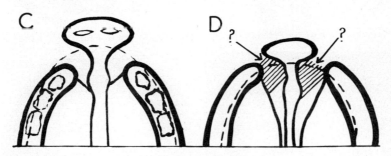

FIG. 2, 5

(A) The position of the maxillary segments at birth in the bilateral condition. (B) The same condition with the inclusion of anterior palate repair at lip operation. (C) Relapse which can occur where the premaxillary segment is not united to the lateral elements at lip repair. (D) This shows incomplete reduction but suggests anterior palate should be closed in order to avoid major relapse.

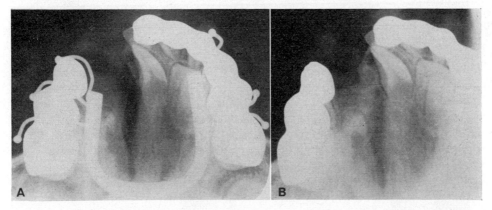

FIG. 2, 6

(A) Radiographs of the maxillary arch and palate of a child of $3\frac{1}{2}$ years of age, showing the anterior palate defect deliberately left at time of primary lip and palate repair. Repair of the anterior palate will now be carried out, and chip bone graft inserted in defect. (B) Condition 18 months later showing spontaneous derotation of the central incisor adjacent to the line of cleft.

PS C 2

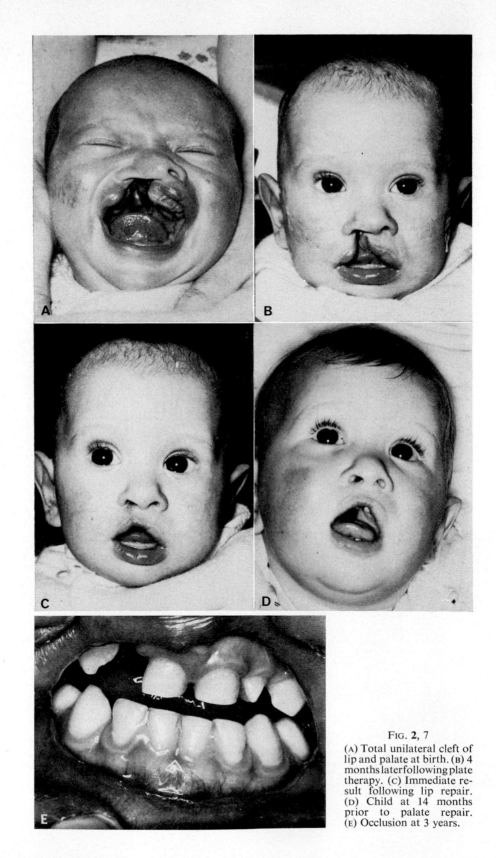

FIG. 2, 7

(A) Total unilateral cleft of lip and palate at birth. (B) 4 months later following plate therapy. (C) Immediate result following lip repair. (D) Child at 14 months prior to palate repair. (E) Occlusion at 3 years.

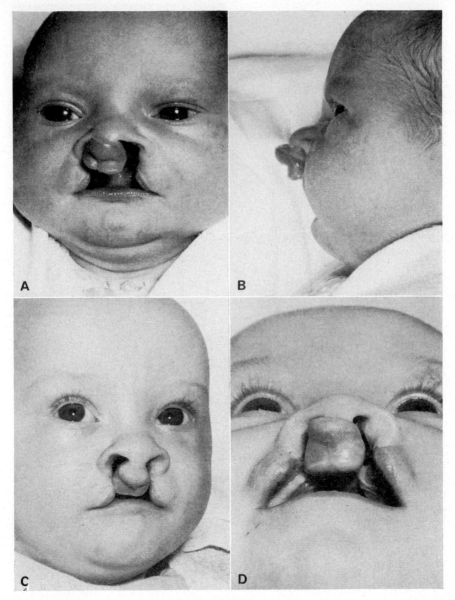

FIG. 2, 8

(A and B) Bilateral condition at birth. (C and D) Condition following plate therapy. Note the better position of the premaxilla in relation to the lateral segments.

the lip. Since the permanent incisor teeth are not too far developed at this stage, once the graft has organised, they will in most cases derotate and move into the area of the graft (Fig. 2, 6A and B).

In the bilateral condition (Fig. 2, 5A and B) where a complete line-up of the segments

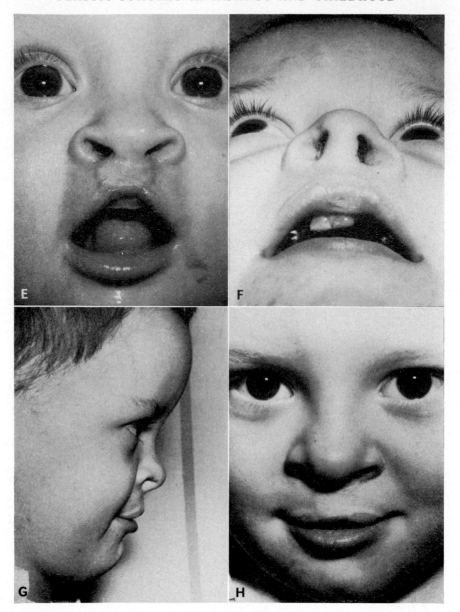

FIG. 2, 8 (*contd.*)

(E) Immediate result following lip operation. (F, G and H) Later result following a Millard (1960) fork flap elevation.

has been obtained, anterior palate repairs are carried out at the time of lip repair to stabilise the premaxilla.

Where complete line up has not been obtained before lip operation (Fig. **2**, 5D) the original approach was to proceed as with the unilateral clefts and not carry out anterior palate repair at the time of lip repair. Experience has shown that there is then a considerable risk of the premaxilla growing forward (Fig. **2**, 5c) so that at the time of palate repair there may be relapse of the position of the segments. For the last four years it has been found best to close the anterior palates in all cases of complete bilateral cleft lip and palate at the primary repair of the lip. In some cases this has led to a degree of 'collapse' of the anterior ends of the lateral segments much of which has been corrected by later orthodontic therapy.

Following early presurgical correction of the displaced maxillary segments the need for bone grafting has been minimal. Soft tissue closure of the anterior palate has produced satisfactory stabilisation of the segments so that it would appear that one of the principal benefits of bone grafting is to provide additional supporting bone in which to align the canine and central incisor adjacent to the line of cleft (the lateral incisor being malformed or frequently absent). Though this may be an idealised treatment, practical considerations, from the dental standpoint (such as the standard of dental health the patient is prepared to maintain, lack of desire for long orthodontic treatment and distance of the home for an orthodontic centre) puts a severe restraint on this approach in the Liverpool Unit. Confronted with this oft-repeated dilemma, the practical compromise has been to accept soft tissue repair of the anterior palate in the knowledge that a small denture may well have to be fitted later.

Figures **2**, 7 and **2**, 8 show a typical unilateral and a bilateral condition treated as outlined above.

W. R. Burston

ACKNOWLEDGMENTS

The writer wishes to thank Miss Isabella Forshall, Consultant Paediatric Surgeon and Mr R. P. Osborne and Mr D. O. Maisels, Consultant Plastic Surgeons for permission to publish their treated cases and also for their generous help, encouragement and interest in this work over the years.

REFERENCES

Burston, W. R., Kernahan, D. A. & Stark, R. B. (1960). A morphological basis for the analysis and treatment of the cleft lip and cleft palate condition. *Trans. int. Soc. plast. Surg.*, 2nd congr., 1959, pp. 9-14. Edinburgh: Livingstone.

Latham, R. A. (1969). The pathogenesis of the skeletal deformity associated with unilateral cleft lip and palate. *Cleft Palate J.* **6**, 404-414.

Latham, R. A. & Burston, W. R. (1964). The effect of unilateral cleft of the lip and palate on maxillary growth pattern. *Br. J. plast. Surg.* **17**, 10-17.

McNeil, C. K. (1954). *Oral and Facial Deformity*. London: Pitman.

Millard, D. R. (1960). *Plastic reconstr. Surg.* **25**, 595-605.

CHAPTER III

DEFORMITIES OF THE JAWS

AETIOLOGY OF JAW DEFORMITIES

Malformations of the maxillo-mandibular region can be classified into three groups: congenital, anlage-induced, and acquired. It is, however, difficult to differentiate clinically these conditions, particularly the first two groups.

Congenital malformations. These are present at birth. In spite of this, the clinical picture may not be very clear at birth, but may develop to a significant deformity during growth. This is especially true of craniosynostoses, dysostoses, and certain craniofacial syndromes. On the other hand it is possible that at birth an impressive clinical picture may be present which tends to correct itself partially with growth, as is the case with extreme retrognathia found in the Pierre Robin syndrome.

Anlage-induced deformities. These malformations of the maxillo-mandibular region are seldom readily identifiable at birth. These conditions are usually noted at a later date when either an under- or over-growth of a particular jaw region occurs. This is often the case in instances of retromaxillism and mandibular retrusion, as well as open bite and cases of maxillary and mandibular protrusion and others.

Acquired deformities. Such deformities of the facial region originate either through disease or the influence of external factors. These external factors can be the direct source of the deformity, e.g., following fractures, infections, or surgical procedures. On the other hand, other external factors such as irradiation or orthodontic appliances can lead to facial deformities appearing during the growth period.

In many conditions anomalies of other structures are present, particularly of the face and facial skeleton, in addition to the deformities of the jaw regions. Classical examples of this are the craniosynostoses and dysostoses, as represented by Crouzon's and d'Apert's diseases and the so-called first branchial arch syndrome. Similar combinations are also found with acquired conditions—particularly post-traumatic— as well as in certain instances of anlage-induced malformations of the jaw regions. A classical example of the latter is micro- or retro-mandibulism, in which in addition to the retruded position of the lower jaw one often finds maxillary anterior protrusion, a 'hook' nose and protruding ears. It is obvious that acquired jaw deformities can be caused not only by direct involvement of the mandible and maxilla, but also by conditions affecting the associated soft and hard structures. Examples of this are the deformities which follow irradiation of the facial structures in childhood, or after trauma or surgical procedures. The severe deformity which results when cleft-lip/cleft-palates are repaired early in infancy must be classified as acquired—although actually a combination of congenital and acquired malformations.

The discussion of therapy will be limited mainly to the management of malformations of the maxillo-mandibular region. The treatment of other deformities of the hard and soft tissue structures of the cranio-facial region will be mentioned only when their management is requisite to the correction of the jaw deformities.

CONSEQUENCES OF JAW DEFORMITIES

Malformations of the maxillo-mandibular region produce various disturbances.

Functional disorders. Particularly noteworthy are disturbances of mastication, speech, respiration, and in certain instances vision.

Disturbances of appearance. In that the cranio-facial skeleton constitutes the 'framework' for the face, any malformation of the jaws produces disturbances of the facial appearance.

Psychological problems. As a result of functional disorders and facial appearance, many patients with maxillo-mandibular deformities also display psychological disturbances. Above all, these patients feel inhibited. Severe psychological alterations may develop, which with early correction of the jaw deformity often disappear. When correction is not performed prior to the beginning of the third decade of life, the psychological alteration may become partially irreversible.

Problems with employment. Another consequence of the disturbances described above are the limitations in the area of professional development. Certain positions may be closed to these patients in spite of adequate intellectual or manual ability.

Problems in private life and social adjustment.

INDICATIONS FOR TREATMENT AND TREATMENT OBJECTIVES

The following indications for treatment are derived from the above described consequences of maxillo-facial deformities: (1) functional, (2) aesthetic-psychological and (3) social.

The treatment objective is the restoration of a normal appearance and function. In general the correction of jaw deformities is planned on the basis of restoration of a normal intermaxillary relationship. In many, but not all, instances it is possible to achieve at the same time a satisfactory or good aesthetic result. For the patient, because of the psychological and social factors involved, the aesthetic result is at least equally as important as the functional: in fact the aesthetic result is often more important than the functional result. Recognizing this, our planning for correction of jaw deformities is now based primarily on the facial form which it is desired to achieve. As one can surgically reposition tooth-bearing jaw segments in any direction, it is generally possible to achieve both the desired aesthetic result and functional improvement.

GENERAL CONSIDERATIONS REGARDING TREATMENT

It must be absolutely clear to anyone treating malformations of the maxillo-facial region that the bony skeleton constitutes the 'framework' of the face. Therefore in planning for the correction of facial anomalies the basic rule is 'first the bone, then the soft-tissue structures' (Pichler, 1948).

The management of malformations of the jaw regions in children is different from that in adults in that procedures are carried out in growing jaws with an incompletely formed dental apparatus. In this respect then the following points require special mention.

The presence of continuing growth. With continuing growth, depending on the age of the patient, it is possible that the malformation may not be fully developed. The result of correction of a condition in a 6-year-old child for example can be so altered, either through expected additional growth or delay in the growth, that the procedure was of no value. Therefore, the operator must be aware of the general growth tendency of the affected jaw region for which correction is planned, and he must also know what the probable appearance of this clinical condition will be at the completion of growth. On this basis one can decide at which age the necessary surgical procedures should be performed.

The influence of neighbouring soft-tissue structures on jaw growth. There is no doubt that the musculature of the jaw region can influence the growth of the jaw bones and significantly affect their final form. Typical examples of this would be masseteric hypertrophy, which causes the formation of prominent mandibular angles, and macroglossia, which often leads to an open-bite condition. There is also little doubt that soft tissue scars, regardless of origin, can significantly influence the growth of the jaws.

Growth disturbances caused by surgery. It should be clear to the surgeon that certain procedures may considerably affect the growth of the jaws. For one thing, elevation of the periostium appears to cause a significant growth disturbance in the form of a local hypoplastic reaction. For another there is no doubt that scarring caused by surgical procedures can markedly reduce the future growth of the jaw. The severe mutilation of the jaws seen in patients operated on as children for cleft-lip or cleft-palate conditions is certainly more a result of the surgery than of hereditary hypoplasia. Although the maxilla reacts more severely in this respect than the mandible does, surgery on either jaw should be delayed as long as possible for the reasons given above.

The furtherance of growth through normal function. In contrast to the above-described interferences in jaw growth caused by surgery, surgery can in certain cases assist in allowing normal growth to occur. In this respect surgery which is intended to correct the jaw deformity and which also makes normal function possible is of the utmost importance. For example, it is known that ankylosis of the temporo-mandibular joints resulting from destruction of the head of the condyle by infection or trauma always produces a 'bird-face' deformity, and likewise, a subtotal jaw resection causes a deformity of the remaining jaw and surrounding soft tissue when no provision for normal function is made. Nevertheless, in patients with bilateral temporo-mandibular joint ankylosis when normal mandibular movement can be achieved relatively early by means of neoarthrosis, the underdeveloped mandible may participate in future growth or even recover its own lost growth potential (Trauner, 1954). Similarly, in cases of subtotal maxillary or mandibular resection the preservation of normal function reduces the danger of growth disturbance. This can be achieved, following a *maxillary* resection procedure, if a functional, perfectly constructed prosthesis is employed. This prosthesis must support the soft tissues and prevent their shrinkage. Naturally, such an appliance must be altered to comply with the growth of the remaining maxilla. In instances of *mandibular* resection, normal function can be retained by means of appropriate splinting or by maxillo-facial appliances. One should as soon as possible, preferably at the same operation, restore the mandible with a free bone-graft to ensure normal mandibular movements.

Surgical access to the jaws. As it is most likely to be improvement in facial appearance which motivates the patient to seek treatment, nothing should be done in any of the treatment which would further detract from the facial appearance; therefore, whenever possible the intraoral approach should be employed so as to avoid external incisions and subsequent scarring. Another advantage of the intraoral approach is that possible injury to important anatomical structures, above all the facial nerve, is avoided. Naturally, one cannot utilize the oral approach in every case, but this applies only in instances of malformations of the upper half of the facial skeleton. For the occasionally necessary access to the region of the temporo-mandibular joint, we employ the tragus margin incision. This incision can be extended superiorly and anteriorly as required.

Injury to the tooth buds. Corrective procedures performed on the jaws of young children can lead to a loss of tooth buds, and the loss of these undeveloped teeth produces a disturbance of growth of the jaw in the affected region. This applies more to the maxilla than it does to the mandible. Therefore if at all possible one should postpone osteotomy in the tooth-bearing jaw regions whenever the osteotomies would cause injury to the tooth-buds.

Problems with splinting. All osteotomies in the jaw regions are synonymous with jaw fractures. Therefore the principles of splinting are the same as those which apply to jaw fractures (Chap. VII). Osteotomies which involve mobilization of only a segment of the alveolar process, without loss of continuity of the basilar bone, can be treated as alveolar process fractures without the use of intermaxillary fixation. Osteotomies which cause a loss of continuity of the body of the jaw, however, require fixation in the new relationship. This is best achieved with intermaxillary fixation. Depending on whether a long-surface osteotomy or a short-surface osteotomy is involved, the duration of the intermaxillary fixation will range from three weeks to two months.

The type of splint employed depends upon the status of the dentition and which facilities are available to the operator by the dental laboratory. With a good dentition, multiple loop wiring can be quite adequate. In partially edentulous cases and in those in which segments of alveolar process are to be mobilized, various types of splints produced by the dental laboratory ensure the most satisfactory results.

Guidance of jaw growth and development by means of orthodontic treatment. An abnormal position of the teeth in the jaw can cause jaw malformation. It is self-evident that such a deformity should be treated as soon as possible orthodontically. Orthodontic treatment with the use of appropriate appliances can force a patient to bite into a desired position. As a result of this, remodelling occurs, and at the termination of growth a normal form and position of the mandible can result. Orthodontic appliances can also be used to eliminate an excessive tongue pressure or to ensure the required degree of mouth opening.

In many instances of maxillo-mandibular deformities, anomalies of tooth position are also present. If one is to achieve the best possible end result, postsurgical orthodontic care will be necessary. In other instances pre-operative orthodontic treatment may be required in order to provide a pre-operative condition which would allow surgery to achieve an acceptable aesthetic and functional result.

Prosthetic techniques. In terms of percentage, the goal of surgery in most instances of jaw deformities, with only a few exceptions, is not only an improvement of form but also function. Mastication, being the significant function of the region, should never be neglected in total planning. The individual involved in planning must take into consideration both the possibilities and limitations of dental prosthetics, recognizing that in certain cases prosthetic appliances may be valuable during the course of treatment. This applies to the previously-described use of prosthetic appliances in cases of resection as well as to postsurgical rehabilitation with crown and bridge or prostheses.

I. ANLAGE-INDUCED JAW DEFORMITIES

A good understanding of the diagnosis and treatment of anlage-induced maxillo-mandibular deformities is a prerequisite in the planning and treatment of the (usually more severe) congenital and acquired jaw deformities. Therefore, these particular deformities will be first considered.

There exist tried and proven classical operative techniques for correcting the simpler forms of these jaw deformities. The more complicated types are usually instances of combinations of the simpler forms. They can seldom be corrected with a single surgical procedure, and require a combination of surgical approaches.

Aetiology and clinical appearance

Anlage-induced differ from congenital malformations in that at the time of birth they are usually not recognizable. The family history, however, frequently reveals many such similar deformities present either in the parents or in closer relations. This is particularly true of prognathism, which is known in German-speaking areas as the 'Habsburger' chin. It is also true of maxillary protrusion, mandibular retrusion, and patients with deep overbite. The only exception seems to be the condition of open bite.

These anomalies should not be considered malformations in the usual sense of the word, but are either deformities of the jaw, e.g., maxillary protrusion or the various forms of open bite, or are positional anomalies of almost normally developed jaws. Examples of the latter are mandibular protrusion, distal occlusion and retromaxillism. Nevertheless, under certain circumstances it is possible to speak of a large or a small jaw, an opinion based both on a comparison with average jaw size, or the relative size of one jaw to the other in the same patient.

Orthodontic treatment

Most of the anlage-induced jaw anomalies display an obvious deviation from normal occlusion. Orthodontists have studied these clinical pictures closely and classified them exactly. Through early orthodontic treatment it is possible to guide jaw growth, so it is therefore understandable that practically all of these cases are within the treatment domain of the orthodontist. Orthodontic care should be started as soon as possible: in certain cases in the primary dentition, in others in the mixed dentition stage. Surgical treatment is indicated only in those instances in which orthodontic care was not successful or was neglected.

Timing of surgical treatment

Surgery is seldom performed in these cases before the completion of eruption of permanent teeth, i.e., 12 to 14 years of age. In individual cases under certain circumstances one would wait until the final completion of growth, i.e., 17 to 20 years of age. In instances when a malformation or deformity appears to cause behavioral disturbances or psychological alterations, however, one should be prepared to correct the deformity at an earlier age than indicated above—even at 12 years it may be necessary to accept a partial relapse, which could be corrected again at a later date.

Treatment planning

The basic problem in the correction of these conditions is that whilst the desired profile line must be achieved, at the same time an exact occlusion must be obtained.

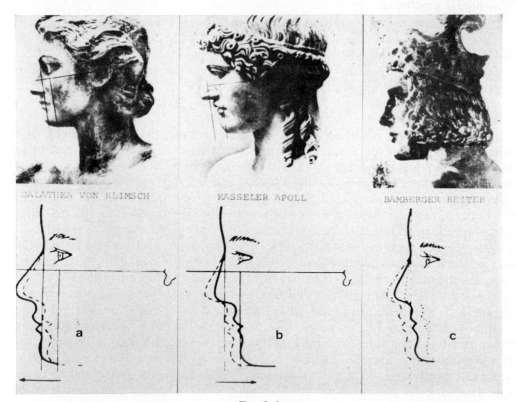

FIG. 3, 1

Normal profile lines according to A. M. Schwarz (from Kirchner, L. in: K. Schuchardt, *Fortschritte der Kiefer- und Gesichtschirurgie*, Bd. VII, George Thieme Verlag, Stuttgart, 1961): (A) Forward projecting face. (B) Backward receding face. (C) Middle (average) value face.

To facilitate planning we utilize a 1:1 profile photograph, upon which the desired profile is drawn. This profile line is placed over the tracing of a cephalogram which allows the determination of which jaw segment should be moved in which direction, and how many millimeters. These jaw movements are performed in vitro by cutting plaster models mounted on specifically designed articulators (Obwegeser, 1964b). With this technique the likelihood of the surgery to achieve the desired profile is evaluated on the basis of the resulting occlusion. When a successful result would seem unlikely, this technique furnishes one with the possibility of finding another method which is then checked for its effect on the profile line by means of the tracing of the cephalogram.

In planning, one always endeavours to achieve one of the classical profile lines (Schwarz, 1951): the projecting face, average-value face, and the receding face (Fig. **3**, 1). The surgeon must decide with the patient which facial form is most desirable.

CLINICAL TYPES AND APPLICABLE OPERATIONS

Mandibular protrusion

It is important to distinguish whether the protrusion is skeletal or alveolar.

SKELETAL MANDIBULAR PROTRUSION (PROGNATHISM)

There are many operative methods available for the correction of mandibular protrusion. The most important are as follows.

Ostectomy in the body of the mandible (Fig. **3**, 2). Whether these procedures are carried out in a 'step-fashion' (Eiselberg, 1907; Pichler, 1948; Converse, 1952 and others) or employing a vertical 'block-ostectomy' (Blair, 1915; Dingman, 1944 and others), the intraoral route is always indicated (Aller, 1917; Ernst, 1934 and others). The disadvantages of this procedure are that the body of the mandible is shortened in a dentulous area—an undesirable location—and that the contents of the mandibular canal are preserved only with difficulty. Another problem exists in the fact that the cut bone surfaces at the osteotomy site do not always fit well after the mandible is immobilized. In addition, there is no correction of the obtuse angle of the mandible.

Ostectomy at the angle of the mandible. This procedure produces better functional and aesthetic results and allows correction of the oblique gonial angle. It has, how-ever, disadvantages similar to the ostectomy of the body when performed as a 'block-ostectomy'. These disadvantages can be circumvented by the procedure depicted in Figure **3**, 3, in which, after removal of the buccal cortex, it is possible to free the contents of the mandibular canal, thus allowing ostectomy of the lingual cortex. When this has been done bilaterally, the mandible is immobilized in its pre-planned relationship to the maxilla. The buccal cortex is then shortened and returned as a free graft overlying the cancellous surface of both segments. It is fixed in position with transosseous wiring. With the utilization of this bridging graft, it is of little consequence whether the lingual cortical segments are well-adapted or not.

Osteotomy in the ramus. There are many possibilities for osteotomy in the ramus. Most surgeons have abandoned the extraoral horizontal osteotomy (superior to the

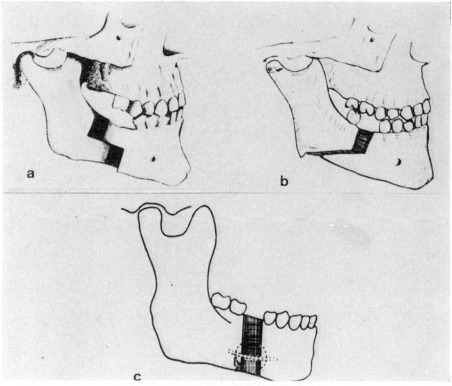

FIG. 3, 2

Various types of body ostectomy for correction of mandibular protrusion or retrusion: (A) Step ostectomy (osteotomy) after Eiselsberg-Auffenberg. (B) Step ostectomy (osteotomy) after Pichler (1948). (C) Vertical ostectomy (osteotomy) after Brown-Lindemann-Ernst-Dingman.

lingula) (Babcock, 1909; Hogemann and Wilmar, 1967) as well as the blind osteotomy with the Gigli saw (Kostečka, 1931). This latter procedure, however, may produce good results when carried out intra-orally (Ernst, 1927) and employing direct wiring of the fragments (Skaloud, 1951). The newer operative methods tend to employ an osteotomy line which produces wide bony surfaces, thus providing for an early consolidation of the fragments in their new position.

Sagittal splitting of the ramus. This procedure (Fig. 3, 4) is the extreme form of such long surface osteotomy (Obwegeser, 1957, 1964a). The diagrams represent an oral view following reflection of the peri-

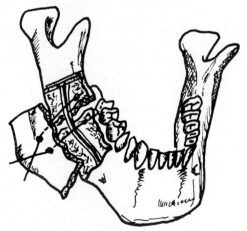

FIG. 3, 3

Obwegeser's technique for ostectomy at the mandibular angle via the oral route for correction of mandibular prognathism and open bite.

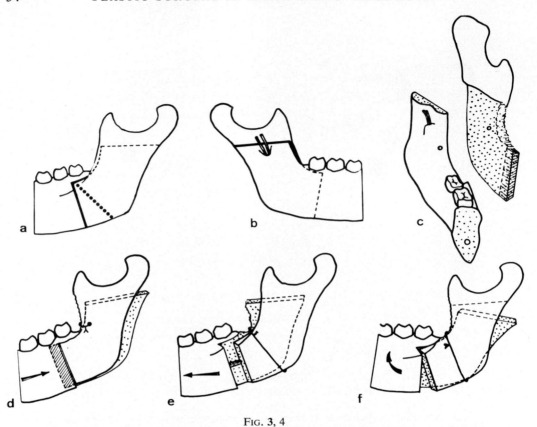

FIG. **3**, 4

Obwegeser's sagittal splitting procedure in the ascending ramus via the oral route (A–C), for correction of mandibular prognathism (D), distal occlusion (E), open bite (F) and asymmetry of mandible.

osteum of the anterior margin and lateral surface of the ramus, as well as the region superior to the lingula: a specifically designed retractor (Fig. **3**, 5) protects the lingual soft-tissues. Utilizing a dental drill a portion of the lingual oblique ridge is removed to furnish visual access to the entire medial surface of the ramus superior to the lingula. The lingual cortex is cut in this region with a Lindemann burr. The buccal cortex is cut from the region of the second molar to the mandibular angle (Obwegeser, 1957) or in a vertical fashion to the lower border of the mandible (Dal Pont, 1961). The incision line directed toward the angle is recommended when it is necessary to correct a flat gonial angle. The vertical incision, on the other hand, offers the advantage of wider bone surfaces. The lingual-superior and the buccal-inferior osteotomy sites are joined along the lateral cortex by a series of burr holes which are connected with a Lindemann burr. The ramus is split with a wide osteotome, being careful to protect the contents of the mandibular canal. Following this the attachment of the internal pterygoid muscle is completely freed from the ramus fragment, in a manner similar to that in which the masseter was separated from the buccal surface. When the attachments of both muscles are

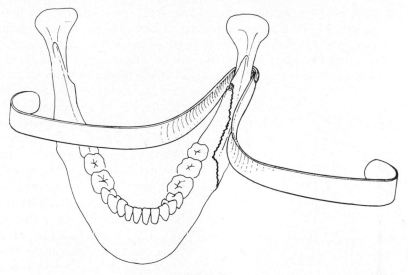

Fig. 3, 5
Obwegeser's special retractors inserted for protection of soft tissues during the sagittal splitting procedure.

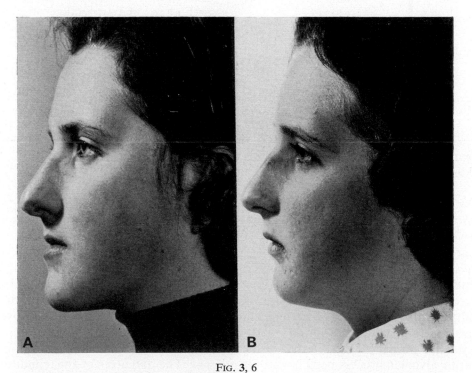

Fig. 3, 6
A 13-year-old girl with skeletal mandibular protrusion before and after correction with the sagittal splitting procedure of the ramus. No change in the postoperative intermaxillary relationship after 10 years.

detached the body of the mandible is completely free, and it can then be moved either anteriorly or posteriorly (Fig. **3**, 6) as desired. It can also be moved asymmetrically and rotated superiorly or inferiorly. The bony fragment is fixed in the desired occlusal relationship with intermaxillary wiring. We always also employ a circummandibular or interosseous wire to ensure good adaptation of the fragments and to make certain that the condylar heads are retained in the depths of the glenoid fossae. The latter is particularly important when this method is employed to bring the body of the mandible forward to correct distal occlusion cases. Many authors who also employ this operative method in correction of prognathism do not use bone wiring. We leave the intermaxillary fixation in place for a minimum of three weeks to a maximum of six weeks.

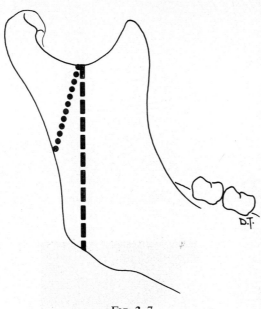

FIG. **3**, 7
Oblique and vertical osteotomy of the ramus through submandibular approach.

Oblique or vertical osteotomy of the ramus from the lateral approach. (Thoma, 1961; Robinson, 1960; Shira, 1961). This is a simple and good operative method for the correction of prognathism (Fig. **3**, 7). This procedure is usually performed from the extraoral, submandibular approach.

All ostectomy and osteotomy procedures for the correction of prognathism have a high percentage (about 55 per cent) of tendency toward relapse when performed before the cessation of growth (Freihofer, 1970). Psychological reasons, however, can still constitute an indication for their performance during late childhood as already described.

ALVEOLAR MANDIBULAR PROTRUSION

In this type of class III malocclusion the alveolar process appears to have been 'pushed forward' along a normal or somewhat too short mandibular base. This situation is clearly seen in the profile, in that the underlip is positioned too far anteriorly, while the chin prominence is either in its proper position or somewhat retruded with respect to the upper jaw. The retrusion of the entire mandible in correction of this apparent prognathism could under certain conditions produce a result regarded as just within normal limits as regards occlusion. It would, however, concurrently produce a retrusion of the chin prominence; and it would not correct the relative protruded relationship of the underlip. Therefore in these cases only the anterior alveolar process need be retropositioned. The diagnosis of this condition is readily made from the cephalogram.

One tooth bilaterally is extracted, usually the first premolar, and the anterior

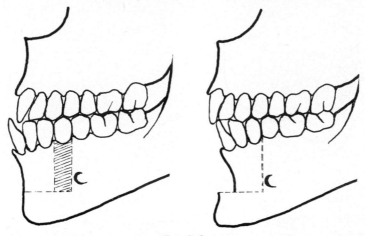

Fig. **3**, 8

Sketch for correction of alveolar mandibular protrusion; the first bicuspid of either side is extracted.

alveolar process is sectioned so as to include the teeth from the basilar portion of the mandible, and to allow its posterior repositioning (Hullihen, 1900; Köle, 1959b) (Fig. **3**, 8). The horizontal bone incision must be placed far enough from the root apices to avoid endangering the vitality of the teeth. Surgical access for the osteotomies is provided by an incision in the vestibular mucosa. The model procedure furnishes information of how many millimeters the anterior alveolar process must be retropositioned, and whether it is also necessary to lower it. When this last is required, a horizontal segment of bone must also be removed. The necessity for vertically splitting the alveolar process in the middle (Obwegeser, 1968), in order to produce a suitable arch form is also demonstrated by the model procedure. The blood supply to the separated segment is provided by the lingually attached musculature and mucosa.

Microgenia

The term microgenia will be interpreted here to mean only the small chin prominence, not the retrusion of the entire lower jaw. It is also presumed that the occlusion is normal, and that only the chin prominence is not far enough forward, or is somewhat retruded.

Correction is usually with onlays of bone, cartilage, or synthetic material. We no longer accept the extraoral approach to the chin region. In that this condition is really a shortening of the body of the mandible in the anterior region, the logical treatment is to achieve an elongation by advancing the lower border. The extraorally-performed advancement employing an attached muscle pedicle, as described by Hofer (1942), does not improve the ugly chin/neck contour. Because of this we advance the lower border as a free segment from the intraoral approach (Obwegeser, 1957, 1958) (Fig. **3**, 9). By dividing the horseshoe-shaped bone segment in the middle, one can alter the arch form of the chin prominence, or correct an asymmetry. The direction of the osseous incision used to separate the lower border is naturally dependent upon which direction one desires to move the chin prominence. Because

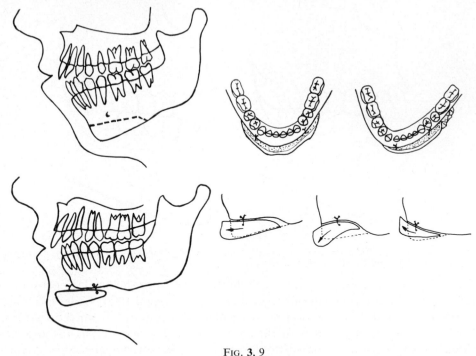

Fig. 3, 9

Obwegeser's intraoral sliding genioplasty for correction of microgenia and other deformities of the chin.

of this it is possible simply to advance a retruded chin, or when necessary, additionally to reduce or increase the height of the chin. In instances of an extremely high chin which is in a retruded position, it is recommended to place the chin margin in front of the mandible (Converse, 1952) (Fig. **3**, 10). The fixation of the chin prominence is accomplished with direct wiring.

Mandibular retrusion

Retrusion of the lower jaw is most often involved with a simultaneous shortening of the body of the mandible. In contrast to prognathism, in which the gonial angle is oblique, in this condition the mandibular angle almost forms a right angle.

To lengthen the body of the mandible one can employ the same 'step-form' osteotomy methods (Eiselsberg, 1907; Pichler, 1948; Converse *et al.*, 1952, 1964) which also have application for correction of prognathism. Gaps in the mandibular body must be filled with bone of course.

The significant disadvantages of the 'step-form' body osteotomy procedures were discussed under the description of their application for the correction of prognathism. Another disadvantage is that one must gain additional mucosa to cover the bone-grafted defect present at the crest of the alveolar ridge.

Today the sagittal splitting of the ramus (see Fig. **3**, 4) is generally accepted as the best method for the correction of mandibular retrusion. When so employed a vertical cut is made in the lateral cortex in the molar region. As already mentioned, direct

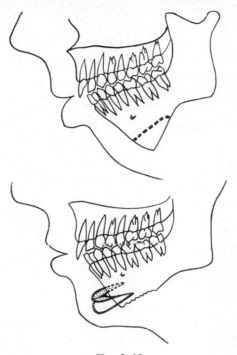

FIG. **3**, 10
Converse's technique for reduction of height
and simultaneous increase of prominence of
chin.

wiring (circummandibular) must be used to ensure that the condylar head is actually maintained in the depths of the glenoid fossa.

The 'bird-face' condition

The so-called bird-face condition is one without common aetiology, but recognized nevertheless clinically-therapeutically as a vast uniform problem. It is a deformity which may be anlage-induced or arise as a secondary condition, but the findings are similar whether the condition results from a congenital failure of development, or, as is more often the case, from a growth disturbance caused by ankylosis of the temporo-mandibular joint. The ramus always appears short. More impressive, however, is the shortening of the body of the mandible, both in its anterior and posterior regions.

The occlusion, however, seldom displays the degree of distal displacement that one would expect on the basis of external appearance. Treatment consists in lengthening the body of the mandible in the distal part in order to achieve an acceptable occlusion. Additionally, the anterior region of the mandibular body, i.e., the chin region, is advanced to correct the usually severe microgenia.

Advancement of the body of the mandible with the ramus sagittal-splitting procedure, and simultaneous one- or two-step advancement genioplasty has shown its value as a standard method for correction of the bird-face condition (Figs. **3**, 11 and

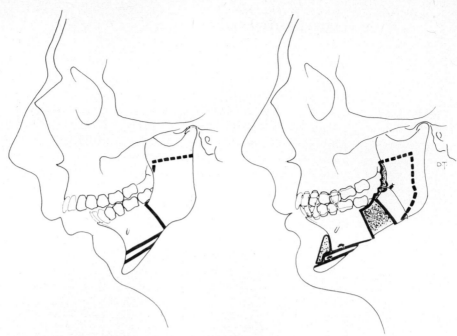

FIG. 3, 11

Obwegeser's procedure for correction of bird-face condition used for elongation of mandibular body by the sagittal splitting procedure and elongation of prominence of chin by one or double step genioplasty procedure.

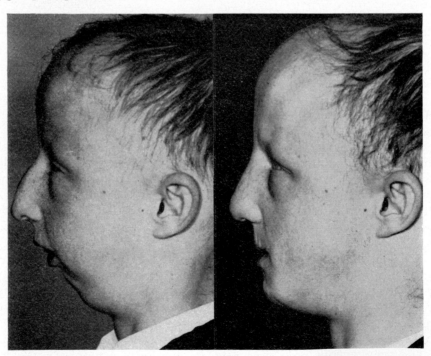

FIG. 3, 12

Correction of bird-face condition in a case of Hallermann-Streiff syndrome achieved by the procedure demonstrated in Figure 3, 11 plus a nasal reduction, performed in two operations.

3, 12). When insufficient mandibular length is gained with these procedures, supplementary advancement of the chin may be necessary, sometimes using bank or autoplastic bone at the site of the osseous incision.

Mandibular asymmetry

Mandibular asymmetry comes into the same category as 'bird-faced' deformity and has many causes with a wide range of clinical appearances. Two classical conditions with similar aetiology, but clinically readily distinguishable, must be specially discussed.

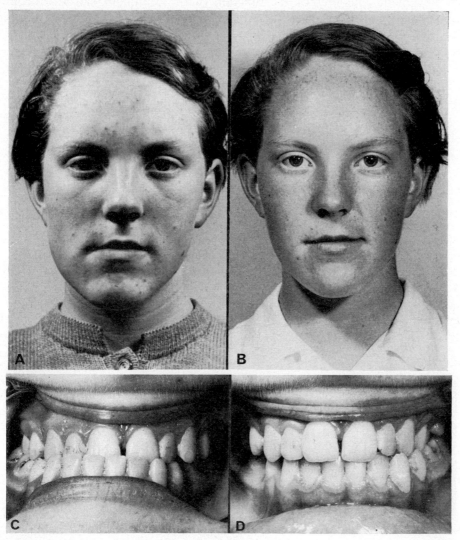

FIG. 3, 13

Case of asymmetrical prognathism corrected by unilateral sagittal splitting procedure: (A and C) Outward appearance and occlusion before the operation. (B and D) Outward appearance and occlusion after the operation.

Asymmetrical prognathism. This is manifestly caused by a unilateral hyperactivity of the condylar growth centre. In this condition the mandible is displaced to the opposite side, causing the mandibular dentition to appear horizontally displaced, but not inclined. Radiographically only a lengthening of the condylar neck is noted on the affected side. This condition is generally arrested with the conclusion of growth, and sometimes earlier. As soon as no further changes in occlusion are noted, the condition can be corrected with either a unilateral or bilateral sagittal splitting of the ramus (Fig. 3, 13). Correction utilizing a partial condylectomy destroys not only the protrusive movement, and thereby the function of the joint, but can also produce a severe deformative arthrosis of the opposite temporo-mandibular joint. This procedure

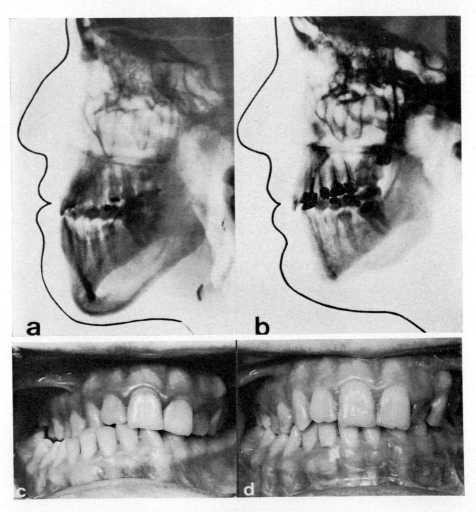

FIG. 3, 14

Case of true condylar hyperplasia with typical occlusal and facial deformity: A and C) Profile X-ray and occlusion before and (B and D) after correction.

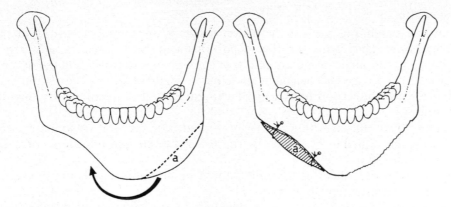

FIG. 3, 15

Transposition of lower border of mandible from hyperplastic to hypoplastic side via the oral route.

is indicated only when the abnormal growth tendency continues over a period of many years without evidence of cessation.

True condylar hyperplasia (Fig. **3**, 14). This produces a special form of distortion of the lower facial half: the teeth appear to be proclined, as though they 'desired to follow' the deformation of the mandible and radiographic findings include true enlargement of the mandibular condyle and lengthening of the condylar neck and ramus. The increase in height of the body of the afflicted side and relative lowness of the opposite side is striking. The therapy of this condition consists usually of a partial condylectomy to eliminate the offending condylar growth centre. The mandible should also be placed in the desired intermaxillary relationship. With the condylectomy we prefer also to perform a bilateral sagittal splitting of the ramus. To correct the difference in vertical height between the affected and unaffected sides of the mandibular body we transpose the inferior mandibular margin as a free-graft (Fig. **3**, 15). Usually these cases require supplementary orthodontic treatment.

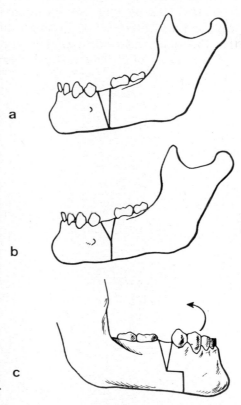

FIG. 3, 16

Various types of V-shaped ostectomy in the body: (A) Blair's procedure. (B) Thoma's procedure. (C) Procedure according to Converse and Shapiro.

The open-bite

Open-bite conditions present the widest range of anatomic variability of the jaw malformations. The cause for this conditions can be located in any region of mandible, e.g., the angle or molar region, or sometimes anteriorly. On the other hand, it can be caused by a displacement of either a segment of, or the entire, maxilla. Therefore, open-bite conditions can be caused by either maxillary or mandibular deformities.

The analysis of this condition in view of its anatomic aetiology is sometimes simple, but more often difficult. The same is true for treatment planning for correction of open-bite conditions.

The following treatment possibilities should be mentioned as being representative of the many variations of the condition.

1. *Rotation of the entire mandible* in the angle region: recommended operative procedures are the sagittal splitting of the ramus and the intraoral angle ostectomy (see Fig. **3**, 3).

2. *The linear osteotomy, or 'V' ostectomy* in the mandibular body (Fig. **3**, 16).

3. *Mobilization of the entire maxilla* utilizing a Le Fort I-osteotomy, and establishing a correct intermaxillary relationship (see retromaxillism, page 9). This presumes that the mandibular occlusal plane is normal.

4. *Lowering of the anterior maxillary region* (see maxillary protrusion, page 66).

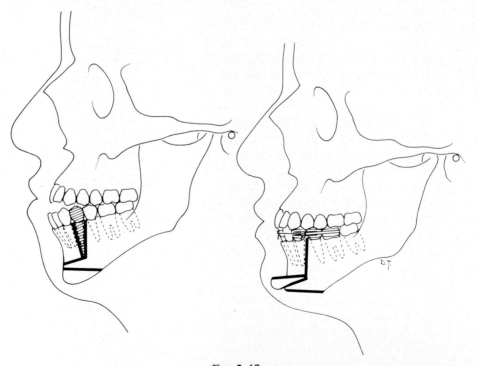

FIG. **3**, 17
Köle's procedure for correction of anterior mandibular open bite.

This is seldom indicated, as the upper lip is seldom sufficiently long to cover the teeth and gingiva.

5. *Elevation of the anterior mandibular alveolar process* and transposing the inferior border of the chin into the resulting defect (Fig. **3**, 17) (Köle, 1959b). This method is the ideal procedure for those cases, in which the inclination of the mandibular occlusal plane is in the premolar region. It is a particularly favourable condition when a prognathic occlusal relationship exists concomitantly, since following bilateral extraction of the first premolars, the lower (mandibular) alveolar process can be separated from the basilar portion of the mandible without danger to the roots of the teeth, and moved superiorly and distally. The segment of chin border which is wedged into the defect permits anterior increase in the chin prominence and a reduction in its height (Fig. **3**, 18). The principle of this procedure is the same as that for moving the lower alveolar process posteriorly.

6. *Raising (or recessing) of maxillary lateral segments.* If an anterior open-bite is caused by the lower level of the maxillary lateral segments, an over-exaggerated maxillary curve of Spee is noted. The logical therapy is to raise the lateral segments. This allows the lower jaw to close further and thus to make contact in the anterior region as well. We perform this procedure at one operation (Fig. **3**, 19) although originally described in two stages by Schuchardt (1955). The model procedure

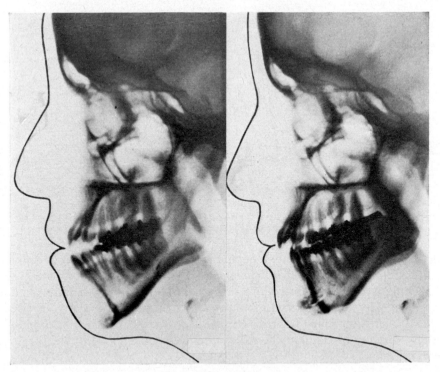

FIG. **3**, 18

Correction of anterior mandibular open-bite with class III occlusion. Correction by Köle's procedure as shown in Figure **3**, 17.

PS D

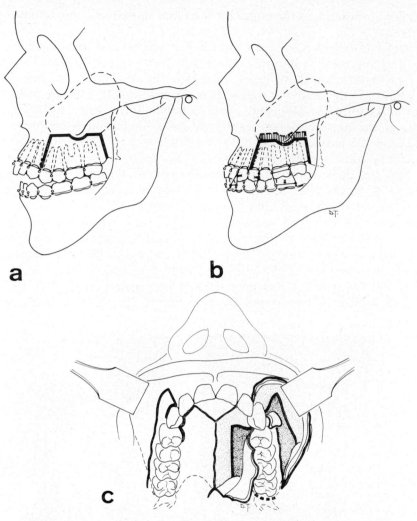

FIG. 3, 19

Sketch of Schuchardt's procedure for raising lateral maxillary segments to correct open-bite (A and B). (C) Obwegeser's incision lines and bone cuts for doing the procedure in one stage.

furnishes information as to the extent of the maxillary segments to be moved, and how many millimeters of superior movement is required.

This ingenious operative procedure brings ideal initial results. The method has, however, a considerable tendency for relapse to occur gradually over a period of years.

The basis of this tendency for recidivism is unexplained. This is in direct contrast to the dependability of results with Köle's previously described operative procedure for the mandible (p. 63).

Maxillary protrusion

Maxillary protrusion is characterized by a distinct enlargement of the angle between the base of maxilla and the upper incisal axis. The alveolar process of the upper incisors appears to be tilted forward, and the teeth themselves often assume a fan-like arrangement. As a result of the labial inclination of these teeth, the upper lip is no longer in a position to cover them. The picture is more conspicuous if it appears in combination with a retroposition of the lower incisors or the whole mandible, and if, in addition, the lower incisors are high-standing so as to bite into the palate. Consequent upon this is the premature loss of the maxillary incisors.

The choice of treatment in childhood is orthodontic correction. Nevertheless, mention of the possibility of surgical approach is being made, since the movement of the front segment of the superior alveolar process might be necessary for many reasons (Fig. **3**, 20). Sectioned study casts furnish the necessary information as to direction and extent of movement. Based on clinical and radiological examination, the necessary teeth for extraction are determined on the dental casts. These teeth are then removed on models and the casts so sectioned as to bring the middle portion of

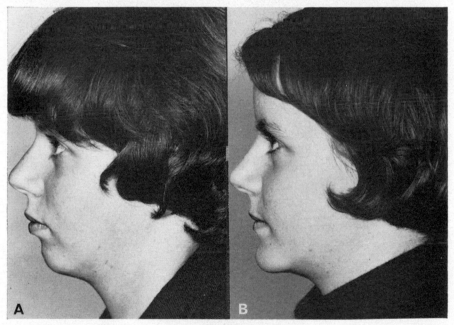

FIG. **3**, 20

Case of maxillary protrusion and retrogenia corrected according to Wassmund's procedure (Fig. **3**, 21) and author's genioplasty-procedure (Fig. **3**, 9).

the maxilla backwards. The surgical mobilization of this middle piece is achieved by the following bone cuts: a vertical osteotomy on each side of the marked-out strip of bone to be removed. The bone-cut leads from the alveolar process into the canine fossa. Since the protruding alveolar process is not moved back in a parallel direction but tilted, the strip of bone to be removed is cut convergent toward the canine fossa. The vertical bone cuts are then connected through a horizontal osteotomy meeting at the piriform aperture. The overlying mucosa and periosteum in this area are not severed; but only tunnelled. On the palatal side, the bone strips are removed and the

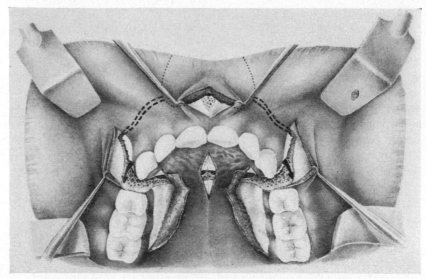

FIG. **3**, 21
Wassmund's procedure for correction of maxillary protrusion.

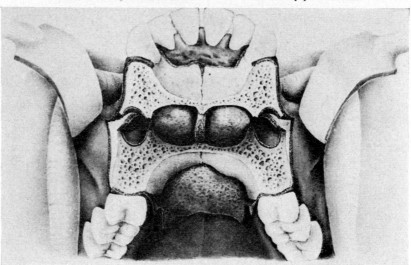

FIG. **3**, 22
Wunderer's procedure for correction of maxillary protrusion.

cut connected. Finally the segment is separated from the nasal septum. The only sure nutritional source of this central segment is now the vertibular muco-periostal covering. An additional source of nutrition can be achieved by undermining the palatal mucosa (Wassmund, 1935) (Fig. **3**, 21), but on the other hand, the operation is made less complicated by detaching the whole palatal soft tissue (Wunderer, 1962) (Fig. **3**, 22). Where the central segment is to be displaced cranially, bone has to be correspondingly removed from the nasal septum. Splinting for immobilization for six weeks is necessary but demands no intermaxillary fixation.

Retromaxillism and Micromaxillism

The outward appearance of the too-small maxilla is very similar to that of the backward positioned but otherwise normal maxilla. Both present a picture of class III occlusion, and outwardly therefore they present the picture of mandibular skeletal protrusion. On the one hand, such a situation could be corrected by backward movement of the mandible as in the correction of prognathism. At the best, a straight or backward-sloping face is achieved. If the face is round and the mandible broad before operation, the above procedure is not advisable: a better approach would be to bring the maxilla forward. The forward movement of the maxilla using the method

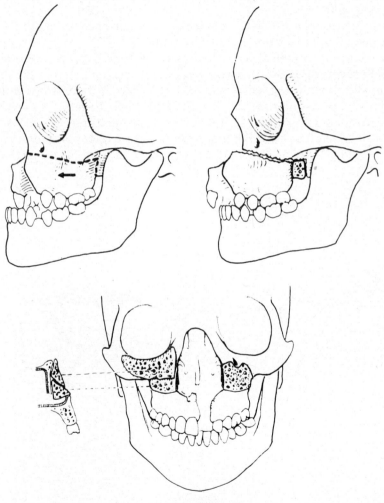

Fig. 3, 23
Obwegeser's technique for correction of retromaxillism in a unilateral cleft case. Large and small maxillary segments are moved independently according to the desired occlusion.

of Le Fort I-osteotomy (Axhausen, 1934; Schuchardt, 1942) has established itself as a routine method in various centres only in the last few years (Obwegeser, 1965, 1969b; Hogemenn, 1967).

Osteotomy of the maxilla combined with a transverse cut on the palate (Gillies, 1957; Converse, 1964) appears to be more complicated than complete forward movement of the maxilla.

We mobilize the upper jaw in one sitting by making a circular bone cut and at the same time severing the nasal septum as well as the connection between pterygoid process and maxillary tuberosities. When this is achieved, the maxilla must be so freed that surgical forceps can be used to bring it to the desired position without traction. A circular vestibular incision of mucosa and periosteum gives the necessary access to the maxilla.

Experience has taught us that a tendency to recurrence is relatively greater in cases where the maxilla was not completely mobile.

To avoid recurrence we also wedge in a piece of bone between the tuberosity and the pterygoid process (Fig. 3, 23). There is always a resultant step in the region of the canine fossa, and in almost all cases bone is put in here if there is not sufficient bone contact to ensure good union. In cases with steps up to 10 mm, we have used deep-frozen banked bone with success, but where the steps are up to 20 mm and over, we use spongiosa from the iliac crest. Although this bone is in open communication with the maxillary sinus, in general healing has been complete without reaction (Gillies, 1954).

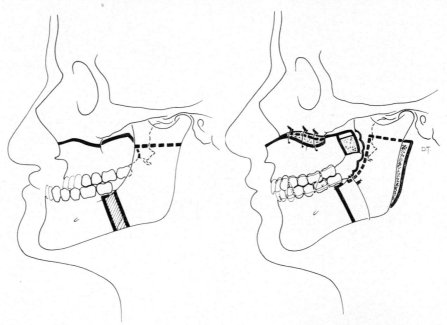

FIG. **3**, 24

Obwegeser's technique for correction of cases with extreme class III occlusion. One-stage operation for moving the maxilla forward according to the procedure demonstrated in Figure **3**, 23 and moving the mandible backward using the sagittal splitting procedure of the rami as demonstrated in Figure **3**, 4.

Intermaxillary fixation for three or four weeks is sufficient to retain the achieved occlusion. An additional interskeletal suspension is necessary during this period. Results obtained with this procedure are aesthetically and functionally very satisfactory.

Extreme retrusion of the maxilla and protrusion of the mandible

The outward appearance and occlusion of those cases with extreme retroposition of the maxilla and protrusion of the mandible is that of extreme mandibular prognathism. If correction of such a combined deformity is made exclusively through forward movement of the upper jaw or backward movement of the lower jaw, the aesthetic result is almost always never satisfactory and there is also a great tendency for relapse to occur.

We move the maxilla forward using the Le Fort I-osteotomy procedure and at the same sitting move the mandible back by the intraoral sagittal split of both rami (Obwegeser, 1970b) (Fig. **3**, 24). This combination appears to give us the best aesthetic and functional results (Fig. **3**, 25).

Since the lower half of the facial skeleton carrying the teeth has been completely mobilized, its fixation in any chosen location is possible. In positioning it in its new place, special attention must therefore be exercised to bring the occlusal plane into its proper locale.

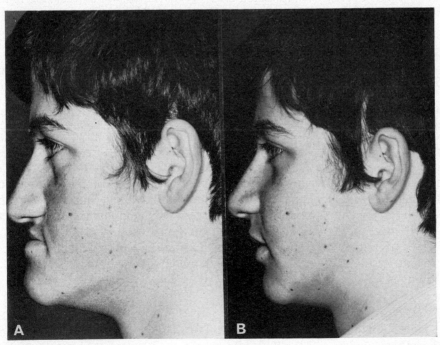

FIG. **3**, 25

Juvenile patient with extreme class III occlusion before and after correction using the technique demonstrated in Figure **3**, 24.

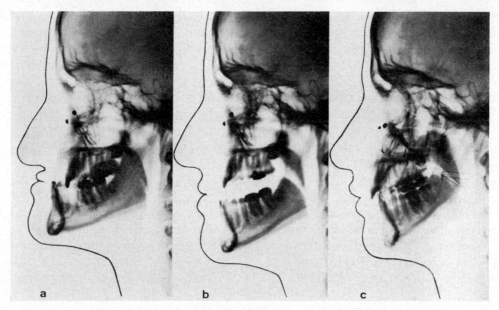

FIG. 3, 26

Cephalometric X-rays of the patient in Figure 3, 25: (A) before operation, with mandible in centric occlusion, (B) before operation, with mandible in resting position, (C) after operation, with mandible in centric occlusion. Note supplementary increase of vertical height of maxilla.

This procedure also allows for an additional elongation or shortening of the height of the middle third of face (Fig. 3, 26). The interskeletal suspension and intermaxillary fixation are likewise worn for three or four weeks.

Combined anomalies

Apart from the anomalies of the jaws described under the previous headings, a large number of cases present diagnostically a combination of these anomalies. It is therefore evident that surgical intervention must include a combination of the operative procedures. Wherever possible the various surgical interventions are carried out in one sitting. In many cases it must be admitted, however, that several operations are necessary in order to accomplish the best results. The operative treatment should always remain in an acceptable relation to the final result. On the other hand, the planning of treatment of these combined anomalies will be dictated to a much larger extent by the surgeon's imaginative acumen than in the case of the classical jaw anomalies.

Macroglossia

True macroglossia may cause deformation of the jaws and the problems related to this must, therefore, be included along with those of other jaw anomalies. Surgical reduction of the tongue is a necessity if the jaw deformity is to be treated with success, and this rule holds whether the jaw treatment is orthodontic or surgical. In the past, we have often reduced the tongue, not only in genuine macroglossia, but also in pseudomacroglossia and tongue-thruster, and especially in mandibular prognathism and open bite. Experience has taught us that the tongue is only seldom guilty for recurrences after surgical correction of jaw deformity, and that most jaw anomalies do not show any tendency for recurrence when diagnosis, proper indication for operation, and surgical technique are right, even if the tongue is relatively large. (For the surgical correction of macroglossia see page 121).

II. CONGENITAL JAW DEFORMITIES

Pierre Robin syndrome

Pierre Robin syndrome (see also page 19) is the only congenital deformity which, because of jaw malformation, can threaten life soon after birth. The causative factor is the pronounced mandibular micrognathism and resultant glossoptosis which, in conjunction with the cleft in the palate, can obstruct the respiratory tract.

It is known that this mandibular micrognathism generally disappears spontaneously within two to three years and surgical intervention is therefore not necessary.

Congenital trismus

Congenital lack of opening of the mouth is to be differentiated clinically from hypoplasia and aplasia of the temporo-mandibular joint, which still permits opening of the mouth. Whereas the malformation is more or less radiologically distinct in the latter, normal conditions may be found in the X-rays of the temporo-mandibular joints of cases with congenital trismus. Mandibular growth does not appear to be disturbed in spite of hindrance of mouth opening.

In those cases of partial congenital trismus which do not respond to exercises and forcible opening of the mouth we have always deferred any surgical intervention in order to avoid disturbance in growth. Aetiology of the disease seems to be unknown.

Craniofacial synostosis

The main problems of this disease (alternatively known as Crouzon's disease or Apert's disease) are discussed in Chapter III. The retroposition of the zygomatico-maxillary complex is more or less obvious but becomes more prominent with age. In some cases it is possible to bring the upper jaw into a good functional occlusion by moving the maxilla forward using the Le Fort III-osteotomy technique of Tessier (1967). Sometimes, however, an additional Le Fort I-osteotomy is necessary, either at the same sitting or during a second operation (Obwegeser, 1969b) (Fig. 3, 27). Such surgery should be postponed until the danger of damage to maxillary tooth germs is non-extant. In individual cases orthodontic regulation of the maxillary dental arch may be desirable or even necessary before surgical intervention.

The same problem is present in post-traumatic cases.

PS D 2

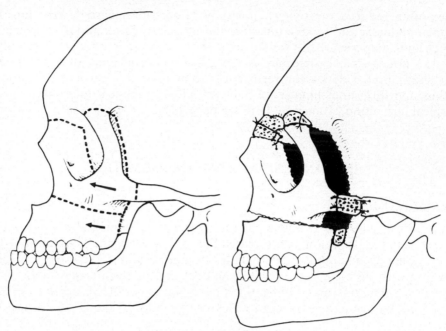

Fig. 3, 27

Combined Le Fort III and Le Fort I-osteotomies for correcting unequal degree of retrodisplacement of the face. (From H. Obwegeser: Surgical corrections of small or retrodisplaced maxillae, *Plast. reconstr. Surg.* **43**, 351. 1969.)

Mandibulo-facial dysostosis (Treacher-Collins syndrome)

The jaw malformations occurring in mandibulo-facial dysostosis of Treacher-Collins (see also page 100) are as follows. Hypoplasia of the whole of the lower jaw, and especially both rami which are strikingly thin and short. The articulating joints are also hypoplastic, and show to some extent changes similar to those seen in oto-mandibular dysostosis. The angle of the jaw is obtuse. The mandible is retrognathic and the chin high and retracted, so that the body of the mandible appears concave on the lower border (Fig. 3, 28). An open bite can also occur as a result of the mandibular malformation. The maxilla is hypoplastic and the dental arch is often crowded like that of the mandible. Still more pronounced is the zygomatic hypoplasia.

Maxillo-facial treatment consists primarily in the closure of the palatal cleft which is often present. As soon as permanent teeth are erupted, orthodontic treatment should be instituted to form the upper and lower dental arch. After complete eruption of permanent teeth, which is at about the age of 14, the jaw deformity can then be corrected through osteotomies as long as the sectioned study casts show that an acceptable occlusion could be reached. Since a forward movement, and sometimes a rotation, of the mandible is necessary to correct the open bite, we use the intraoral sagittal splitting technique. The operation is not easy, because of the anomalous anatomical conditions and especially the extremely thin ramus. In addition to the rotation of the mandible, and sometimes as the only measure of treatment, genioplasty in one or two steps is necessary.

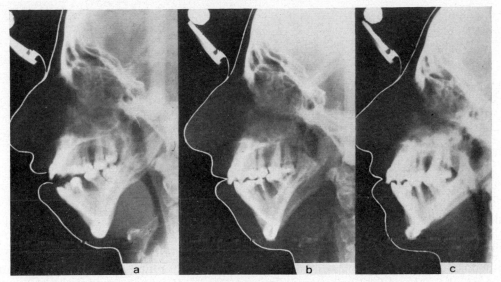

FIG. **3**, 28

Cephalometrics of a case with Treacher-Collins syndrome: (A) before correction of open bite (note the typical concavity of lower border of mandible), (B) after correction of open bite using the sagittal splitting procedure, (C) after supplementary correction of retrogenia and reduction of height of chin with sliding genioplasty according to Figure **3**, 9.

Bone or cartilage onlay is used for reconstruction of the hypoplastic zygoma. The operation is carried out from an intraoral approach and through an incision on the lateral portion of eyebrow.

Otomandibular dysostosis (first and second branchial arch syndrome)

This complex deformity (see also page 291) appears from our records to occur mostly on the right side and limits itself to the lower two-thirds of the face. In one case the deformity of the soft tissue, and especially the external ear, may especially strike the eyes, whereas in another it is the anomaly of the jaw. In its classical manifestation, the lower two-thirds of the bone and soft tissue on the affected side of face are involved.

The deformed side of the face shows a vertical as well as a horizontal hypoplasia of the lower two-thirds of the maxillo-facial skeleton. This hypoplasia may not be marked and onlays only may be necessary for correction. But it could be so pronounced that the upper part of the ramus, including the articulating joint, remains undeveloped.

In its less severe form, the articulating joint usually appears normal radiographically. But in spite of this, forward movement of the mandible is not possible and results in an obvious mandibular deviation to the diseased side when the mouth is opened. The chin is always retruded and the prominence of the chin appears to be shifted to the affected side. As a result of the vertical hypoplasia of this side there is a discrepancy in the occlusal height of the healthy and diseased side in the more pronounced skeletal forms. This results in an obvious oblique occlusal level which

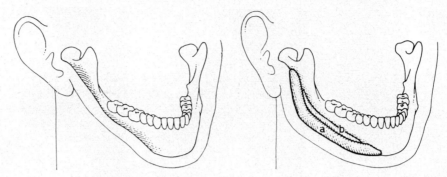

FIG. 3, 29
Correction of unilateral hypoplasia of mandibular body and ramus by multiple onlays.

can readily be demonstrated by biting on a wooden spatula placed between the teeth (Converse, 1964).

Treatment of the asymmetry in the less severe forms produces relatively good results with bone-onlays on the mandible (Fig. **3**, 29), or additionally on the maxilla and zygoma. We now prefer lyophilized preserved cartilage, however, and we place large pieces of this subperiostally, via an oral approach, on the mandible extending upwards as far as to the articulating region. Sometimes it is necessary to repeat the procedure two or three times, partly because enough cartilage may not have been grafted in one operation and partly because resorption of the cartilage has taken place to some extent.

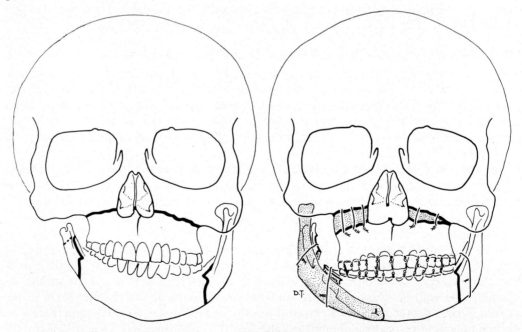

FIG. **3**, 30
Obwegeser's technique for correction of skeletal deformity in otomandibular dysostosis.

Onlays in the more developed skeletal forms of this clinical picture (Longacre *et al.*, 1968) can, in our opinion, only correct the horizontal, but not the vertical hypoplasia —and we think that the correction of the vertical hypoplasia is of primary importance. This we do in one sitting by using a combination of Le Fort I-osteotomy and sagittal splitting of the rami, which then enables us to align the occlusal plane parallel to the pupillary line by rotating the jaws using the healthy tuberosity region as a pivot (Fig. **3**, 30). The resultant wedge-like defect in the upper jaw is filled with a bone graft. Bone wiring keeps them in place and these bone wires also fix the mobilized

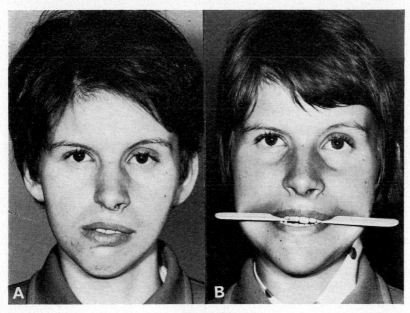

FIG. **3**, 31

Case of otomandibular dysostosis with mainly skeletal deformities before and after correction in two operations. During the first operation the procedure demonstrated in Figure **3**, 30 was applied but without bone grafting to the mandible; during the second operation correction of asymmetry and retrusion of chin was achieved using the technique demonstrated in Figure **3**, 9.

maxilla in its new position. The resultant defect on the ramus of the involved side is bridged with a bone graft. Such a bone graft fulfils the double duty of replacing the missing articulating end of the ramus and of partially correcting the horizontal mandibular hypoplasia. In later operations onlays are placed on the zygoma, lower and upper jaw of the affected side to correct the horizontal hypoplasia of the bony framework. Furthermore, advancement of the chin along with a lateral movement to the healthy side is necessary (Fig. **3**, 31). From an intraoral approach, the chin is advanced in one step as a free transplant (Obwegeser, 1958; Grimm, 1961) or in two steps (Neuner, 1965). Finally, mobilization of the articulating joint is considered. The surgical operation is similar to that done in fibrous ankylosis of the temporo-mandibular joint followed postoperatively by energetic training with orthopaedic apparatus in order to ensure the necessary mandibular movement. After completion of correction of the bone deformities, the soft tissue may then be dealt with, using dermis plus fat either as a pedicle flap or as a free graft.

Other congenital deformities

Some clinical pictures produced by congenital deformities of the lower two-thirds of the facial skeleton have been mentioned, but there are many more in this group. Klein (1968) has afforded a general view of the clinical findings, comparing them one against the other. They are rare and the jaw deformities are similar to the already-described clinical pictures so that they need no separate description as far as treatment is concerned.

III. ACQUIRED DEFORMITIES IN THE REGION OF THE JAWS

External or endogenous noxious agents could lead to arrest of growth in certain regions of the jaws, whereas trauma and surgical intervention could cause a direct displacement of jaw segments; the possibility of cicatricial tissue forming could further hinder growth or normal development of the jaw. On the other hand, osteo-myelitis or radiation injury of bone could give rise to a deformation of the jaw which only becomes fully manifested in the course of further jaw-growth. This also applies to damage done to the growth-zone of the condyles through the influence of other endogenous and exogenous poisons.

It is therefore necessary, during planning of treatment, first to ascertain the cause of the jaw deformity and if possible to eliminate the same. A classical example here is the cicatricial contraction following cervical burns (which is rather similar to the functional hindrance of mandibular movement in ankylosis).

In those cases where the consequences of a preceding injury cannot be eliminated, it must be expected that the jaw deformity will increase in intensity until completion of growth. This applies also partially to the congenital, as well as the constitutionally-induced jaw deformities. In every case therefore it must be decided whether a surgical intervention would eliminate the retarding factor of the growth of jaw, or cause an additional damage to growth.

Ankylosis-induced mandibular micrognathism

Post-traumatic or post-inflammatory ankylosis of the temporo-mandibular joint always leads to a considerable retardation of mandibular growth—usually mainly on the ankylosed side. The result is asymmetry of the mandible. In bilateral ankylosis, both sides of the mandible are underdeveloped, and this gives the patient the characteristic bird-like profile. The extent to which destruction of the temporo-mandibular growth centre can be held responsible for retardation of growth is not known, nor is it known how far functional loss of mandibular movements can be made answerable —or indeed whether both causative factors are guilty. In any case, before correction of a jaw deformity, ankylosis must be eliminated and normal mandibular movement restored. The earlier this is done, the better will be the correction of the jaw deformity.

On the other hand, treatment of temporo-mandibular ankylosis yields good lasting functional results if the treatment is carried on postoperatively with orthopaedic contrivances, and if the patient reliably cooperates. This may in many cases be successful by about 6 years of age (although occasionally even 12 may be regarded as too early). This cooperation generally depends more on the parents than on the child.

Surgical correction of ankylosis-induced jaw deformities is the same as for analogous embryonic anomalies, namely for bird-like profile, mandibular micrognathism or asymmetry. Reconstructive surgery should be delayed until about the age of 12, when intervention does not endanger any tooth-germs.

Post-traumatic jaw deformities

Post-traumatic jaw deformities can generally be corrected with the surgical procedures described under 'Anlage-Induced Deformities'. The problem is proper diagnosis, that is establishment of the site of disruption of the jaw, which helps in the proper choice of osteotomy. For this a sectioned dental cast is very useful in diagnosis and planning. Surgical intervention should be done as soon as possible, if existing dentition allows for exact splinting, and if the procedure does not cause any additional damage to teeth.

Early orthodontic treatment can sometimes make certain surgical intervention unnecessary; it may also be required in pre- and postoperative treatment.

Jaw deformities following irradiation injuries and inflammation

The degree of jaw deformity following irradiation or inflammation of bone and soft tissue is dependent on the site of injury and on the intensity of the noxious influence. It also depends on the age of patient at the time the damage was inflicted, and in individual cases the extent of deformity can therefore only be surmised.

Operative treatment of jaw deformity following irradiation injuries should be delayed as long as possible, and meantime one must be content with surgical intervention aimed purely at eliminating inhibitary factors on growth and improving blood circulation. This waiting period should also be utilized to direct growth with orthodontic appliances and to create favourable conditions for any later surgical treatment.

Functional disturbance of the jaws arising from inflammation, on the other hand, is treated soon after complete healing in order to avoid any jaw deformity consequent upon the functional imbalance (Fig. 3, 32).

Jaw deformities following cleft lip and palate repair

It is known that in cleft lip and palate the maxilla develops almost normally if there is no surgical intervention until growth has ceased. Only the maxillary segment with the cleft shows a minor degree of hypoplasia. Cross-bite and a slight retrusion of the ala nasi on the side of the cleft may persist after growth has ceased. This applies to both sides of the maxilla if the cleft is bilateral. The premaxilla pursues an independent unhindered growth.

The essential maxillary deformities and occlusal disharmony in cleft lip and palate patients are the result of operation during early growth. It appears as if the elevation of the periosteum resulting in circulatory disturbance might be held partly responsible, but the major causative factor in these jaw deformities is definitely the surgically-

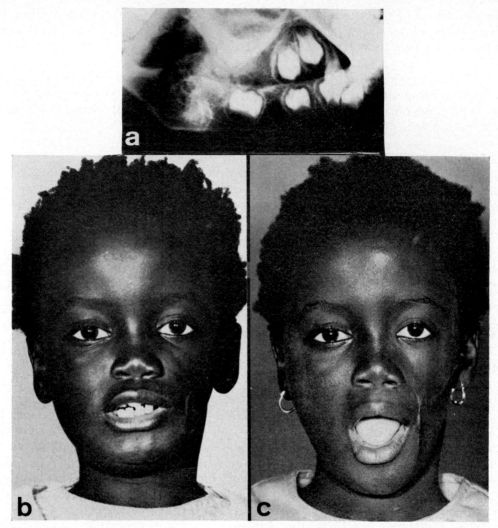

FIG. 3, 32

Case of deformity of lower half of left side of face after noma: (A) X-ray showing bony ankylosis between mandible and maxilla from the semilunar notch to the vicinity of the premolar area; (B) Outward appearance and impossibility of opening of mouth before operation; (C) Outward appearance with normal mouth opening after separating the mandible from the maxilla followed by full thickness skin grafting to the inner side of the cheek and split skin grafting for the raw bone surfaces of mandible and maxilla.

induced scarring in the tissues which hinders normal maxillary growth. An early and constant orthodontic treatment may partially diminish this late damage.

In unilateral and bilateral clefts, one always sees the characteristic late malformations of maxilla; their degree of deformity is largely dependent on the method and quality of the surgery. These cases may also show mandibular deformities similar to those described under the heading of anlage-induced deformities.

Jaw orthopaedic treatment. It cannot be gainsaid that many of the most extreme maxillary mutilations could be avoided through early, constant and good ortho-paedic treatment. Most important, it is capable of moulding the dental arch in individual segments of the jaw. In addition, using proper orthopaedic appliances and within certain limits, remoulding of bone and stimulation of growth are possible. But it must be made clear that these jaw orthopaedic appliances on the maxilla have

their anchor only on teeth, and the jaw segments to be moved can therefore be tilted only in a direction in which the point of rotation lies either near the apex of roots or somewhat higher, as in the so-called forced expansion. Ortho-dontics produces scarcely any essential sagittal movement in the maxillary base, so it is therefore not surprising that, in spite of satisfactory and constant ortho-paedic treatment, some cases manifest gradual disharmony in occlusion and profile during growth (Fig. 3, 33). Even the widening of the maxillary base achieved through forced expansion seems to regress during the course of growth (Rinderer, 1966). Conservative treatment of extreme cases of jaw mal-position by means of orthopaedic ap-pliances followed by secondary osteo-plasty (Johanson and Ohlsen, 1960; Nordin and Johanson, 1955) have long been abandoned by us. We prefer today surgical repositioning of jaw segments in the desired location; of course with previous orthodontic correction of the position of teeth where necessary. Ex-perience gathered from our large num-bers of cases has shown that forceful orthodontic treatment to achieve almost normal occlusion in such cases is func-

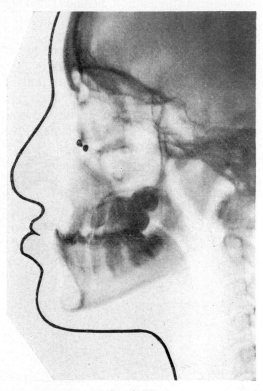

FIG. 3, 33

Cephalometric of unilateral cleft lip and palate de-monstrating a typical class III occlusion caused by micro maxillism in spite of continuous orthodontic treatment; axis of anterior maxillary teeth at good angle to base of maxilla. This is a favourable con-dition for surgical correction of profile and occlusal abnormality.

tionally unfavourable from a masticatory point of view. Furthermore, the facial contour cannot be improved to the desired degree.

It also seems to us to be a draw-back when the patient later requires a surgical improvement of his outward appearance because, after surgical repositioning of jaw segments in their proper place in relation to the rest of the maxillo-facial skeleton, orthodontic treatment of teeth already inclined by previous orthodontics is once again necessary. We therefore work in close collaboration with Professor Hotz, Chief of the Department of Orthodontics, School of Dental Medicine, Zurich, so that in these cases orthodontics brings the teeth of the affected jaw segment into the desired arch, achieving the normal angle of inclination of teeth and alveolar process to the maxillary base.

Those patients who, as far as dentition is concerned, have reached the age for surgery, that is, 13 or 14 years of age, receive orthodontic moulding of the dental arch generally after surgical movement and stabilisation in the correct position of the otherwise mutilated and displaced maxillary segments.

These remarks apply equally to prosthetic rehabilitation of adults with these jaw deformities.

The displaced premaxilla. Displacement of the premaxilla may take place in all directions. Most frequently, it is dorsally displaced or it is too long and tilted to one side. It seems to us to be too short in those cases only in which osteotomy was done in infancy.

The necessary positional correction is achieved with osteotomy of its bony pedicle (Fig. 3, 34). It is then fixed in its new position as in fracture of the alveolar process.

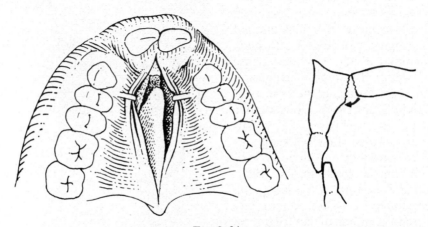

FIG. 3, 34
Technique for repositioning of displaced premaxilla in bilateral cleft.

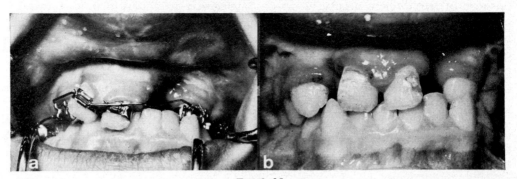

FIG. 3, 35
A case of displaced premaxilla in bilateral cleft: (A) Occlusal situation with orthodontic treatment, showing displacement of maxilla before surgical correction. (B) Occlusal situation after surgical correction of displaced premaxilla using technique illustrated in Figure 3, 34.

We prefer orthodontic bands for this. On the site of the osteotomy of the premaxilla bone contact must be established with the lateral alveolar process and for this bone transplant is necessary. The accomplishment of osteotomy of the premaxilla and implantation of bone and closure of an often V- or Y-residual cleft in one sitting (Perko, 1969) has proved very satisfactory to us. This positional correction of the premaxilla (Fig. **3**, 35) can be instituted soon after eruption of the maxillary incisors

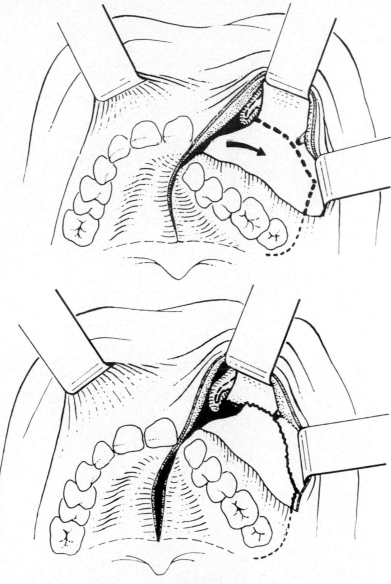

FIG. **3**, 36

Gillies's technique for lateral rotation of small maxillary segment with reopening of cleft in collapsed upper arch of an operated case with unilateral cleft lip and palate.

if bone is implanted and if continuous orthopaedic postoperative care can be vouched for.

Movement of smaller maxillary segment. If, in unilateral cleft, only the smaller maxillary segment is dislocated, what is necessary is only its repositioning into proper occlusion. To achieve this, we make the segment so mobile that it can be correctly placed in its axial inclination to the maxillary base, and at the same time in its inter-

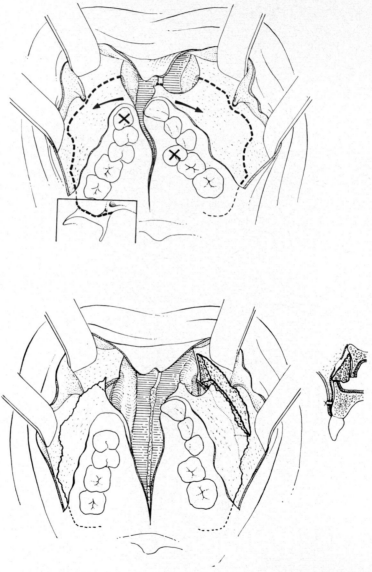

Fig. 3, 37

Gillies's technique for reconstruction of a normal maxillary arch in a case of an operated unilateral cleft lip and palate with collapse of the small and large segment.

maxillary relationship (Fig. **3**, 36). We sever the segment in the canine fossa from a vestibular approach. If necessary the cleft is re-opened. Separation of this segment from the pterygoid process is often necessary. The source of nutrition is the palatal sheath. In its new position, the segment is fixed to the rest of the maxilla with a splint and bone defects are filled with bone grafts.

Occasionally, extreme mobilization is not necessary and a lateral rotation with the tuberosity region as a pivot is sufficient (Gillies and Rowe, 1954).

The re-opened cleft can be closed in a second operation with a simultaneous secondary osteoplasty.

If the lateral segments of the maxilla in a bilateral cleft are mutilated and displaced, but the premaxilla is in proper position, the above-described procedure should be done on both lateral maxillary segments in one sitting. Splinting is carried to the stable premaxilla. To secure proper occlusion additional intermaxillary fixation and interskeletal suspension are necessary.

Movement of smaller and larger maxillary segments in unilateral cleft. If in a uni lateral cleft lip and palate the smaller and larger maxillary segments are to be altered

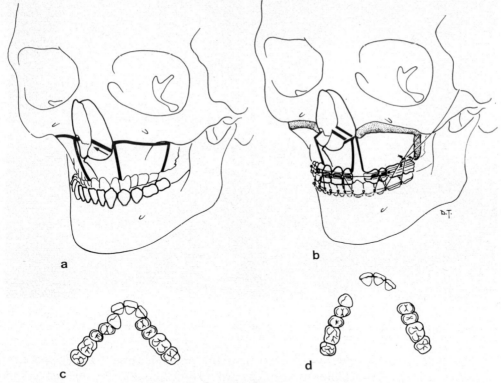

FIG. 3, 38

Author's technique for correction of retromaxillism and reconstruction of normal upper arch in a case of severe maxillary deformity after closure of bilateral cleft lip and palate in early childhood: (A) Heavy lines indicate bone cuts of lateral segments and premaxilla. (B) Situation after independent forward and lateral movement of all 3 maxillary segments. Dotted areas indicate inserted bone grafts. (C and D) Configuration of upper arch before and after correction.

in form and position, this is done in one sitting. The procedure is practically that of Le Fort I-osteotomy with re-opening of the cleft, so that both maxillary segments could be individually placed in the desired occlusion (Obwegeser, in press) and bone grafts again inserted in the gaps (Fig. 3, 37).

Intersegmental and intermaxillary fixation help to secure the segments in their new position. Additional interskeletal suspension is necessary.

Movement of maxilla in three parts. Dislocation of lateral maxillary segments and premaxilla is prevalent in bilateral cleft, and occasionally unilateral cleft presents a similar occlusal picture although there is no cleft of the alveolar process on one side.

Establishment of proper occlusion, and therefore reconstruction of the maxillary arch, demands complete mobilization of all three maxillary segments, their independent movement to the new position (Fig. 3, 38) and fixation. The lateral maxillary parts get their nourishment from palatal soft tissue. The premaxilla is cut from the palatal

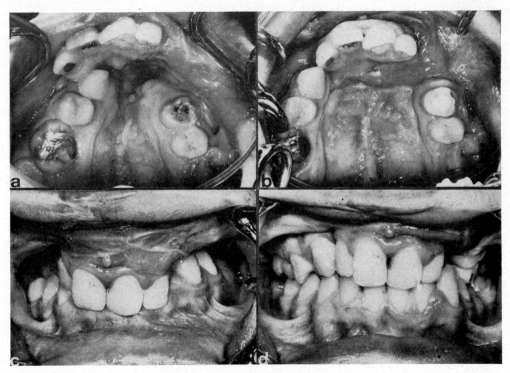

FIG. 3, 39

Maxillary deformity with remaining cleft in a bilateral cleft lip and palate in a patient 16 years old, before (A and C) and after (B and D) correction in two operations.

side, and its source of vascular nutrition is from the vestibular mucosa. The procedure is therefore a Le Fort I-osteotomy with forward advancement of the maxilla in three segments. Splinting is the same as for Le Fort I-osteotomy. Closure of the re-opened cleft and bony stabilization of the fragments with one another is done in a second operation (Fig. 3, 39).

Deformation of upper and lower jaw in the anterior region only. Isolated cases show

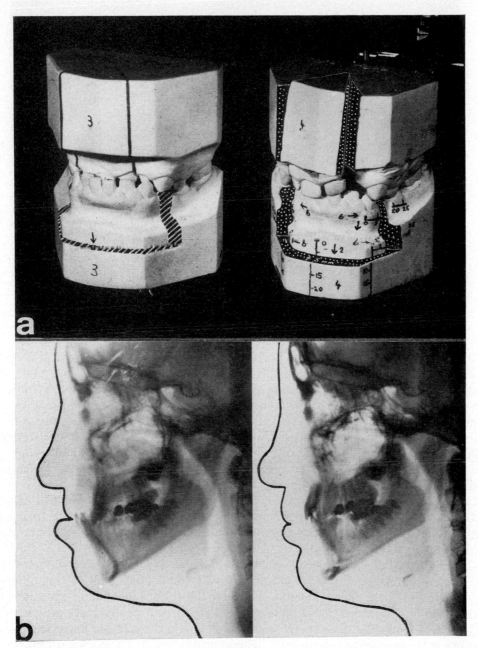

Fig. 3, 40

Pseudoprognathism in juvenile unilateral cleft lip and palate. (A) Pre-operative occlusion, and operation-model with osteotomy lines. (B) Cephalometrics before and after anterior movement of frontal maxillary segment and posterior movement of frontal mandibular segment.

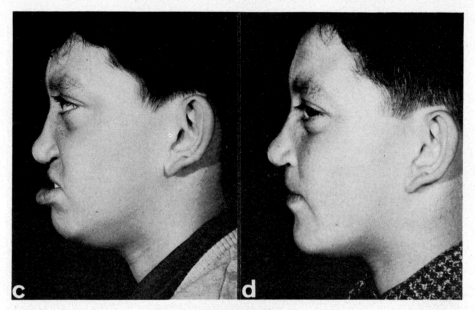

FIG. 3, 40 (*contd.*)
(c and d) Outward appearance of the same case before and after operation.

a distinct retrusion of the middle portion of the maxilla (it could involve a uni- or bi-lateral cleft) and a simultaneous protrusion of the anterior mandible. Outwardly these cases present the appearance of pseudoprognathism with extreme ectropion of the lower lip (Fig. **3**, 40). An osteotomy of premaxilla and forward advancement, combined simultaneously with backward movement of the anterior segment of the mandibular alveolar process often bring a satisfactory intermaxillary relationship. The retracted upper lip and the ectropion of the lower lip follow the movements of the upper and lower alveolar process. In this way, the desired occlusion is achieved, and on the other hand the profile is greatly improved.

In a second operation, the premaxilla which has been moved forward must be stabilized to the lateral alveolar processes using a secondary osteoplasty (if it could not be done during the first operation because of the difficulty of the necessary mobilization of soft tissues).

Extreme maxillary retrusion and mandibular protrusion. In uni- and bi-lateral cleft one sometimes comes across an extreme prognathic profile, such as was described above without cleft. The difference between these and the anlage-induced cases is that the individual maxillary segments in cleft lip and palate cases are extremely collapsed. The maxilla must therefore be advanced in three parts. Because of profile reasons, it is expedient to move back the mandible as well. The backward movement of the mandible may be limited only to the lower anterior alveolar process, or the whole mandible in toto. In rare cases a combination of backward movement of the whole mandible and the anterior mandible alveolar process is necessary. Sometimes an additional genioplasty—either forward or backward sliding—is necessary.

Most of these cases have, of course, reached the sixteenth birthday or are slightly older.

Other postoperative jaw deformities

Out of the wide range of possible postoperative jaw deformities, we shall select only three groups for description.

Maxillo-facial deformity following partial resection of maxilla. Several types of tumour could necessitate a partial resection of maxilla in early childhood. To avoid disturbance in speech and masticatory function, as well as for the aesthetic effect, prosthesis rehabilitation is essential because of the resultant maxillary defect. Such so-called resection-prostheses must be so anchored on remaining teeth that these are not damaged. The prosthesis closes the defect against the nose and antrum, and also

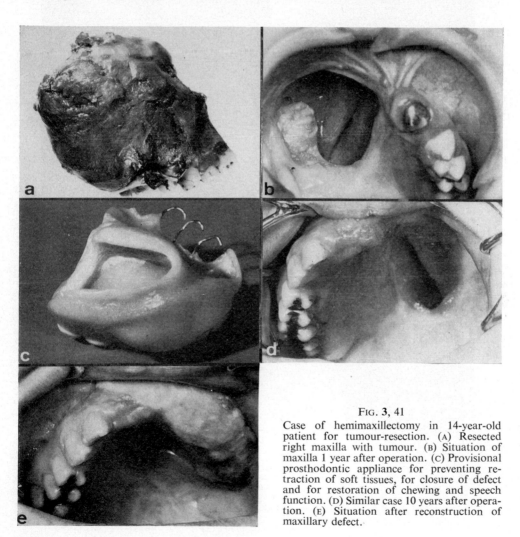

FIG. 3, 41

Case of hemimaxillectomy in 14-year-old patient for tumour-resection. (A) Resected right maxilla with tumour. (B) Situation of maxilla 1 year after operation. (C) Provisional prosthodontic appliance for preventing retraction of soft tissues, for closure of defect and for restoration of chewing and speech function. (D) Similar case 10 years after operation. (E) Situation after reconstruction of maxillary defect.

gives support to the soft tissue, moulding it as well. It creates at the same time the best conditions for later reconstruction of the defect (Fig. **3**, 41).

Jaw deformities following resection of mandible. Resection of part of the mandible without adequate splinting of the rest of the mandible leads to its deviation towards

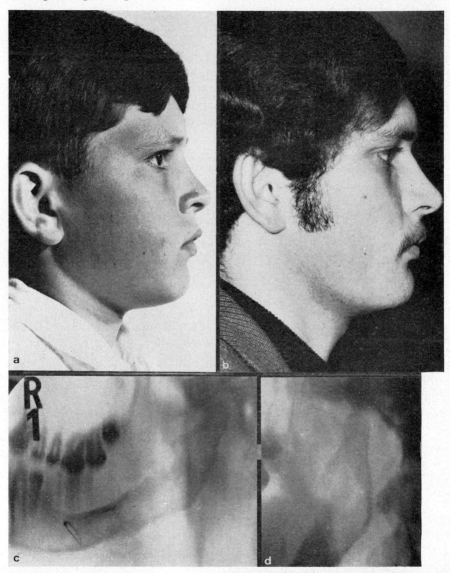

FIG. **3**, 42

Case of simultaneous resection and reconstruction of mandibular ramus and part of the body via the oral route. It also demonstrates growth of bone graft. (A) Patient's profile soon after operation at the age of 12. (B) Patient's profile 8 years later. (C) Bone graft 5 years after operation with reconstructed condyle and spontaneous reformation of a coronoid-like bony process. (D) Same reconstructed ramus moving normally forward to the articular tubercle.

the resected side and thus to grave occlusal and aesthetic disturbance. The remaining part of the mandible continues to develop independent of the usual functional occlusal stimulus, and everything must therefore be done to bring the remaining mandibular teeth into proper occlusion with the maxillary teeth. This is only very seldom possible with the help of jaw orthopaedic splinting contrivances. The best solution appears to us to be the immediate reconstruction of the defect, followed by energic postoperative treatment using orthopaedic appliances to achieve normal mandibular movement: occlusion and the shape of the mandible can be thus secured. If satisfactory function is achieved, the bone transplant seems to grow with the rest of the mandible (Fig. 3, 42). In nonmalignant and semimalignant tumours, operation is possible without external incision (Obwegeser, 1966). The important point is the removal of the jaw segment invaded by tumour along with the soft tissue belonging to it, as far as radical surgery demands it, and fitting in of a piece of bone moulded according to the resected mandible—and finally securing central occlusion. Exact suture of oral mucosa, avoiding dead space, is self-understood. Appropriate splints with sliding mandrels and a jaw orthopaedic appliance are necessary for postoperative functional treatment.

Jaw deformities following systemic diseases. Among the systemic disorders, fibrous dysplasia leads readily to jaw deformities in childhood. In minor cases, no treatment is necessary; it comes to spontaneous healing, as is well known in cherubism. In cases where fibrous dysplasia has brought about extreme jaw deformity, a surgical

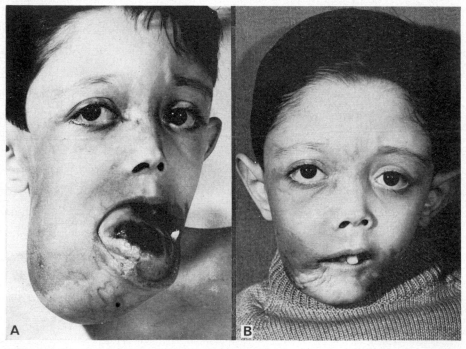

FIG. 3, 43

Deformity of mandible and maxilla in a case of generalized fibrous dysplasia before and after correction of mandibular deformity via the oral route.

modelling correction may be necessary because of psychological and aesthetic reasons —sometimes even when the prognosis is poor (Fig. 3, 43).

HUGO L. OBWEGESER

ACKNOWLEDGEMENTS

I am very grateful to my co-workers Dr A. L. Nwoku, Dr G. Pedersen and Dr R. Gerhard (the latter two Lt. Col. of the US Army, Dental Corps) for their invaluable assistance in correcting the English in this paper.

I would also like to express my gratitude to my co-worker Dr Perko for permission to use the illustrations of the case in Figure 3, 12, in whose operation he participated.

REFERENCES

ALLER, T. G. (1917). Operative treatment of prognathism. *Dent. Cosmos*, **59**, 394.

AUFFENBERG, F. (1906). Osteoplastische Verlängerung des Unterkiefers bei Mikrognathie. *Arch. klin. Chir.* **79**, 594.

AXHAUSEN, A. (1934). Die Behandlung veralteter, disloziert geheilter Oberkieferbrüche. *Dt. Zahn- Mund- u. Kieferheilk.* **1**, 334.

BABCOCK, W. W. (1909). Surgical treatment of certain deformities of jaw associated with malocclusion of teeth. *J. Am. med. Ass.* **53**, 833.

BLAIR, V. P. (1915). Instances of operative correction of malrelation of the jaws. *Int. J. Orthod. Dent. Child.* **1**, 395.

BROWN, J. B. (1946). Facial asymmetry and malocclusion from hypoplasia of the mandible. *Plastic reconstr. Surg.* **1**, 284.

CONVERSE, J. M. (1964). *Reconstructive Plastic Surgery*, Vol. II. Philadelphia: Saunders.

CONVERSE, J. M. & SHAPIRO, H. H. (1952). Treatment of developmental malformations of the jaws. *Plastic reconstr. Surg.*, Baltimore, **10**, 473.

DAL PONT, G. (1961). Retromolar osteotomy for the correction of prognathism. *J. Oral Surg. Anes Hosp. dent. Serv.* **19**, 42.

DINGMAN, R. O. (1944). Surgical correction of mandibular prognathism, an improved method. *J. Oral Surg.* **30**, 683.

EISELSBERG, A. VON (1907). Ueber Plastik bei Ektropium des Unterkiefers. *Münch. med. Wschr.* **54**, 36.

ERNST, F. (1927). In *Die Chirurgie*. Ed. Kirschner & Nordmann. Vol. IV, Part I. Berlin-Wien.

ERNST, F. (1934). Ueber die chirurgische Beseitigung der Prognathie des Unterkiefers (Progenie). *Dt. zahnarztl. Wschr.* **37**, 949.

FREIHOFER, H. P. (1970). Ergebnisse kieferorthopädischer Operationen beim Jugendlichen (in press).

GILLIES, H. D. (1957). In *The Principles and Art of Plastic Surgery*. Ed. Gillies, H. D. & Millard, R. London: Butterworth.

GILLIES, H. D. & ROWE, N. L. (1954). L'ostéotomie du maxillaire supérieur envisagée essentiellement dans les cas de bec-de-lièvre total. *Rev. Stomat.* **55**, 545.

GRIMM, G. (1961). Die intraorale Operation der asymmetrischen Kinnregion. *Fortschr. Kiefer- u. Gesichts-Chir.* Bd. VII. Stuttgart.

HOFER, O. (1942). Die operative Behandlung der alveolaren Retraktion des Unterkiefers und ihre Anwendungsmöglichkeit für Prognathie und Mikrogenie. *Dt. Zahn- Mund- u. Kieferheilk.* **9**, 121.

HOGEMANN, K.-E. (1951). Surgical orthopaedic correction of mandibular protrusion. *Acta chir. scand.* Suppl. 159.

HOGEMANN, K.-E. & WILMAR, K. (1967). Die Vorverlagerung des Oberkiefers zur Korrektur von Gebissanomalien. *Fortschr Kiefer- u. Gesichts-Chir.* Bd. XII.

HULLIHEN, S. R. (1900). Case of elongation of the under jaw and distortion of the face and neck, caused by a burn. *Dent. Cosmos*, **42**, 287.

JOHANNSEN, B. & OHLSSEN, A. (1960). Die Osteoplastik bei Spätbehandlung der Lippen-Kiefer-Gaumen-Spalten. *Arch. klin. Chir.* **295**, 876.

KIRCHNER, L. (1961). Die Bedeutung der Gesichtsproportionen für die Wiederherstellungschirurgie. *Fortschr. Kiefer- u. Gesichts-Chir.* Bd. VII.

KLEIN, D. (1968). Genetic factors and classifications of craniofacial anomalies derived from a perturbation of the first branchial arch. In *Craniofacial anomalies: Pathogenesis and Repair*. Ed. Longacre, J. J. Pitman Co./Lippincott Co.

KÖLE, H. (1959a). Surgical operations on the alveolar ridge to correct occlusal abnormalities. *Oral Surg.* **12**, 277.

KÖLE, H. (1959b). Formen des offenen Bisses und ihre chirurgische Behandlung. *Dt. Stomat.* **9**, 753.
KÖLE, H. (1965). In *Chirurgische Kieferorthopädie.* Ed. Reichenbach, Köle & Brueckl. Leipzig: Barth.
KOSTEČKA, F. (1931a). Die chirurgische Therapie der Progenie. *KorrespBl. Zahnärzte,* **55**, 223.
KOSTEČKA, F. (1931b). Die chirurgische Therapie der Progenie. *Zahnärztl Rdsch.* **40**, 669.
LINDEMANN, A. Leitfaden der Chirurgie und Orthopädie des Mundes und der Kiefer. Leipzig 1938–1954.
LONGACRE, K. L. *et al.* (1968). The surgical management of first and second branchial arch syndrome. In *Craniofacial anomalies: Pathogenesis and Repair.* Ed. Longacre, J. J. London: Pitman.
NEUNER, O. (1965). Chirurgische Orthodontie. *Schweiz. Mschr. f. Zahnheilk.* **75**, 940.
NORDIN, E. & JOHANSON, B. (1955). Freie Knochentransplantation bei Defekten am Alveolarkamm nach kieferorthopaedischer Einstellung der Maxilla bei Lippen-/Kiefer-/Gaumenspalten. *Fortschr. Kiefer-u. Gesichts-Chir.,* Bd. I, 168.
OBWEGESER, H. (1957). In Trauner, R. & Obwegeser, H. The surgical correction of mandibular prognathism and retrognathia with consideration of genioplasty. *Oral Surg.* **10**, 677.
OBWEGESER, H. (1958). Die Kinnvergrösserung. *Öst. Z. Stomat.* **55**, 535.
OBWEGESER, H. (1964a). The indications for surgical correction of mandibular deformity by the sagittal splitting technique. *Br. J. oral Surg.* **1**, 157.
OBWEGESER, H. (1964b). Der offene Biss in chirurgischer Sicht. *Schweiz. Mschr. Zahnheilk.* **74**, 668.
OBWEGESER, H. (1965). Eingriffe am Oberkiefer zur Korrektur des progenen Zustandsbildes. *Schweiz. Mschr. Zahnheilk.* **75**, 365.
OBWEGESER, H. (1966). Simultaneous resection and reconstruction of parts of the mandible via the intraoral route. *Oral Surg.* **21**, 693–705.
OBWEGESER, H. (1968). Die Bewegung des unteren Alveolarfortsatzes zur Korrektur von Kieferstellungs-anomalien. *Dt. Zahnärztl. Z.* **23**, 175.
OBWEGESER, H. (1969a). Die Bewegung des unteren Alveolarfortsatzes zur Korrektur von Kieferstellungs-anomalien. *Dt. Zahnärztl. Z.* **24**, 5.
OBWEGESER, H. (1969b). Surgical correction of small or retrodisplaced maxillae. The 'dish-face' deformity. *Plastic reconstr. Surg.* **43**, 351.
OBWEGESER, H. (1970a). Zur Korrektur der Dysostosis otomandibularis. *Schweiz. Mschr. Zahnheilk.* **80**, 331.
OBWEGESER, H. (1970b). Die einzeitige Vorbewegung des Oberkiefers und Rückbewegung des Unterkiefers zur Korrektur der extremen 'Progenie'. *Schweiz. Mschr. Zahnheilk.* **80**, 547.
OBWEGESER, H. (1970c). Surgical Correction of Maxillary Deformities. In *Cleft Lip and Palate.* Ed. Grabb, W. C., Rosenstein, S. W. & Broch, K. R. Boston: Little, Browns (in press).
PERKO, M. (1966). Gleichzeitige Osteotomie des Zwischenkiefers, Restspaltenverschluss und Zwischen-kieferversteifung durch sekundäre Osteoplastik bei Spätfällen von beidseitigen Lippen-Kiefer-Gaumenspalten. *Dt. Zahn- Mund- u. Kieferheilk.* **47**, 1.
PERKO, M. (1969). Die chirurgische Spätkorrektur von Zahn- und Kieferstellungsanomalien bei Spalt-patienten. *Schweiz. Mschr. Zahnheilk.* **79**, 19 + 179.
PICHLER, H. (1948). In *Mund- und Kieferchirurgie,* Bd. II. Ed. Pichler, H. & Trauner, R. Wien: Urban & Schwarzenberg.
RINDERER, L. (1966). The effects of expansion of the palatal sutures. *Trans. Eur. orthod. Soc.* 1–18.
ROBINSON, M. (1960). Open vertical osteotomies of the rami for correction of mandibular deformities. *Am. J. Orthod.* **46**, 425.
SCHUCHARDT, K. (1942). Ein Beitrag zur chirurgischen Kieferorthopädie unter Berücksichtigung ihrer Bedeutung für die Behandlung angeborener und erworbener Kieferdeformitäten bei Soldaten. *Dt. Zahn- Mund- u. Kieferheilk.* **9**, 73.
SCHUCHARDT, K. (1955). Formen des offenen Bisses und ihre operativen Behandlungsmöglichkeiten. *Fortschr. Kiefer- u. Gesichts-Chir.*
SCHWARZ, A. M. (1951). *Lehrgang der Gebissregelung,* Bd. I. Wien: Urban & Schwarzenberg.
SHIRA, R. B. (1961). Surgical correction of open-bite deformities by oblique sliding osteotomy. *J. Oral Surg. Anesth. Hosp. dent. Serv.* **19**, 275.
SKALOUD, F. (1951). New surgical method for correction of prognathism of the mandible. *Oral Surg.* **4**, 689.
TESSIER, P. (1967). Ostéotomies totales de la face: syndrome de Crouzon; syndrome d'Apert. Oxycéphalies; scaphocéphalies; turricéphalies. *Annls Chir. Plast.* **12**, 273.
THOMA, K. H. (1945). Deformities of the jaws. A comparison of two methods of treating apertognathia. *Am. J. Orthod.* **31**, 248.
THOMA, K. H. (1961). Oblique osteotomy of the mandibular ramus. *Oral Surg.* **14**, Suppl. 1.
TRAUNER, R. (1954). Personal communication.
WASSMUND, M. (1935). *Lehrbuch der Praktischen Chirurgie des Mundes und der Kiefer,* Bd. I. Leipzig: Meusser.
WUNDERER, S. (1962). Die Prognathieoperation mittels frontal gestieltem Maxillafragment. *Öst. Z. Stomat.* **59**, 98.

CHAPTER IV

VERTICAL AND OBLIQUE FACIAL CLEFTS
(ORBITO-FACIAL FISSURES)

The term orbito-facial fissure emphasises the importance of the orbital aspect—as distinct from the cheek and lip aspect—which plays such an important part in the

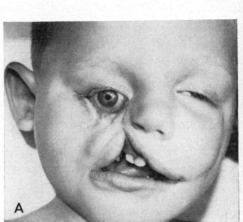 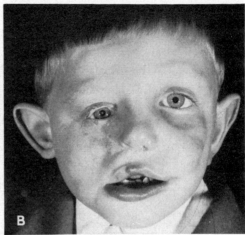

Fig. 4, 1
Vertical facial cleft. (A) Pre-operative. (B) Postoperative.

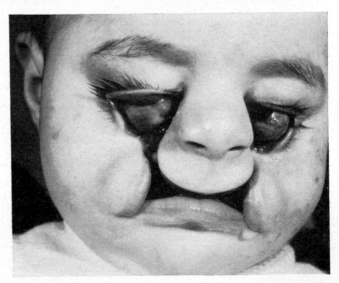

Fig. 4, 2
Double vertical facial cleft.

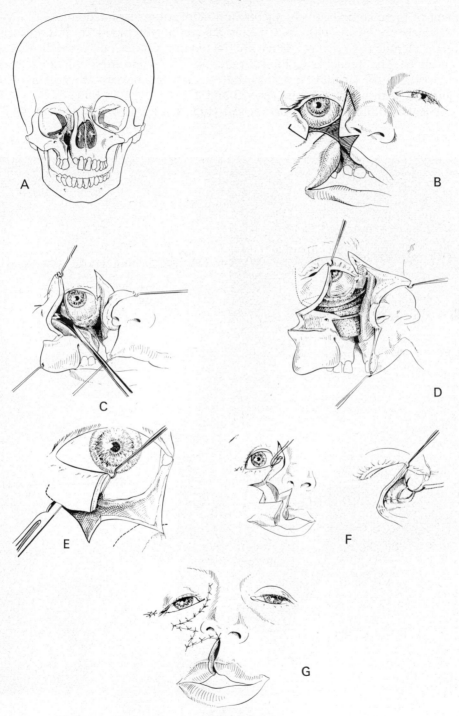

FIG. 4, 3
Surgical correction of vertical facial cleft (see text).

treatment of these comparatively uncommon deformities. Isolated colobomas of the eyelid (which are dealt with in Chapter X) are not included in this discussion, nor does it include partial clefts which are treated in a similar but less radical manner to total clefts. The Treacher-Collins (Franchescetti) Syndrome is included because of similarities in the orbital deformity, but median facial clefts do not involve the orbit and are dealt with elsewhere (pp. 33 and 271).

The essential difference between vertical (Fig. **4**, 1) and oblique (Figs. **4**, 4 and

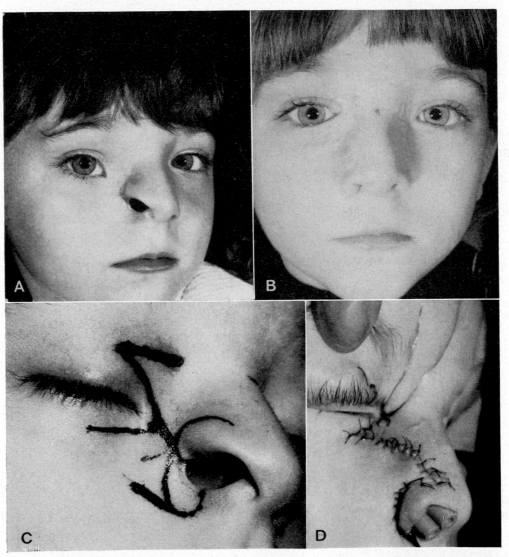

FIG. **4**, 4

Oblique facial cleft. (A) Pre-operative. (B) Postoperative. (C and D) Design of flaps.

4, 5) facial clefts is that in the former the cleft runs vertically from the orbit to the palate through the maxilla itself, leaving the lateral wall of the nose intact, whilst in the latter the cleft runs obliquely from the orbit into the nasal aperture so that the lateral wall of this last is defective in its lower part. (It is of interest that in the facial fissure associated with mandibulo-facial dysostosis the maxilla is cleft lateral to the infero-orbital canal.)

Both clefts have some characteristics in common, viz: a gap in the lower lid or at the medial canthus; displacement (usually downwards) of the medial and lateral

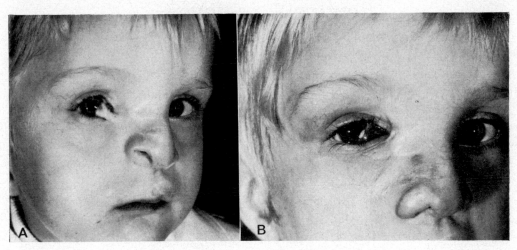

FIG. 4, 5
Oblique facial cleft showing pterygium involving cornea.

canthi; abnormalities of the lacrymal passages; hypoplasia of the ala of the nose (and even of the whole nose—particularly in the oblique cleft); a cleft of the lip, and perhaps a cleft of the maxillary alveolus.

As far as similarities in the underlying skeletal defects are concerned, in both types there is a fissure of the margin and floor of the orbit with an increase in the vertical height and a decrease in the transverse width of the orbit.

The lid coloboma is always towards the medial side but shows minor differences between the two types. It is lateral to the punctum in the vertical cleft, and in the oblique cleft there is very poor formation of the medial canthal ligament with almost non-existent lacrymal crests.

In both types of cleft the deformity is on rare occasions bilateral (Fig. **4**, 2) and in these patients the middle third of the face projects forward with a tendency to produce a beaked nose effect.

The differences, apart from the difference in the position of the maxillary cleft already noted, are mainly as follows: in the vertical type the orbital floor is practically absent, and the eye is displaced markedly downwards into the gap. In both types there is a vertical shortage of tissue between the orbit and the mouth or nose

PS E

associated with hypoplasia of the maxilla, but whereas the cleft of the lip in the vertical type is lateral to the nose, in the oblique type there is a true hare lip.

There may be associated deformities such as microphthalmia, epibulbar dermoids, or pterygia (Fig. **4**, 5), and in some cases the whole of the deformity as described above may not be present so that there may be intervening closed areas and partial clefts only are present.

OPERATIVE CORRECTION

Surgery (Fig. **4**, 3) should deal with all deformities at one stage and should have six objectives:

1. Fill the gap in the maxilla and orbital floor with a bone graft. (This of course reduces the size of the orbit—but see (5) below.)

2. Correct the coloboma of the eyelid, and reconstruct the lacrymal passages, with reposition and re-attachment of the medial canthal ligament—and possibly the lateral canthus also.

3. Increase the vertical length of the soft tissue of the cheek by Z-plasty.

4. Close the cleft of the lip by one of the standard techniques.

5. Expand the orbit by displacing the lateral wall outwards (not always possible, especially in young children).

6. In oblique clefts (Figs. **4**, 4 and **4**, 5) restore the lateral wall of the nose by a perichondro-mucous flap from the septum.

Secondary operations may be required to improve the position of the canthi (particularly the lateral, to correct ptosis or upper lid colobomas), and to carry out further work on the nose as is done in true lip and palate clefts.

TREACHER-COLLINS (FRANCHESCETTI) SYNDROME

In this form of mandibulo-facial dysostosis (Fig. **4**, 6), first described by Treacher-Collins without emphasising the bilaterality of the condition as did Franchescetti at a later date, various deformities may be present including: a deficiency of the lower lids at the junction of the lateral and central thirds; malar hypoplasia with a downward displacement of the grossly underdeveloped malar bones; downward displacement of the lateral canthi with an anti-mongoloid slant of the palpebral fissures, and also a corresponding downward displacement of the lateral end of the eyebrow and the superior external angle of the orbital margin; deformities and failure in development of the ears; a high arched palate; increase in size of the pre-auricular scalp area (side-burns); mandibular hypoplasia; and, rarely, an actual cleft of the maxilla itself as in facial clefts.

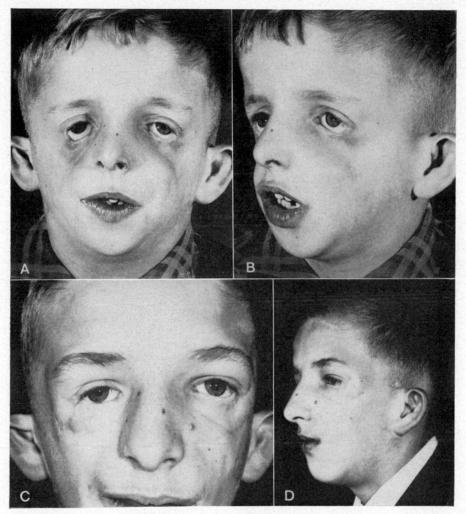

FIG. 4, 6
Treacher-Collins syndrome (see text). (A and B) Pre-operative. (C and D) Postoperative.

The orbits are shortened in the lateral direction and lengthened in the vertical diameters as with facial clefts, and as in patients with bilateral facial cleft there is a prominence of the central part of the frontal bone and fronto-nasal process with a degree of forward projection of the nose—which is exaggerated by the malar hypoplasia.

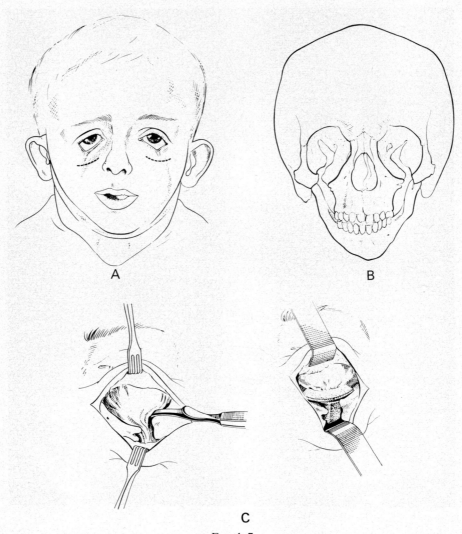

FIG. 4, 7

Correction of Treacher-Collins syndrome with filling of cleft in maxilla by bone graft.

Operative correction

Surgery aims at transposing the lateral canthi upwards (after division of the orbital septum and freeing of the lid from the maxilla), closure of the colobomas of the

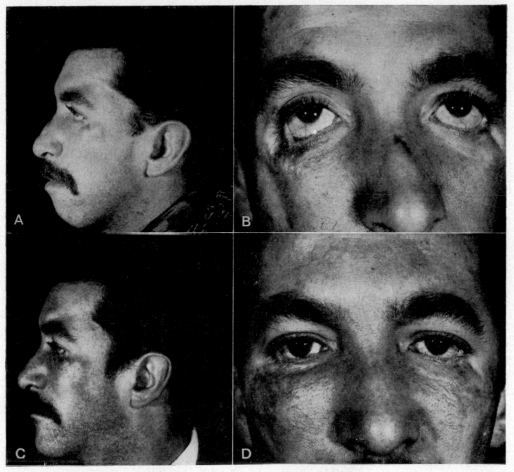

FIG. 4, 8
Treacher-Collins syndrome showing marked lower lid coloboma.

lower lids, building up of the malar prominences and closing any maxillary defect with bone grafts (Fig. **4**, 7 and 8) and reduction of the 'beak' nose.

P. TESSIER

REFERENCES

FRANCESCHETTI, A. & ZWAHLEN, P. (1944). Un syndrome nouveau: la dysostose mandibulo-faciale. *Bull. schweiz. Akad. med. Wiss.* **1**, 60.
TESSIER, P. (1967). *Entretiens sur la Chirurgie Orbito-cranienne.* Paris.

CHAPTER V

LIPS, TONGUE AND FLOOR OF MOUTH

THE LIPS

Congenital defects

The subject of *cleft lip* is considered in Chapter I of this volume and that of *macrostoma* in the same chapter under 'Rare Facial Clefts'.

MICROSTOMA

Microstoma may be congenital or acquired. The plastic surgeon most often encounters this condition in its milder form as it is associated with the cleft palate patient who has a small mandible. It may be difficult to insert the mouth gag and obtain sufficient room to operate with ease (Fig. **5**, 1). Such patients do not have a cosmetic problem, indeed it requires a considerable degree of narrowing of the mouth to produce a cosmetic disability. More severe degrees of bilateral underdevelopment of the mandible may be associated with more significant degrees of microstoma (Figs. **5**, 2 and **5**, 3).

Acquired microstoma is usually a result of some form of burning, but may also be produced by extensive excisional lip surgery. Electrical burns are the commonest cause of microstoma in a paediatric population (Fig. **5**, 4). The involvement is frequently eccentric due to involvement of one corner of the mouth. Corrosives when

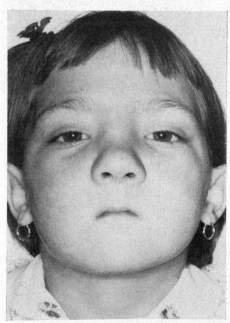

FIG. **5**, 1
Microstoma. The patient had a cleft palate.

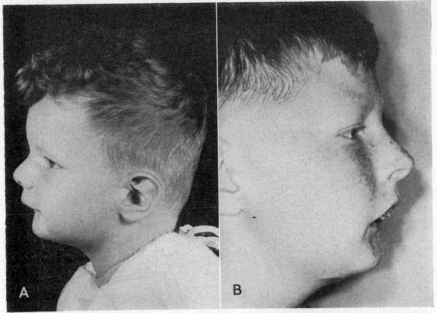

FIG. **5**, 2

(A) Microstoma. A more severe degree associated with some hypoplasia of the tongue and the mandible. (B) The patient at 10 years of age undergoing orthodontia for severe class II malocclusion and after one mental autogenous onlay bone graft procedure.

held in the mouth, instead of being swallowed, produce diffuse scarring which can result in microstoma (Fig. **5**, 5).

Treatment depends on the degree of involvement. Surgical intervention for congenital microstoma may first be requested by a dentist because of his inability to work in the mouth. Asymmetrical microstoma will require surgical intervention for lesser degrees of involvement than will symmetrical microstoma, because the deformity is more obvious. Acquired microstoma often indicates earlier operation than congenital microstoma.

If the involvement is diffuse, one or other buccal sulcus will be obliterated and this should be corrected before the commissures are reconstructed. Lesser degrees of sulcus obliteration can be corrected by local rotation flaps of mucous membranes. More extensive involvement requires reconstruction by medium thickness free skin grafts and the Esser inlay technique.

Oral commissure reconstruction for microstoma is often relatively unsatisfactory because it is difficult to reduplicate the complex contours of the corner of the mouth. The best line to transect the cheek must first be decided. The anaesthetic equipment should not be allowed to distort the lip while this is being measured and marked. As the cheek is being transected, care is taken to preserve two flaps at the lateral end of the incision, a very small skin flap based slightly below and a somewhat larger mucous membrane flap based slightly above. Judicious amounts of scarred muscle are excised before mucosa is rotated out for suturing to white lip. It is better to under-correct then over-correct because a microstoma is less unsightly than a macrostoma.

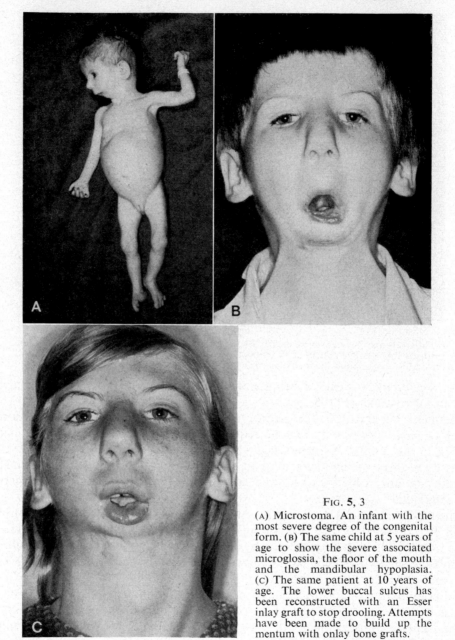

Fig. 5, 3

(A) Microstoma. An infant with the most severe degree of the congenital form. (B) The same child at 5 years of age to show the severe associated microglossia, the floor of the mouth and the mandibular hypoplasia. (C) The same patient at 10 years of age. The lower buccal sulcus has been reconstructed with an Esser inlay graft to stop drooling. Attempts have been made to build up the mentum with onlay bone grafts.

MACROCHEILIA

Macrocheilia may be apparent or real, generalized or localized, congenital or acquired, specific or non-specific.

Apparent macrocheilia is due to dental or facial bone disproportion, or relative tightness of one lip making the other look large. Class II dental malocclusion may

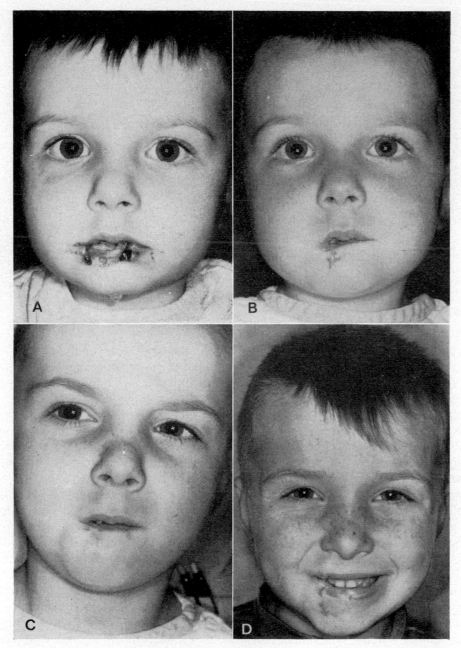

Fig. 5, 4

Electrical burn of mouth. (A) Ten days after the injury. (B) Eight weeks following the injury demonstrating spontaneous healing. (C) Two years after the injury following local procedures to the scar inside and outside of the mouth, and right commissure reconstruction. The patient still had considerable microstomia and asymmetry on opening the mouth. (D) Following Abbe cross-lip pedicle flap from the upper lip to the lower lip. The patient has better mouth balance, particularly on opening.

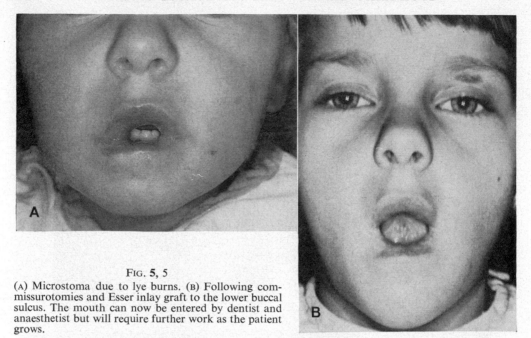

FIG. 5, 5

(A) Microstoma due to lye burns. (B) Following com-
missurotomies and Esser inlay graft to the lower buccal
sulcus. The mouth can now be entered by dentist and
anaesthetist but will require further work as the patient
grows.

make the upper lip seem large (Fig. **5**, 6), while class III dental malocclusion with
or without true mandibular prognathism will make the lower lip seem large. Correction of the malocclusion or the facial bone disproportion improves the apparent lip
prominence.

Prominence of the lower lip is common in cleft lip patients, due to relative tightness
of the upper lip. Severe degrees of protuberance may require wedge excision. Lower
lip fullness and upper lip tightness can be improved spectacularly by an Abbe or
cross-lip pedicle flap. Lesser degrees of lower lip prominence may be improved by
transverse elliptical excisions of lower lip mucous membrane.

Congenital reduplication of the lip is rare. Either lip may be involved. The inner
reduplicated segment is excised. The congenital thick or hypertrophied lip is usually
a diffuse non-specific overgrowth of all the lip elements (Fig. **5**, 7). This condition is
commoner and more acceptable in the Negro race. It is less acceptable to Causasians.
Excisional treatment is not as satisfactory because the involvement is diffuse.
Judicious transverse longitudinal wedge excision of mucous membrane, glandular
elements and muscle, with suitable tapering and line length discrepancy corrections
will give satisfaction to some patients. Rarely are external incisions justifiable.

Congenital soft tissue tumours, including capillary haemangioma (port wine stain),
arterio-venous lesions, lymphangioma (Fig. **5**, 8), neurofibroma and lipomatosis
may produce macrocheilia. Involvement is usually diffuse and therefore cannot be
completely eradicated. Through and through excisions may be necessary for very
gross involvement, but in general the external incisions produce as much deformity
as the original lesion did. Excisions from the mucosal aspect of the lip may be
sufficient to satisfy patient and surgeon.

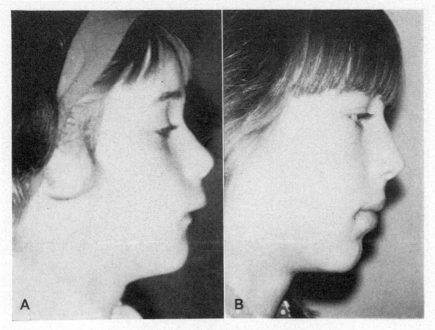

FIG. 5, 6

(A) Macrocheilia—apparent due to class II malocclusion. (B) The same patient following maxillary and mandibular orthodontia. (Courtesy Dr R. B. Ross, Division of Orthodontia, Department of Dentistry, The Hospital for Sick Children, Toronto.)

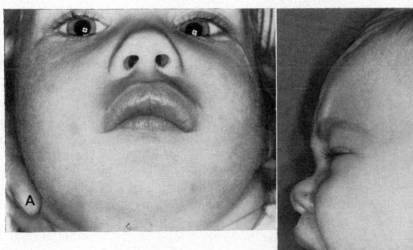
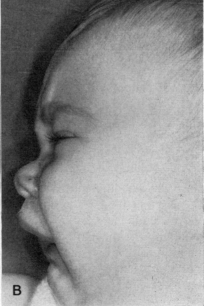

FIG. 5, 7

Macrocheilia, congenital, diffuse, non-specific. This degree may become acceptable by 6 years of age. If it does not, a transverse longitudinal wedge excision of mucous membrane and deeper elements may be necessary.

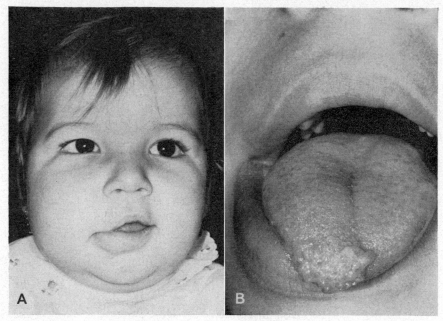

FIG. 5, 8

(A) Macrocheilia—asymmetrical specific associated with regional facial hypertrophy.
(B) The tongue of the same patient has a lymphangioma suggesting that the lip and face deformities are produced by the same lesion.

Laceration of the lip, even small puncture wounds, in children may be followed by localized areas of lip thickening. Children frequently heal with excessive connective tissue production. The surgeon must wait for as much resolution of this tissue as possible, a process which may take two years. Residual protuberant areas are then excised, staying on the mucosal aspect of the lip as much as possible. Elliptical excision on lip mucosa must be tapered out a considerable distance into normal mucous membrane.

WEBS AND FRENULI

Normally there is a well-developed midline upper lip frenulum and a smaller midline lower lip frenulum. There may be in addition paired lower lip frenuli in the first bicuspid regions. An upper lip frenulum which is thicker and shorter than normal and particularly one which extends onto the hard palate, may cause spreading of the upper central permanent incisor teeth. This tendency may be decreased by a Z-plasty lengthening of the band, with excision of excessive submucosal tissue close to the alveolar bone.

Stout frenuli may be present across the lower buccal sulcus continuing onto the floor of the mouth and even onto the tongue (Fig. 5, 9). This condition is usually associated with abnormal or missing teeth and with tongue abnormalities. This complex may be part of the Psaume syndrome. Again Z-plasty procedures to the lower webs and V-Y lengthening procedures to the base of the tongue will decrease web tension and provide better tongue mobility.

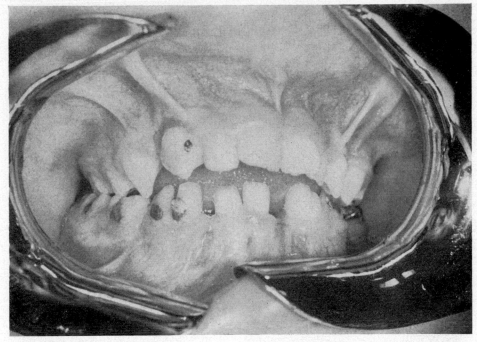

FIG. 5, 9

Lip webs or frenuli. Although shown in the upper sulcus, they are also present in the lower sulcus. There are congenitally hypoplastic teeth.

MANDIBULAR LIP PITS

The mandibular lip pit anomaly is usually associated with cleft lip, or occurs in cleft lip-cleft palate families. This complex is inherited as if due to a single dominant gene with variable expressivity. The pits may be single or double, superficial dimples or deep sinuses. The treatment is transverse elliptical excision including the sinus openings and tracts. All the involved mucous membrane must be excised or the sinus will recur (Fig. 5, 10).

EPIGNATHUS

Teratoid lesions are occasionally found in the region of the upper and lower jaws anteriorly and are usually associated with lip and jaw defect (Fig. 5, 11). Tissue representative of ectoderm, mesoderm and entoderm will be present. Malignant change has been reported. Excision of the lesion and reconstruction of the associated defects is indicated.

Injuries

LACERATIONS

The principles of wound care are the same for adults and children. General anaesthesia is necessary for the adequate care of many children's wounds when local anaesthesia might be satisfactory for a similar wound in an adult. It is often only in this way that adequate cleansing, regional antisepsis, judicious debridement and

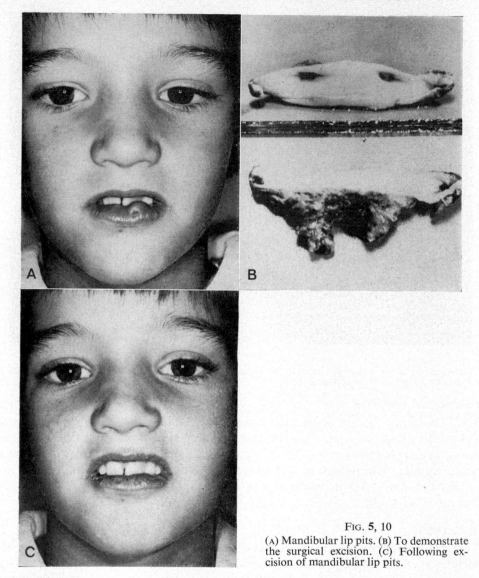

FIG. 5, 10
(A) Mandibular lip pits. (B) To demonstrate the surgical excision. (C) Following excision of mandibular lip pits.

haemostasis can be obtained. The mucocutaneous line must always be approximated accurately. This is difficult to find laterally in small children's lips.

Children produce more fibrous tissue than adults and resolve this more slowly than adults. Lacerations of the lip are prone to develop a fullness of the red lip which frequently never resolves and must be revised by trimming—usually in a transverse elliptical manner.

DOGBITES

There is still controversy whether dogbite wounds should be closed primarily. It

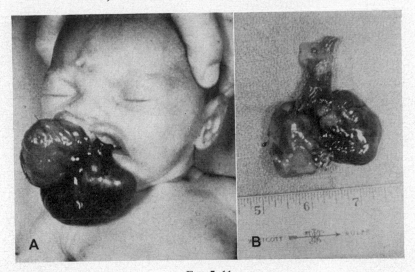

FIG. **5**, 11

(A) Epignathus or teratoma of the premaxilla. (B) Excised surgical specimen.
(Courtesy Dr James T. Mills, Dallas, Texas, and Year Book Medical Publishers
Incorporated, Chicago, *Paediatric Surgery*, 1962, p. 1157.)

is the experience of The Hospital for Sick Children, Toronto, that dogbite wounds
seen within the first eight hours may be closed primarily, provided they are thoroughly
cleansed. It is difficult to cleanse the isolated deep puncture wound and very occasionally it may be wise to leave such a wound open. Rabies and tetanus prophylaxis
measures, in keeping with local hospital rules, should be instituted.

BURNS

Flame burns commonly produce ectropion of lips (Fig. **5**, 12). Free full-thickness
or thick partial-thickness skin grafts are the commonest method of reconstructing
the deformity. Partial recurrence in the young patient is common, requiring re-
operation. It is sometimes possible to use regional local rotation flaps from the labial-
facial skin folds, particularly for asymmetric ectropion. Larger upper neck bipedicled
visor flaps may be useful if that donor region is not burned, and particularly, if both
upper and lower lips are involved.

Electrical burns frequently involve the full thickness of the lip. Their primary
management is still controversial. Early excision and reconstruction has not been
satisfactory in our hands. It is impossible to decide on the line of demarcation between
living and dead tissue. We prefer to allow the necrotic tissue to separate spontaneously. Parents or nurses must be alerted for the possibility of secondary haemorrhage between the fifth and tenth days. The defect is allowed to heal and then resolve
for 6 to 12 months, before starting reconstruction (Fig. **5**, 4).

The buccal sulcus, if obliterated, should be reconstructed first. Narrow bands of
obliteration may be corrected by local rotation flaps of regional buccal mucosa. Long,
narrow based flaps of mucous membrane will survive. Wide obliteration will require
release by incision and resurfacing by medium-thickness free skin graft. The skin is

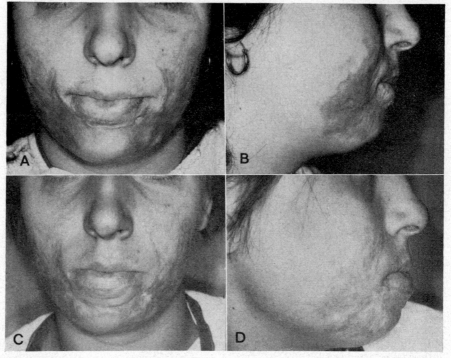

FIG. 5, 12
Ectropion of lower lip. (A and B) Pre-operative. (C and D) Following release of lip and free full thickness skin graft.

applied to dental compound that has been moulded to the size and shape of the released defect. This skin-covered stent is sutured into the defect in such a way that it will remain there from 7 to 10 days.

The commissures of the mouth frequently require reconstruction (see microstoma, p. 102). Occasionally various forms of cross-lip pedicle flap will give a worthwhile result in terms of the balance between deformity correction and donor site scarring.

Infections

Chronic fissures and ulcers of the oral commissure and lips are common in childhood. They are almost always nonspecific. They may be self-inflicted by tongue habits or be a manifestation of impetigo. The rare condition of keratodermia (see Scleroderma, Chapter 39) is sometimes first manifested by commissure fissures (Fig. 5, 13). Broad spectrum topical antibiotic application and the avoidance of finger picking and tongue rubbing is usually effective.

Pyogenic granuloma (Fig. 5, 14) occurs after a trivial break in the skin and presents as a small discrete raised red friable mass, closely resembling a haemangioma. The lesions bleed profusely when disturbed. They respond effectively to electrocoagulation.

The more diffuse inflammatory processes about the lips are not common but can be grossly destructive. Some prefer to group these under the broad heading of *noma, gangrenous stomatitis* or *cancrum oris*. The possibility of reactions to viruses,

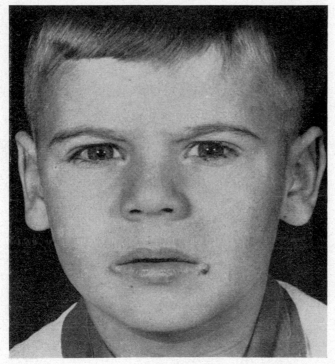

FIG. 5, 13

Chronic lip commissure fissures produced by keratodermia. The patient also had hyperkeratosis plantaris et palmaris.

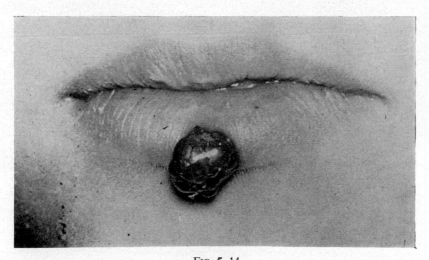

FIG. 5, 14

Pyogenic granuloma of lip. The lesion responded well to superficial excision for biopsy purposes followed by electrocoagulation of the base.

particularly varicella, should always be considered. Meningococcal infections, when associated with meningococcaemia, may produce specific oral lesions as well as extremity gangrene. Purpura fulminans, probably produced by intravascular thrombosis following another infection, may have areas of oral ulceration, as well as extremity gangrene. The original infection may have been relatively mild, such as a pharyngitis, although purpura fulminans is more common after meningococcal and haemophilus influenza infections.

The causative factor of gangrenous stomatitis may be less specific. The patient was

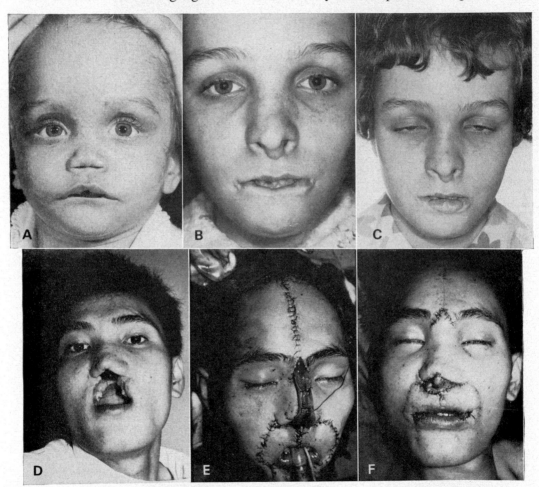

FIG. 5, 15

(A) Gangrenous stomatitis. There has been loss of columella, much of the mucosa of the upper and lower lips together with a considerable portion of the margin of the lower lip. (B) Following inner arm costal cartilage reinforced pedicle flap reconstruction of the columella and Esser inlay graft reconstruction of the upper and lower buccal sulci. Demonstrating a residual marginal defect of the lower lip. (C) Following a cross-lip pedicle flap of scarred upper lip mucous membrane to the lower lip. (D) Noma in a young adult. Loss of columella, upper lip and anterior palate, alveolus and septum. (E) Repair of upper lip by double rotation flaps. Repair of palate by turn-over palatal flaps with upper layer formed by forehead flap. (F) Columella and septum reconstructed from forehead flap pedicle. (Courtesy J. C. Mustardé and Children's Medical Relief International, Saigon for Figs. D, E and F.)

frequently debilitated prior to the severe systemic infectious illness. The destruction may be widespread involving lips, oral mucosa, nose, maxilla and palatine bones to varying degrees (Fig. **5**, 15). Early identification of a predominating organism and its antibiotic sensitivities, followed by prompt systemic specific antibiotic therapy, is the best early treatment measure. Reconstructive procedures must be delayed until the defects have healed and resolved considerably. Reconstruction needs will vary markedly with the residual deformity and may include buccal sulcus, partial or full thickness lip, columella and alar reconstruction. The inner arm pedicle graft is a useful reconstructive measure in a child. It is advisable to avoid forehead or facial donor site scars in children. As the child grows up he frequently becomes at least as concerned about visible donor site scars as his parents were about the original deformity. In older children and young adults, however, forehead and cheek flaps may be utilized with less obvious resultant scars (Fig. **5**, 15D, E and F).

Tumours

BENIGN

Benign tumours of the lips are not premalignant to the degree that adult benign lesions are. Papillomata, verrucae and mucous cyst (Fig. **5**, 16) are treated by simple

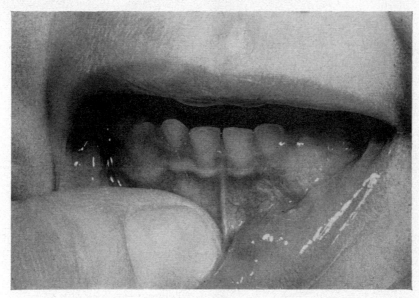

FIG. **5**, 16
Mucous cyst of lower lip.

excision. Brown pigmented *naevi* are frequently present at birth, but may appear later in life. They may be removed because of the fear of malignant change, although this is a remote possibility. It is more common to consider their removal for aesthetic reasons, therefore the plastic surgeon must be certain the results of his surgery will be less obvious than the original benign lesion. Excision and resurfacing with a free full thickness skin graft is probably the safest measure for larger lesions. The colour

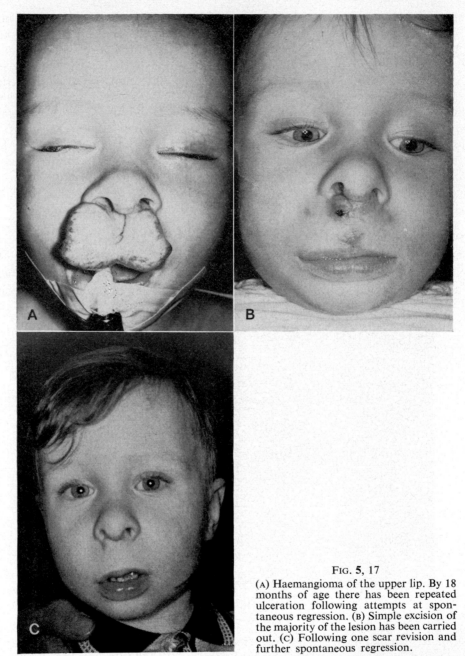

FIG. 5, 17

(A) Haemangioma of the upper lip. By 18 months of age there has been repeated ulceration following attempts at spontaneous regression. (B) Simple excision of the majority of the lesion has been carried out. (C) Following one scar revision and further spontaneous regression.

match will be best if mastoid post auricular skin or neck skin is used. Even a neck donor site incision may concern a grown-up female paediatric patient. Local rotation flaps give excellent colour and texture match but the donor region incisions must be inconspicuous. Cervical pedicle flaps, sometimes tunnelling under intervening normal skin, should be considered. However, these tend to produce a bulkiness in the reconstructed area which can be as great a concern to the patient as the sometimes undesirable quality of a free full-thickness skin graft.

The *haemangioma* is the commonest paediatric lip tumour. It has a definite tendency to regress spontaneously in approximately four years time, although the tendency is not as great for the lip as for other areas of the body. Spontaneous resolution, when too rapid, may be associated with ulceration (Fig. **5**, 17). Parents should be encouraged to wait for the possibility of spontaneous regression whenever possible, although some will not accept this. In such cases the lesion should be excised or materially

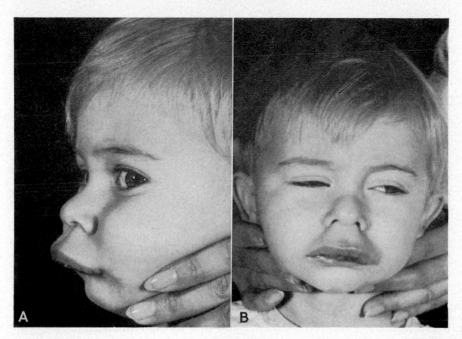

FIG. 5, 18

Lymphangioma of upper lip producing diffuse macrocheilia. The possibility of spontaneous regression is less for this lesion than for haemangioma. One should try to wait for four to six years for this possibility but surgical reduction probably will be necessary.

decreased in bulk, once it has passed through its rapid growth. This should be done without producing excessive surgical deformities.

Lymphangiomata of the lip rarely regress spontaneously and present a greater surgical problem (Fig. **5**, 18). Efforts should be directed toward decreasing lip bulk without adding significant surgical deformities.

MALIGNANT

Malignant tumours restricted to the lip are extremely rare in children. We have seen only one at The Hospital for Sick Children, Toronto, a 4-year-old boy (Fig. **5**, 19) with a rapidly developing sarcoma which was treated by wedge resection. The patient developed upper cervical disease within one year which was treated by

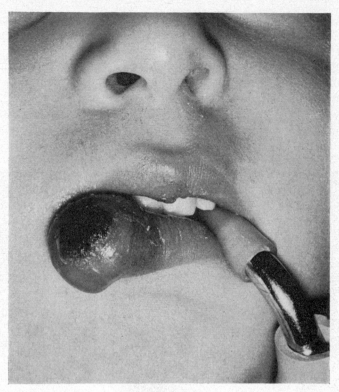

FIG. 5, 19

Sarcoma of the lip. Rapid onset at 4 years of age but appearing like a
haemangioma. Treated by wedge resection and subsequent suprahyoid lymph node dissection when glands appeared with long survival. (Courtesy Year Book Medical Publishers Incorporated,
Chicago, *Paediatric Surgery*, 1962, p. 1161.)

suprahyoid dissection and has been alive and well for 13 years. It is more common for
the lip to be involved with sarcoma, or rarely carcinoma, from surrounding regions
such as the cheek or the floor of the nose although even these tumours are rare.

THE SPECTRUM OF MALIGNANT TUMOURS OF THE HEAD AND NECK IN CHILDREN

It was felt that a better appreciation of the head and neck malignant tumour picture
could be obtained if the total experience of a large children's hospital was reviewed.
During the 15-year period 1951 to 1965 inclusive there were 434 patients admitted
to The Hospital for Sick Children, Toronto with malignant tumours presenting in
the head and neck. If those with intracranial tumours (276) and retinoblastomas (62)
are excluded, the remaining 96 patients represent less than 0·03 per cent of the total
hospital admissions during that period.

The age range was from birth to 16 years. The sexes are equally affected in all age
groups. The frequency-age distribution histogram reveals peaks in the first (somatic
soft tissue sarcoma) and sixth years (lymphomas) of life (Fig. 5, 20). This pattern is
the same for childhood cancer in general.

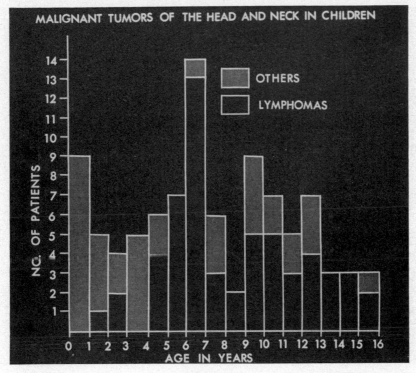

FIG. 5, 20

The frequency-age distribution of malignant tumours of the head and neck at The Hospital for Sick Children in Toronto.

Anatomically (Fig. 5, 21) 59 malignant tumours were in the neck, most being lymphomas. The other neck tumours during the study period were 3 neuroblastomas (primary) and 3 thyroid carcinomas.

Ten patients had soft somatic tissue tumours of the face; three were fibrosarcomas, two undifferentiated sarcomas, two secondary neuroblastomas, one rhabdomyosarcoma, one malignant haemangiopericytoma, and one lymphosarcoma.

There were eight intraoral tumours of varied origin: three rhabdomyosarcomas, two reticulum-cell sarcomas, one epidermoid carcinoma, one undifferentiated sarcoma and one lymphosarcoma.

There were seven orbital tumours; two undifferentiated sarcomas, two rhabdomyosarcomas, one fibrosarcoma, one lymphosarcoma, one malignant melanoma.

Although five tumours were diagnosed clinically as bone tumours, only one of these, an occipital chordoma, could be classified pathologically as such. The others were: undifferentiated sarcomas (two of the maxilla, one of the cervical spine) and a secondary neuroblastoma of the maxilla.

The nasopharynx was the site of four malignant tumours (three undifferentiated sarcomas and one lymphoepithelium).

There were three facial skin tumours (two basal cell carcinomas and one malignant melanoma).

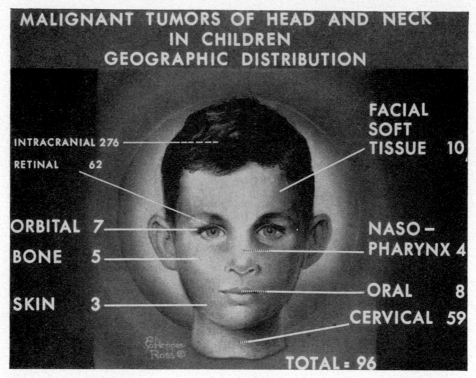

FIG. 5, 21

The geographical distribution of malignant tumours of the head and neck seen at The Hospital for Sick Children, Toronto. (Courtesy the Editor, *Plastic and Reconstructive Surgery*, **44**, 256.)

Surprisingly there was only one malignant parotid tumour during this study period, a girl with lymphosarcoma, alive and well after superficial parotidectomy for 13 years. We have seen others before and after this study period.

The primary tumours were classified according to their embryonic layer of origin; 8 were of ectodermal or neuroectodermal origin, 81 of mesodermal origin and 4 of entodermal origin. There were no malignant teratomas.

Of the eight patients with ectodermal tumours, two had neuroblastoma, primary in the neck. One patient with a malignant melanoma of the iris and ciliary body is free of tumour six years after treatment. The other malignant melanoma had been originally diagnosed as a 'juvenile' (benign) but two months later metastatic malignant melanoma was found in a lymph node excised from the submandibular region.

Among the 81 patients with tumours of mesodermal origin 58 had lymphoma, 29 Hodgkin's disease, 20 lymphosarcoma and 9 reticulum cell sarcoma. Four of the patients who had Hodgkin's disease appeared cured (3- to 14-year follow-up) and seven still have disease. Three of the patients who had lymphosarcoma are cured (8, 13 and 14-year follow-ups) and one who had reticulum cell sarcoma is well 11 years after treatment.

In the group of patients with various other sarcomas, two of the six patients with rhabdomyosarcoma and two of the four patients with fibrosarcoma survive. The patient with the haemangiopericytoma and the one with chordoma died from intracranial extension of the tumour.

In the group of patients with tumours of entodermal origin, two teenage girls with thyroid carcinoma have survived more than five years. A 1-month-old infant with thyroid cancer and a 13-year-old girl with lymphoepithelioma died.

Lymphomas in childhood may occur as a localized form of disease. If so they are curable by wide surgical excision and post-operative radiation.

The paucity of intra- and extra-oral epidermoid carcinoma in childhood is worthy of note as is the relatively high frequency of orbital, nasopharyngeal and soft tissue sarcomas. The difficulties with the microscopic diagnosis of the latter group of tumours are many. Early diagnosis, pre-operative or postoperative radiation and radical surgery are indicated. The prognoses are not universally grave.

The majority of the childhood head and neck malignant tumours in this study were lymphomas (60 per cent), the next largest group had other soft somatic tissue sarcoma (25 per cent) The mortality in both of these groups was high (80 per cent) compared to the patients with tumours of ectodermal or entodermal origin (mortality 25 to 40 per cent). There are other malignant tumours of the head and neck, such as malignant teratoma, parathyroid and parotid carcinoma, plasma-cytoma, the so-called branchiogenic carcinoma, reported in the literature previously observed in this hospital but not encountered during the 15-year study period.

THE TONGUE

Congenital defects

ANKYLOGLOSSIA (TONGUE TIE)

Tongue tie is habitually suspected by parents of newborns because of their fear of impaired speech. Parents should be reassured and encouraged if the frenulum is not grossly short. Later, if the child does develop an anterior articulation defect which can be attributed to faulty tongue tip movement, the frenulum should be lengthened.

More severe degrees of tongue tie should be treated early. Simple transverse section of the frenulum with or without longitudinal closure will be sufficient for most cases. The most severe degrees are usually associated with hypoplasia of the tongue and the mandible. They will require lengthening by Z-plasty or V-Y procedures. Occasionally there is so much hypoplasia of the floor of the mouth that free skin graft reconstruction must be resorted to.

MICROGLOSSIA

It is often difficult to tell whether a tongue is small or retroplaced. Glossoptosis is more common. Microglossia does occur in severe deformities involving the mandible and the floor of the mouth (Fig. 5, 22). Such cases frequently have a generalized articulation speech defect. Any attempt to mobilize the tongue surgically will be of value.

MACROGLOSSIA

Macroglossia may be produced by generalized hypertrophy or hemihypertrophy.

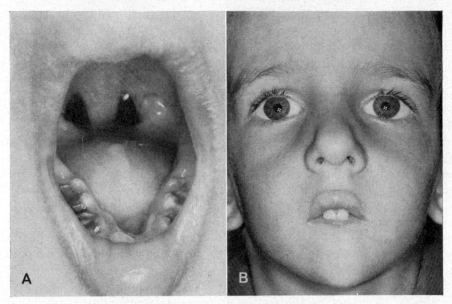

FIG. 5, 22

(A) Microglossia—the most severe degree of this anomaly. One is looking at the floor of the mouth with a sessile noduel of tongue mucosa in its centre. The small remnant of tongue cannot be visualized. It is situated posteriorly just distal to the epiglottis. Note the maxillary collapse. (B) Extra-oral view of the same patient, showing the small mouth.

It may be non-specific, when there is an overgrowth of all the tongue tissues, or it may be specific, when the enlargement will be due to haemangioma, lymphangioma or neurofibroma.

Generalized non-specific macroglossia is often associated with mongolism, mental retardation, cretinism or Wrestler's syndrome, but also may occur in a child normal in every other way. It is important to wait until up to 4 years of age to see if the tongue will be accepted inside the mouth. If, by then, there is no sign of acceptance and the tongue tip is developing glossitis, surgical reduction should be undertaken. The tongue is held forward by progressively placed stay sutures from the tip to the foramen caecum region. Symmetrical marginal wedge excisions are carried out with the cutting cautery. The resulting defects are sutured. If the tongue is not accepted inside the mouth following this procedure, it may be repeated in one to two years time or a deep wedge may be excised from the midline of the tongue. The lingual and hypoglossal nerves must be spared.

Hemihypertrophy or asymmetrical enlargement of the tongue, if due to haemangioma, may improve with time. Spontaneous improvement is less likely to occur with lymphangioma (Fig. 5, 23) and never occurs with neurofibroma. The involved area is excised, again protecting the nerves.

PIERRE ROBIN SYNDROME

Glossoptosis or posterior displacement of the tongue, combined with micrognathia and often with an associated cleft palate is known as the Pierre Robin syndrome (see

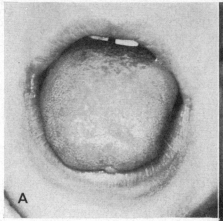

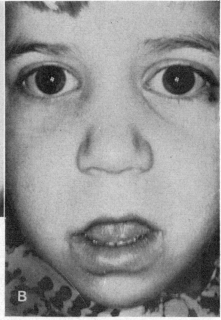

FIG. 5, 23

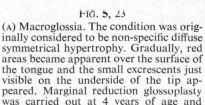

(A) Macroglossia. The condition was orig-inally considered to be non-specific diffuse symmetrical hypertrophy. Gradually, red areas became apparent over the surface of the tongue and the small excrescents just visible on the underside of the tip ap-peared. Marginal reduction glossoplasty was carried out at 4 years of age and histological examination demonstrated diffuse lymphangiomatosis. (B) The characteristic open mouth deformity which is extremely aggravating to parents.

also p. 19). Inspiratory obstruction and failure to thrive due to sucking and degluti-tion difficulties are common features of the condition. Aspiration is the very great fear of all responsible for the care of these neonates.

Glossoptosis and micrognathia improve with time and for this reason most cases can be managed conservatively, but with prodigious nursing care. Positioning the baby on its side or even face down will frequently improve the airway. Nursing the baby upright in one arm, or occasionally while lying on one side, but always spending a great deal of time with the baby will frequently tide the baby over until its own intrinsic muscle action takes over.

Surgical intervention is necessary in only a small proportion of our patients. It is usually necessary when the ptosed tongue is noted to lock in the cleft palate. A traction tongue tip suture is used as a clinical trial to see if holding the tongue forward materially improves the airway. Sometimes this measure is all that is necessary, otherwise a modified Beverley Douglas operation is done: a midline incision is made on the undersurface of the tongue, floor of the mouth, buccal sulcus and mucosal aspect of lower lip. Book flaps are turned out on both the undersurface of the tongue and the floor of the mouth-labial components of this incision. The raw surface of the tongue is opposed to that of the floor of the mouth and the lip and the edges of the book flaps are sutured. Further tension reduction is necessary in the form of a horizontal mattress suture passed through the tongue and lower lip, tying this over buttons on the upper surface of the middle third of the tongue and the midzone of the outer aspect of the lower lip. The tongue has a tendency to separate from the lip about the time general improvement has occurred. Permanent tongue-lip adhesions must be separated when the lower incisor teeth are starting to erupt.

A recently described operative procedure is that of holding the tongue forward while a Kirschner wire is placed through one mandibular angle, across the base of the tongue and out the other mandibular angle.

Patients who do not respond to forward positioning of the tongue and have primarily respiratory problems will require tracheostomy. Perinatal tracheostomy should be done, whenever possible, by an expert. When carried out electively, this procedure should be combined with bronchoscopy. Tracheostomy tubes must usually be left in for a long time and their presence does not favour early tongue and mandible development. Gastrostomy is occasionally resorted to if failure to thrive persists.

The tongue of Pierre Robin syndrome patients becomes normal and the mandible develops to normal limits. The patients frequently end up with a straight profile but usually have some class II malocclusion with dental crowding in the permanent dentition.

DROOLING

Drooling occurs normally in many babies, particularly those with a small mandible. It usually clears spontaneously with growth, development and learning. Two types of patients, certain cerebral palsy patients and those with Worster Drought syndrome have persistent drooling after 4 years of age. An operation has been described recently which is worthy of consideration for the latter group of patients. Stenson's duct and its orifice are transferred submucosally to a point posterior to the posterior tonsillar pillars. If this procedure produces worthwhile decrease in drooling it can then be followed by resection of both submaxillary glands.

BIFID TONGUE

Various types and degrees of notching or bifiding of the tongue may occur. This anomaly is commonly a manifestation of the Psaume syndrome (Fig. 5, 24). The deformity is lessened by incising the margins of the notch or cleft and directly suturing

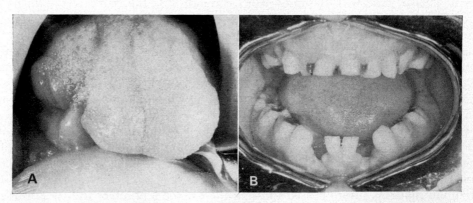

FIG. 5, 24

(A) Bifid tongue. The tongue is notched asymmetrically. This was part of the Psaume syndrome.
(B) The alveolar and dental defects of the same patient. Buccal sulcus webbing was also present.

the resulting two superior and the two inferior edges. Occasionally this can be combined advantageously with a Z plasty manoeuvre.

Injuries

Puncture wounds and flap lacerations of the tongue are common once children commence to toddle. Small lacerations involving only one surface heal well without suturing. Through and through lacerations tend to produce a bifid tongue and those with large torn flaps should be sutured.

The tongue rarely suffers significantly from chemical or electrical burns.

Tumours

BENIGN

Dermoid cysts commonly present on the inferior surface of the tongue and the floor of the mouth (Fig. **5**, 25). Direct excision, staying close to the cyst wall with the tongue well controlled by stay sutures is effective treatment. The papilloma and the fibroma occur occasionally in childhood.

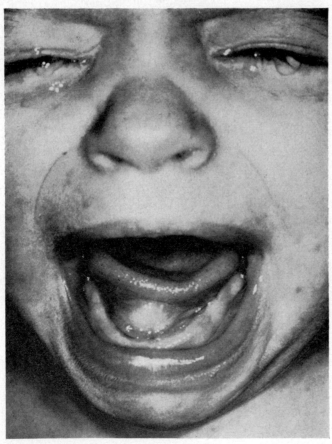

FIG. **5**, 25

Dermoid cyst. There is involvement of the tongue and the floor of the mouth.

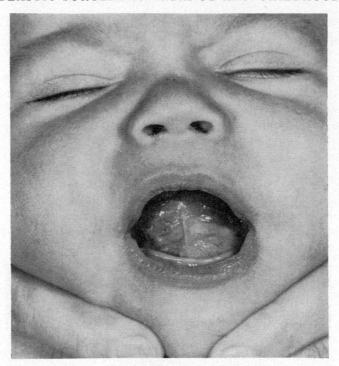

FIG. 5, 26

Fibrosarcoma of tongue and floor of mouth. The lesion was present at birth. It was removed by a wide local resection at 10 days of age. Histologically the lesion was of low grade malignancy. There has been no recurrence for 12 years.

Lingual thyroid occurs as a swelling in the vicinity of the foramen caecum. An investigation must be carried out to determine if the patient has cervical thyroid tissue. The lesion is excised by retracting and controlling the tongue with multiple stay sutures. Postoperative hypothyroidism is readily controlled by thyroid replacement therapy.

Haemangioma, lymphangioma and neurofibroma should be excised as described for macroglossia (p. 122). Granular-cell myoblastoma has a peculiar predilection for the upper respiratory and digestive passages and has been described in the tongue. Complete surgical excision and careful follow-up is indicated.

MALIGNANT

Ectodermal malignant tumours do not occur in children but mesodermal lesions do (Fig. 5, 26), as described above under lip tumours.

FLOOR OF MOUTH AND BUCCAL MUCOSA

Congenital

RANULA

Ranula is a descriptive term for any cystic swelling of the floor of the mouth

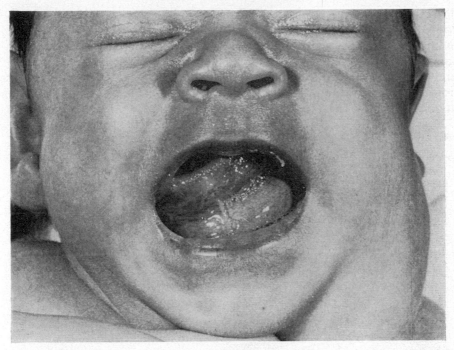

FIG. 5, 27

Ranula. Lymphangiomatous complex ranula with involvement of both the floor of the mouth and the neck. This was treated by separate extra-oral and intra-oral excisions.

(Fig. 5, 27). The condition may be simple or complex. The simple form is relatively localized and is a superficial dilated segment of a blocked sublingual duct. The complex form burrows deeper into the submaxillary region and may be salivary gland, branchiogenic or lymphangiomatous in origin. The ranula usually presents as a slow growing softly fluctuant clear or bluish swelling in the floor of the mouth. Occasionally the swelling presents in the submandibular region, but will be palpable in the mouth on bimanual examination.

Some ranulae will resolve spontaneously, but if this does not occur in two to three months time they should be treated surgically. The operator should approach the lesion intraorally and attempt to excise it, having in mind that marsupialization is adequate treatment for simple ranulae and is preferable to deep relatively blind dissection in the floor of the mouth or submaxillary region. The thin wall of the lesion frequently predicates marsupialization. Complex ranulae require separate, or occasionally, combined intra- and extra-oral excisions.

Infections

LUDWIG'S ANGINA

The rapidly spreading infection of the floor of the mouth and the submaxillary region has been called this because of its tendency to strangle or suffocate. It is produced by an infected mandibular molar tooth, wound or ulcer in the floor of the mouth. The streptococcus is commonly the predominating causative organism but mixed organisms are usually present. Treatment is by early massive broad spectrum antibiotics without waiting for cultures or antibiotic sensitivity studies. Cases not responding to this treatment will require tracheostomy and deep incision and drainage of the submaxillary area. *Peritonsillar abscess* and *retropharyngeal abscess* are rarely encountered in this era of early antibiotic treatment of children's throat infections. Incision and drainage are indicated with great care being taken to avoid aspiration of pus.

GANGRENOUS STOMATITIS, NOMA OR CANCRUM ORIS

This condition has been dealt with under the section on lips.

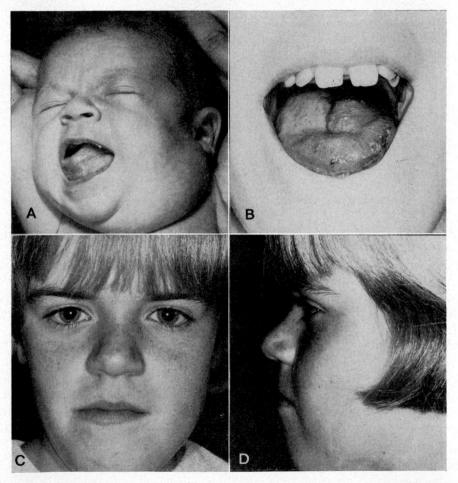

FIG. 5, 28

(A) Lymphangioma with extensive involvement of the floor of the mouth, treated by separate intra-oral and extra-oral excisions. (B) Residual involvement of the tongue which required a central excision to decrease bulk and a marginal excision to remove troublesome localized areas of glossitis and haemorrhage. (C and D) Mandibular overgrowth tends to occur with these patients with or without radiological evidence of lymphangiomatous involvement of the mandible.

Tumours

Tumours of this area are similar to and frequently blend with tumours of the tongue and lip and even those of the submaxillary region. The *papilloma* and *mucous cyst* are treated by simple excision.

Lymphangioma (*cystic hygroma*) (Chap. 36) is the commonest childhood tumour involving the floor of the mouth. It is usual for there to be involvement of the widely surrounding regions and structures (Fig. **5**, 28). These complex cases require judicious but radical surgical treatment. The surgeon must be satisfied with approaching one area at a time and dealing with that area thoroughly, yet sparing important structures such as the facial, hypoglossal and lingual nerves. The first approach should be where the maximum presentation of the lesion is—either intra-oral or submandibular. Several months later, when the usually extensive postoperative reaction has subsided, the next major area of presentation should be approached.

Meticulous oral hygiene and dental prophylaxis must be insisted upon. Failure to do this will result in returning bouts of acute lymphangitis in the residual tumour. Mandibular overgrowth frequently becomes evident as the years go by. This may be due to either direct lymphangioma involvement of the mandible or to increase tissue mass and blood supply to the area. Inferior border and mental mandibulectomy may be necessary, or, horizontal ramus resections. The latter procedure should be deferred until the child is older if at all possible.

W. K. LINDSAY

REFERENCES

BIRDSELL, D. C. & LINDSAY, W. K. (1969). Malignant tumours of the head and neck in children. *Plastic reconstr. Surg.* **44**, 255–260.
PALETTA, F. X. (1966). Lymphangioma. *Plastic reconstr. Surg.* **37**, 269.
PSAUME, J. (1957). A propos des anomalies fascalies associées à la division palatine. *Annls Chir. plast.* **2**, 2–11.
THOMSON, H. G., JUCKES, A. W. & FARMER, A. W. (1965). Electrical burns of mouth in children. *Plastic reconstr. Surg.* **35**, 466–477.
WOOLF, R. M., GEORGIADE, N. & PICKRELL, K. L. (1960). Micrognathia and associated cleft palate (Pierre Robin syndrome). *Plastic reconstr. Surg.* **26**, 199.

CHAPTER VI

TUMOURS OF THE JAWS IN CHILDHOOD

In view of the rarity of benign and malignant neoplasms of the jaws in childhood and the comparative frequency with which other swellings occur during this period of life, the term 'tumour' in the context of this chapter will be taken to mean swelling. Swellings of the jaw during childhood will be discussed under the following headings: (1) Inflammatory (*a*) acute (*b*) chronic, (2) Cystic, (3) Hamartomatous, (4) Neoplastic (*a*) benign (*b*) malignant, (5) Bony dysplasia, (6) Unknown aetiology, e.g. histiocytosis 'X'.

INFLAMMATORY LESIONS

ACUTE INFLAMMATORY LESIONS

Acute inflammatory lesions of the jaws in childhood are common and may be subdivided into those of dental or non-dental origin.

Lesions of dental origin

Acute dentoalveolar abscess and/or cellulitis of the soft tissues around the mandible and maxilla are common during childhood subsequent to carious exposure of teeth, pulpitis and infection proceeding from an infected necrotic pulp. Whilst this process is common, it is not as frequently seen as might be pre-supposed from the number of infected and non-vital teeth that are seen during early childhood, particularly in the deciduous dentition. The reasons for this are twofold, and depend on the one hand on the virulence of the invading organism and on the other hand on the resistance of the host to the infection. The majority of dental infections during childhood are due to the streptococcus viridans type organism which is of comparatively low virulence, and the resistance of the child to infection is considerable owing to the very high vascularity of the jaws during this period of growth. Should the child's general resistance be lowered by some inter-current infection such as an exanthematous fever, a previous chronic infection in association with a non-vital or infected tooth may become acute.

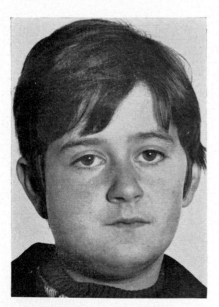

FIG. 6, 1
Girl aged 8 years with an acute suppurative right submandibular lymphadenitis, the primary infection spreading from an infected lower deciduous molar.

Local trauma to the previously chronically infected tooth may also swing the balance in the direction of an acute spreading infection. The presentation of the child with an acutely painful swollen face (Fig. **6**, 1) is not unusual. Evidence of suppuration with fluctuation may be already evident and there will be an associated tender lymphadenopathy in the regional lymph nodes. A pyrexia of 38·3° to 39·4°C (101° to 103°F) is frequently associated with these lesions. If the swelling is predominantly due to cellulitis then the initial treatment will be with appropriate antibiotics, but should suppuration and abscess formation predominate then removal of the offending tooth, plus incision and drainage under general anaesthesia would usually be required, supported perhaps with appropriate antibiotic therapy.

Lesions of non-dental origin

A fairly common lesion seen in the region of the jaws during childhood may be termed cervico-facial suppurative lymphadenitis. In these cases the teeth may be perfectly sound and no dental cause may be seen for a lesion which, whilst being predominantly submandibular in origin, may extend up above the lower border of the mandible. These lesions tend to be extremely tender and indurated with an outline which is difficult to discern. Associated pyrexia of 37·7° to 38·8°C (100° to 102°F) is common. The most frequent cause for such lesions is the coagulase positive staphylococcus aureus. Infected lesions on the face, particularly around the nose and in the anterior nares, are occasionally associated with such swellings. Should the child present early in the condition, prior to suppuration and evidence of fluctuation, suitable antibiotic therapy may bring about a resolution. Because so many of the staphylococci that cause these lesions may be penicillin insensitive, some other antibiotic may be more appropriate, e.g. cloxacillin or erythromycin. Once suppuration and fluctuation are evident, extra-oral incision and drainage will be required. The causes of acute cervico-facial lymphadenitis, other than those due to staphylococcus pyogenes infection, may be found associated with acute stomatitis, e.g. herpes simplex infection or, infrequently, with such rare conditions as cat-scratch fever.

Acute osteomyelitis

Acute osteomyelitis of the maxilla occurs essentially during the neonatal period and early infancy. It may result either from local trauma with associated infection or haematogenous spread from an infective lesion elsewhere. The latter is not infrequently seen in cases of staphylococcal pyoderma where the child may have multiple staphylococcal lesions on the skin and in the conjunctivae. Haematogenous spread in these cases may result in a lesion in the maxilla. Such haematogenous lesions frequently commence in the first deciduous molar region of the jaw resulting in the destruction of the tooth germ for this tooth and rapidly leading to suppurative lesions pointing into the mouth, onto the face, and into the orbit. The prognosis for this previously almost fatal condition has been radically altered since the advent of antibiotic therapy but it should be emphasised that the organism responsible is generally a *penicillin resistant* staphylococcus. Acute osteomyelitis of either jaw can occur later in childhood, being more frequently seen in the mandible as an extension of infection from a dental source. Such a complication is comparatively rare and occurs in children who are considerably debilitated from some other cause.

CHRONIC INFLAMMATORY LESIONS

Lesions of dental origin

Chronic inflammatory lesions of dental origin are extremely common, particularly in the deciduous dentition during childhood, being derived from a carious exposure of the pulp with subsequent infective necrosis and periodontal involvement by the invading organism. The clinical manifestations of such a chronic infection are the commonly seen gum-boil or chronic abscess, or the somewhat less frequently seen so-called granulomatous epulis (Fig. **6**, 2).

The lesions heal following the extraction of the infected tooth or after appropriate endodontic therapy of the tooth with subsequent resolution of the infection.

Another chronic lesion of dental origin may be seen in cases of infection of the tooth germ of successional teeth subsequent to infection of the deciduous predecessor. Continued suppuration from the tooth socket with jaw swelling subsequent to the extraction of deciduous teeth should indicate the possibility of an infected tooth

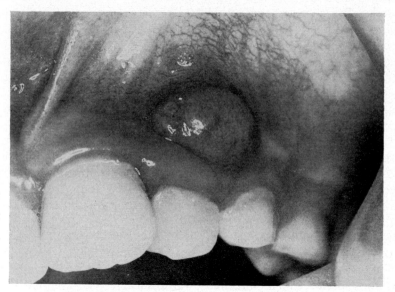

FIG **6**, 2

Epithelialised granuloma obscuring an apical sinus from an infected and non-vital ⌊2. Pulpal necrosis had resulted from accidental trauma to the tooth.

germ. The radiographic examination in these cases shows total loss of the lamina dura around the tooth germ with a wide area of bony rarefaction. Occasionally in these cases an occlusal view will show a subperiosteal reaction to the infection in the form of a thin involucrum.

EPULIDES

Localised forms of chronic irritation and inflammation are probably responsible for a number of circumscribed lesions of the gingival tissues known as epulides; these are only occasionally seen during childhood and are comparatively rare under the age of 10 years. The following types of epulis in childhood have been described:

Fibrous epulis. This presents as a localised pedunculated or sessile swelling of the gingival tissues in childhood mainly confined to the incisor regions. The lesion has a smooth well-keratinised surface of normal gingival colour unless traumatised by the opposing teeth. The corium consists of a mass of firm fibrous tissue interspersed with chronic inflammatory cells (Fig. **6**, 3).

Whilst in adult life an obvious source of chronic irritation is frequently present to account for these lesions, e.g. the sharp edge of a carious cavity, a faulty restoration

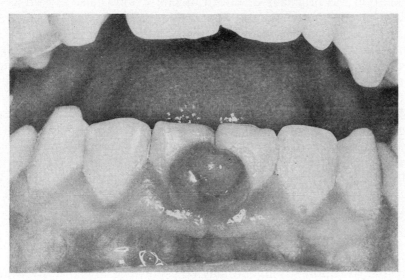

FIG. **6**, 3

Well developed fibrous epulis derived from the inter-dental tissues between 1|1 in a child aged 11 years.

or dental calculus, in childhood these lesions occur without observable cause. A conservative local excision of the lesion, combined with currettage, will usually effect a cure.

Giant cell epulis. (Peripheral giant cell reparative granuloma.) Giant cell epulides occur only rarely during childhood as a sessile or pedunculated maroon-coloured swelling of the gingiva a few millimetres to 1·5 cm in diameter. These lesions are almost always situated in the arch proximal to the first permanent molar, and spring from the gingiva or periodontal ligament. Trauma is thought to be the causative factor for these lesions and they are no longer considered to be neoplastic. Histologically the lesions are composed of a vascular granulomatous tissue infiltrated with multinucleated giant cells, red blood cells, and are covered by a layer of epithelium.

These epulides proliferate rapidly, bleed easily with minor trauma, and tend to recur unless the local excision is very carefully undertaken.

CHRONIC PERIOSTITIS

The periosteum of the child possesses a high osteogenic potential which implies that it will lay down bone to a greater extent and under less favourable conditions than is the case in an adult. Chronic subperiosteal infection of a low degree of pathogenicity will result in the elevation of the periosteum by infected granulation tissue and this, in turn, stimulates the periosteum to lay down new bone. After such a layer has been formed the infection may permeate through this layer and the process will be repeated, often several times, so that a number of laminae of bone arranged parallel to the cortical plate of the jaw will be seen in a radiograph. Clinically a hard bony mass, resembling an osteoma, can be palpated.

This condition was originally described by Garré and is also known as periostitis ossificans or productive periostitis. The radiographical appearance of so-called 'onion-skin' laminae can give rise to an erroneous diagnosis of neoplasm.

Treatment consists of an intraoral reflection of the overlying muco-periosteum and the radical removal of all new bone together with infected granulation tissue down to, and including, the original outer plate of the bone.

Lesions of non-dental origin

Tuberculous lesions. Primary tuberculosis in the mouth is a rare cause of chronic swelling around the jaws. The primary tuberculous lesion in the mouth is said to be a painless lesion and frequently to be sited in the region of an exfoliated or previously extracted tooth. In association with the chronic ulcer are enlarged, hard, firm, only moderately tender lymph nodes. In these cases appropriate tuberculin testing and biopsy of the lesion will establish the diagnosis.

CYSTIC LESIONS

Cysts of the jaw during childhood may be subdivided into the following groups: (1) Eruption cyst, (2) Dental cyst, (3) Dentigerous cyst, (4) Developmental cyst and (5) Primordial cyst.

Eruption cyst

Eruption cysts may be associated with the eruption of both the deciduous and permanent dentitions.

Deciduous dentition. True cysts of eruption associated with the deciduous dentition are comparatively rare and said to be developed either from the epithelial glands of Serres, remnants of the dental lamina overlying the erupting teeth, or from the reduced enamel epithelium after cessation of amelogenesis. These rare eruption cysts of the deciduous dentition are frequently mistaken for the more commonly seen eruption haematoma. The latter is caused by bleeding into the gingival tissues during tooth eruption. Distinction between the two conditions may be readily made by means of transillumination. In the case of the haematoma the lesion is opaque whilst the cyst transilluminates brilliantly.

Permanent dentition. Eruption cysts associated with the permanent dentition may be either derived as in the deciduous dentition or may commonly be due to a dentigerous cyst bursting through the bone into the soft tissues and presenting as a rapidly developing swelling of the jaw. Treatment in both eruption cysts of the deciduous and permanent dentitions may be expectant. Occasionally the cyst may burst spontaneously with complete resolution. However, if treatment is required owing to failure of spontaneous resolution or due to discomfort in the deciduous dentition, an elliptical portion of mucosa overlying the erupting tooth and including the cyst wall should be removed, whilst in the permanent dentition marsupialisation of the cyst either under local or general anaesthesia can be undertaken. In both cases successful eruption of the teeth subsequent to treatment can be expected.

Dental cyst

Dental cysts form essentially at the apex of infected and non-vital teeth both in the deciduous and permanent dentitions. Teeth may have been rendered non-vital as a result of trauma or subsequent to a carious exposure and infection of the dental pulp. Spread of infection from the pulp into the periapical tissues may occasionally lead to cystic degeneration occurring in the epithelial remnants present in the periodontal tissues. Such lesions may present as slowly developing painless lesions of the jaw overlying the apex of the infected tooth. In the case of the deciduous dentition

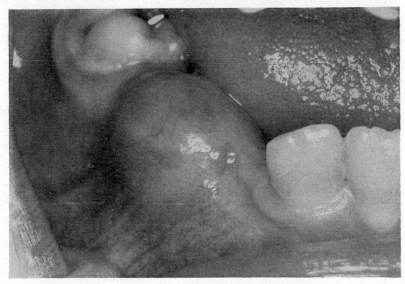

Fig. 6, 4

Residual dental cyst of the right mandible. This lesion was probably derived from an apical dental cyst associated with a non-vital, infected, deciduous molar which had previously been extracted.

such dental cysts may enclose the crowns of the underlying permanent successor (Fig. 6, 4) and therefore become by definition dentigerous cysts. The treatment of such conditions in childhood involves either the surgical removal of the cyst together with the overlying infected tooth, unless the latter can be conserved by endodontic therapy and root filling, or marsupialisation of the cyst as described below. The former technique is particularly indicated when cysts are associated with the permanent dentition.

Dentigerous cysts

Dentigerous cysts may form, as stated above, from dental cysts on infected non-vital deciduous predecessors (Fig. 6, 5) or alternatively the cyst may develop from the reduced enamel epithelium overlying the crowns of developing teeth after the cessation of amelogenesis. In the latter instance the tooth most frequently affected during early childhood by such cystic degeneration is the displaced maxillary canine. The treatment of the dentigerous cyst usually involves marsupialisation of the cyst which allows subsequent eruption of the tooth. Marsupialisation involves excision of the overlying mucoperiosteum, bone, and cyst lining as far as the maximum diameter of the cavity. This is packed for 10 days until the cyst lining which remains heals in continuity with the surrounding mucosa.

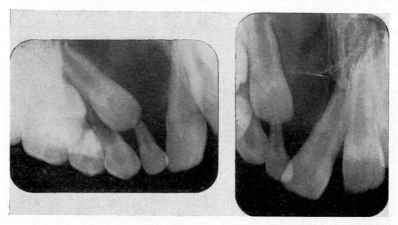

FIG. 6, 5

Radiograph showing well-defined area of rarefaction overlying B⌋ and involving the unerupted 2⌋. A dentigerous cyst which was found to be present at operation probably derived from the infected and non-vital B⌋. Note the displacement of 21⌋ by the cystic lesion and internal resorption of the root canal in B⌋.

Developmental cysts

Developmental cysts are said to be derived from the inclusion of epithelium at the line of junction of developing portions of the mesoderm during the formation of the jaws. The types of developmental cyst described and seen during childhood are the extra-osseous nasolabial cysts and cysts of the incisive papilla, the intra-osseous naso-palatine cysts, median cysts of the palate, globulo-maxillary cysts and, more rarely, the median mandibular cyst. Such cysts cause gradually increasing non-tender swelling of the jaw and displacement of the adjacent teeth. In the case of the naso-labial cyst, the cyst forms in an extra-osseous site in the upper labial sulcus and elevates the alar margin, whereas the naso-palatine, median palatine, and globulo-maxillary cysts of the maxilla cause bony swelling and, in the latter instance, displacement of developing teeth. The globulo-maxillary cyst forms most frequently between the upper lateral incisor and canine teeth, but more rarely, may occur between the lateral and central incisors. The naso-palatine cyst is derived from epithelium in the

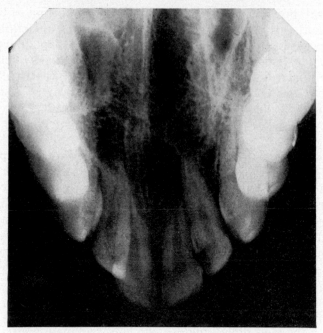

FIG. 6, 6

Radiograph showing the location and pattern of rarefaction produced by a naso-palatine cyst. As the lesion was mainly confined to the left side of the palate it did not give the typical 'heart-shaped' appearance.

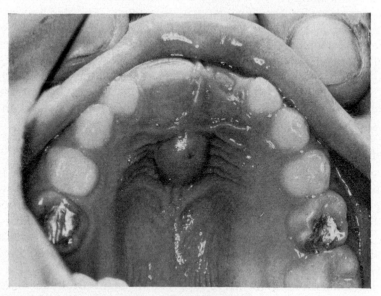

FIG. 6, 7

A cyst of the palatine papilla. Note the punctum from which fluid could be expressed.

PS F 2

naso-palatine canal, presents as a swelling in the anterior portion of the hard palate, and radiographically is seen as a large area of well-defined rarefaction with a typical heart-shaped appearance (Fig. **6**, 6). Cysts of the incisive papilla are extra-osseous lesions and present as mid-line swellings of the palate immediately behind the incisor teeth. Such lesions may show evidence of a small punctum from which a salty-tasting fluid may be expressed (Fig. **6**, 7). These developmental cystic lesions cannot be treated by marsupialisation and must be excised in their entirety.

Primordial cysts

Primordial or keratogenic cysts are derived from the odontogenic epithelium which would normally give rise to a developing tooth. The most usual site for primordial cysts is the lower third molar region but they have been reported in other regions of the jaw, e.g. the lower incisor region. Multiple keratocysts of the jaws have been reported in association with Gorlin's syndrome (basal cell skin tumours, bifid ribs and sometimes medulloblastoma). Cysts of this nature are particularly liable to recur following surgical removal, and follow-up examination over a prolonged period is essential.

HAMARTOMAS

Hamartomas of the jaws presenting during childhood may be divided into haemangiomas, lymphangiomas and odontomes.

Haemangiomas

Haemangiomas leading to swelling of the jaw are usually of the cavernous variety. Such lesions may involve the jaws as part of a more extensive lesion sometimes involving the soft palate, pharyngeal and basal regions of the skull (Fig. **6**, 8). More rarely haemangiomas may be central in origin and give rise to gradual swelling of the jaw as development proceeds. Such haemangiomas involve the roots of teeth, and should these teeth be extracted with subsequent rupture of the central haemangioma, a torrential haemorrhage is likely, which may prove to be fatal. Haemangiomas involving the jaws should, therefore, be treated with the utmost care. Tooth extraction adjacent to such lesions should be avoided at all costs.

Lymphangiomas

Lymphangiomas of the cheeks, tongue, or floor of the mouth may involve the maxilla or mandible during childhood giving rise to quite massive facial swelling and considerable deformity. Such lesions show the typical sago-grained appearance in the mouth (Fig. **6**, 9) and, if involving the buccal sulci in the mandibular or maxillary region, may make it virtually impossible to anaesthetise teeth with local anaesthetic solutions during restorative procedures. Presumably the local anaesthetic solution is entrapped by the lymphangiomatous tissue and cannot be diffused into the underlying bone where it can anaesthetise the nerve supply to the teeth. Both haemangiomas and lymphangiomas tend to grow during the normal period of childhood and cease growth at adolescence.

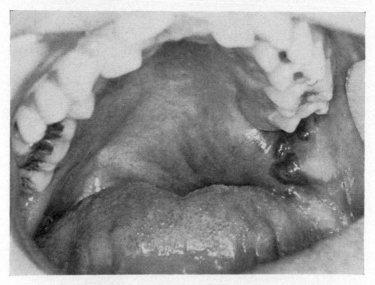

Fig. **6**, 8

Cavernous haemangioma which involved the soft palate, pharyngeal wall, cheek and extended beneath the base of the skull. A possible extension of the lesion into the left maxillary tuberosity gave rise to considerable concern when |7 became cariously exposed. To avoid the possibility of a fatal haemorrhage on extraction of this tooth, it was conserved by endodontic therapy and root filling.

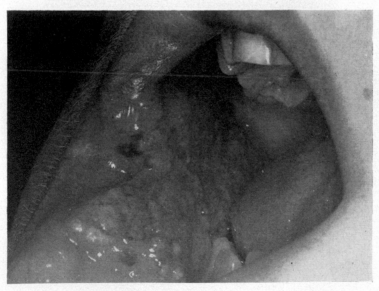

Fig. **6**, 9

A massive lymphangioma involving the right cheek and right side of the mandible in a boy of 10 years.

Odontomes

Odontomes causing swelling of the jaws may be of the following varieties: (1) Cystic (invaginated odontome), (2) Compound composite odontome and (3) Complex composite odontome.

Odontomes are formed as a result of the unco-ordinated and excessive growth of dental formative tissue.

Cystic odontome. Invagination of the dental epithelium into the developing tooth

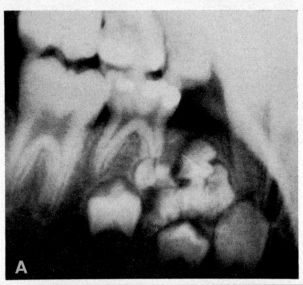

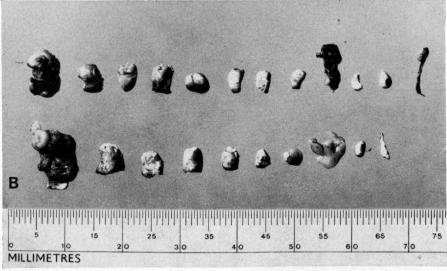

FIG. 6, 10

(A) Radiograph showing a developing compound composite odontome in the right mandibular premolar region. Note the displacement of developing teeth. (B) During operation 22 separately calcified denticles were obtained.

germ leads to a dens in dente malformation. A more gross example of the invaginated odontome gives rise to the so-called cystic odontome.

Compound composite odontome. These lesions are composed of a multiplicity of small denticles within a common follicular sac (Fig. **6, 10**). Such lesions have been recorded as containing anything from 20 to 250 denticles.

Complex composite odontome. In this case the developing anomaly consists of a mass of dental tissue containing enamel, dentine and cementum, all fused together in one lump, within the follicular sac. Such lesions may measure several centimetres in diameter. Both the compound composite and complex composite odontomes may present during childhood as gradually developing non-tender bony-hard lesions of the jaws. Radiographs show the typical malformation with the displacement of the surrounding developing teeth. Whilst the invaginated odontome frequently occurs from the developmental anomaly of a tooth in the normal series, particularly the upper lateral permanent incisor, the composite odontome is more frequently derived from odontogenic epithelium which would not have given rise to teeth in the normal series. These entirely benign developmental lesions require surgical removal together with the residual follicular tissue, successful treatment resulting in the eruption of the surrounding teeth.

NEOPLASTIC LESIONS

Embryological considerations and classification

During the sixth week of intra-uterine life the oral ectoderm grows downwards into the underlying mesoderm and divides into inner and outer processes. The latter later participates in the separation of the lips and cheek from the jaws, thus forming the labial and buccal sulcus, whereas the former, or dental, lamina develops by differentiation into the enamel organ of the teeth. Condensation of the mesoderm adjacent to the bell-shaped ectodermal enamel organ gives rise to the dentine papilla which forms the main core of the tooth and, in the region of the roots, differentiation of cells into cementoblasts results in the formation of the specialised form of bone termed cementum which covers the root surface. At an early stage in development, fibroblasts differentiate to enclose the tooth germ in a fibrous sac or follicle.

At about the same time, epithelial ingrowth of the oral ectoderm into the adjacent mesoderm gives rise to the formation of the major salivary glands, and also to the minor glands which are distributed widely throughout the oral mucosa, particularly in the palate.

From this brief description it will be observed that a considerable amount of ectodermal and specialised mesodermal tissue is enclaved or buried within the jaw bones, and aberrant growth of such tissues can give rise to neoplasms peculiar to the region of the jaws. Misplaced odontogenic epithelium does not possess the ability to lay down enamel in the absence of specialised mesodermal dentine-forming cells. If these are present, hard mixed odontomes result of the type already described, such as the complex and compound composite varieties. In the absence of dentinogenesis the residual epithelium, in most cases, lies dormant throughout life but may be stimulated into non-neoplastic proliferation resulting in cyst formation of the types which have already been mentioned, or neoplastic change of a benign or malignant nature which is essentially of odontogenic origin. Occasionally both ectodermal and mesodermal odontogenic tissues proliferate in a neoplastic fashion without differentiating to the point where enamel and dentine can be formed, or mesodermal tissue of odontogenic origin may also undergo neoplastic change in which case no dentine formation takes place.

Apart from those of odontogenic origin, the neoplasms commonly encountered in the rest of the body, with obvious exceptions related to specialised tissues, occur in the oral cavity either as primary or secondary tumours. Only those tumours which are peculiar to childhood will be considered. With this limited account of the embryological and developmental processes involved, it is possible to classify neoplasms of the odontogenic tissues in the following manner:

1. *Arising from odontogenic ectodermal tissue*
   Ameloblastoma (adamantinoma)
   Adenoameloblastoma
   Calcifying epithelial tumour
   Primary endosteal (embryonic) carcinoma
2. *Arising from odontogenic ectodermal and mesodermal tissue*
   Ameloblastic fibroma
   Ameloblastic sarcoma
3. *Arising from odontogenic mesodermal tissue*
   Odontogenic fibroma
   Odontogenic myxoma

Ameloblastoma

This neoplasm, otherwise known as adamantinoma or multilocular cyst, is very rare in childhood and most multilocular radiographical appearances in this age group are due to other causes. The tumour gives rise to a slow-growing painless expanding swelling of the jaw and is located approximately ten times more frequently in the mandible than the maxilla. Both outer and inner plates are expanded and the roots of adjacent teeth may be resorbed by contrast with a cyst of dental origin where the outer plate is generally selectively thinned and root resorption does not usually take place. Aspiration biopsy of an ameloblastoma gives little or no fluid and scanty cholesterol crystals, whereas a cyst has abundant fluid and is full of shining cholesterol crystals. The correct diagnosis, however, must rest upon histological examination of biopsy tissue.

Treatment should be conservative and consist of careful removal of all epithelial lining surrounding the cyst-like spaces together with a margin of the adjacent bone, followed by packing of the residual cavity and healing by granulation and secondary epithelialisation. Radical resection is contra-indicated since most lesions occur in the region of the angle and ramus and severe interference with growth and development of the jaw would ensue from an excessively aggressive surgical policy in this region. Recurrence is possible if removal is inadequate, but the neoplasm is slow-growing and every attempt should be made to defer further surgery until development has been completed. Metastasis does not occur, the clinical pattern of behaviour being similar to a basal-cell and not a squamous-cell carcinoma.

Adenoameloblastoma

This possible variant of ameloblastoma, although rare, is more likely to occur in childhood than ameloblastoma, the usual age of incidence being in the 11- to 13-year-old age group. It is generally monocystic and, radiographically, closely resembles a dentigerous cyst. There is a slow, progressive, painless swelling more often in the upper jaw and usually located in the canine or first premolar (bicuspid) region. The size rarely exceeds 2 to 3 cm in diameter. The important difference is that simple enucleation will effect a cure and recurrence is very improbable. Histologically the columnar cells are arranged in a tubule-like pattern resembling ducts or acini although the adenoid appearance is considered by Lucas (1964) to be an abortive attempt at the formation of an enamel organ rather than an origin from glandular tissue.

Calcifying epithelial tumour

This tumour, described by Pindborg (1958), is not unlike an ameloblastoma with calcium deposited in concentric masses around the epithelial cells. It does not appear to have been reported in childhood.

Primary endosteal carcinoma

A few cases have been reported where a poorly-differentiated squamous-cell carcinoma appears to have arisen *de novo* from within the medullary cavity of the mandible, and the origin is thought to be from enclaved epithelial rests (Campelia and Boyle, 1943). Although initially responsive to radiotherapy, recurrence is probable and resection is advisable.

Ameloblastic fibroma

This is a rare neoplasm resulting from the simultaneous proliferation of both ectodermal and mesodermal elements of the enamel organ and the dentine papilla respectively. It closely resembles an ameloblastoma radiographically and clinically but occurs more commonly in the pre-adolescent age group (Fig. 6, 11). Growth of the tumour may, however, be rapid in the later stages and can give rise to a false suspicion of malignant change to an ameloblastic sarcoma which is extremely rare.

The neoplasm expands, but does not invade, the bone and displaces adjacent developing teeth. Treatment is by simple enucleation from an intra-oral approach, the mass shelling out quite easily. The condition is benign and does not recur if adequately removed but care must be taken to ensure that no loculi or extensions remain behind.

Odontogenic fibroma

This neoplasm arises from the fibrous follicle surrounding a developing tooth and is most commonly observed in relation to a molar tooth at the angle of the mandible, usually at the beginning of the second decade. There is considerable expansion of the bone with displacement of adjacent teeth. Whereas, in the case of the ameloblastic

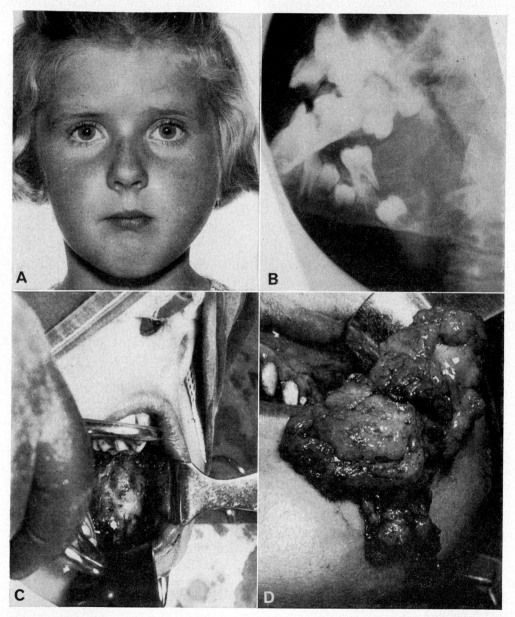

FIG. 6, 11

(A) Expansion of the left ramus in a child aged 7 years. The swelling had been present for one year and had increased rapidly during the preceding 3 months. (B) Lateral oblique radiograph of the mandible of the patient shown in (A). Note the displacement of the developing second molar tooth. (C) View at operation following reflection of the overlying muco-periosteum. (D) Appearance of tissue during enucleation.

fibroma, there is an equal distribution of ectodermal and mesodermal tissues, in the case of the odontogenic fibroma the tumour mass is composed almost entirely of loosely arranged young fibroblasts in which only an occasional mass of epithelial rests of odontogenic origin can be detected. Treatment is by surgical enucleation from an intra-oral approach taking care to avoid damage to adjacent teeth and neuro-vascular structures.

Odontogenic myxoma

The association of this neoplasm with unerupted or missing teeth, its frequency in childhood, and the presence of odontogenic epithelium on many occasions is suggestive of a dental origin. The lesion tends to present more commonly in the first molar region and is a slowly growing, painless swelling which appears, radiographic-ally, as a multilocular 'soap-bubble' radiolucent defect. The neoplasm is particularly infiltrative and wide local removal must be undertaken if recurrences are to be avoided. Metastasis does not, however, take place and the condition is essentially benign in character.

Non-odontogenic tumours of special interest in childhood

There are certain primary and secondary neoplasms which are of particular interest in childhood and which require brief mention. The histogenesis and aetiology of many of these is still debatable.

Pigmented tumour of the jaw in infancy. This is a circumscribed swelling, often occurring in the premaxillary region, which presents during the first three months of life and rarely occurs after the first year of life. Radiographically the radiolucency resembles a cyst and the particular point of interest histologically is the presence of melanin particles within the cytoplasm of cuboid cells lying in a connective tissue stroma. The rate of growth is variable but may be aggressive and rapid, thus giving rise to a false impression of malignancy. Adjacent developing deciduous teeth are displaced widely. The lesion has been described as a melanotic variant of adamanti-noma and attempts to explain the origin of the melanin pigment have led to sugges-tions of a melanotic progonoma or retinal anlage tumour or misplaced sensory neuroectoderm from Jacobson's vomeronasal organ.

The important point, from the surgical aspect, is that these rare tumours are benign and respond to simple surgical excision, and radical surgery or radiotherapy are contra-indicated.

Congenital epulis of the newborn. This is generally a pedunculated swelling, 1 or 2 cm in diameter, covered with smooth mucosa arising from the anterior part of the upper jaw and present at birth. It should be treated by simple excision and does not recur. The swelling is of considerable academic interest from the histological point of view as the large polyhedral cells containing fine eosinophilic granules closely resemble a myoblastoma, although there is evidence to suggest an origin from atypical fibroblasts or, alternatively, neural tissue.

Familial white folded dysplasia. Although not a tumour, in the sense of a swelling, this condition, sometimes termed congenital white spongy naevus, requires mention in order that a distinction may be drawn between the white appearance of the mucosa in this harmless lesion and the appearance of leucoplakia observed in adults. The affected area, which often occurs symmetrically on either side of the lingual fraenum or on the buccal mucosa, is thrown up into thick white folds with a wrinkled surface. The lesion may be present at birth or develop slowly, reaching its maximum around adolescence and, thereafter, remaining static. Histologically the predominant feature is parakeratosis with a marked 'basket-weave' pattern. The condition is harmless and no treatment is indicated.

Hereditary fibromatosis gingivae. The teeth, in this condition, are buried beneath a mass of fibrous tissue, covered with normal epithelium which is derived from the gum. In many cases hypertrichosis is also present. It is a benign condition and careful excision, which may have to be repeated, will expose the teeth which will then be functional and aesthetically more pleasing. The condition should not be confused with the enlargement of the interdental papillae resulting from the prolonged use of Epanutin (Diphenylhydantoin).

Fibro-osseous neoplasms. Ossifying fibroma and fibro-osteoma occur in childhood and can cause gross disfigurement by expansion and distortion of the jaws. These lesions are encapsulated and can be separated from the adjacent normal bone. Resection or mutilating surgical procedures are unnecessary and the majority of cases are amenable to an intraoral approach, the affected area of the jaw being carefully 'de-gloved' by an extensive incision in the sulcus which enables the muco-periosteum to be widely reflected over the tumour area.

Neurofibromatosis. The oral cavity can be affected as part of a generalised neurofibromatosis, the mucosa being the site of separate pedunculated swellings or diffusely thickened. When the tongue is affected, macroglossia may be extreme and require surgical reduction. Plexiform neurofibroma of the trigeminal nerve gives rise to elephantine distortion of the affected side of the face and treatment, by plastic surgery, is extremely difficult and necessitates many operative procedures.

Rhabdomyosarcoma. This highly malignant tumour generally occurs in children during the first decade of life and forms a firm polypoid mass beneath the mucous membrane. It can present in almost any part of the oral cavity with some predilection for the tongue and floor of the mouth. Histologically, cross-striation in the tumour cells may be seen. Treatment is primarily by radiotherapy and local excision but the prognosis is poor.

Lymphosarcoma. Burkitt (1958) described a special type of lymphosarcoma arising in African children which occurs within definite geographical limits which appear to be determined by climatic factors. The disease does not occur in those areas where the temperature falls below 15·5°C (60°F), this being, in turn, dependent upon variations in local altitude. The responsible agent has not been positively identified but is thought to be a virus transmitted by an insect vector. The condition is responsible for 50 per cent of all malignancies in the area and in approximately the same percentage of cases a tumour of the jaw is the presenting symptom. The mass enlarges very rapidly and causes gross distortion of the features. A swift and dramatic response may result from the use of cytotoxic drugs such as cyclophosphamide, but death from wide-spread metastases generally ensues within a few months. Surgery is contra-indicated.

Giant-cell reparative granuloma. The true osteoclastoma of bone is extremely rare in the jaws. It does not occur in childhood and those cases, in the past, which were diagnosed in this way were, in reality, examples of what Jaffe (1953) has termed giant-cell reparative granuloma. Radiographically one or more radiolucent defects similar to a cyst may be noted but the well-demarcated laminar outline is absent (Fig. **6**, 12). Clinically there is expansion of the jaw, with loosening of teeth and some dull pain at intervals. There may be tenderness on deep palpation. Histologically the

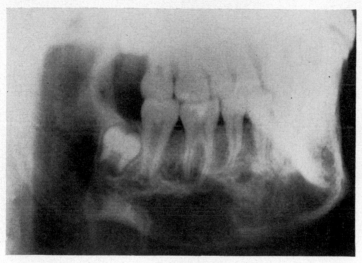

FIG. **6**, 12

Lateral oblique radiograph of the mandible in a boy aged 13 years. Note the irregular margin of the radiolucent defect.

predominant tissue is fibrous and the giant cells, which are not as large or multi-nucleated as in an osteoclastoma, are relatively poorly distributed throughout the mass. These are closely related to areas of haemorrhage and contain haemosiderin particles.

The condition is thought to be due to an abnormality of bone formation related possibly to repeated minor intramedullary haemorrhages of unknown aetiology. The condition is benign and should never be confused with any sarcomatous condition. Treatment is by simple curettage but the diffuse nature of the process may result in some tissue being left behind to form a further focus of bone malformation. In this case the curettage should be repeated and, under no circumstances, is any radical surgery indicated. Any patient exhibiting giant-cell lesions of the jaws should be investigated biochemically to exclude the possibility of hyperparathyroidism.

Teratoma. These rare tumours may be found in the new-born child and may fill the entire oral cavity. The neoplasm generally arises from the region of the sphenoid bone or palate. The larger masses are incompatible with life as the result of respiratory obstruction.

Metastatic neoplasms. These are uncommon in childhood but may result from a primary neuroblastoma of the adrenal, generally of the left side (Fig. **6**, 13) or from a

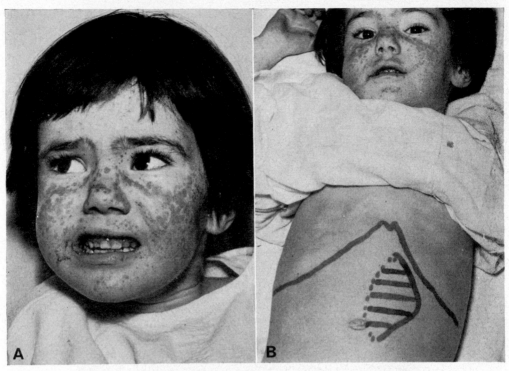

FIG. 6, 13

(A) This girl, aged 4 years, was referred for a swelling at the right angle of the mandible which had been present for 3 weeks and was increasing rapidly. Note the contrast between the pigmentation of the freckles and the pallor of the skin. The haemoglobin was only 33 per cent. (B) The outline of the tumour mass in the left hypochondrium. This had erroneously been treated for 9 months in the belief that it was due to tuberculous abdominal glands.

nephroblastoma or Wilms' tumour. Treatment is palliative by radiotherapy and a good initial response obtained, but the condition, at this stage, is invariably fatal.

BONY DYSPLASIAS

There exists a group of fibro-osseous lesions affecting the facial bones which are not neoplastic in nature, and which have no associated hyperparathyroidism. Apart from a slight increase in the alkaline phosphatase level, the blood chemistry is normal. Previously these conditions were termed osteitis fibrosa along with many other conditions of a similar fibro-osseous nature but with a very different aetiology. There is no evidence of an hereditary or familial background and the fibro-osseous changes cease when skeletal growth is completed.

Although others had previously described the salient features of the condition, Albright *et al.* (1937) have subsequently been credited with a syndrome consisting of fibro-osseous lesions of the bones, light brown pigmentation of the skin, and sexual precocity. This combination of signs is, however, uncommon by comparison with those cases of fibro-osseous change unaccompanied by the other factors. Lichtenstein

(1938) recognised this to be the case and designated the condition polyostotic fibrous dysplasia of bone. Further research lead to the acceptance of the fact that the condition often existed in a single or monostotic variety and was sometimes confined to the facial bones as facial fibrous dysplasia.

Clinically the maxilla, or less frequently the mandible, undergoes a slow uniform expansion commencing at about 11 years of age except in Albright's syndrome when the changes often start as early as 5 years of age. A more pronounced deformity is evident after puberty and the condition becomes relatively static about 17 years of age. The teeth in the affected area become tilted out of position from displacement of their roots. There is no pain or tenderness and it is some time before the patient

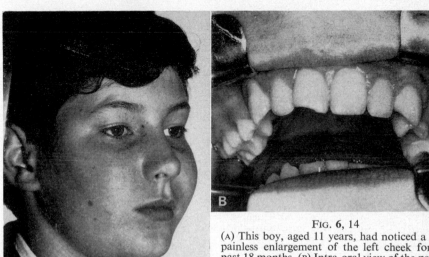

FIG. 6, 14

(A) This boy, aged 11 years, had noticed a slow painless enlargement of the left cheek for the past 18 months. (B) Intra-oral view of the patient shown in (A) demonstrating bony enlargement of the left maxilla.

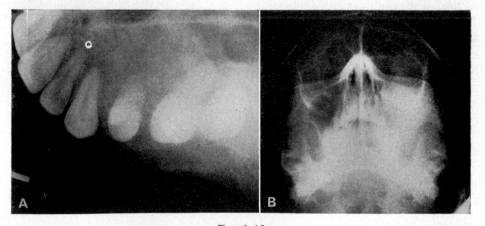

FIG. 6, 15

(A) Occlusal view of the maxilla shown in Fig. 6, 14B illustrating disappearance of the lamina dura and replacement of the normal trabecular pattern of the bone with a 'ground glass' appearance. (B) Occipitomental radiograph of the patient shown in Fig. 6, 14A.

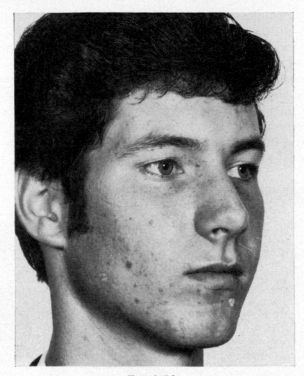

FIG. 6, 16

Appearance of the patient shown in Fig. 6, 14A at 16 years
of age after intra-oral reduction of the fibrous dysplastic
mass of bone.

realises that there is a distortion of the features and seeks advice (Fig. 6, 14). The
radiographic appearances are variable according to the stage of maturity of the
condition. The condition is a developmental dysplasia of the bone and, as such, tends
to be confined to one or more individual bones and not to extend beyond their
anatomical confines or to cross the midline. Areas of mottled radiolucency are
observed which may coalesce to create a uniform 'ground-glass' effect. In the smaller
intra-oral film this may be replaced by a stippled 'orange-peel' effect. The cortex of
the mandible becomes thinned and the entire bone assumes a 'swollen' appearance.
Disappearance of the lamina dura around the teeth may also be noted (Fig. 6, 15).

Treatment is surgical and is achieved by paring down the excess bone from an
intra-oral approach after 'de-gloving' the jaw by the technique previously described.
Operation should be deferred until skeletal growth has mainly been completed since
premature interference may stimulate the dysplastic process and cause a recurrence
(Fig. 6, 16). Radiotherapy should never be employed not only because it is ineffective,
but also because there have been cases of malignant change following its application.

Cherubism

This curious condition, first described by Jones (1933) and also termed familial
multilocular disease of the jaws, is thought by some authorities to be a variant of

fibrous dysplasia but evidence to this effect is not entirely conclusive. Children affected by this dysplasia of bone growth develop swellings of the mandible and, later, the maxilla at about 2 to 4 years of age which are caused by the formation of fibrous masses in the medullary portion of the bone which expand the jaw extensively and displace the erupted and unerupted teeth to a marked degree. The distortion of the cheeks and displacement of the globe of the eye result in the exposure of a greater than normal amount of sclera beneath the iris creating the impression of an upturned eye which reinforces the 'cherubic' appearance (Fig. **6**, 17A). The condition is painless and tends to reach its maximum development just before puberty so that, with further growth and development of the face, the distortion becomes relatively less apparent.

Radiographically there are multiple areas of radiolucency scattered throughout the jaws with marked displacement of the tooth germs. The condition is familial and is thought to be due to a dominant gene of variable expressivity.

Histologically the predominant tissue is fibrous with a collection of giant cells mainly at the periphery of the lesion. These are grouped around areas of haemorrhage and are filled with haemosiderin particles, these also being found in the submandibular lymph nodes which are enlarged.

The distortion of the features usually causes the patient to seek surgical treatment

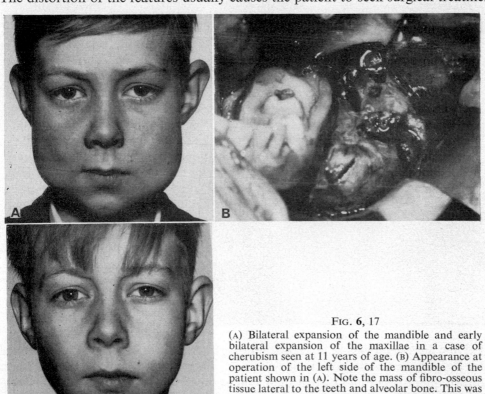

FIG. **6**, 17

(A) Bilateral expansion of the mandible and early bilateral expansion of the maxillae in a case of cherubism seen at 11 years of age. (B) Appearance at operation of the left side of the mandible of the patient shown in (A). Note the mass of fibro-osseous tissue lateral to the teeth and alveolar bone. This was removed by a chisel and the contour of the mandible trimmed to normal. A similar procedure was carried out in the other affected areas. (C) Appearance one year later.

and this should not be withheld on the grounds that spontaneous improvement will take place in late adolescence. Such improvement is only relative and never adequate. Since the maximum disfigurement is reached about 11 years of age, treatment should then be instituted and consists, like fibrous dysplasia, in a simple intra-oral paring down or removal of the abnormal fibro-osseous masses (Fig. **6**, 17B and C). Recurrence is unlikely and, as in the case of fibrous dysplasia, radiotherapy should never be employed.

HISTIOCYTOSIS 'X'

The disturbances of the reticuloendothelial system which were previously separately described under the headings of Hand-Schüller-Christian's disease, Lettere-Siwe disease, and Eosinophilic Granuloma are now considered to be variants of the same

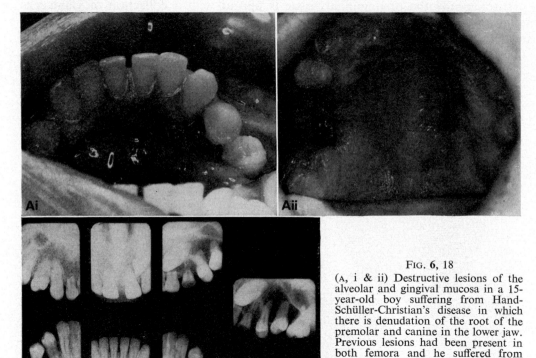

FIG. **6**, 18

(A, i & ii) Destructive lesions of the alveolar and gingival mucosa in a 15-year-old boy suffering from Hand-Schüller-Christian's disease in which there is denudation of the root of the premolar and canine in the lower jaw. Previous lesions had been present in both femora and he suffered from diabetes insipidus. (B) Radiographs of the jaws of patient seen in (A) showing great destruction of bone around the roots of many teeth.

underlying disease process of unknown aetiology and they have recently been grouped under the generic heading of Histiocytosis 'X'—the letter 'X' signifying the, as yet, unknown quantity common to all these conditions.

The oral manifestations consist of swelling and necrosis of the alveolar portion of the jaws and loosening of the teeth (Fig. **6**, 18), sometimes accompanied by signs of constitutional disturbance such as mild pyrexia and leucocytosis. Biopsy shows the presence of a granulomatous-like lesion with a preponderance of eosinophils and lipoid-laden histiocytes or 'foam' cells. Curettage of the affected area and removal of the loose teeth is the only surgical treatment indicated.

N. L. ROWE AND G. B. WINTER

REFERENCES

ALBRIGHT, F., BUTLER, A. M., HAMPTON, A. O. & SMITH, P. (1937). *New Engl. J. Med.* **216**, 727.
BURKITT, D. (1958). *Br. J. Surg.* **46**, 218.
CAMPELIA, C. M. & BOYLE, P. E. (1943). *Am. J. Orthodont.* **29**, 299.
JAFFE, H. L. (1953). *Oral Surg.* **6**, 159.
JONES, W. A. (1933). *Am. J. Cancer,* **17**, 946.
LICHTENSTEIN, L. (1938). *Arch. Surg.* **36**, 874.
LUCAS, R. B. (1964). *Pathology of the Oral Tissues.* London: Churchill.
PINDBORG, J. J. (1958). *Cancer, N.Y.* **11**, 838.

CHAPTER VII

TRAUMATIC LESIONS OF THE JAWS AND TEETH

INJURIES TO THE TEETH

Maxillo-facial trauma during childhood commonly results in injury to the anterior teeth. The immediate treatment of such injury is frequently neglected owing to concern about the associated soft tissue and bony lesions; this in turn may result in unnecessary complications and the need for prolonged dental treatment. A discussion of these dental injuries may be divided into those lesions which involve the deciduous or primary dentition, mainly during the pre-school years, and those involving the permanent dentition later in childhood.

Traumatic lesions of the deciduous dentition

Injuries to the deciduous dentition occur most frequently between the ages of $1\frac{1}{2}$ and $2\frac{1}{2}$ years (Schreiber, 1959). At this time the majority of children are learning to walk and in the process not infrequently fall, banging themselves against the floor or a projecting object. The face and upper anterior teeth are commonly traumatised by this process. The lower anterior teeth are less frequently involved by trauma unless the child falls whilst sucking a dummy or similar comforter. The lips, tongue and gingival tissues around the teeth may be bruised or lacerated. Due to the comparative softness of the premaxillary bone in these very young children the commonest injury seen in the deciduous dentition is one of displacement of teeth. This may result either in an intrusion of the tooth into the premaxillary bone, a loosening or partial dislocation with lingual or labial displacement or a total avulsion.

Intrusion of maxillary deciduous teeth into the premaxilla at this age may be so gross as to displace the tooth completely out of sight beneath the swollen gingival tissues. Careful inspection of the injured site is required with gentle palpation in the labial sulcus which will reveal the bulge of the submerged crown beneath the gingival tissues. Radiography is sometimes possible in a cooperative child and this will confirm the presence of the displaced tooth. Primary treatment of such lesions consists of parental reassurance and the prescription of a mild antiseptic paint to prevent infection, such as 0·5 per cent dequalinium chloride (Dequadin paint) applied with a cotton bud. Intruded teeth not infrequently re-erupt in the subsequent weeks and may reach full eruption in four to six months. In a very young child with incomplete root formation these intruded teeth may retain normal vitality after re-eruption. Calcific degeneration or necrosis of the pulp are common sequelae to the re-eruption of intruded teeth once root formation is complete, in children over $2\frac{1}{2}$ or 3 years of age.

Partial dislocation of deciduous teeth may require immediate treatment, particularly if the teeth are displaced lingually preventing normal occlusion and mastication. In these circumstances manipulation by gentle pressure with a piece of sterile gauze between the thumb and index finger will re-position the teeth in the arch. The child is then given a soft diet for a day or two and rarely requires the teeth to be splinted. Severe labial displacement of deciduous teeth may result in fracture of the alveolar plate and a tearing of the mucosa. In such circumstances, immediate extraction of the tooth may be required.

Total avulsion of deciduous teeth is fortunately less common than other forms of displacement as it results in the greatest damage to the overlying permanent successors (Ravn, 1968). Failure to locate such avulsed teeth should suggest the possibility of pulmonary aspiration, and chest radiography arranged as a precaution.

Fractures of the crowns and roots of deciduous teeth are comparatively rare and far less common than in the permanent dentition. Minimal fractures of the crowns of deciduous teeth may occur occasionally but when extensive these coronal fractures will almost invariably involve the pulp. Such an incident with a very young and apprehensive child will necessitate immediate extraction. Root fractures, particularly those involving the coronal portions of the root are also indicative of early extraction. Simultaneous surgical removal of the apical portions of the fractured root is necessary to prevent later interference in the eruption of the successional permanent teeth. Fractures in the apical portion of the root do not indicate immediate extraction and usually heal without event.

Trauma to deciduous teeth such as those enumerated above may lead to complications in the successional permanent teeth which include the following conditions. (1) Hypocalcification

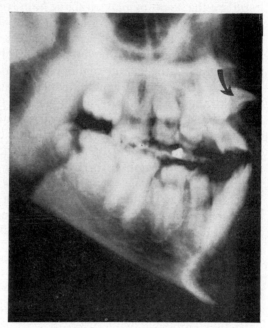

FIG. 7, 1

Dilacerated upper central incisor prior to surgical removal.

and hypoplasia of the crown. (2) Dilaceration of the crown, root or crown-root junction (Fig. 7, 1). (3) Arrested root growth and pulpal calcification. (4) Retarded, mal-, or non-eruption of permanent successors which may be the result of a failure of resorption of highly infected non-vital deciduous teeth. (On rare occasions these infected deciduous teeth may stimulate dental cyst formation which may then involve the crowns of overlying permanent teeth, preventing their eruption.) The treatment for such a condition will be the removal of the retained deciduous tooth and marsupialisation of the cyst, which generally results in eruption of the overlying teeth. Many of these complications are commonly seen in clinical practice and this should suggest the necessity for warning parents of their possible occurrence later in childhood.

Traumatic lesions of the permanent dentition

Estimates for the prevalence of injury to anterior teeth in school children between the ages of 5 and 15 years in Britain vary between 4 and 9 per cent and occur more commonly in boys than girls (Gelbier, 1967). The teeth most frequently traumatised during these incidents are the upper incisors either as a result of direct trauma or to indirect trauma from the lower teeth when the jaws are rapidly and forcibly closed together. The skeletal relationship of the jaws is of aetiological importance and children with protruding upper anterior teeth have a greater likelihood of damaging these when involved with facial trauma. The majority of facial injuries during childhood are the result of play either at home or in school. Approximately 12 per cent of traumatic injuries to anterior teeth (Gelbier, 1967) occur as a result of organised contact sports such as football and cricket and the remainder are due to automobile and bicycle accidents. The latter probably represents about 15 per cent of such injuries during the school years (Winter and Kernohan, 1966).

Injuries to the upper permanent anterior teeth are frequently associated with traumatic lesions of the lips, tongue and gingival tissues. These may be limited to minor abrasions and bruising but occasionally result in extensive and deep lacerations of the soft tissues. These lacerations should be carefully inspected for foreign material, such as fractured crowns of teeth, and where necessary an immediate suture repair undertaken, using non-absorbable material rather than catgut to minimise scarring. In taking the history it is important to obtain an accurate estimate of the time that has elapsed since the teeth were traumatised, and to discover whether previous trauma has occurred to the teeth in the same region. In this respect a history of other accidental trauma to the child is relevant as it may indicate some degree of accident proneness.

EXAMINATION

In examining the injured teeth it is important to inspect the degree of tooth loss, particular emphasis being given to whether or not there is a pulpal exposure. The degree of tooth mobility can be ascertained by careful digital examination; increased mobility indicating the possibility of either root fracture or subluxation with or without coincidental alveolar fracture. Alteration to the colour of teeth may be of diagnostic importance. Immediate coronal discolouration may be indicative of intra-pulpal haemorrhage but not necessarily of pulp death. A greyish discolouration of the crown in a tooth traumatised months or years prior to examination may, however, indicate a non-vital tooth. Certain special investigations, including the following, are necessary to aid diagnosis:

Transillumination of teeth. Increased opacity of teeth subsequent to trauma suggests changes in the pulp space indicative of either a non-vital pulp or perhaps a degenerating and calcifying pulp.

Testing the vitality of teeth. A simple and useful test is to apply cold to the surfaces of teeth. Should the tooth be unduly sensitive to cold it may indicate a degree of hyperaemia or inflammation of the underlying pulp whereas a reduced or non-existent response may indicate a degenerative or non-vital pulp, but all pulp tests of teeth in children rely on the subjective response of the child and therefore in this respect are unreliable. One particular trap for the unwary is found in recently traumatised teeth.

These teeth may fail to respond to any form of pulp testing because of the so-called condition of pulp concussion. This, however, is a reversible state and some 4 to 6 weeks later the tooth may respond quite normally to pulp tests. Unless otherwise indicated, treatment of recently traumatised and apparently non-vital teeth should be deferred until repeat pulp testing can be arranged 4 to 6 weeks later.

Dental radiography. This may give the following information: (1) the degree of root formation may be ascertained, (2) the possibility of root fracture may be confirmed, (3) coincident alveolar or jaw fractures may be seen and (4) other pathological conditions in association with traumatised teeth may be visualised, e.g. areas of apical rarefaction indicating a chronic inflammatory granuloma or dental cyst.

MANAGEMENT

Without going into details of the actual dental treatment employed, the management of fractures of the permanent teeth may be summarised as follows:

Fractures of teeth involving enamel only

The primary treatment required is to smooth the enamel surface and to treat associated soft tissue injury. Such teeth, however, must be kept under constant review from the point of both continued pulp vitality and pathological processes occurring both in the pulp and surrounding periodontal structures.

Fractures involving enamel and dentine

When recently injured teeth are seen in which a considerable area of exposed dentine is present, emergency treatment to cover the latter is required. The reasons for this are two-fold. Firstly, the child may suffer undue discomfort from extremes of temperature and other irritants on the exposed vital dentine surface; secondly, continued irritation of the underlying pulp via the immature dentine may result in irreversible pulpitis and pulpal necrosis.

Fractures involving the pulp

The immediate treatment of teeth in which pulpal involvement has occurred (Fig. 7, 2) will depend largely on the age of the child and the maturity of the dentition. When root formation is incomplete and the apex widely open, in patients seen within 72 hours of trauma, the usual form of treatment is a vital pulpotomy. In cases in which root formation is complete at the time of injury the most appropriate form of therapy will be a total pulpectomy in which the entire pulp is extirpated and the root canal subsequently filled with an occlusive material.

Fractures involving the root

Where the coronal half of the root is involved in the fracture line, often by extensive oblique fractures of the crown but occasionally by transverse fractures of the root, the prognosis, because of involvement or proximity of the epithelial attachment, is extremely poor. It is essential to ensure that the entire root is removed, the apical portion requiring a surgical approach. In fractures involving the apical half of the

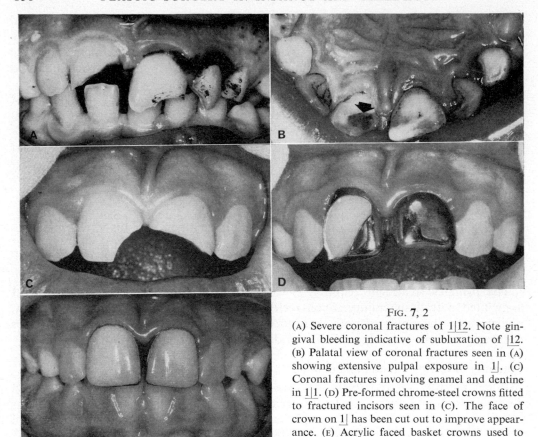

FIG. 7, 2
(A) Severe coronal fractures of 1|12. Note gingival bleeding indicative of subluxation of |12. (B) Palatal view of coronal fractures seen in (A) showing extensive pulpal exposure in 1|. (C) Coronal fractures involving enamel and dentine in 1|1. (D) Pre-formed chrome-steel crowns fitted to fractured incisors seen in (C). The face of crown on 1| has been cut out to improve appearance. (E) Acrylic faced basket crowns used to restore coronal fractures of 1|1.

root, the prognosis is much improved: in these cases increased mobility of the tooth usually necessitates emergency splinting (with figure-of-eight wiring between adjacent teeth, using 0·4 mm soft stainless steel or copper wire, or by burnishing a sheet of lead or aluminium foil onto the surfaces of the teeth), if technical assistance is not immediately available and early sophisticated splinting is not possible. This emergency splinting is generally replaced in 24 to 48 hours by a more carefully constructed acrylic splint (Fig. 7, 3). In cases where multiple teeth are injured or in which there is an associated alveolar or other bony fracture, cast silver splints (Fig. 7, 4), an arch bar or Risdon's method (Hamilton, 1967) may be more appropriate to gain adequate immobilisation. Fractured roots usually heal by fibrous union but on occasions this may be aided by calcific repair between the fractured ends of the root (Fig. 7, 5). These reparative processes between the root ends will only occur when adequate immobilisation is effected, when there is no excessive distraction of the root ends, and when the site of fracture remains free from infection.

Subluxation and complete avulsion of teeth from the socket

Subluxation of teeth requires emergency treatment. The teeth should be repositioned

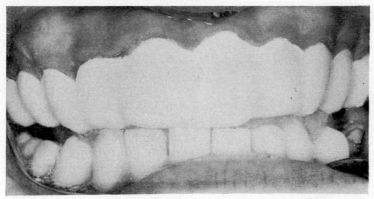

FIG. 7, 3
Acrylic splint covering the upper teeth.

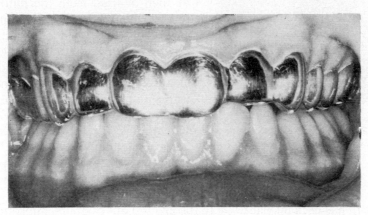

FIG. 7, 4
Silver cap splint.

in the arch by digital pressure under local analgesia and an appropriate splint provided. Such teeth frequently become non-vital and require root canal therapy and root filling at a later date; this is particularly the case when root formation is complete at the time of injury (Fig. 7, 6A and B).

In cases where complete avulsion of teeth has occurred from the socket a decision for reimplantation will have to be rapidly reached. Such a decision will be influenced by the state of root formation of the avulsed tooth, by the time the tooth has been out of the mouth and by such other factors as the presence or absence of crowding in the arch or other form of malocclusion. Where a decision to reimplant is reached the prognosis will be determined by two factors:

1. In cases where the root is immature, the apex widely open and the tooth reimplanted in the socket within a few minutes of injury the prognosis is good. Provided appropriate splinting is immediately undertaken the pulp may succeed in being re-vascularised and re-innervated and the root to continue formation, although the coronal portions of the pulp will usually undergo calcific degeneration. Circum-

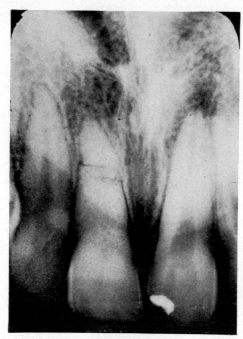

FIG. 7, 5

Root fracture of ⌐1 showing evidence of partial calcific repair and total calcific degeneration of the pulp.

stances such as these may be obtained when immature teeth are avulsed in operating theatres by the misuse of a laryngoscope or Boyle-Davis gag.

2. In other cases of tooth avulsion where root formation is complete and where the tooth has been out of the mouth for periods in excess of 30 minutes the prognosis for reimplantation is not as good. Almost invariably after reimplantation in these cases root resorption occurs. However, this may be an exceedingly slow process and may take a period of more than 10 years to destroy the root. Prior to the reimplantation of such avulsed teeth the pulps should be removed via an access cavity in the palatal aspect of the crown and the pulp space restored with a continuous metallic point, e.g. silver point. The tooth should then be cleansed with a sterile brush under running water and the root disinfected by immersion in chlorhexidine solution at 40°C for 15 minutes. Under appropriate local analgesia the blood clot may be removed from the socket and the tooth reimplanted.

Adequate splinting along the lines suggested above should then be undertaken. Prophylactic antibiotic therapy with oral penicillin may be implemented and in cases where the tooth has been displaced on to the ground out of doors, appropriate tetanus prophylaxis undertaken. In cases where, subsequent to the avulsion of an incisor, a decision is reached against reimplantation two alternative forms of treatment remain. The first is to retain the space, provide a temporary partial denture and replace

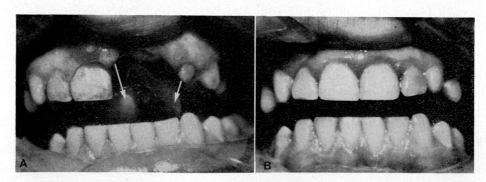

FIG. 7, 6

(A) Lingual displacement of ⌐12 following a severe blow. (B) Eighteen months after repositioning ⌐12 seen in (A) and root filling both teeth.

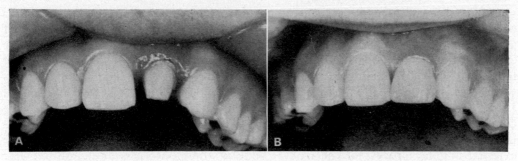

FIG. 7, 7

(A) Subsequent to avulsion of |1, |2 has been moved mesially and prepared for a jacket crown. (B) Jacket crown fitted to |2 seen in (A) to simulate a central incisor. Incisal edge of |3 has been ground flat.

this in early adult life with a fixed bridge. The second is to close the space orthodontically and crown an adjacent tooth to simulate the missing member (Fig. 7, 7A and B).

Outlined above are the principal ways in which permanent teeth may be damaged by trauma but it is possible to get combinations of such injury in any one patient. For example, coronal fractures of the enamel may be associated with apical fractures of the root. In such cases a combination of treatment methods will be required.

FRACTURES OF THE FACIAL BONES

The prevalence of fractures of the facial bones in childhood is low by comparison with adults, in spite of a generally impetuous nature and adventurous spirit which combine to encourage participation in physical activities with little thought for the immediate consequences. Although falls are commonplace, they are usually from a small height and the momentum gained, being the product of a small bodily mass and low velocity, is relatively minor in degree before the moment of impact (Rowe, 1968).

The principal reason, however, for the disparity in the prevalence of facial fractures between the child and the adult lies in the significant differences between the relationship of the neurocranium and the facial skeleton, which in turn arise from the differential rates of growth of the brain and the masticatory apparatus during the early years of life. At birth, the brain is relatively advanced in its development and during the first two years of life triples in volume, subsequently slowing down in its rate of growth until, after the seventh year, the annual increment is extremely small so that approximately 90 per cent of the final volume has been attained by ten years of age (Sicher, 1948). During the second year of life, in association with the development of the deciduous dentition, the facial bones not only commence to overtake the cranium in rate of growth but maintain a progressive development until about 21 years of age.

The antra and paranasal air sinuses are rudimentary at birth and do not attain any significant size until the deciduous teeth have been replaced by the permanent teeth, thus permitting a greater degree of pneumatisation of the maxillary antra and, at the

PS G

same time, promoting a more powerful masticatory force with its associated stimulus to the development of the facial bones. It will be noted, therefore, that at the age of approximately ten years there is not only an emergence of the facial skeleton from the cranial base but also a change from an almost solid structure packed with developing tooth germs to a tubular type of mandible occluding with an upper jaw which is separated from the skull base by a series of extensive air-filled bony cavities (Rowe, 1969). At this stage of growth and development the upper jaw transmits the masticatory force to the skull via the vertical pillars formed medially by the fronto-maxillary and fronto-nasal conjunctions, and laterally by the zygomatic bone with the external angular process of the frontal bone at the fronto-zygomatic suture. The upper and lower orbital margins act as 'tie rods' to these pillars, further support being provided by the arch of the palate.

The net effect is to provide great strength to resist a force applied along the axes of the teeth but little resistance to a blow from an anterior or antero-lateral direction such as would be encountered in a frontal impact on the upper jaw or a lateral blow upon the malar prominence. It is at this age, therefore, that fractures of the middle third of the facial skeleton are first encountered, such injuries being almost unknown in the early years of childhood unless gross violence has been applied. In such cases the relative prominence of the frontal bone almost invariably results in a fracture in this area, often with fatal results. McCoy *et al.* (1966), in a series of 86 children with fractures of the facial bones, showed that 35 cases (40·8 per cent) had sustained other skull fractures.

Scott and Symonds (1967), in pointing out that the cranium increases in size four-fold compared to the twelve-fold increase in size of the facial bones, stress that the growth of the nasal septum is the primary factor in the downward and forward movement of the facial skeleton. Severe injury to this structure in childhood is liable to lead to a failure of projection of the middle third of the facial skeleton and the development of a 'saddle-shaped' nasal bridge.

The principal growth centre of the mandible consists of an area of hyaline cartilage situated beneath the fibrous tissue which covers the articular surface. Growth must, therefore, take place only in a downward and forward direction apart from any increase in thickness resulting from appositional bone growth. Blackwood (1965) has shown that, by the twentieth week of foetal life, large vascular canals appear in the mandibular condyle which are present at birth and persist until the second or third year of life after which they progressively diminish. Hunsuck (1968) has analysed the micro-circulatory architecture of the mandibular condyle in young Rhesus monkeys using micro-injection techniques of silicone self-polymerising rubber and has confirmed the abundant blood supply to this structure during the early phase of life. The gross morphology of this structure also changes from a short thick stump to its more definitive form with a relatively slender neck and well-delineated sub-articular and pre-osseous zones about the age of 7 years. A severe blow directed along the long axis of the mandible before 3 years of age tends to burst open the thin-walled highly vascular condyle and cause an intra-capsular comminuted fracture with haemarthrosis and gross disorganisation of the growth cartilage. A similar blow, at a later age, causes only a 'green-stick' type of extra-articular or sub-condylar fracture comparable, in many ways, to the type of fracture sustained by the adult. The former injury has a poor prognosis, as will be discussed later, but the latter type of injury is self-correcting as growth proceeds.

The relative infrequency of fractures of the facial bones in children is supported by the statistical evidence shown in Table 7, 1.

Table 7, 1

Author	Age group	Total in Series	Percentage
Schuchardt *et al.*, 1960	0–10 years	1,566	6·1
McCoy *et al.*, 1966	0–14 years	1,500	6·0
Rowe and Killey, 1968	0–11 years	1,500	5·1
Fickling, 1968	0–12 years	1,000	6·0
Donaldson, 1961	0–11 years	335	5·3
Hagan and Huelke, 1961	0–10 years	319*	6·2
Halazonetis, 1968	0–11 years	147†	4·0

* Mandibular fractures only.
† Single fractures of the angle and condyle only.

Below the age of 5 years the prevalence is significantly less, as the figures in Table 7, 2 indicate.

Table 7, 2

Author	Age group	Total in Series	Percentage
MacLennan, 1956	0–5 years	187	1·0
Donaldson, 1961	0–5 years	335	1·0
Hagan and Huelke, 1961	0–5 years	319	1·2
Rowe and Killey, 1968	0–5 years	1,500	0·87
Halazonetis, 1968	0–5 years	147	0·68

In the region of the middle third of the facial skeleton the prevalence, as might be anticipated from the anatomical and development factors previously mentioned, is very low. In the series published by Schuchardt *et al.* (1966), in the age group 0 to 10 years, there were only 28 cases out of a total of 2,901 fractures of the facial bones, a prevalence of 0·96 per cent MacLennan (1957) quotes a level of 0·25 per cent, and Rowe and Killey (1968) observed only three Le Fort type fractures and four zygomatic bone fractures which, combined, give a prevalence of 0·46 per cent in a total of 1,500 cases. It is significant that these injuries all occurred within the 7- to 11-year-old age group.

It would probably be reasonable to assume, from a consideration of the figures quoted above, that in general terms the average prevalence is:

Fractures of the mandible below 5 years   1 per cent.
Fractures of the mandible 6 to 11 years   5 per cent.
Fractures of the middle third 0 to 10 years   0·5 per cent.

It will be evident that the experience of any one person, even in a lifetime in a maxillo-facial unit, must be limited.

There are certain other features of fractures of the jaws in children which must be briefly mentioned and, together with what has already been described, these may conveniently be summarised as follows:

1. A greater prominence of the frontal bone with a rudimentary development of the frontal sinus.

2. A lesser degree of prominence of the facial bones with an incomplete development of the paranasal air sinuses (Fig. 7, 8).

3. The presence of multiple growth centres permitting a greater degree of elasticity following trauma.

4. A high degree of vascularity of the bones with an associated high osteogenic potential.

5. The presence of the developing teeth and, at certain ages, the incomplete root formation associated either with resorption of the deciduous teeth or the partial formation of the permanent teeth (Fig. 7, 9).

6. The adaptability of the alveolar bone associated with the presence and eruption of the teeth.

7. Emotional and psychological problems associated with childhood.

Treatment

Before considering treatment in detail, it will be helpful to sub-divide patients into four groups based upon the state of the dentition at the time of injury since this profoundly influences the methods chosen for immobilisation of the jaws.

Table 7, 3

Age group	Dental development
0–2 years	Before completion of the eruption of the deciduous dentition.
2–4 years	Before the roots of the deciduous *incisor* teeth show marked resorption. Many permanent teeth are, however, already partly formed.
5–8 years	Before the roots of the deciduous *molar* teeth are in an advanced state of resorption or the roots of the permanent incisor teeth are adequately developed.
9–11 years	Before eruption of the premolar teeth but after adequate formation of the roots of the permanent first molar and incisor teeth. In this group, development of the antra and paranasal air sinuses may predispose to fractures of the middle third of the facial skeleton following trauma in this region.

The problem of finding suitable teeth to act as anchorage points in the fixation of fractures of the jaws is frequently complicated by the premature loss, or partial destruction by caries, of the deciduous dentition. Cautious excavation of the superficial caries and the insertion of a temporary sedative dressing of zinc oxide and cloves, mixed to a stiff paste, may permit retention, for the period of fixation, of an otherwise useless tooth.

General principles of treatment

These are essentially similar to those in the adult, namely fixation of the fragments in their correct alignment with the teeth in correct occlusion until union has taken place. However, it should be appreciated that the degree of precision required in the child is not as great as in the adult since the replacement of the deciduous teeth by

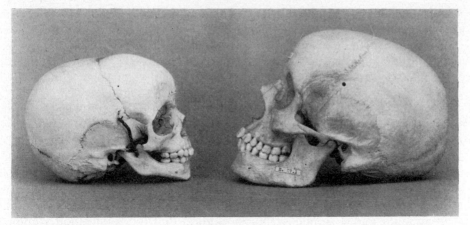

FIG. 7, 8

A comparison between the relative degree of development of the calvarium and facial bones in a child aged 2 years and an adult.

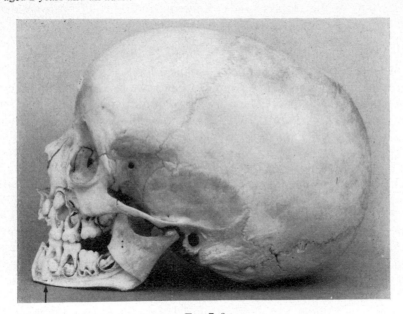

FIG. 7, 9

The skull of a child aged 5 years sectioned to show the state of the deciduous and permanent dentitions. Note the close proximity of the root of the developing permanent lower canine tooth to the lower border of the mandible, as indicated by the arrow.

the permanent teeth, or the further eruption of the latter, will, owing to the adaptive potential of the alveolar bone, bring about a considerable degree of self-correction should alignment or articulation not be perfect. None the less, this does not imply that thorough fixation is not required; indeed, the child will tend to loosen most types of apparatus more readily than the adult and considerable care and ingenuity must be exercised in the design and application of methods of jaw fixation. Fortunately, as the result of the high degree of osteogenic activity, union takes place in about half the time taken for an adult most mandibular fractures being firm in three or four weeks. In the middle third of the facial skeleton the time is only slightly reduced since, for reasons already mentioned, such injuries tend to occur at a relatively later age. Again, three or four weeks fixation is generally adequate.

Tracheostomy must be approached with extra caution, should this be required, in view of the high position of the innominate vein in the child and it is easy to make the error of incising the first tracheal ring with subsequent post-operative stenosis.

Vomiting of gastric contents is more prone to occur and gastric lavage may be indicated. Blood loss may be difficult to estimate clinically and compensatory vasoconstriction is well marked in the child. It is sometimes overlooked that a loss of 200 ml in a child of 3 years of age is equivalent to a loss of approximately a litre of blood in an adult and it should be borne in mind that the total blood volume in a child of that age is little more than 1,000 ml.

In temperate climates, with good nursing facilities, the problem of dehydration rarely arises but, in the tropics, under limited conditions of postoperative care, a child with the jaws immobilised, and with a fretful disposition, must be observed very carefully for this complication.

Methods of immobilisation

Aged 0 to 2 years. A fracture in this age group is generally the result of severe violence such as an automobile accident. The teeth are of no practical use in the fixation of the fragments. Condylar fractures are not treated; if a sub-condylar 'greenstick' type of injury has been sustained this can confidently be expected to straighten itself out as further growth proceeds. If an intracapsular comminuted type of fracture has occurred, every effort should be made to keep the jaws moving in order to avoid the complication of ankylosis. This is more liable to occur with the bilateral than the unilateral fracture.

As far as the remainder of the mandible is concerned, there are basically two types of fracture to consider. The first is where the fracture is in the tooth-bearing portion, and it occurs in practice usually in the region of the symphysis. The fracture should be treated essentially as an edentulous problem and, if laboratory facilities are available, the technique advocated by MacLennan (1956) is excellent. A pre-fabricated acrylic Gunning-type splint, which is a simple 'horse-shoe' shape, is adapted to fit on its under surface by a *thick* layer of softened gutta-percha, and is pressed down over the lower teeth and alveolus following manual disimpaction and reduction of any displacement. The splint is retained in place by two circumferential wires placed on either side of the fracture line. These wires, of 0·5 mm diameter soft stainless steel, can easily be passed around the lower border of the mandible by attaching the end to a curved abdominal needle of suitable size. The point of the needle enters the lingual sulcus and, keeping close to the bone, emerges through the skin at the lower border of the mandible. A short length is pulled through and the needle re-enters the skin puncture to pass upwards on the outer aspect of the jaw and emerge through the labial or buccal sulcus. When both ends have been pulled upwards, taking care not to kink the loop at the lower border as it enters the tissues, a few sawing movements will ensure that the wire is in contact with the bone. The two ends are then twisted together over the top of the acrylic splint thus anchoring it to the mandible. The splint and wires remain in position for three weeks. To remove the wires, they are partly untwisted, cut low down at the point where the buccal or labial portion enters the tissues and, with a swift movement, the wire, grasped by a haemostat at the point where the ends are twisted together, is withdrawn. A short general anaesthetic may be required and antibiotic cover is desirable to eliminate any infection drawn into the deep tissues by this manoeuvre.

The second type of fracture which must be considered is one where the fracture has occurred proximal to the tooth-bearing area, i.e. through the angle, and it will be evident that such a fracture necessitates immobilisation of the mandible for union to occur satisfactorily unless recourse is made to an open reduction and the insertion of a trans-osseous wire. If an external scar is to be avoided, a very satisfactory method of control is to proceed as before but to modify the acrylic splint to incorporate blocks in the molar region, hollowed out to accommodate soft gutta-percha on the occlusal aspect which will occlude with the upper teeth or alveolus, thus stabilising the bite. Immobilisation of the lower jaw is achieved by naso-mandibular wires (Thoma, 1943). A small incision is made in the upper labial sulcus on either side of

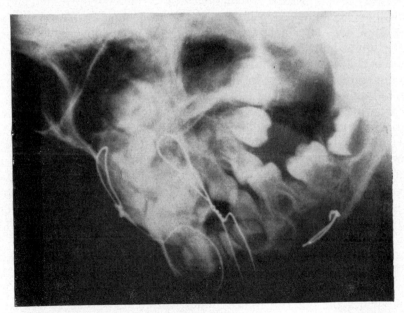

FIG. 7, 10

The patient, aged 18 months, sustained a bilateral fracture of the body of the mandible, externally compound on the left side. In this location, a trans-osseous wire was inserted and circumferential (perimandibular) wires passed in the canine region and twisted tightly down on to the alveolar bone. Wires were also passed through the pyriform aperture bilaterally and one end threaded beneath each circumferential wire before being twisted together with the other end. In this manner, the mandible was immobilised to the upper jaw. Union was complete within three weeks. This is a very simple, but effective, method.

the fraenum and the margin of the pyriform aperture of the nose exposed. This margin is considerably thicker in the child than in the adult and forms a good secure point of anchorage. The nasal mucosa is reflected for about 1 cm and a hole approximately 1 mm in diameter is drilled through from the outer aspect of the bony aperture, being located approximately 1 cm from the free margin. A length of 0·5 mm diameter soft stainless steel wire is threaded through and the end brought back out of the space between the bone and the reflected mucosa. The wound is then closed with black silk sutures. One of the two ends is passed beneath the circumferential wire at the point where it is twisted over the top of the splint, and tightened with the other end after bringing the mandible up to occlude, via the acrylic blocks and gutta-percha inserts, with the upper jaw. A similar procedure on the other side effectively immobilises the lower jaw (Fig. 7, 10). Removal of the wires is achieved in a very similar manner to the circumferential wire, by cutting one end and pulling the wire through by swift traction upon the other end.

Aged 2 to 4 years. Provided that there is a sufficient number of well-formed deciduous teeth free from gross decay, control of the fragments can usually be achieved by wiring around the teeth. The most simple method is to pass a length of 0·4 mm diameter soft stainless steel wire through the interdental space, and around the lingual or palatal aspect of the tooth, to emerge through the next interdental space. The two ends of the wire are then twisted together, leaving about 3 cm of twisted end emerging between the lips. A similar procedure is carried out around a corresponding tooth in the opposite jaw and, after an adequate number of teeth have been treated in this manner, the upper and lower lengths of twisted wire, following reduction of the fracture and occlusion of the teeth, are themselves twisted together to effect immobilisation. Better stability is achieved if the wires can be arranged in a criss-cross pattern rather than straight up and down.

If there are wide gaps in the dentition, an arch bar may be required, or, if facilities are available, cap splints can be used. The latter, however, are avoided if possible since the cementing on of the splints and their subsequent removal and cleaning of the teeth necessitates a great deal of cooperation between the operator and the child. There is no objection to the use of trans-osseous wiring provided that the wires are placed low down through the cortical bone to avoid the drill penetrating through the developing permanent teeth. It is, however, prudent to avoid this technique in the canine region owing to the extremely deep location of the developing tooth germ (Fig. 7, 9).

If the fracture is within the tooth-bearing area of the mandible, a single one-piece lower cap splint, despite its other shortcomings, may often be the best method since this clearly avoids immobilisation of the lower jaw. If there is any doubt about the security of the cement fixation two circumferential wires should be passed to avoid loosening of the splint (Fig. 7, 11). As has been pointed out, a *minor* degree of displacement following removal of the splint is acceptable with the knowledge that this will rapidly be corrected by further alveolar growth and eruption of teeth.

Aged 5 to 8 years. It is between these ages that the greatest problem arises with regard to the fixation of the bone fragments. This results from the fact that the anterior teeth are of little or no use owing to resorption of the roots of the deciduous teeth,

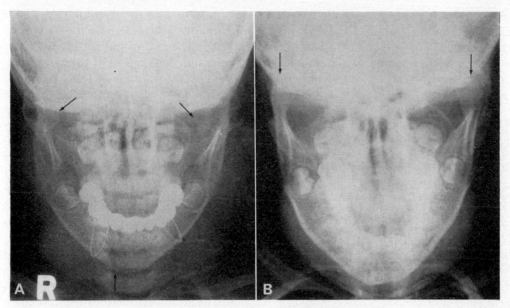

FIG. 7, 11

(A) This child, aged 3 years, has sustained a fracture in the right canine region associated with a 'green-stick' type of fracture of the right condylar neck and a complete fracture dislocation of the left condyle. The mandibular teeth are covered with a cast silver/copper alloy cap splint, fixation being reinforced by bilateral circumferential (perimandibular) wires. The mandible was not immobilised. (B) The patient seen in (A), aged 7 years. Both condyles are morphologically and functionally normal.

or incomplete formation of the roots of the permanent teeth which would be avulsed if they were used for anchorage. Reliance must be placed essentially upon the deciduous molar teeth but, unfortunately, these have often been lost or destroyed by dental decay. The pattern of tooth loss may be such that lower molars have no opposing teeth in the upper jaw and *vice versa* so that the establishment of the occlusion is extremely difficult and stability of the fragments very precariously achieved.

These difficulties can generally be overcome by constructing a partial upper Gunning-type splint incorporating occlusal blocks in conjunction with a similar type of apparatus in the lower jaw, the exact design being dependent upon the precise location of the tooth loss.

The lower splint is secured by circumferential wires and the upper splint is maintained in position by being 'sandwiched' between the lower splint and the palate, immobilisation of the mandible to the bone of the pyriform aperture having been effected in the manner previously described. An alternative method of fixing the upper splint to the maxilla is to process into the acrylic a small loop of wire in the first molar region. Wires are passed around the zygomatic arches (circum-zygomatic) and attached to the loop on the splint. The technique employed is to make a small stab incision through the skin just above the point where the frontal process of the zygomatic bone and the temporal process originate. A slightly curved needle with a sharp point and an eye in the end (a 'J'-shaped post-mortem needle can be used) is passed *deep* to the zygomatic bone. After threading the wire (0·5 mm diameter soft stainless steel) the needle is withdrawn through the mouth and the wire detached. Another needle is threaded with the upper end of the wire and passed through the same skin wound but manipulated so as to pass over the *outer* aspect of the zygomatic arch and down into the mouth to emerge through the same point in the buccal sulcus. The needle is pulled through and the wire detached, leaving a loop outside the skin over the zygomatic arch which is carefully manipulated down by traction on the two ends emerging from the mouth. A few sawing movements of the wire will carry the loop down on to the bone. Owing to the acute bend in the wire, care must be taken not to manipulate the wire too much otherwise it will break, and it should also be recognised that the arch, in the child, is fragile and easily cut through by the wire if excessive force is employed.

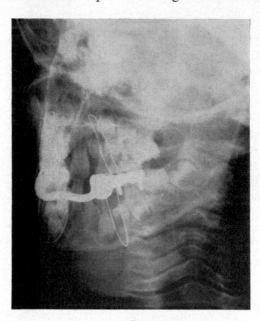

FIG. 7, 12

A bilateral fracture at the angle of the mandible controlled by a cast silver/copper alloy cap splint which covers the deciduous teeth only. In this child, aged 7 years, the lower anterior teeth have been by-passed with a lingual bar owing to their incomplete state of root development, and fixation was reinforced with circumferential wires. Immobilisation of the lower jaw has been achieved using wiring through the margins of the pyriform fossae.

In some cases, a cast metal cap splint can be used as an integral part of the appliance incorporating the acrylic blocks in the molar region provided that the deciduous teeth are sound, but a cap splint must *not* be applied to the permanent incisor teeth—which must be by-passed with a lingual or palatal bar (Fig. 7, 12).

Aged 9 to 11 years. In these cases the development of the roots of the permanent incisor and first molar teeth has proceeded to the point where they can safely be employed for fixation. Trans-osseous wiring, particularly in the externally compound fracture, is also useful.

In those rare instances when a Le Fort type fracture, separating the upper jaw from the cranial superstructure, has occurred it will be found that a plaster of Paris headcap is difficult to apply satisfactorily in the child owing to the lack of development of the frontal sinus and occipital protuberance. It is generally preferable, having united the upper and lower jaws by the best available method, to immobilise by internal skeletal fixation, probably better referred to as a suspension of the mandible sub-cutaneously to some point above the level of fracture of the upper jaw. In practice, this generally means that circum-zygomatic wiring is employed for the low-level Le Fort I or the pyramidal Le Fort II type of fracture. In the case of the high-level Le Fort III fracture or cranio-facial dysjunction, suspension is achieved by utilising the zygomatic process of the frontal bone as a point of anchorage.

An incision through the outer end of the eyebrow provides access to this structure and a small hole of 1 mm diameter, or slightly larger, is drilled through from the outer aspect to the orbital surface, the tissues on the inner aspect being suitably protected. A 25 cm length of 0·5 mm soft stainless steel wire is threaded through the hole and brought back so that the two ends, passed through the eye of a suitable introducer, can be passed down behind the zygomatic bone along the plane of dissection employed in the Gillies' temporal approach for elevation of that bone, inclining forward to emerge through the upper buccal sulcus in a manner similar to that which has been described in relation to circum-zygomatic wiring. One end of this suspension wire is passed underneath the circumferential (peri-mandibular) wire used to secure the mandibular splint or arch bar and twisted together with the other end after placing the united upper and lower jaws into their correct vertical relationship with the base of the skull. The upper jaw is, therefore, 'sandwiched' between the lower jaw, suspended from the zygomatic process of the frontal bone, and the skull base. Removal of the suspensory wire is facilitated by passing a short length of wire beneath the portion crossing the zygomatic process of the frontal bone and twisting this up tightly before closing the soft tissues. This withdrawal wire is cut short where it emerges through the incision and curled into a small loop which can be covered with a small dressing. After three weeks, when union is generally present, the lower ends of the suspensory wires are cut where they emerge into the buccal sulcus, and traction upon the withdrawal wire will then pull the suspensory wire out through the site of the original incision.

Separation of the fronto-zygomatic suture or inferior orbital margin, occurring as part of a fracture of the zygomatico-maxillary complex, is generally an indication for the insertion of a trans-osseous wire, as in the case of an adult, and, very rarely, a graft, preferably of autogenous cartilage or bone, may be required to restore a 'blow-out' type of fracture of the orbital floor (see p. 188).

DISTURBANCE OF DEVELOPMENT OF THE FACIAL BONES

The infrequency with which severe injury occurs to the region of the middle third of the facial skeleton and the problem which is generally encountered in endeavouring to follow up such cases makes an accurate assessment of the long-term results very difficult to obtain. According to McCoy et al. (1966), it is only the more severe type of naso-ethmoidal or orbital injury which persists into adult life as a residual deformity although, as already noted, interference with the growth of the nasal septum from a variety of causes has been shown to result in a lack of downward and forward growth of the upper jaw.

Injury to the mandibular condyle, however, is relatively more frequent, and the end-results have been studied in considerable detail both in humans and, experimentally, in monkeys. Walker (1960) and Boyne (1967) have convincingly demonstrated that surgically created fracture dislocations of the condyle in the young Macaca Rhesus monkey will, under the influence of functional modelling resorption and bone apposition, result in the re-formation of a morphologically and functionally normal structure. This research is substantiated in humans by clinical reports by Blevins and Gores (1961), Rakower et al. (1961), Kaplan and Mark (1962),

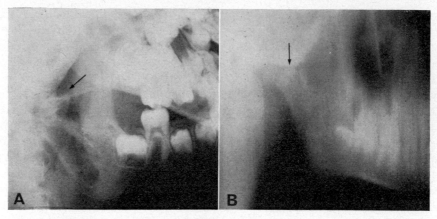

FIG. 7, 13

(A) Antero-medial fracture dislocation of the right condyle in a child aged 7 years. (B) A tomogram of the patient whose radiograph is depicted in (A), taken three years later at the age of 10 years. Note the effective degree of remodelling of the condyle. Active movement was encouraged following fracture and the subsequent jaw movements were normal.

MacLennan and Simpson (1965) and Rowe and Killey (1968) (Fig. 7, 13). Unless there is gross lateral displacement or mechanical interference with mandibular movement, there is no indication for open reduction and immobilisation of a fractured con-

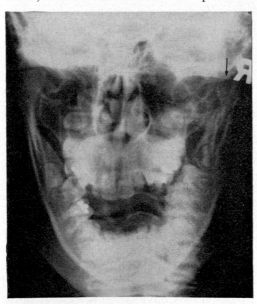

FIG. 7, 14

This patient, aged 11 years, sustained an intra-capsular comminuted fracture of the condyle at 3 years of age. The arrow indicates the failure of growth in the sub-articular area and it will be observed that the mid-line of the mandible has already deviated towards the affected side.

dyle. The results obtained by conservative treatment, particularly those where muscle training is adopted to encourage the child to close the mouth with the teeth in their correct centric relationship, are extremely satisfactory and, with further growth and development, a very satisfactory end result can be anticipated (Rowe, 1960).

The intracapsular comminuted fracture involving severe disorganisation of the articular surface, which is liable to occur before 3 years of age, does carry a poor prognosis since this injury results in an arrest of the cartilaginous growth in the immediate sub-articular region (Fig. 7, 14). Greer Walker (1957) investigated 50 cases demonstrating arrest in development of the condyle and noted that 14 out of 39 unilateral cases and 5 out of 11 bilateral cases were due to trauma. He also observed that only 2 of the 14 unilateral cases exhibited limitation of opening whereas *all* of the

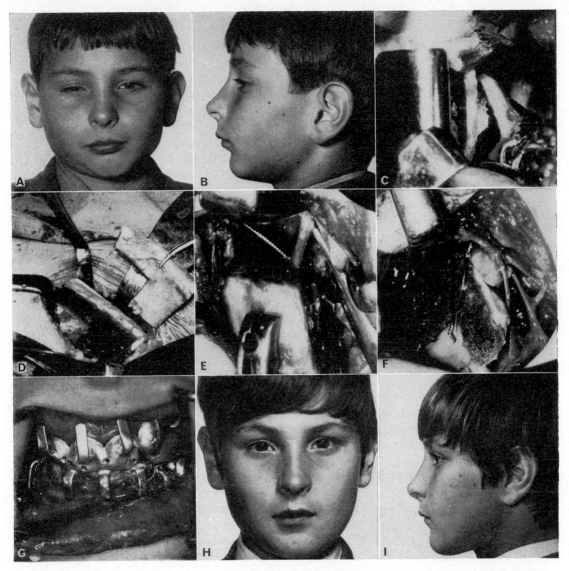

Fig **7, 15**

(A) This patient, aged 12 years, received an intra-capsular comminuted fracture of the left condyle at 2 years of age. Although there was no ankylosis, the interference with the growth centre has resulted in a deviation of the chin towards the affected side. Some secondary distortion of the upper jaw is already apparent. (B) In the profile view, early recession of the chin may be seen. (C) Advancement of the mandible with elongation of the left ramus necessitates division of the right (normal) ramus in order to prevent displacement of the condyle and disturbance of the occlusion on that side. This intra-oral view shows the right ramus after sectioning in the sagittal plane by the Obwegeser/Dal Pont technique. (D) A cortico-cancellous section of bone is taken from the outer aspect of the iliac crest, the precise pattern being determined pre-operatively from X-rays and a model replica of the jaws. (E) The left ramus has been exposed from a sub-mandibular approach. A horizontal cut passes above the level of the mandibular foramen to reach the angle. In this view the cut ends have been separated to the desired degree and the haemostat, placed deep to the inferior dental neurovascular bundle, demonstrates the location and integrity of this structure. (F) The bone graft, with the cancellous surface facing outwards, has been wired into position. (G) The cast metal cap splints incorporate a pre-operatively planned block of acrylic which has been interposed between the separated occlusal surfaces of the splints on the left side. This degree of open bite results from elongation of the ramus, and the block takes all stress off the graft during the healing phase. This takes approximately six weeks. (H) Appearance two years postoperatively. (I) Profile view. The incision line should be planned, as shown, to occupy the optimum position *after* elongation of the ramus.

bilateral cases were severely affected. The failure of growth, in the unilateral cases, results in a deviation of the chin towards the affected side with retrognathism and, in the bilateral cases, the classical 'bird-face' deformity ensues with the mid-line of the chin centrally placed but associated with a severe degree of retrognathism. The tongue, in both cases, being unaffected tends to guide the erupting teeth into occlusion and there is considerable compensatory adjustment in dental position possibly through the adaptability of the alveolar bone. The apices of the teeth, being situated upon an asymmetrical or insufficiently developed basal bone, cause the tips or occlusal surfaces of the teeth to be 'fanned' outwards and proclinated by the action of the tongue.

The only treatment of any value for the intracapsular comminuted fracture is to avoid immobilisation and to keep the jaw moving in the hope of preventing ankylosis. If this complication should supervene, and when the condition is well established after a year or more, a condylectomy should be performed. This operation should not be deferred until adult life in the belief that there will still be some growth activity left. This is not the case, and a far better appositional bone growth will result from a functional jaw with well-developed muscles than an inactive ankylosed jaw with atrophic muscles.

Whether a condylectomy is performed or not, there will inevitably be a progressively developing asymmetry and failure of forward growth of the chin unless surgical treatment is undertaken to correct this deformity. In the past, and in the majority of cases at the present time, the view has been taken that treatment must be postponed until adult life when an attempt is made to camouflage the deformity by means of bone or cartilage onlays or epithelial inlays in the buccal or labial sulcus and the provision of a suitably-contoured intraoral prosthesis. Although quite good results are obtainable by this means, the secondary twisting of the middle third of the facial skeleton arising from the interference with the downward and forward growth of the maxilla, which is blocked by the short under-developed ramus, still persists and is often associated with a tilting of the anterior nasal spine and twisting of the nasal skeleton and cartilages. Under these circumstances, it will be clear that any radical attempt to re-orientate the basal bone of the mandible would result in a posterior open bite with the teeth thrown out of occlusion unless, additionally, a maxillary osteotomy were to be performed.

The current view, therefore, is that an attempt should be made, generally at the time that the deciduous teeth are being shed and the permanent premolar teeth will erupt, to elongate the short ramus by osteotomy and the insertion of a bone graft. The normal ramus must also be sectioned to allow a pivotal point for rotation around the coronal plane. The resultant open bite in the molar region is controlled orthodontically and is eliminated by alveolar bone growth carrying the erupting teeth into position (Fig. 7, 15). A further graft may be required after the post-pubertal burst of growth activity subsides. Promising results have been obtained from this technique but further time is required before a final analysis of the effects can be adequately assessed. (See also Chapter III under 'Acquired deformities in the region of the jaws', p. 78.)

N. L. ROWE AND G. B. WINTER

REFERENCES

BLACKWOOD, J. H. (1965). *J. Anat.* **99**, 551.
BLEVINS, C. & GORES, R. J. (1961). *J. oral Surg. Anesth. Hosp. dent. Serv.* **19**, 392.
BOYNE, P. J. (1967). *J. oral Surg. Anes. Hosp. dent. Serv.* **25**, 300.
DONALDSON, K. L. (1961). *N.Z. dent. J.* **57**, 56.
FICKLING, B. W. (1968). Personal Communication.
GELBIER, S. (1967). *Br. dent. J.* **123**, 331.
HAGAN, E. K. & HUELKE, D. F. (1961). *J. oral Surg. Anesth. Hosp. dent. Serv.* **19**, 93.
HALAZONETIS, J. A. (1968). *Br. J. oral Surg.* **6**, 37.
HAMILTON, A. F. (1967). In *Transactions of the 2nd Congress of the International Association of Oral Surgeons.* Ed. Husted, E. & Hjørting-Hansen, E. p. 333, Copenhagen: Munksgaard.
HUNSUCK, E. E. (1968). *J. oral Surg.* **26**, 449.
KAPLAN, S. I. & MARK, H. I. (1962). *Oral Surg.* **15**, 136.
MACLENNAN, W. D. (1956). *Br. J. Plast. Surg.* **9**, 125.
MACLENNAN, W. D. (1957). *Archs Dis. Childh.* **32**, 492.
MACLENNAN, W. D. & SIMPSON, W. (1965). *Br. J. plast. Surg.* **18**, 423.
MCCOY, F. J., CHANDLER, R. A. & CROW, M. L. (1966). *Plastic reconstr. Surg.* **37**, 209.
RAKOWER, W., PROTZELL, A. & ROSENCRANS, M. (1961). *J. oral Surg. Anesth. Hosp. dent. Serv.* **19**, 517.
RAVN, J. J. (1968). *J. Dent. Child.* **35**, 281.
ROWE, N. L. (1960). *Int. dent. J. Lond.* **10**, 484.
ROWE, N. L. (1968). *J. oral Surg.* **26**, 505.
ROWE, N. L. (1969). *J. oral Surg.* **27**, 497.
ROWE, N. L. & KILLEY, H. C. (1968). *Fractures of the Facial Skeleton*, 2nd ed. Edinburgh: Livingstone.
SCHREIBER, C. K. (1959). *Br. dent. J.* **106**, 340.
SCHUCHARDT, K., BRICHETTI, L. M. & SCHWENZER, N. (1960). *Stoma* **13**, 159.
SCHUCHARDT, K., SCHWENZER, N., ROTTKE, B. & LENTRODT, J. (1966). *Fortschr. Kiefer- u. Gesichts-Chir.* **11**, 1.
SCOTT, J. H. & SYMONDS, N. B. B. (1967). *Introduction to Dental Anatomy*, 5th Ed. Edinburgh: Livingstone.
SICHER, H. (1948). *Oral Anatomy*, London: Kimpton.
THOMA, K. (1943). *Am. J. Orthod. oral Surg.* (Oral Surg. Sect.), **29**, 433.
WALKER, D. G. (1957). *Dent. Pract. dent. Rec.* **7**, 160.
WALKER, R. V. (1960). *Am. J. Surg.* **100**, 850.
WINTER, G. B. (1966). *Br. dent. J.* **120**, 249.
WINTER, G. B. & KERNOHAN, D. C. (1966). *Br. dent. J.* **120**, 564.

CHAPTER VIII

OSTEITIS OF THE MAXILLA

As a result of the successful treatment of septicaemia in the newborn, more small infants are living long enough to show clinical evidence of haematogenous osteitis. (We prefer the term 'osteitis' to 'osteomyelitis' as the marrow plays no important part in the disease.)

While osteitis of the maxilla most commonly affects neonates and infants in the first few months of life it is occasionally seen in older children (most commonly in those suffering from Down's syndrome). The patient is usually referred to hospital with a diagnosis of orbital cellulitis (Fig. 8, 1). True orbital cellulitis in infancy and

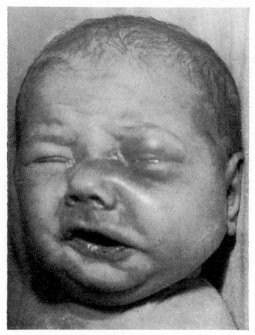

FIG. **8**, 1
Typical appearance in neonatal osteitis of maxilla.

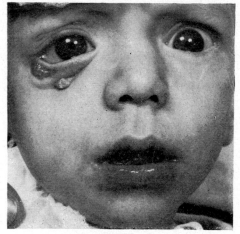

FIG. **8**, 2
Osteitis of right maxilla. Pus has been allowed to point at lower lid with sinus formation leading to underlying sequestra. This happened only once in a series of 24 patients.

childhood almost always follows infection of a peri-orbital haematoma. In the early stages, radiography reveals little apart from soft tissue oedema although sequestrum formation may show in the later stages of the disease. Pus may discharge through the nose, the alveolar sulcus or through the palate and incision should be made at the appropriate site. If at all possible pus should *not* be allowed to point below the eye, as incision there and possible subsequent extrusion of the sequestrum (Fig. **8**, 2) will lead to unsightly ectropion (Fig. **8**, 3). The primary teeth erupt earlier on the diseased

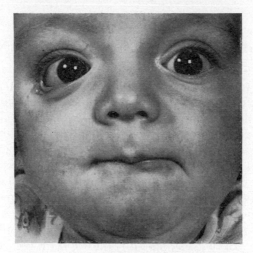

FIG. 8, 3
Same patient one month later. Sequestra have
been extruded and ectropion is developing.

side (presumably due to hyperaemia) and there is no damage to the permanent teeth.

In the infant the infection is commonly due to a coagulase positive staphylococcus resistant to penicillin and is treated with ampicillin and cloxacillin (in Britain Ampiclox Neonatal is a convenient specific formulation of these two antibiotics). We have found no improvement in our results following direct instillation of antibiotics into the maxilla. Rarely the infecting organism is streptococcal and such infection is readily controlled by penicillin and the sulphonamides.

W. M. DENNISON

SELECTED BIBLIOGRAPHY

CAVANAGH, F. (1960). Osteomyelitis of the superior maxilla in infants. *Br. med. J.* 1, 468.
DENNISON, W. M. (1967). *Surgery in Infancy and Childhood*, 2nd ed. Edinburgh: Livingstone.
TAYLOR, W. O. G. (1959). Osteitis of the maxilla in sucklings. *Trans. Ophthal. Soc. U.K.* 79, 355.

CHAPTER IX

FAICAL INJURIES IN CHILDREN*

Children are exposed to injuries as are adults and facial injuries are no exception. Children ride with their parents in automobiles and are victims of crashes. Athletic activities are responsible for many facial injuries in the older child. The vast canine population subjects the child to dog-bites often resulting in considerable soft tissue disorganization and loss. Facial injuries in children are considered separately in this text because of special problems which arise in treatment. Soft tissue injuries and fractures may require special techniques due to difficulties in obtaining the co-operation of young children. Another aspect of facial injuries in children is that which results from the influence of trauma upon facial development. A facial deformity due to trauma in a child is the result not only of the displacement of bony structures due to fracture, but also to faulty development resulting from the injury. Developmental malformations seen in young adolescents and adults are often the result of early childhood injury.

BIRTH INJURIES

The mechanical strains and stresses of birth when delivery is prolonged or aided by instrumental means may lead to a wide variety of facial injuries. Fortunately, most of the injuries are mild and the effects are transient. Deviation of the septum has been attributed to forced deflection during birth. More severe injuries have been attributed to forceps compression of the soft tissues and bones of the face resulting in permanent facial scars, and of the bone in the region of the zygomatic arch and temporomandibular joint, resulting in temporomandibular ankylosis with subsequent developmental atresia of the mandible. Because of the lack of development of the mastoid process at birth and the superficial position of the seventh nerve, facial paralysis, due to injury of the nerve by delivery forceps pressure, is also observed.

Injuries to the eye or its adnexa, such as damage to the extraocular musculature, may be caused by intraorbital haemorrhage. Fractures of the body of the mandible due to birth injury are rare. Those seen by the author have been simple linear fractures with little, if any, displacement, healing occurring in a short time without manipulative treatment.

INJURIES IN INFANTS

It has long been suspected that infants fall much more frequently than is generally known. Of 536 infants involved in a study sponsored by the National Safety Council

---

* *Editor's Note:* Fractures of the mandible and maxilla are dealt with in detail in Chapter 7 and secondary deformities following trauma in Chapter 3. A short account of these is included in this Chapter in order to put them in their proper perspective in relation to facial trauma as a whole, and it is felt that the different authors each contribute points of view which make retention of such apparent overlaps of the subject of value to the reader.

(Kravits *et al.*, 1969), 47·5 per cent fell from a high place such as an adult bed, a crib, or an infant dressing table during their first year of life. Some of the infants in the series suffered cranial and intracranial injuries. It can be assumed that facial trauma occurring in such falls in infants while not frequently resulting in fractures, because of the elasticity of neonatal bones, may be sufficient to interfere with growth centres and explain some of the developmental malformations of the face observed in later years.

INJURIES IN CHILDREN

SOFT TISSUE INJURY

Soft tissue wounds in children heal rapidly and therefore require primary suture early. Such wounds tend to heal with considerable hypertrophic scarring; discouraging results often require later secondary repair of the scar. Scars in children usually soften and lose their red colour with the passage of time, thus becoming less noticeable; they tend to widen, however, as the face grows. It is wise to mention this possibility to the parents, advising them that later secondary surgery may be necessary. Densely scarred areas may require reconstructive procedures, for such untreated areas may interfere with subjacent bony growth, particularly in the area of the mandible.

Loss of soft tissue of the face by avulsion or thermal burns is remedied by transplantation. Loss of portions of the nose are adequately repaired, in many cases, by composite auricular grafts which show a high propensity of success in children. Subtotal or total loss of the nose has not been observed by us. Lewin (1955) has described the reconstruction of the nose in an infant.

FRACTURES

Considerable trauma is required to produce a fracture in a child because of the relative elasticity of the bony structures which are not yet calcified. The fractures suffered by children are similar to those incurred in adults, but these are influenced by the fact that in young children and infants some suture lines are not yet closed. Despite satisfactory healing and consolidation, fractures of the jaws may also cause derangement of developing tooth follicles and faulty eruption of teeth. The influence of the fracture on growth centres of the jaws may result in development malformation.

Emergency treatment

Arrest of haemorrhage and provision of an adequate airway are emergency measures that apply to the facially injured child as well as the adult. Because of the small size of the laryngotracheal airway in the child, oedema of the laryngeal mucous membrane or retroposition of the base of the tongue can produce a sudden obstruction. A suture placed through the tongue permits forward traction and relief of obstruction. Although treatment in a steam room and the administration of corticosteroids can relieve symptoms of laryngeal obstruction, there should be no hesitancy in performing a tracheotomy in a child with fractured mandible or maxilla who is unconscious or who is showing increasing respiratory distress.

Fractures of the facial bones

INCIDENCE

The incidence of facial bone fractures in children varies according to various reports. In our series of mandibular fractures, children's fractures represented approximately 10 per cent in the age group between 4 and 11 years. In a series reported by Panagopoulos (1957), fractures of all facial bones in children represented only 1·4 per cent of the entire series. Pfeifer (1966) reviewing a series of 3,033 cases of facial bone fractures noted that only 4·4 per cent of these cases had occurred in children in the age group extending to the age of 10 years; in the age group extending to 14 years, the incidence was 11 per cent; in the age group extending from 11 to 20 years of age, the incidence increased to 20·6 per cent. McCoy et al. (1966) had 86 fractures in children in a series of 1,500 cases of facial bone fractures, an incidence of 6 per cent in the age group extending from 6 months to 14 years. Rowe and Killey (1955) reported that in a series of 500 cases of fracture, the incidence of mandibular fractures in children was 1·2 per cent in the age group 0 to 5 years and 4·4 per cent in the age group extending from 6 to 12 years.

SPECIAL ASPECTS

While the fundamental principles of treatment of these fractures do not differ materially from the treatment of fractures in adults, special aspects should be emphasized.

1. In this age group, the developing permanent teeth occupy most of the body of the mandible. This anatomic characteristic must be taken into account if interosseous fixation is to be employed in order to avoid injuring the tooth buds of the permanent teeth. The wires must be placed near the lower border of the mandible. The roots of the deciduous teeth are gradually being resorbed and between the ages of 5 and 9 years, because of the mixed dentition, the frequent absence of teeth and the poor retentive shape of the crowns of deciduous teeth, it is often difficult to utilize the dentition for fixation.

2. The reparative process in children is rapid; loose, displaced fragments become quite adherent to one another within three or four days of the injury. At this time, fragments are difficult to manipulate and must be loosened under general anaesthesia before reduction of the fracture is possible.

3. The developing bone predisposes to the characteristic 'greenstick' type of fracture. The elasticity of young bone explains the lower basic frequency of such fractures than in the adult. When fracture does occur, however, fractures involving the body of the mandible frequently show a considerable degree of displacement and the fracture lines tend to be long and oblique, extending downward and forward from the upper border of the mandible. This obliquity of the fracture line is quite different from that observed in the adult where the direction of the fracture line is usually downward and backward.

4. Fractures of the condyle which involve the base of the neck of the condyle are

often of the 'greenstick' variety and are not usually accompanied by disturbance of the temporomandibular joint. The high level fracture must always be viewed with concern in the young child because of the possibility of secondary growth anomalies from damage to the condylar growth centre.

Temporomandibular joint injury may lead to ankylosis. The following example is characteristic: a 3-year-old boy was examined following a fall on the chin. No apparent injury could be found on clinical and radiological examination. Six months later, the child had developed marked limitation of motion of the mandible due to partial ankylosis of the right temporomandibular joint. Resection of the head of the condyle restored mandibular function.

Topazian (1964) reported that trauma, most frequently a traumatic force applied to the point of the chin in children under 9 years of age, was responsible for approximately one-third of the cases of temporomandibular ankylosis in a personal series of 44 cases and in 185 cases culled from the literature. Fortunately many injuries and fractures in the condylar area of the mandible in children are not followed by ankylosis and growth disturbances.

A progressive straightening of the neck of the condyle is observed after fractures in which bony contact between the fragments has been maintained. Pfeifer (1966) noted that in fracture dislocations with loss of the contact between the fragments, there was a shortening of the ramus on the fractured side and asymmetry of the mandibular arch. In these cases, resorption of the condyle was observed with the formation of a new joint. In none of these cases did ankylosis occur, although deviation upon opening of the mouth was frequent due to the shortening of the affected side.

A case which was brought to our attention (Gregory, 1957) is that of a girl, aged 8 years, who sustained a subcondylar fracture of the mandible on the right side when she fell while riding on her bicycle. Roentgenographic examination revealed a marked medial displacement of the right condyle (Fig. 9, 1A); the teeth were wired in occlusion by means of intermaxillary wire (Fig. 9, 1B). Consolidation was completed with the head of the condyle at right angles to the ramus (Fig. 9, 1C). The patient had no trouble in masticating food but there was a deviation of the mandible to the affected side when the mouth was opened wide. She was instructed to stand before a mirror and exercise her jaw daily. Radiographs taken three years later (Fig. 9, 1D) show nearly normal position of the condyle, satisfactory growth, position, and function of the mandible.

Temporomandibular ankylosis and mandibular hypoplasia appear to be the consequence of damage to the articular cartilage on the head of the condyle. Varying degrees of anatomical disruption of the condylar process, overriding of fragments, comminution, do not appear to be the responsible factors in causing temporomandibular ankylosis. Prior to the age of 5 years, the condylar neck is less developed, the bony tissues are soft and more susceptible to a 'crush' type of injury; after the age of 5, the condyle will, in all probability, fracture at the neck. The 'crush' type of injury may cause the condylar cartilage to sustain the main damage. The condylar cartilage being the major factor in mandibular growth, mandibular hypoplasia results when it is injured (Walker, 1957).

5. Fractures involving the body of the mandible frequently involve the permanent

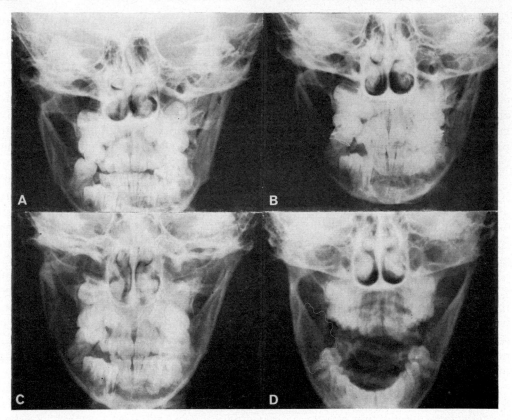

FIG. 9, 1

Radiographic follow-up of a subcondylar fracture in an 8-year-old child treated conservatively. (A) Fracture of the neck of the condyle on the right side with angulation medially. (B) Intermaxillary fixation has been established. (C) Appearance of the fractured bone after early consolidation. (D) Three years later the vertical position of the condyle has been resumed.

tooth follicles but it is seldom necessary to remove these. Eruption of the permanent teeth may be delayed and the teeth may show varying degrees of damage following consolidation of the fracture.

6. Children are not expected to be cooperative and even minor manipulative work, such as intermaxillary wiring or the making of wire loops or buttons, should be performed under general anaesthesia. A few children, however, if the need for treatment is carefully explained to them, do become remarkably cooperative and these procedures can then be done under sedation which may also be required prior to radiographic examination.

TREATMENT

Methods of reduction and fixation. Methods of reduction, both immediate and progressive, are similar to those employed in the adult. Methods of fixation, however, depend upon the presence of teeth with retentive crowns, a factor which varies with the age of the child and the state of evolution of the dentition.

Intermaxillary fixation may be difficult to insure because of the poor retentive quality of the teeth. Circumferential wiring around the body of the mandible and around the maxillary alveolar process constitutes an excellent means of intermaxillary fixation in the child. The maxillary wire is passed through the pyriform aperture into the floor of the nose and downward through the palate, thus surrounding the alveolar area of the maxilla without interfering with the tooth buds of the second dentition. Transalveolar wiring can be used in the older child after the eruption of the second dentition. At this later age, however, the dentition may be adequate for intermaxillary dental fixation.

Every effort should be made in the child to provide rapid and effective treatment; reduction and fixation should be accomplished in one operation whenever possible.

The cable arch-wire (Fig. **9**, 2) is useful as an emergency fixation appliance followed later by a band and arch appliance, if the teeth permit retention of the appliance. Direct interosseous fixation, placing the wire near the lower border of the mandible in order to avoid injuring the tooth buds (see Fig. **9**, 7) or transalveolar interosseous wiring can be employed after exposing the ends of the fractured bone when the teeth do not permit retention of splints or wires.

Internal wiring fixation of the maxilla may be indicated; healing is so rapid in children that a simple headgear appliance may be adequate to maintain cranial and intermaxillary fixation (Fig. **9**, 3).

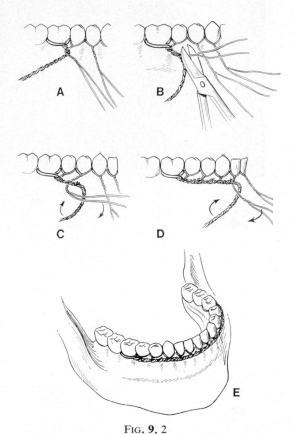

FIG. **9**, 2

The cable arch-wire technique. (A) A heavier gauge wire is twisted around a molar tooth and upon itself. (B to D) Wires twisted around each individual tooth are also twisted around the cable arch-wire. (E) The cable arch completed.

Delayed treatment. If reduction has been delayed and cannot be achieved through simple manipulation, the fibrous tissue which forms rapidly in children between the ends of the fragments is incised and loosened in order to regain mobility of the fragments. A stout needle or trocar establishes a hole through the alveolar process of the distal and proximal fragments. Fine stainless steel wire is then passed from the buccal to the lingual side across the fracture line, and returned from the lingual to the buccal side. The fragments are manipulated into normal position and the ends of the

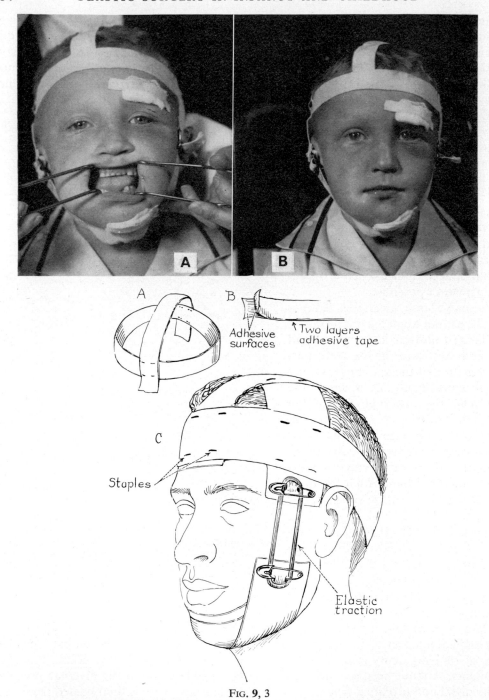

FIG. 9, 3

(A and B) Simple headgear for maxillary fracture fixation in children. (C) The appliance is made of two juxtaposed layers of adhesive tape. Elastic bands between the safety pins provide sufficient pressure to ensure maxillary consolidation.

wire are twisted together. The twisted ends are bent close to the alveolar process and left long enough to protrude through the gingival tissue.

Although this procedure occasionally may cause injury to unerupted teeth, little damage has occurred in our cases. Even though one or more teeth must be sacrificed eventually, less harm ensues than would occur if the jaw fragments were permitted to heal in a distorted position which may lead, in children, to greater deformity than in adults.

The bones of the middle third of the face

Because of the higher degree of elasticity of the facial bones in young children and the lesser degree of development of the middle third of the face in relation to the frontal and cranial area, middle third fractures are rare in comparison to fractures in the adult. Maxillary, naso-orbital, and orbital blow-out fractures are observed and in children submitted to an unusually strong traumatic force frontal bone and telescoping naso-orbital fractures are associated with middle third fractures.

FRACTURES OF THE MAXILLA

The typical Le Fort lines of fracture are rarely seen in children's fractures. Low maxillary (Le Fort I) fractures and pyramidal (Le Fort II) are occasionally encountered.

Problems with fixation are similar to those encountered in the treatment of mandibular fractures because of the presence of poorly retentive teeth. Additional problems in establishing fixation are caused by the luxation and loosening, fracture or avulsion of the teeth, particularly the anterior teeth which are particularly exposed to injury. The cable-arch can be attached to the remaining teeth and in the older child bands may be applied to selected erupted permanent teeth.

Internal wire fixation is an excellent means of fixation in the older child. In the younger child internal fixation to the frontal bone or to the orbital rim may be unsatisfactory because of the relatively poor development of these structures, which consist of soft bone; the wire tends to cut through the bone when placed under tension. Internal wire fixation to the edges of the pyriform aperture, which consists of thicker and stronger bone, is a preferable method.

Rapid fabrication of an acrylic splint in the operating room, with quick curing acrylic resin, while other fractures of the middle third of the face are being treated, will provide an appliance which is held by wire fixation to the edge of the pyriform aperture.

It must be emphasized that fractures of the facial bones in children consolidate readily and rapidly. A simple headgear (Fig. 9, 3) may be all that is required to provide cranial fixation of the fractured maxilla in the young child.

NASAL AND NASO-ORBITAL FRACTURES

Fractures of the nasal skeleton in children are more frequent than fractures of the maxilla and zygoma. The nasal bones in children are separated in the mid-line by a suture line. The open-book type of fracture, with overriding of the nasal bones over the frontal process of the maxilla, is a frequent type of fracture due to the presence of this suture line between the nasal bones. Nasal bone fractures heal rapidly in children, frequently with overgrowth of bone and hypertrophic callus resulting in widening of the bony dorsum of the nose. Fractures and dislocations of the septal cartilage are frequent and haematoma of the septum is always a serious complication in children, not only because of nasal obstruction which results from widening of the septum but also because of the possibility of saddling, which occurs along the dorsum due to loss of cartilage produced by pressure necrosis or a septal abscess.

Treatment of nasal bone fractures in children is similar to that of fractures in adults. Under general anaesthesia, an elevator is placed into the nasal fossa and elevates the fractured fragments which are further realigned by external manual palpation. A splint of plaster or dental compound is placed over the nose for a few days.

Special care should be taken to drain a septal haematoma, a collection of blood between the septal framework and the covering mucoperichondrium and muco-periosteum, a frequent occurrence in children. An L-shaped incision extending through the mucoperiosteum over the vomer is made along the floor of the nose and extends forward and then vertically upward through the mucoperichondrium over the septal cartilage. The flap of mucous membrane thus outlined is raised and the haematoma evacuated. The dependent position of the incision assures drainage and thus prevents a recurring collection of blood. When the septal framework is fractured, the haema-toma may collect bilaterally on both sides of the septal cartilage. A portion of the septal cartilage should be removed in order that the two areas of haematoma com-municate; a bilateral incision through the mucoperiosteum covering the vomer at the base of the septal framework assures dependent drainage and prevents recurrence of the haematoma.

Naso-orbital fractures in which the nasal bones are pushed back into the inter-orbital space with involvement of the fronto-ethmoidal structures can best be treated by the 'open-sky' method. Open reduction through lateral incisions which may be joined, for better exposure, by an incision extending horizontally across the root of the nose is desirable in such complicated fractures. The comminuted bones are exposed, realigned, and maintained by transosseous wiring (Fig. **9**, 4). This type of direct approach can prevent the subsequent sequela of a traumatic telecanthal and saddle-nose deformity. Naso-orbital fractures are often associated with a blowout fracture of the orbital floor (Fig. **9**, 5).

Flattening of the nasal dorsum, often combined with thickening of the nasal septum, results in marked nasal obstruction which may require early corrective pro-cedures in children. The deformity, characterized by depression of the dorsum with widening of the nasal bridge, may require correction for psychological reasons.

Children who have suffered comminuted nasal bone fractures may show develop-mental deformities years later even though they had correct treatment following the accident. The deformities have consisted in flattening of the nasal dorsum, widening of the bony skeleton by hypertrophic callus, and varying degrees of nasomaxillary recession.

One of the major problems is interference with the nasal airway caused by deviation and thickening of the septum. Many of these children become mouth breathers and

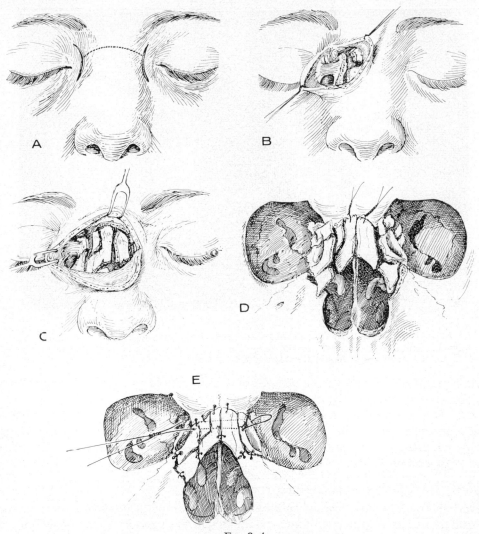

FIG. **9**, 4

The open-sky approach in naso-orbital factures. (A) Outline of lateral incisions which may be joined by transverse incision (dotted line). (B) Exposure obtained by lateral incision. (C) Exposure obtained when additional transverse incision is made. (D) Illustrates direct interosseous wiring of fragments. (E) Direct interosseous wiring and through-and-through transosseous wiring.

may suffer from chronic rhinitis and sinusitis. Surgical intervention is required to relieve the obstruction and treatment should not be postponed until the child has reached adolescence for fear of interfering with nasal growth. If such impairment of growth does occur, it is the result of the trauma producing the fracture. Surgical procedures to relieve obstruction should be conservative, if at all possible, consisting in thinning the septal cartilage, straightening it after incising the cartilage at selected points, resecting vomerine spurs and replacing the vomer and nasal spine in the midline after osteotomy. If necessary, one should not hesitate to do a submucous resection

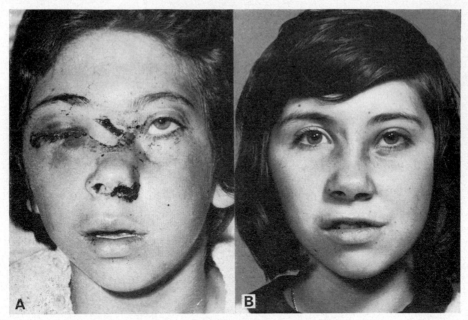

FIG. 9, 5

(A) Comminuted compound naso-orbital fractures with blowout fracture of the right orbit following automobile accident. (B) Appearance after reduction and fixation of naso-orbital fracture and treatment of blowout fracture of the right orbit.

of the septal framework if such a procedure is necessary to restore the airway. Young children should be checked for adenoid hypertrophy.

Flattening or saddling of the nasal dorsum may be treated by costal cartilage or bone grafting to relieve the deformity with the understanding that definitive surgery will be required during adolescence. Nasomaxillary deformities are discussed on page 195 (see Fig. 9, 10).

ZYGOMA AND ORBITAL FLOOR FRACTURES

Zygoma fractures are rare in children and occur mostly in older children. Considerable force is required to fracture the resilient zygoma of the child and the fracture usually takes the form of a fracture-dislocation. Lack of complete union at the frontozygomatic suture also explains the frequency of this type of fracture. Treatment is similar to that of zygoma fractures in the adult.

Orbital fractures in children are observed following automobile accidents and are often characterized by a separation of the frontozygomatic junction in the lateral orbital wall with downward displacement of the floor. This type of unilateral craniofacial detachment is more frequent in the child than the Le Fort III bilateral craniofacial dysjunction. Treatment consists of direct interosseous wire fixation.

The mechanism of production of orbital blowout fractures is similar to that of fractures in adults. We have observed blowout fractures in children caused by the throwing of a snowball, another child's fist, tennis balls, and from other causes. The maxillary sinus is small in the young child and the floor of the orbit is concave, dipping downward from the rim of the orbit, an anatomical characteristic that can mislead the surgeon into an erroneous diagnosis of orbital floor collapse. Despite the small size of the maxillary sinus, escape of orbital contents through the fractured floor occurs and causes enophthalmos. Restoration of the continuity of the orbital floor is the method of treatment, as it is in the adult. We do not advocate packing the maxillary sinus as a modality of treatment of blowout fractures, and it would appear to have only a rare application in children's fractures.

Comminuted fragments should be carefully preserved in children as they consolidate very rapidly in a realigned position. The release of the entrapped orbital contents into the area of the blowout which can then be covered by a small alloplastic implant is followed by rapid return of ocular rotary movements. Children appear to have rapid recuperative ability, following a blowout fracture, to restore the full range of extraocular muscle function, a recuperative ability which recalls that observed following flexor-tendon repair in children.

INJURY TO THE FACIAL NERVE

Facial nerve branch section distal to the anterior borders of the parotid gland does not require suture of the nerve as spontaneous regeneration will restore facial nerve function. Facial nerve section medial to the anterior border of the parotid gland requires exposure and identification of the cut ends of the nerve and suture approximation. Excellent results are obtained because of the higher potential of nerve regeneration in the child (Önne, 1962).

DEVELOPMENTAL MALFORMATIONS OF THE FACIAL SKELETON DUE TO TRAUMA

Many developmental malformations can be attributed to trauma in early childhood. Trauma may have a nefarious effect on the growth of bone in postnatal life similar to that of the defective gene during prenatal development. In many cases, it is difficult to ascertain whether the deleterious effect on growth and development occurred before or after birth.

In order to understand some of the developmental deformities resulting from injury, a review of facial development follows.

Postnatal growth of the mandible

The mandible, small at birth, is destined to grow both by development of the alveolar process which accompanies the development of the teeth and by bone growth.

John Hunter (1835–1837) demonstrated the mode of growth of the mandible. He applied the discovery of Duhamel (1734) who had studied the growth of bone by feeding madder to animals. The observation that madder, a root of a plant, had the property of acting as a vital stain for living bone cells, had been described by Belchier (1738). Belchier fed some of his fowls with madder and noted that living bones were stained red by the madder.

Hunter fed two young pigs on a madder diet for a month. He sacrificed one of the pigs at the end of the month and retained the other for an additional month on ordinary food before sacrificing it. Hunter found that the appearance presented by these two bones met his expectation in the most exact manner. What had been the condyle and the posterior border of the mandible during the madder period were now included in the substance of the ramus, surrounded by new bone forming the new condyle and a new posterior border of the ramus, which had grown during the period in which the pigs had not received madder. The madder-stained bone was almost completely removed by absorption from the anterior border of the ramus. Hunter concluded that growth of the bone is due to the addition of bone on the extremity of the mandible, combined with absorption of bone in other areas (Keith, 1919).

The recognition of condylar growth centres (Charles, 1925; Brodie, 1931) confirmed Hunter's original findings and have shown that the forward projection of the mandible is a consequence of this posterior growth. Elongation of the mandible involves continued additions of bone at each condyle and along the posterior border of the ramus. This posterior appositional growth is only one of the many major movements associated with total growth as all of the different positions of the bone participate in the growth process (Enlow, 1968). In addition to the centres of growth, increase in size is the result of surface apposition, the local contours of the mandible constantly undergoing changes as a result of relocation and remodelling, and resorptive and depository activities.

Growth of the condyle is the result of endochondral ossification in the epiphysis. Microscopic examination of human material (Orban, 1944; Rushton, 1946) showed chondrogenic, cartilaginous and osseous zones. The condyle is capped by a narrow layer of avascular fibrous tissue which contains connective tissue cells and a few cartilage cells. The inner layer of this covering is chondrogenic, giving rise to hyalin cartilage cells which form the second or cartilaginous zone. Destruction of the cartilage and ossification around the cartilage scaffolding can be seen in the third zone. The cartilage of the head of the mandible is not similar to the epiphyseal cartilage of a long bone for it is not interposed between two bony parts, and it is not similar to articular cartilage because the free surface bounding the articular space is covered by fibrous tissue.

Developmental malformation of the mandible from trauma is varied but is most severe when temporomandibular ankylosis and mandibular hypoplasia result from damage to the articular cartilage on the head of the condyle prior to the age of 5 years (Walker, 1957).

Postnatal growth of the nasomaxillary complex

The skeleton of the midfacial area is formed from membrane, with the exception of the nasal cartilaginous capsule. These bones grow in a complex manner in a variety of regional directions.

The growth and development of the nasomaxillary complex has been studied by numerous anatomists. Among early studies are those of Disse (1889), Peter (1913), Stupka (1938), who was concerned with developmental anomalies, and Negus (1958) with the comparative anatomy. Recent studies in animals and man, using vital staining and anatomical sections and cephalometrics, include those of Scott (1953–1963), Baume (1968) and Enlow (1968). The anteroposterior growth of the nasomaxillary complex is related in utero, and also after birth, to the growth of the basal cranial cartilages and their synchondroses. The intersphenoidal and the septo-ethmoidal synchondroses show signs of activity until adulthood. At birth the nasal septum is continuous with the cartilages of the cranial base. Around the first year, the perpendicular plate of the ethmoid starts to ossify from the mesethmoid centre. At 3 years of age, there is bony union between the ethmoid and the vomer. The bony structures of the nasomaxillary area then follow a complex process of growth which has been reviewed in detail by Enlow.

There is not only a forward and downward growth of the maxilla, but a constant remodelling of the multiple regional parts. The main steps in this development include a displacement away from the cranial base, a posterior enlargement corresponding to the lengthening of the dental arch, and an anterior resorption of the malar region. The nasal vaults grow forward and laterally, the descent of the premaxillary area occurs by resorption on the superior and anterior surface of the nasal spine and by bony deposition on the inferior surface.

Considerable controversy has arisen over the role of the septum in the growth of the nasomaxillary complex and over the implications of trauma in causing abnormal growth of the area. Scott, reminding us that the midfacial area is formed by membrane with the exception of the cartilaginous nasal capsule, considers the septum to be the driving force in the growth of the midfacial area. Scott's hypothesis has been supported by Baume (1961), Wexler and Sarnat (1961, 1965), Sarnat and Wexler (1966) and Sarnat (1969).

This hypothesis has been questioned by Moss (1968), who considers that nasal roof collapse occurs as a result of septal destruction or removal, in accordance with the mechanical requirements of framed structures.

The role of trauma in interfering with growth and development of the midfacial area appears to be difficult to determine. In making a comparison with another facial area, namely the mandibular, one finds a considerable disparity between the extent of damage suffered by the condylar area and the extent of the ensuing maldevelopment. In some cases of fracture of the condylar area in children, complete restoration of anatomical form occurs without interference with growth and development; in other cases, what appears to be minor damage results in mandibular hypoplasia. Much depends, apparently, upon the extent of damage to the condylar cartilage (Walker, 1957).

RECONSTRUCTIVE SURGERY FOLLOWING TRAUMA IN CHILDREN

Facial scars

In reconstructive surgery in children, certain features in the treatment of the child differ from that of the adult, not only in the approach to the treatment of scars resulting from trauma, but also in the technique and choice of grafts.

Children present a vast array of deformities resulting from facial trauma. Hypertrophic scarring is frequent following soft tissue wounds in children. After primary suture, it is wise to allow a period of four to six months to elapse before considering secondary repair of the scar. The child is then examined at the end of this interval and a decision is taken whether or not to effect the secondary repair. It may be advisable to allow a further period of time to elapse in order to permit softening of the scars and flattening of the hypertrophy.

The age of the child must also be considered. It is preferable to wait until the age of 5 or 6 years when the child can offer better co-operation. It is not necessary, however, to delay the treatment until early adolescence. Paediatricians will often advise the parents to wait until adolescence before undertaking the repair of the scars. In most cases, there does not seem to be an indication for this delay. Early repair minimizes the danger of psychological trauma. The longer the period of time which ensues between the repair and adolescence, the greater the chance of progressive improvement in the appearance of the scar through the passage of time and the less conspicuous the scar may be after the achievement of growth.

The principles of scar repair are similar to those which apply to adults. Scar contractures must be relieved by Z-plasty procedures or other flap transfers or by skin grafting. Skin sutures should be removed early in children in order to prevent cross-hatching scars from the sutures, the so-called stitch marks. Because of difficulties in the management of small children, buried catgut sutures are a useful means of approximating wound edges in primary wound suture or secondary scar repair. Reinforcement of the wound by means of 'steristrips' is a useful aid. The continuous intradermal pullout suture, usually employing a nylon suture is another technique which is particularly applicable to children. These techniques of wound suture have the added advantage of avoiding stitch marks.

Skin grafts

Because the skin of children is thinner than that of adults, the removal of grafts of excessive thickness may result in a full-thickness defect in the donor areas. Grafts should, therefore, be cut thinner in children than in adults. Grafts in infants should not be thicker than 0·25 mm (0·010 in); in children to the age of 6 years 0·30 mm (0·012 in); in older children 0·40 mm (0·016 in). Grafts in children are always sufficiently thick because of the marked contraction of the skin after its removal.

Bone grafts

Because the donor site of iliac bone is cartilaginous in children, the rib constitutes a better donor area of bone grafts. Costal bone is cancellous in children and constitutes a better quality bone transplant than in the adult in whom it is formed mostly of cortical bone. Subperiosteal removal of the bony rib (Longacre and de Stefano, 1957) permits spontaneous regeneration of the rib. This regeneration provides a veritable living bone bank and is particularly useful when large quantities of bone are required. Large cranial defects, for example, can be repaired by this technique. The rib is split longitudinally and the two halves of the rib are laid side by side over the defect. Costal bone is also available for repair of traumatic defects of the mandible, the floor of the orbit, the nose or the zygomatic area. In older children a limited amount of bone is available and the technique advocated by Robertson and Baron (1946) can be employed. In this technique, the bone is sectioned below the cartilaginous crest of the ilium which is thus left undisturbed. The cartilaginous portion of the crest is incised along its junction with the body of the iliac bone, and is raised upward thus preserving the origin of the abdominal muscles. The insertion of the abdominal muscles is undisturbed; the cartilage is thus not separated from the muscles of the trunk. The major portion of the blood supply is preserved. Cancellous bone can be removed from the centre of the bone after separation of the cortical surfaces. The iliac crest is then replaced in its original position.

Composite grafts

Because of the high degree of vascularization of the tissues of the child, composite grafts from the auricle constitute a favourable means of reconstructing defects about the nose. Repeated grafts can be employed and a secondary composite graft can be overgrafted over the preceding composite graft in order to provide a satisfactory contour. The prior graft is abraded and the subsequent graft is placed over the abraded area.

The defect in the auricle resulting from the removal of the composite graft can usually be repaired by direct approximation of the edges of the auricular wound.

TREATMENT OF MANDIBULAR MICROGNATHIA

Traumatic damage to the condylar head may be sufficient to result in temporomandibular ankylosis either unilateral or bilateral. Sufficiently severe injury, without resulting in temporomandibular ankylosis, may affect mandibular growth. When the damage sustained is bilateral, a fairly symmetrical atresia of the mandible results (Fig. 9, 6). The patient develops a 'bird-face' profile, the protrusion of the maxillary teeth contrasting with the retruded position of the mandibular teeth. When the damage sustained is unilateral, shortening of the ramus and body of the mandible is limited to one side only. The patient's chin is deviated toward the affected side and the body of the mandible on the unaffected side is flattened leading the uninitiated observer to conclude that the major deformity is on the unaffected side. Relief of temporomandibular ankylosis should be provided as early as possible. Unilateral or bilateral temporomandibular arthroplasty restores mandibular movement and permits mastication.

Correction of the micrognathic deformity, either bilateral or unilateral, is achieved by means of elongation osteotomy in the body of the mandible. Bone grafting is also necessary in conjunction with the elongation osteotomy in order to provide bony continuity and to add bulk to the undersized mandible. These procedures have been achieved in our series of cases by means of an intraoral approach (Converse, 1963).

Elongation osteotomy of the body of the mandible is a procedure limited to those patients who have already erupted their second dentition, as the presence of the deciduous teeth in the body of the mandible precludes the use of this technique. For this reason, the correction of mandibular micrognathia has been performed during the adolescent years.

The technique consists of a step osteotomy which extends through the body of the mandible anterior to the mental foramen in order to avoid interrupting the continuity of the inferior alveolar nerve (Fig. 9, 7). The integrity of the mental nerve branches is respected. The horizontal branch of the step osteotomy extends close to the lower

PS H

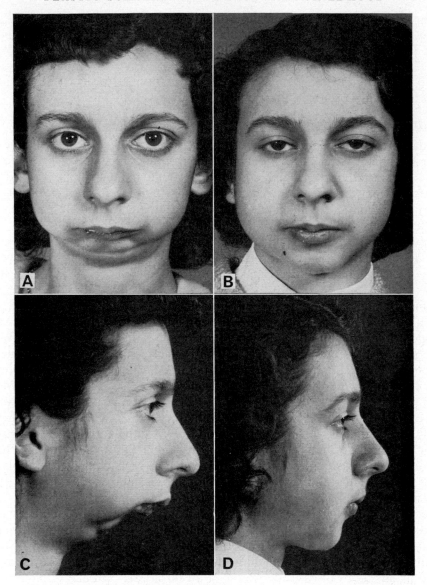

FIG. 9, 6

Micrognathia from injury in early childhood. (A and C) Appearance of the patient prior to relief of temporomandibular ankylosis and elongation of the body of the mandible. (B and D) Postoperative appearance following elongation procedures illustrated in Fig. 9, 7.

border of the mandible in order to avoid entering the inferior alveolar canal. After advancement of the anterior mandibular segment, bone grafts are packed within the interstices between the bone fragments and onlay bone grafts are placed over the line of osteotomy. Intermaxillary fixation is established during the period of consolidation.

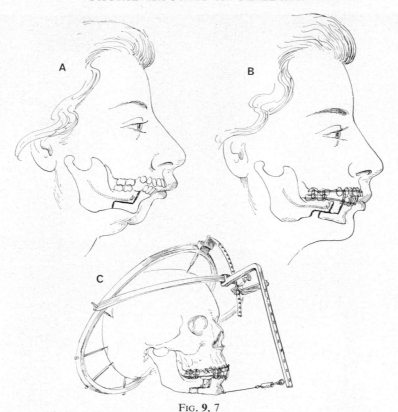

FIG. **9**, 7

Technique of elongation osteotomy in micrognathia. (A) Outline of osteotomy.
(B) Advancement obtained by step-osteotomy. (C) Illustrating the forward
traction exerted through a cranially fixed 'halo' appliance.

One should particularly avoid and advise against intempestive orthodontic treatment which may modify the position of the dentition to conform to the malformed mandible and greatly complicate subsequent surgical treatment. Of what useful purpose is the achievement of a satisfactory occlusion between the teeth of the upper and lower jaws when surgical elongation will, of necessity, produce malocclusion? Such ill-advised pre-surgical orthodontic treatment should be averted by co-ordinated observation and future planning by both the orthodontist and the surgeon during the pre-surgical phase.

Bilateral vertical section of the ramus of the mandible, advancement of the body of the mandible into more satisfactory dental occlusal relationships, the addition of split-rib grafts to the atresic mandibular ramus—these procedures have been done in some of our recent cases between the ages of 6 and 9 years old in order to minimize the deformity and simplify the dental occlusal problem and lessen the magnitude of the definitive surgery required during adolescent years.

TREATMENT OF NASOMAXILLARY HYPOPLASIA

Since Dieffenbach (1845) described a V-Y procedure to lengthen the nose, forehead

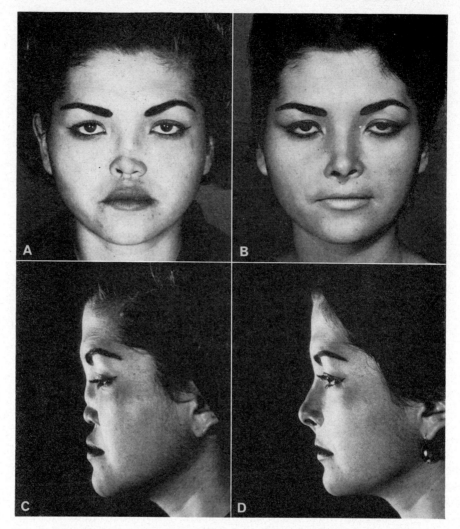

FIG. **9**, 8

(A and C) Appearance of patient with nasomaxillary hypoplasia following irradiation in childhood. (B and D) Postoperative appearance following nasomaxillary skin graft inlay technique.

flaps have been employed to provide additional cutaneous covering for the fore-shortened nose. Providing additional nasal lining was also recognized as a necessity and local turnover hinge flaps and nasolabial flaps were used for this purpose. Gillies, in 1923, described the nasomaxillary skin graft inlay technique for the correction of the nasomaxillary hypoplasia of the syphilitic nose. The patient shown in Figure **9**, 8 received radon seed irradiation for recurrent epistaxis at the age of 8 years resulting in a developmental deformity of the nasomaxillary area similar to that observed in congenital syphilis. The technique employed, modified from Gillies' original technique, has been previously described (Converse and Jeffreys, 1951; Kazanjian and

Converse, 1959). Briefly stated, it consists in approaching the nasomaxillary area through an oral vestibular incision, freeing the attachments of the nose to the edge of the pyriform aperture and the soft tissues over the adjacent maxillary area. The cartilaginous portion of the nasal septum is usually destroyed in these cases. The inadequate constricting nasal lining is incised, thus permitting a wide expansion of the volume of the cartilaginous nose. The extensive intra- and peri-nasal raw area is covered by a split-thickness graft maintained on a dental compound mould which greatly expands the nasomaxillary soft tissues. Thus, an excess of skin graft is introduced and compensates for subsequent contraction. After an interval of 10 days, the dental compound mould is replaced by an acrylic prosthesis which is progressively reduced until the definitive contour of the nasomaxillary area is obtained. The reduction is done over a period of 10 to 12 weeks. This technique provides adequate contour restoration, but has the undoubted disadvantage of obliging the patient to wear a permanent support prosthesis.

To obviate this disadvantage, Kazanjian (1948) utilized a median forehead flap which he introduced through a transverse incision immediately below the level of the lower border of the nasal bones; bilateral nasolabial flaps can also provide adequate lining in the older patient.

A small amount of nasal lengthening can also be obtained by repeated addition of conchal cartilage in the region of the nose. Dingman and Walter (1969) have lengthened the foreshortened nose by the addition of nasal lining and cartilaginous support by means of a composite graft from the auricular concha.

Kazanjian (1937) appears to have been the first to utilize the tissue lining the bony bridge of the nose to obtain additional lining for nasal elongation purposes: the lateral cartilage is detached from its insertion under the nasal bones, the mucoperiosteum is elevated from the nasal bones as high as possible, a transverse incision then permits sliding the lining tissue downward and the raw surface under the nasal bones is left to undergo spontaneous epithelialization. Edgerton (1966) utilized this principle in a patient with a foreshortened nose.

These procedures, although producing an elongation of the nasal pyramid, do not correct the adjacent maxillary recession. Coughlin (1925) placed costal cartilage grafts over the maxilla through an external incision around each external naris, as well as over the dorsum of the nose to correct the 'dish-face' deformity. Bone grafts introduced through an intraoral approach were also utilized for this purpose (Converse, 1954).

In order to find a solution to the problem of naxomaxillary hypoplasia which would provide elongation and an increase in size of the undeveloped nose and also correct the maxillary deformity, the following procedure was developed.

Pyramidal naso-orbito-maxillary osteotomy

The principles of the operation (Figs. 9, 9 and 10) are the following: (1) the foreshortened nasal septal framework must be resected as it will oppose nasal lengthening; (2) the nasal bones are separated from the frontal bone and the line of osteotomy is extended backward along the medial wall of the orbit to a point situated posteriorly to the lacrimal groove; (3) the line of osteotomy extends downward on each side through

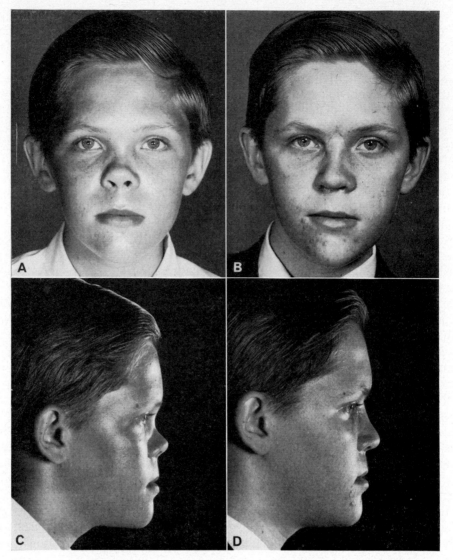

FIG. **9**, 9

(A and C) Appearance of patient with nasomaxillary hypoplasia resulting from septal abscess in childhood. (B and D) Postoperative appearance following naso-orbito-maxillary osteotomy as illustrated in Fig. **9**, 10.

the floor of the orbit, lateral to the lacrimal groove, through the infraorbital rim, maxilla, and alveolar process between the premolar teeth; (4) the hard palate is cut across horizontally. The central nasomaxillary block is then displaced downward and forward. Dental arch continuity and fixation of the advanced maxillary segment are maintained by an orthodontic-type fixation appliance and the gaps between the bone fragments are filled with bone grafts, a bone graft also providing nasal dorsal support and contour.

Exposure of the nasal framework and medial orbital skeleton is obtained by means of a trap-door incision, triangular in shape with its apex at the glabella (Fig. **9**, 10A); this incision provides additional skin coverage by means of a V-Y advancement (Fig. **9**, 10F). The incisions extend downward laterally over the frontal processes of the maxilla. Subperiosteal exposure of the framework of the nose and exposure of the nasal cartilages is thus obtained by the retraction of the flap and the exposure is extended downward to the base of the pyriform aperture on each side (Fig. **9**, 10B). The periosteum is then elevated from the bone over the lacrimal groove and the medial wall of the orbit exposed backward over the lamina papyracea of the ethmoid. The medial palpebral ligament and the lacrimal sac are reflected laterally with the orbital contents.

A submucous resection of the entire septal framework is done through an L-shaped incision through the mucoperichondrium near the caudal end of the septal cartilage. The cartilaginous portion of the nose, released from the restrictive influence of the septum, becomes more extensible. Exposure of the area of junction of the lateral cartilages with the nasal bones is obtained by reflecting the trap-door flap downward. The lateral cartilages are now separated from the undersurface of the nasal bones. The mucoperiosteum underlying the nasal bones is undermined as far upward as possible and is then incised transversely (Fig. **9**, 10B). At this point, it is noted that by placing the thumb and index finger on each side of the columella near the tip of the nose, it is possible to draw the nasal structures downward, the structures situated beneath the nasal bones sliding downward thus producing appreciable nasal lengthening (Fig. **9**, 10C). Further lengthening is obtained by raising the vestibular lining of the alar cartilages and incising through the loose connecting tissue joining alar and lateral cartilages (Fig. **9**, 10E). The short nose can thus be lengthened appreciably.

The operation is now completed by the pyramidal osteotomy. A horizontal osteotomy is done at the nasofrontal junction through the thick bony layer formed by the nasal bones and underlying the nasal process of the frontal bone. The cribriform plate lies posteriorly and is not involved in the osteotomy. The line of osteotomy is continued laterally along the upper portion which constitutes the lateral wall of the ethmoid sinus of the medial wall of the orbit, above the lacrimal groove to the lamina papyracea. The line of osteotomy then extends vertically downward to the medial portion of the floor of the orbit, and forward, lateral to the lacrimal groove, medial to the infraorbital foramen thus preserving the infraorbital nerve downward through the anterior wall of the maxillary sinus, and through the alveolar process between the first and second bicuspid teeth (Fig. **9**, 10G).

A mucoperiosteal flap is raised from the palatine vault exposing the hard palate and the hard palate is cut across transversely into the floor of the nose (Fig. **9**, 10H). The stable posterior portion of the maxilla provides a strong abutment and the orthodontic bands on the molar teeth are stable posterior points of fixation. The entire nasomaxillary segment is then advanced into a Class II dental occlusal relationship and the position is maintained by the orthodontic-type appliance. The forward movement of the pyramidal segment is also accompanied by a downward movement and the lacrimal sac and nasolacrimal duct participate in the downward and forward displacement of the nose (Fig. **9**, 10J).

The gaps in the facial skeleton are filled with fragments of cancellous iliac bone. A

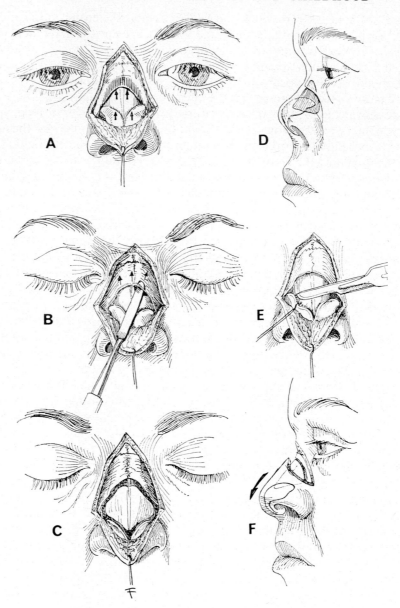

FIG. 9, 10

Nasomaxillary hypoplasia. Elongation of skeletal framework. (A) Arrows indicate usual overlapping of nasal bones and alar cartilages over the upper laterals. (B) Detaching the upper laterals and mucoperiosteum from under the nasal bones. (C) After the lining tissues have been severed transversely under the nasal bones they can be drawn downward to elongate the lining. (D) Diagram of hypoplastic nose. (E) Further elongation is obtained by separating the alars from the upper laterals and sliding the alars down. (F) Sketch of elongation obtained by (E).

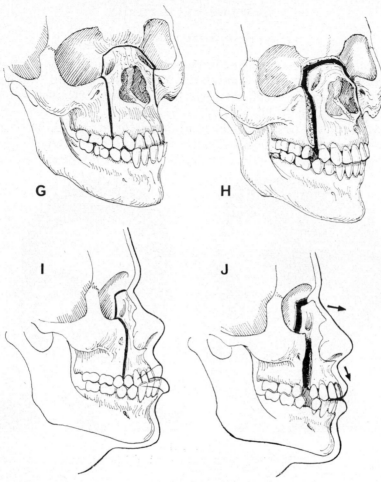

FIG. **9**, 10 (*contd.*)

(G to J) Nasomaxillary hypoplasia. Elongating the bony nasomaxillary complex by the naso-orbito-maxillary osteotomy technique. After moving the central segment forward and downward, the bone gaps are filled with bone grafts and the position of the segment is maintained by orthodontic fixation. Note that the line of osteotomy severs the medial wall of the orbit posterior to the lacrimal fossa.

thin layer of cancellous bone is placed over the bony gaps in the lamina papyracea. Fragments of bone are wedged into the bony gap at the nasofrontal area and in remaining gaps in the medial portion of the orbit and over the maxillary sinus. Wedges of bone are placed in the open spaces in the hard palate and alveolar process. The operation is completed by placing an iliac bone graft over the dorsum of the nose. The upper portion of the bone graft is maintained by wire fixation at the nasofrontal area and the distal tip of the bone graft is placed between the domes of the alar cartilages which are sutured to each other over the bone graft.

J. M. CONVERSE

PS H 2

ADDENDUM TO CHAPTER IX

THE FORESHORTENED NOSE

Foreshortening of the nose may be found in patients with bilateral congenital cleft of the lip and palate, or it may occur in otherwise normal patients who have suffered a severe injury to the nose in infancy—with subsequent interference with the growth of the nasal septum (Fig. **9**, 11).

The shortness of the nose becomes more apparent in the second decade of life when the rest of the face is growing rapidly, and the comparatively simple technique to be described for lengthening the nose should probably not be carried out until late

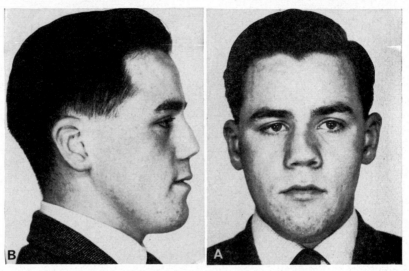

FIG. **9**, 11
Short nose following trauma in childhood.

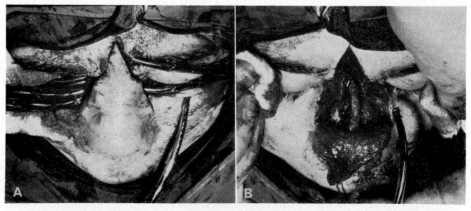

FIG. **9**, 12
Technique of lengthening nose. (A) Skin incision running up as a Λ to glabella. (B) Nasal skin turned down. Double saw-cut to free nasal bones from septum. Nasal bones infractured.

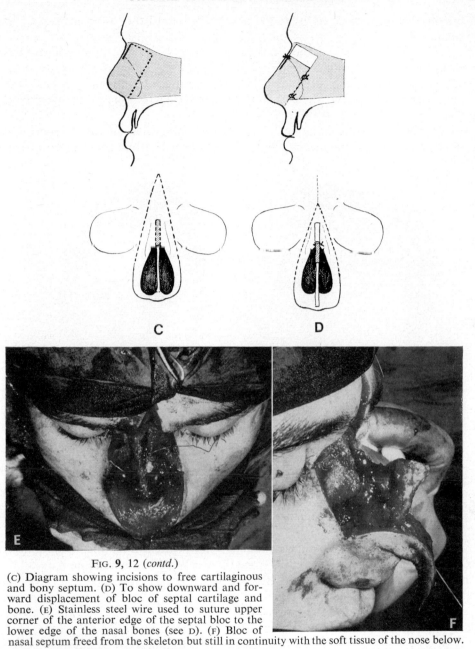

Fig. **9**, 12 (*contd.*)

(C) Diagram showing incisions to free cartilaginous and bony septum. (D) To show downward and forward displacement of bloc of septal cartilage and bone. (E) Stainless steel wire used to suture upper corner of the anterior edge of the septal bloc to the lower edge of the nasal bones (see D). (F) Bloc of nasal septum freed from the skeleton but still in continuity with the soft tissue of the nose below.

adolescence to allow the maximum growth of the nose to take place. As the essence of the operation is a downward and forward slide of a rectangular bloc of septum the presence of cartilaginous septum, even if underdeveloped, is essential.

The steps of the operation are as follows:

1. A 'V' incision is made around the upper three-quarters of the nose (Fig. **9**, 12A),

and the nasal skin is raised up from the nasal bones until the lower edge of the latter are reached. The nasal mucosa on the inner aspect of the nasal bones is stripped away from these latter for the distance it is proposed to lower the nose: the mucosa is incised at the upper limit of dissection, and horizontally along the lateral wall of the nose above the level of the turbinates. The flaps of mucosa thus formed will serve to line the nasal skin flap and the raw area inside the nasal bones will re-epithelialize in time.

2. A vertical saw-cut is made in the nasal bones on either side of the septum (Fig. **9**, 12B and C lower). A fine osteotome is driven inwards along the septum at the top

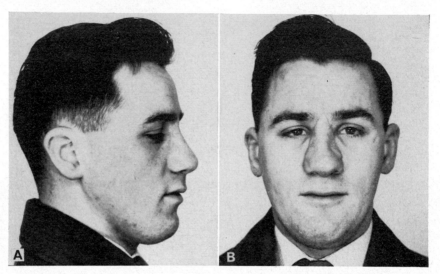

FIG. **9**, 13

Appearance of the nose two years postoperatively. Note the return of some of the deformity of the nasal bones, particularly on the left side, and the rather obvious V-Y scar line in the glabellar region.

of the saw-cuts at the root of the nose and at the same angle as the lower free border of the septal cartilage.

3. A vertical section of the septum is now made with scalpel and osteotome from a point just behind the anterior nasal spine obliquely upwards in a line parallel to the external bridge line and unites with the horizontal section in (3) (Fig. **9**, 12C, upper, and F).

4. The alar bases and soft tissue of the cheek and upper lip are freed from the underlying maxilla so that the nose can be moved downwards.

5. The septal bloc is displaced downwards forward and fixed by stainless steel wire anteriorly, and by catgut posteriorly (Fig. **9**, 12D and E).

6. The mucosal layer is sutured to the overlying skin and the glabellar defect closed as a Y (Fig. **9**, 13). A plaster of Paris splint is applied for one week.

J. C. MUSTARDÉ

BIBLIOGRAPHY
BAUM, L. J. (1961). The postnatal growth activity of the nasal cartilage septum. *Helv. odont. Acta*, **5**, 9.

BAUM, L. J. (1968). Patterns of cephalofacial growth and development. A comparative study of the basi-cranial growth centres in rat and man. *Int. dent. J. Lond.* **18**, 489.

BELCHIER, J. (1738). An account of the bone of animals being changed to a red colour by aliment only. *Phil. Trans. R. Soc.* **39**, 287.

BRODIE, A. G. (1931). On the growth pattern of the human head. *Am. J. Anat.* **68**, 209.

CHARLES, S. W. (1925). The temporomandibular joint and its influence on the growth of the mandible. *J. Br. dent. Ass.* **46**, 845.

CONVERSE, J. M. (1954). Technique of bone grafting for contour restoration. *Plastic reconstr. Surg.* **14**, 332.

CONVERSE, J. M. (1963). The intra-oral approach in the treatment of jaw malformations. In *Modern Trends in Plastic Surgery*, *1*, ed. Gibson, T. London: Butterworth.

CONVERSE, J. M. & JEFFREYS, F. E. (1951). The nasomaxillary epithelial inlay for dish-face deformity. *J. oral Surg.*, **9**, 183.

COUGHLIN, W. T. (1925). A new procedure for the relief of facies scaphoidea—'dish-face'. *Surgery, Gynec. Obstet.* **40**, 332.

DIEFFENBACH, J. F. (1845). *Die operative Chirurgie*. F. S. Brockhaus, Leipzig.

DINGMAN, R. O. & WALTER, C. (1969). Use of composite ear grafts in correction of the short nose. *Plastic reconstr. Surg.* **43**, 117.

DISSE, J. (1889). Die Ausbildung der Nasenhöhlen nach der Geburt. *Arch. Anat. Physiol.* (Suppl.), **29**, 54.

DUHAMEL, H. L. (1734). Quatrième mémoire sur les os. Dans lequel on se propose de rapporter de nouvelles preuves qui établissent que les os croissent en grosseur par l'addition de couches osseuses qui tirent leur origine du périoste. *Communs Acad. R. Sci.* **56**, 87.

EDGERTON, M. T. (1966). Surgical lengthening of the external nose to correct congenital or traumatic arrest of nasal growth (an operation of value in treating nasal deformities of cleft lip and palate). *Plastic reconstr. Surg.* **38**, 320.

ENLOW, D. H. *The Human Face*. An account of the postnatal growth and development of the craniofacial skeleton. New York: Harper & Row.

GILLIES, H. D. (1923). Deformities of the syphilitic nose. *Br. med. J.* **2**, 977.

GREGORY, T. G. (1957). Personal communication.

HUNTER, J. *The Works of John Hunter*. Edited and published by James F. Palmer, London, 1835.

KAZANJIAN, V. H. (1937). Plastic repair of deformities about the lower part of the nose resulting from loss of tissue. *Trans. Am. Acad. Ophthal. & Oto-lar.* **42**, 338.

KAZANJIAN, V. H. (1948). Nasal deformities of syphilitic origin. *Plastic reconstr. Surg.* **3**, 517.

KAZANJIAN, V. H. & CONVERSE, J. M. (1959). *The Surgical Treatment of Facial Injuries*. 2nd ed. p. 749. Baltimore: Williams and Wilkins.

KEITH, A. (1919). *Members of the Maimed*. London: Oxford University Press.

KRAVITS, H., DRIESSEN, G., GOMBERG, R. & KORACH, A. (1969). Accidental falls from elevated surfaces in infants from birth to one year of age. *Pediatrics*, Report of the National Childhood Injury Symposium. **44**, p. 869.

LEWIN, M. L. (1955). Total rhinoplasty in infants—report of a case of Waterhouse-Friederischsen syndrome. *Plastic reconstr. Surg.* **15**, 131.

LONGACRE, J. J. & DE STEFANO, G. A. (1957). Observations on the behaviour of autogenous split-rib grafts in reconstruction of extensive defects of the cranium and face. *Plastic reconstr. Surg.* **20**, 281.

McCOY, F. J., CHANDLER, R. A. & CROW, M. L. (1966). Facial fractures in children. *Plastic reconstr. Surg.* **37**, 209.

MOSS, M. L., BROMBERG, B. E., IN CHUL SONG & EISENMAN, G. (1968). The passive role of nasal septal cartilage in midfacial growth. *Plast. & Reconstr. Surg.* **41**, 536.

NEGUS, V. (1958). *The Comparative Anatomy and Physiology of the Nose and Paranasal Sinuses*. Baltimore: Williams and W'lkins.

ÖNNE, L. (1962). Recovery of sensibility and sudomotor activity in the hand after nerve suture. *Acta chir. scand.* Suppl. 300.

ORBAN, B. (1944). *Oral Histology and Embryology*. St. Louis: Mosby.

PANAGOPOULOS, A. P. (1957). Management of fractures of the jaws in children. *J. int. Coll. Surg.* **28**, 806.

PETER, K. (1913). *Atlas der Entwicklung der Nase und des Gaumens beim Menschen*. Jena: Fisher.

PFEIFER, G. (1966). Kieferbrüche im Kindesalter und ihre Auswirkungen auf das Wachstum. *Fortsch. Kiefer- u. Gesichts-Chir.* **11**, 43.

ROBERTSON, I. M. & BARON, J. N. (1946). A method of treatment of chronic infective oteitis. *J. Bone Jt Surg.* **28**, 19.

ROWE, N. L. & KILLEY, H. C. (1955). *Fractures of the Facial Skeleton*. Edinburgh: Livingstone.

RUSHTON, M. A. (1946). Unilateral hyperplasia of the mandibular condyle. *Proc. R. Soc. Med.* **39**, 431.

SARNAT, B. G. (1969). Experimental surgery as an aid to clinical practice: The septo-vomeral region. Paper read at the 23rd Annual Meeting of the American Society of Maxillofacial Surgeons, San Francisco.

SARNAT, B. G. & WEXLER, M. R. (1966). Growth of the face and jaws after resection of the septal cartilage in the rabbit. *Am. J. Anat.* **118**, 755.

SCOTT, J. H. (1953). The cartilage of the nasal septum. *Br. dent. J.* **95**, 37.

SCOTT, J. H. (1956). Growth of facial sutures. *Am. J. Orthod.* **42**, 381.

SCOTT, J. H. (1951). Studies in facial growth. *Dental Pract.* **7**, 344.

SCOTT, J. H. (1958). The growth of the human skull. *J. dent. Ass. S. Afr.* **13**, 133.

SCOTT, J. H. (1959). Further studies on the growth of the human face. *Proc. R. Soc. Med.* **52**, 263.

SCOTT, J. H. (1963). The analysis of the facial growth from fetal life to adulthood. *Angle Orthod.* **33**, 110.

STUPKA, W. (1938). *Die Missbildungen und Anomalien der Nase und des Nasenrachentaumes*, pp. 1–319. Vienna: Springer.

TOPAZIAN, R. G. (1964). Etiology of ankylosis of temporomandibular joint: analysis of 44 cases. *J. oral Surg. Anes. Hosp. dent. Serv.* **22**, 227.

WALKER, D. G. (1957). The mandibular condyle. Fifty cases demonstrating arrest in development. *Dent. pract.* **7**, 160.

WEXLER, M. R. & SARNAT, B. G. (1961). Rabbit snout growth. Effect of injury to septovomeral region. *Archs Otolar.* **74**, 305.

WEXLER, M. R. & SARNAT, B. G. (1965). Rabbit snout growth after dislocation of nasal septum. *Archs Otolar.* **81**, 68.

CHAPTER X

THE ORBITAL REGION

Epicanthal folds and telecanthus

An epicanthal fold is defined as 'a semi-lunar fold of skin running downwards at the side of the nose with its concavity directed to the inner canthus' (Duke-Elder, 1952). Such folds may be present at birth, may appear shortly after birth, or may result from contraction of scars in the canthal area. Treatment of the latter type of epicanthal fold by Z-plasty is no different from that in the adult and will not be considered here. Of the folds which are present in babies and young children, it should be appreciated that only about 3 to 4 per cent of such folds are actually present at birth, and the majority of epicanthal folds seen in young children appear within the first few weeks of life and gradually disappear after the third or fourth year. These latter, minor folds, do not require any surgery and probably disappear as a result of the forward growth of the nose. A number of patients with true congenital folds may not require operation but in a few of them the apparently broad appearance of the base of the nose will call for surgical correction (Fig. **10**, 10). Sometimes, particularly if the fold is more pronounced on one side, patients will be referred because of an apparent squint, when no squint in fact is present. Epicanthal folds may occur as a single abnormality or may be found in conjunction with other deformities in the orbital region, such as ptosis, telecanthus (increase in width between the medial canthi) and shortness of the palpebral aperture at both lateral and medial canthi—resulting in blepharophimosis (Fig. **10**, 1, 2 and 3).

Many operations have been described for dealing with simple epicanthal folds, and the main principle has been to break up the line of the fold using small flaps or Z plasties. The technique first published by the writer in 1959 was, however, designed not only to deal with the fold itself but also to correct any degree of telecanthus which might be present at the same time. The technique has the additional merit that any resultant scars pass *through* the canthus itself and therefore it is not possible for a secondary cicatricial epicanthal fold to form at a later date. Although originally described for patients with epicanthus and telecanthus the operation can be used equally well when only epicanthus is present (Fig. **10**, 10), or indeed when only telecanthus is present (Fig. **10**, 11). The design of the flaps is carried out in exactly the same way in all three types of case and any difference in the technique of the operation will be described in the appropriate sections (Mustardé, 1966a).

EPICANTHUS WITH TELECANTHUS

Patients exhibiting these two abnormalities may vary from comparatively mild cases (Fig. **10**, 1) with no other abnormality present to patients with blepharophimosis where the lids are very short and the palpebral aperture narrow in addition

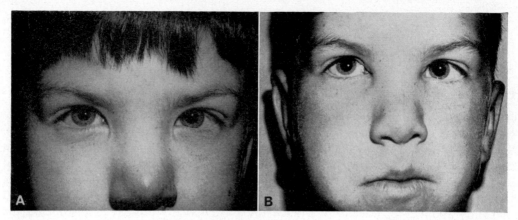

FIG. 10, 1

Epicanthus with moderate degree of telecanthus. (A) Pre-operative appearance. (B) Postoperative appearance.

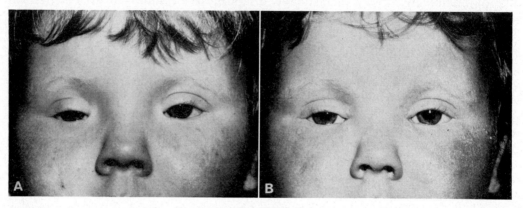

FIG. 10, 2

Epicanthus with marked telecanthus and ptosis (blepharophimosis). (A) Pre-operative appearance. (B) Postoperative appearance.

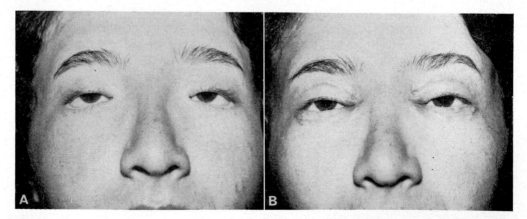

FIG. 10, 3

Blepharophimosis with congenital ectropion of the lower lids. (A) Pre-operative appearance. (B) Postoperative appearance following insertion of full-thickness skin graft in lower lid as well as correction of epicanthus and telecanthus.

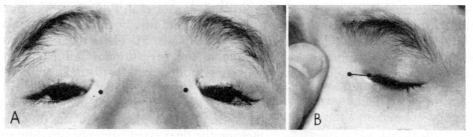

FIG 10, 4

(A) Projected site of new canthi marked on skin. (B) Obliteration of fold: actual canthus marked in.

to the epicanthus and telecanthus. In such patients, there is ptosis of the upper lids (Fig. **10**, 2) and sometimes a displacement medially and downwards of the lateral canthus. Indeed, in very excessive examples of this deformity there may in addition be shortage of skin in the lower lids with the production of ectropion in the outer half of the lid (Fig. **10**, 3). The correction of the epicanthus along with the telecanthus is carried out in all cases in the following manner.

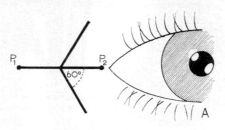

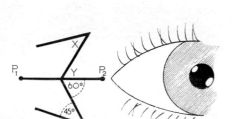

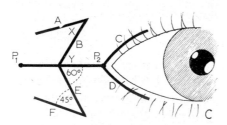

Operative technique

The site of the proposed new canthus is marked on each side halfway between the centre of the pupil and the midline of the nose; let us call this point P_1 (Fig. **10**, 4A). The skin of the nose is pulled forward to obliterate the fold, and the actual canthus (point P_2) is marked (Fig. **10**, 4B). These two points are joined and the line bisected.

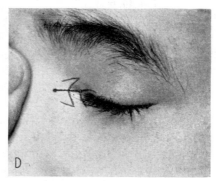

FIG. **10**, 5

(A) Bisection of line between P_1 and P_2; vertical line drawn, at 60° from centre for a distance equal to P_1–P_2 less 2 mm. (B) Backcuts from vertical lines, again equalling P_1–P_2 less 2 mm. (C) A, B, C, and D, E, F all equal P_1–P_2 less 2 mm. Angle $Y = 60°$; angle $X = 45°$. (D) Lines of skin incisions.

present but will give no indication of the function of the levator complex, and the use of a formula such as that of Rycroft where the amount of levator to be resected was based on estimating the number of millimetres of ptosis present and multiplying this by four, can serve only as a rough guide. The final test, as far as patients operated on under general anaesthesia is concerned, is to check that the lid margin lies just above the centre of the pupil at the end of the operation—assuming that the eyes are in the forward gaze position. With the return of tone in the orbicularis muscle once the effect of the anaesthetic has worn off it will be found that the lids will close, or almost close, and the cornea will be covered during sleep when the eye rolls upward. It is more difficult to check the position of the lid when the posterior approach to the levator is used and for this reason, although perfectly satisfactory results may be obtained in degrees of ptosis requiring resection of not more than 15 or 16 mm of levator muscle, where a greater amount of resection than this is required the anterior approach is preferable. A further advantage of the anterior approach in severe cases of ptosis is the greater accessibility of the levator within the orbit when approached from the front (Beard, 1969).

OPERATIVE TECHNIQUE

Anterior approach (Fig. **10**, 14) (Everbusch, 1883)

A traction suture is inserted into the margin of the upper lid at what is considered to be the highest point. An incision is made horizontally across the upper lid at the site of the superior palpebral furrow, about 2 mm above the superior edge of the tarsal plate (Fig. **10**, 14A). The incision should extend almost the whole width of the lid and it is deepened through the orbicularis muscle by a spreading action with scissors. The exposed orbital septum is opened in the same line and the underlying aponeurosis of the levator muscle is identified and cleaned of fat, a considerable pad of which may lie between it and the orbital septum in children. The dissection is carried upwards until at least 20 mm of aponeurosis and levator muscle can be visualised.

Two small vertical incisions 3 to 4 mm in length are made through levator aponeurosis, Müller's muscle and conjunctiva into the upper fornix. The incision should be immediately above the tarsal plate and should lie 10 mm on either side of the traction suture (Fig. **10**, 14B). A ptosis muscle clamp is then passed through these incisions and closed; the tissues are now divided along the lower edge of the clamp immediately above the tarsal plate and the original incisions are extended with scissors in a vertical direction for about 15 mm (Fig. **10**, 14C). The muscle clamp is lifted upwards revealing the conjunctiva on the deep surface of the composite flap, and this is now carefully stripped away from Müller's muscle leaving a small fringe of conjunctiva still held within the grasp of the muscle clamp (Fig. **10**, 14D). (An alternative technique involves dissecting a tunnel between the levator aponeurosis— with its closely applied Müller's muscle—and the underlying conjunctiva: when the muscle clamp is inserted it grasps only the aponeurosis and Müller's muscle so that

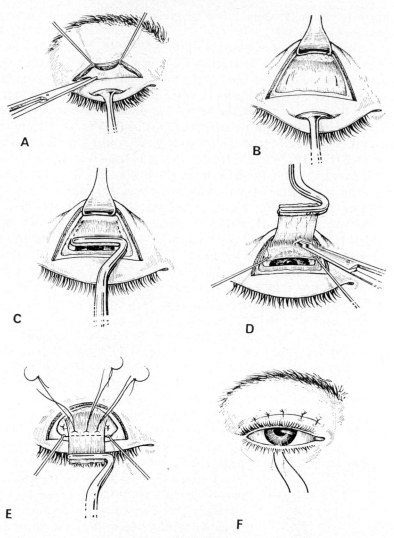

FIG. **10**, 14

Ptosis: **anterior approach**. (A) Incision through skin and orbicularis in position
of desired skin fold. (B) Orbital septum exposed. Incisions carried through into
upper fornix immediately above tarsal plate. (C) Ptosis clamp passed through
incisions and structure divided distal to clamp and along vertical dotted line.
(D) Orbital septum and conjunctiva dissected off from levator flap. (E) Conjunctival wound closed. Levator flap brought forward and sutured to upper edge
of tarsus. Excess levator excised. (F) Skin and orbicularis closed, and lower lid
lifted up by single suture.

the conjunctiva is preserved when an incision is made distal to the clamp and the
muscle and aponeurosis are lifted upwards). If it is found that the lateral horns of the
levator aponeurosis are tethering the flap these should be divided and it will then be
found that the levator muscle can be drawn down freely. Orbital fat may tend to
herniate under the arcus marginalis of the septum but it may be held out of the way

by a Desmarre retractor: it should not be excised in children in order to avoid a hollow appearance of the lid.

The flap of conjunctiva is now sutured to the edge of the tarsal plate and, drawing forward the levator muscle flap by means of the clamp and at the same time pushing the tarsus upwards using toothed forceps the lid margin is brought to lie 1 mm above the centre of the pupil. A reference mark is made with ink on the levator muscle at the point where the upper edge of the tarsus lies directly beneath. Three 4/0 catgut sutures are inserted into the anterior surface of the tarsal plate 3 mm from the superior edge. These sutures are passed through the overlying levator muscle and a provisional tie is made in each (Fig. **10**, 14E). The level of the lid margin is checked and if necessary the sutures are passed through the levator muscle higher or lower as may be required. The excess levator is excised below the catgut sutures. It is unnecessary to close the orbital septum or orbicularis muscle layer and the skin wound may be closed using four or five 6/0 catgut sutures (Fig. **10**, 14F). These fine sutures do not require to be removed—a decided advantage when dealing with small children. The traction suture is removed from the upper lid and a similar type of suture is inserted into the margin of the lower lid so that it may be raised to protect the cornea and keep tension off the sutures fixing the levator muscle to the tarsal plate during the first 48 hours postoperatively. After this, once it is seen that the cornea is covered by the upper lid during sleep, the suture in the lower lid margin may be removed.

Alternative techniques. There have been many techniques published designed to approach the levator from the front but most of them differ only in small details from the procedure described above. One operation which is worthy of mention is that described by Lester Jones (1964). In this operation, in order to avoid interfering with the superior conjunctival fornix, the undermining and transection of the levator muscle takes place some 10 mm above the superior edge of the tarsus and the levator is then drawn downwards over the aponeurosis and Müller's muscle to be shortened and attached to the anterior surface of the tarsal plate.

The writer has recently been experimenting with a technique designed to preserve all of the action of Müller's muscle and of that part of the malfunctioning levator muscle which is normally thrown away. This operation is based on research work which has shown that Müller's muscle, if not denervated, produces an involuntary lift of 2 to 3 mm of the upper lid, a lift which gradually decreases and eventually disappears during fatigue and in sleep. The operation involves taking a tuck in the levator muscle high in the orbit, but is still experimental (Fig. **10**, 15) (Mustardé, 1968a).

FIG. **10**, 15

High levator plication, preserving action of superior tarsal (Müller's) muscle and all of the defective levator.

Posterior approach

The posterior approach to the levator complex has the advantage that it leaves no scar on the outside of the upper lid, but on the other hand the scar on the upper lid may help to produce a more dis-

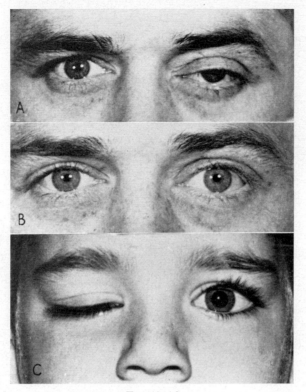

FIG. **10,** 16

(A) Moderate degree of ptosis (unilateral). (B) Following levator resection (Blascovics). (C) Complete ptosis (unilateral). See Figure **10,** 17Q and R for postoperative appearance of this patient.

tinct superior lid furrow and many surgeons feel that, for this reason alone, the anterior approach is to be desired. Apart from this, the posterior approach allows a perfectly satisfactory operation to be carried out for patients with ptosis in which at least 4 mm of movement of the upper lid is present—and it may be effective in a number of patients with even more severe degrees of ptosis (Fig. **10,** 16). In such patients 16 to 18 mm of muscle and aponeurosis must be removed, and this is about the limit of the amount of tissue which can be readily removed by the posterior route.

Technique (Fig. **10,** 17A to R). A silk traction suture is inserted into the proposed highest point of the lid and the lid is then everted over a suitable lid retractor (such as a Desmarre or Mustardé lid retractor, obtainable from Down Bros., England). In order to facilitate the dissection of the conjunctiva from the underlying Müller's muscle it is ballooned off by injection of fluid, preferably local anaesthetic, beneath it. An incision is then made in the conjunctiva immediately proximal to the superior edge of the tarsal plate and the conjunctiva is dissected from the underlying tissue. It is important at this stage to avoid including any of the thin layer of Müller's muscle which lies directly deep to the conjunctiva, but if the ballooning of the conjunctiva has been carried out correctly the layer between this and the muscle should

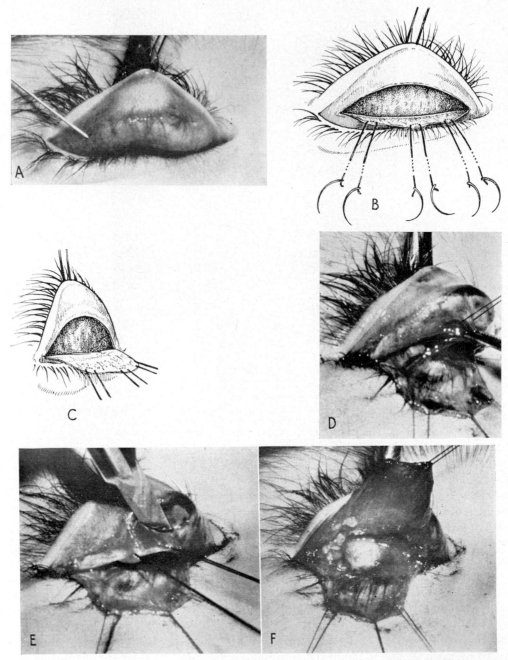

FIG. **10**, 17

Levator and tarsus resection—**posterior approach**. (A) 'Blowing off' conjunctiva from Müller's muscle. (B and C) Conjunctiva dissected off from Müller's muscle. Double-armed sutures inserted from raw surface (see also Figure **10**, 18A). (D) Müller's muscle and underlying levator aponeurosis picked up. First of two silk traction sutures inserted. (E) Freeing the above sutures by incision along upper edge of tarsus (see also Figure **10**, 18B). (F) Levator completely freed from conjunctiva and tarsus (see also Figure **10**, 18C).

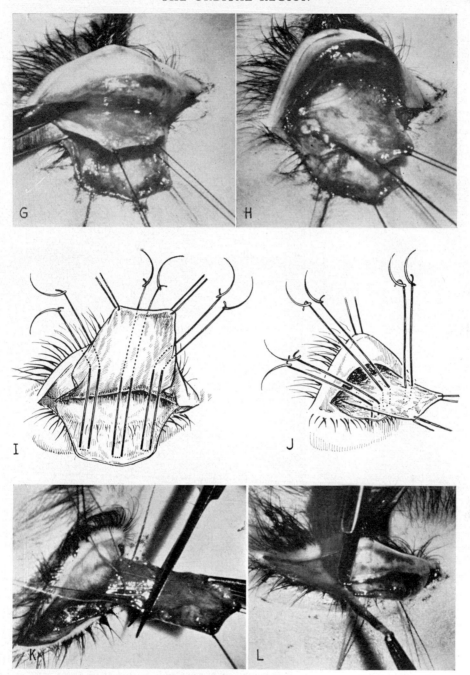

FIG. **10**, 17 (*contd.*)

(G) Sectioning lateral horns of levator aponeurosis. (H) Levator can now be drawn out further. Note reflected orbital septum above. (I and J) Double-armed conjunctival sutures carried through levator at predetermined distance from free edge. (K) Resection of levator peripheral to double-armed sutures. (L) Removal of 2 mm strip of upper edge of tarsus.

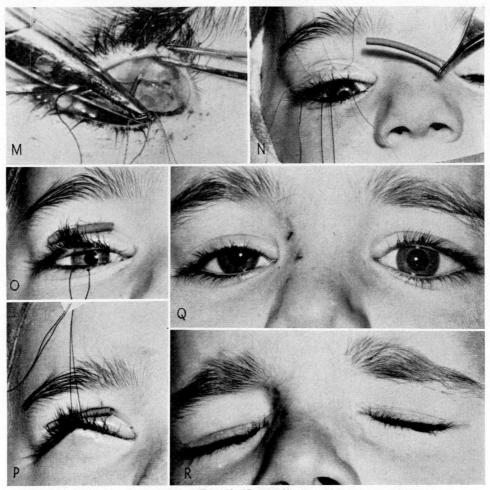

FIG. 10, 17 (contd.)

(M) Double-armed sutures passed through lid at upper cut edge of tarsus (see also Figure 10, 18D).
(N) Double-armed sutures brought out through skin. (O) Sutures tied over rubber tubing (see also
Figure 10, 18E). Traction suture transferred to lower lid. Note level of upper lid, margin. (P) Lower lid
drawn up over cornea. (Q) Three months postoperative appearance. Reasonable opening, but not
quite as high as opposite side. (R) Full closure.

not be difficult to find. Three double-armed 4/0 silk sutures are inserted in mattress
fashion from the raw surface of the conjunctiva 2 mm from the edge and these serve
as traction sutures to help in the further dissection of the conjunctiva from the underlying levator muscle.

The next step is to free Müller's muscle, and the aponeurosis of the levator which
lies deep to it, from the superior edge of the tarsal plate. This may be done by grasping
the muscle and aponeurosis with forceps at two sites, 3 to 4 mm from the superior
edge of the tarsus and about 7 mm on either side of the line of the traction suture.
The 'bite' of tissue held in the forceps is secured with a 4/0 silk suture, which is
knotted. Once the two sutures have been inserted into the muscle and aponeurosis

these latter can now be separated from the superior edge of the tarsus by sharp dissection. An alternative technique is to make a small button-hole through muscle and
aponeurosis at a point 7 mm on either side of the line of the traction suture and to
pass a ptosis muscle-clamp through these button-hole incisions so that the tissues
can be grasped before cutting it free from the edge of the tarsus.

The layer between the levator structures and the orbital septum is opened up with
blunt scissors until the levator can be freely drawn downwards, but it may be found
that the lateral and medial horns of the aponeurosis will prevent adequate mobilisation of the levator complex. These horns should be divided and it will then be found
that the levator can be pulled downwards unhindered so that it can be advanced the
required amount. On the tentative basis of removing 4 mm of levator complex for
every 1 mm of ptosis of the lid when the patient is looking straight forward, the
amount of aponeurosis and muscle to be resected is calculated. In theory 4 mm should
be deducted from the total to account for the tissue lying between the black traction
sutures and the final line of section of the tarsal plate but if the total is greater than
12 mm no deduction should be made. The muscle is marked at the proposed line of
section and the double-armed sutures originally inserted into the conjunctival edge
are passed through the muscle at this line. The stitches on the lateral and medial side
should actually be inserted 2 to 3 mm lower down in the levator so as to produce a
curving edge to the lid margin. The sutures are now carried through the edge of the
tarsal plate and brought out on the skin surface, one at 6 mm from the lid margin and
the other about 2 mm above this. They are lightly tied with a single bight to check
that the level of the lid lies about 1 mm above the centre point of the pupil (again it

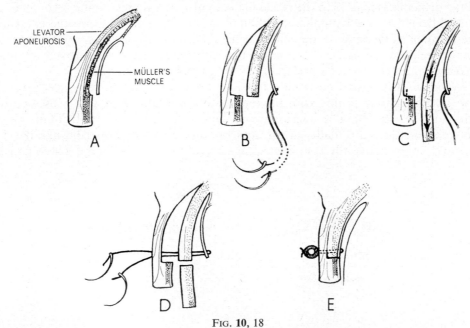

FIG. 10, 18

Levator resection (Blascovics). Sagittal section of upper lid showing relationship of double-
armed sutures to levator aponeurosis and underlying Müller's muscle.

should be stressed that the eyes may be rotated under the influence of the general anaesthetic and this must be taken into account in deciding where the centre point of the pupil should be).

Having ascertained that the sutures are in the correct position—they must of course be re-inserted through the muscle if the level of the lid margin is not satisfactory—the lid is again everted and the excess aponeurosis and muscle is removed. The sutures are loosened on the skin surface and subsequently tied over a small length of rubber tubing 3 mm in diameter (Fig. **10**, 18). The traction suture in the upper lid is removed and a similar type of suture is inserted into the lower lid margin to enable it to be drawn up to cover the cornea and to put the upper lid at rest for 48 hours post-operatively. The three silk sutures tied over the rubber tubing are left in situ for 12 days and are then removed. As with all ptosis operations, oedema of the orbital structures will prevent the final appreciation of the effect of the operation from being made for three to four weeks.

Sling operations

When there is a failure of innervation of the levator muscle, or where it is absent—as in most cases of anophthalmia—or when no significant improvement has been obtained after an attempt to shorten the levator complex, operations on the levator complex will be doomed to failure, and recourse must be had to taking advantage of the ability to raise the eyebrows by contraction of the frontalis muscle in order to produce any movement in the upper lid. The number of techniques for doing this is extremely large and includes the use of every structure in the eyelid, from the skin and the orbicularis muscle to the tarsal plate, in order to achieve some form of attachment of the lid to the frontalis. A different approach is to utilise some extraneous material such as fascia lata, toe tendon, silicone or collagen tape, or nylon sutures in order to achieve the lift, but the latter two substances have not proved altogether satisfactory and the writer's preference is for the use of fascia lata.

Technique. Three small horizontal incisions are made, immediately above the eyebrow, approximately in line with the medial and lateral canthi and with the centre of the lid (Fig. **10**, 19). The incisions must be carried down to the frontalis muscle. Two small incisions are made on the anterior surface of the upper lid about 1·5 cm apart and 3 mm above the lash line, so as to avoid eyelash follicles. These incisions

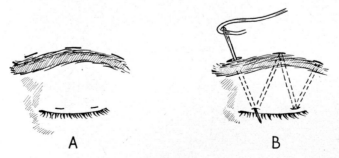

FIG. **10**, 19
(A and B) Fascia-lata sling hitching lid to frontalis muscle.

are made horizontally and carried down to the anterior surface of the tarsal plate. A strip of homograft fascia lata 2 to 3 mm wide and 15 cm long is threaded on a wide-eyed needle and is then woven from one incision to the other in the form of a 'W'. One end of the fascia lata is threaded through and sutured to the frontalis muscle, using fine monofilament nylon and, having raised the lid margin by tightening the sling so that the margin lies 1 mm above the centre of the pupil when the eye is in its normal position, the other end of the fascia lata is similarly secured. The fascia should be anchored to the anterior surface of the tarsal plate with a single suture of 6/0 mono-filament nylon at each lower angle of the 'W' to prevent the loop of fascia gradually becoming drawn up over the surface of the tarsus, with consequent slackening of the sling. Finally, a suture is inserted into the margin of the lower lid which is then drawn upwards to cover the cornea for the first 48 hours. It may be found that the lid will not close completely during sleep after this and the use of the traction suture in the lower lid should be continued for a few more days until a more satisfactory covering of the cornea is obtained. The fascia lata will stretch slightly, as will its attachment to the frontalis, and any slight overcorrection will be overcome within two to three weeks.

COLOBOMA OF THE EYELID

Coloboma of the eyelid, which presents as an actual gap in the lid margin, is a comparatively rare congenital deformity affecting mainly the upper lid and occasion-ally affecting both upper lids in the same individual. Coloboma of the lower lid may be associated with a corresponding coloboma of the iris of the eye, but in the upper lid type it is unusual to find any defect of the eye itself (although opacity and perhaps even partial covering of the cornea by squamous epethelium extending from the upper lid skin may be present). A more severe coloboma of the lower lid may be associated with a facial cleft which involves the lip, cheek and underlying maxilla (Chap. IV).

Upper Lid

In many instances there is little, if any, actual absence of lid substance and the two segments of the lid can readily be approximated. When the gap in the lid is too large to allow direct closure, a full-thickness wedge of tissue from the corresponding lower lid is rotated up on a small pedicle to fill the defect in the upper lid. It must be appreciated that what may appear to be a very large defect may be quite small once the rest of the lid is pulled across.

Technique

Direct closure (Fig. **10**, 20). The edges of the coloboma should be excised, so that the tarsal plate is exposed (it is important that the exposed edge of the tarsus should lie in a line perpendicular to the margin of the lid, to avoid any angulation, and the

PS I

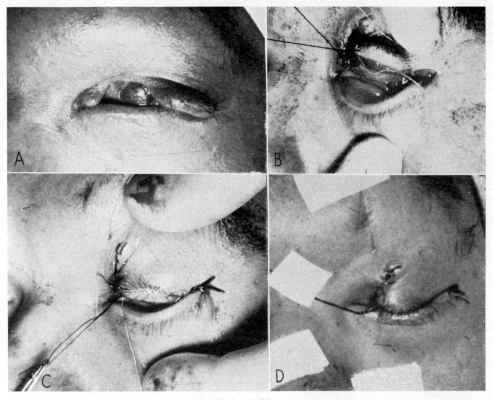

Fig. 10, 20

(A) Congenital coloboma (Mexican Indian). (B) Edges of defect excised. Closure of wound in three layers (a white nylon tarso-conjunctival suture and the suture in the grey line have been inserted). A lateral cantholysis of upper crus of canthal ligament has given adequate relaxation—defect is actually a quarter-plus. (C) Final closure of coloboma. Cantholysis closed by two skin sutures. Note temporary excessive length of lower lid. (D) Monofilament pull-out nylon fixed to skin by squares of adhesive.

lid is closed using the three-layer technique (Fig. **10**, 21). A 6/0 monofilament nylon suture is inserted through the skin above the highest point of the coloboma and, having been brought out through the conjunctiva, the suture is then passed through conjunctiva and tarsus on either side in an over-and-over fashion until the margin of the lid is reached, where the suture is again brought out through the skin. On being pulled tight, this suture will accurately splint the two edges of the exposed tarsal plate together, and a single 5/0 black silk suture may be inserted in the grey line to produce exact apposition of the edge of the margin itself. A number of interrupted 5/0 catgut sutures are used to close the orbicularis, and finally skin sutures of 6/0 nylon or silk are inserted. The continuous nylon suture is fixed to the forehead and the cheek under slight tension, using double squares of adhesive tape, and the single suture in the margin, which has been left 1·5 cm in length, is similarly fixed to the skin of the lid with adhesive tape to prevent it turning in on the cornea. All the sutures are removed at seven days, but if it is found that the continuous nylon suture will not readily pull out it should be left a further four or five days when an attempt may again be made.

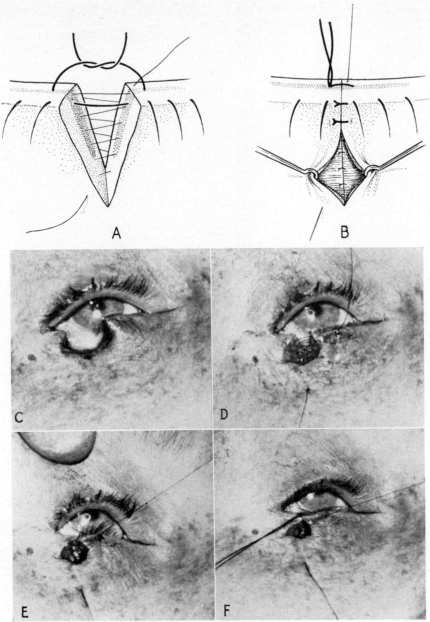

FIG. **10**, 21

Technique for closure of lid wounds. (A) Tarso-conjunctival layer closed by continuous 6/0 monofilament nylon. This gives accurate splinting of the edges of the tarsus. A single 5/0 silk suture is inserted precisely in the grey line on either side. The nylon suture is held under moderate tension by means of double squares of adhesive tape. (B) Closure of orbicularis muscle using 5/0 catgut sutures, and finally skin using 5/0 or 6/0 silk or nylon. (c) Shows closure of small lid defect using the above technique. (D) Continuous 6/0 monofilament nylon inserted in tarso-conjunctival layer. (E) Nylon suture drawn tight. (F) 5/0 silk suture in grey line.

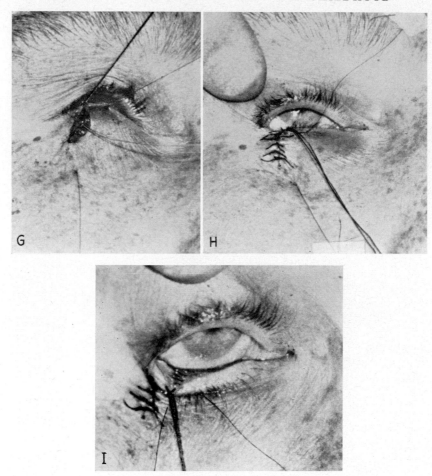

FIG. **10**, 21 (*contd.*)

(G) 5/0 catgut sutures to close orbicularis. (H) 6/0 silk sutures in skin: pull-out nylon fixed by squares of adhesive tape. (I) Lid turned down to show continuous nylon suture 'splinting' the tarsus accurately together.

By this time the suture will be found to be looser and should draw out readily. If the suture has been inadvertently knotted it should be drawn as tight as possible and then cut off flush with the skin: it will retract into the tissues and cause no trouble.

Use of a switch-flap from the lower lid. When it is found that the defect in the upper lid is too great to be closed direct (Fig. **10**, 22A), a switch-flap of lower lid tissue may be designed along the lines laid down for the use of switch-flaps from lower to upper lid in the treatment of lid tumours (Mustardé, 1966b). Ink marks are made on the lower lid corresponding with the defect on the upper lid, and the centre point between the two ink marks is found. This represents the site of the hinge of the switch-flap, and a small full-thickness flap of the lower lid, up to one-quarter of the lower lid in length—depending on the size of the gap to be filled—is designed on one or other side

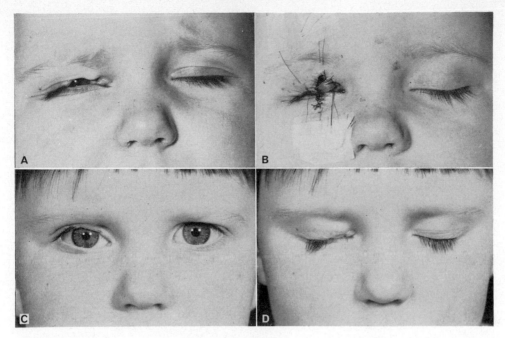

FIG. 10, 22

Large congenital coloboma of upper lid. Upper lid reconstruction using a switch flap turned up on a vascular hinge from lower lid. (A) Original defect. (B) Switch flap turned into defect: vascular hinge divided after two weeks. (C and D) Three months after division of pedicle.

of the hinge as determined by the site of the coloboma. The marginal pedicle, which maintains the blood supply to the lid flap through the marginal vessels must be not less than 4 mm in width. The gap in the lower lid is closed in layers as described above, but without inserting a marginal suture or damaging the marginal vessel, and the small switch-flap is then sutured into the defect in the upper lid, again in three layers (Fig. 10, 22B). After an interval of two weeks the vascular pedicle may be divided and both upper and lower lid margins revised (Figs. 10, 22C and D).

Because the tissues of the lid will stretch considerably, a true absence of up to a half of a lid can be repaired by this technique using a flap of up to a quarter of the lower lid. Larger defects of the upper lid, which would require more than one-quarter of the lower lid to fill the gap, should be repaired using a switch-flap designed in the same manner as for defects in adult lids (Mustardé, 1968b). Such large colobomata must be extremely rare congenital deformities, and the writer has never seen one of this width.

LOWER LID

In the lower lid, if a coloboma cannot be closed direct, a cheek rotation flap should be used to bring in additional tissue, lining the new section of the lid with nasal septal mucosa in the unlikely event of there being insufficient conjunctiva available

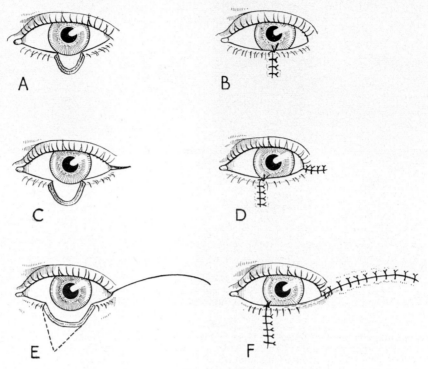

FIG. 10, 23

Loss of lid in vertical direction. (A and B) Small defect, up to a quarter of lid length, closed direct. (C and D) Defect of just over a quarter closed by mobilising lid on lateral side (after dividing lower crus of lateral canthal ligament). (E and F) Defect between a quarter and half. Remainder of lid cannot be closed, even with stretching of tissues. Small amount of additional tissue brought in from lateral side by rotation of cheek.

(Fig. **10**, 23). The closure of the lip defect in patients with a facial cleft (lateral or oblique facial cleft) is carried out as in closure of cleft lip deformities (Chaps. I and IV).

DISTICHIASIS

This is a condition which, though extremely rare, may prove very troublesome and may result in corneal ulceration if no treatment is carried out. Instead of a single row of lashes on the lid margin, two rows, and even three, may be present and the inner row rubs on the surface of the cornea (Fig. **10**, 24). Epilation by electrolysis is of no permanent value and the whole of the posterior lash-bearing area should be excised. The raw area which is left should be covered by a long strip of thick mucosa taken from the nasal septum and held in place by means of a continuous pull-out nylon suture.

ANGULAR DERMOID

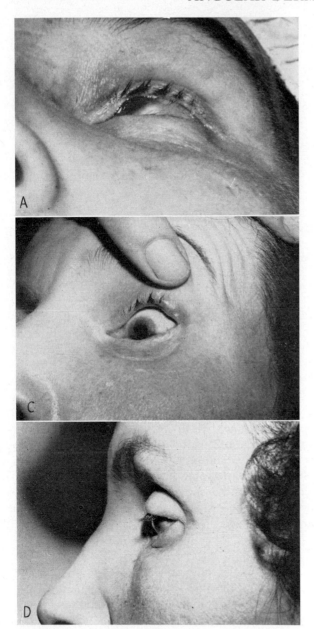

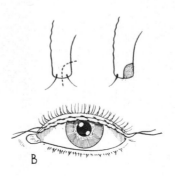

Fig. **10**, 24

Distichiasis. (A) Pre-operative condition showing additional row of lashes rubbing on eyeball. (B) Excision of abnormal lash-bearing area and insertion of graft of nasal septal mucosa. (C and D) Final appearance six months postoperatively.

In this comparatively common congenital abnormality a dermoid cyst is to be found lying beneath or close to the outer one-third of the eyebrow (Fig. **10**, 25). The cyst is generally adherent to the periosteum of the frontal bone and should be approached via an incision running in the line of the eyebrow itself. It will often be found that the cyst is lying in a saucer-shaped depression in the bone. This depression gradually fills out as the child grows.

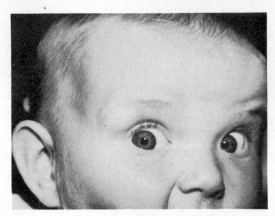

FIG. **10**, 25
Angular dermoid.

CONGENITAL ABSENCE OF THE EYE

Absence of the eye at birth proves on rare occasions to be a true anophthalmos in which there is not even a rudiment of an eye present. More often the condition is that of microphthalmos in which a vestigial eye has actually developed, although it may be microscopic and may be difficult to see clinically. In the latter type of deformity a cyst is often present, and the cyst itself may be more readily discovered. The distinction between the two conditions is not a purely academic one for it would appear that even a small rudimentary eye will usually produce a growth potential in the orbit itself which will result in the development of an orbit which is only about one-fifth smaller than the normal orbit on the opposite side. This is very much in keeping with the 12 to 15 per cent failure of development of an orbit which takes place when an eye has to be removed in early childhood. True anophthalmos on the other hand invariably results in a very considerable degree of failure in the development of the orbit and the facial bones on the same side so that by the time adult life is reached the orbit may be less than half the size of the normal side.

Microphthalmos (Fig. **10**, 26)

Although the orbit may grow to within 80 or even 90 per cent of the normal size the eye socket itself will remain too small to retain a prosthesis, and in such circumstances it is necessary to reconstruct an eye socket which will be large enough for this purpose. Apart from the conjunctiva on the posterior surface of the tarsal plates close to the margin of the lids the rest of the mucosa should be excised and a dissection made in the fat of the orbit towards the orbital margins themselves, as in reconstruction in the usual type of contracted socket (Fig. **10**, 27). In most of the patients with this condition there is a complete ptosis of the upper lid as the levator

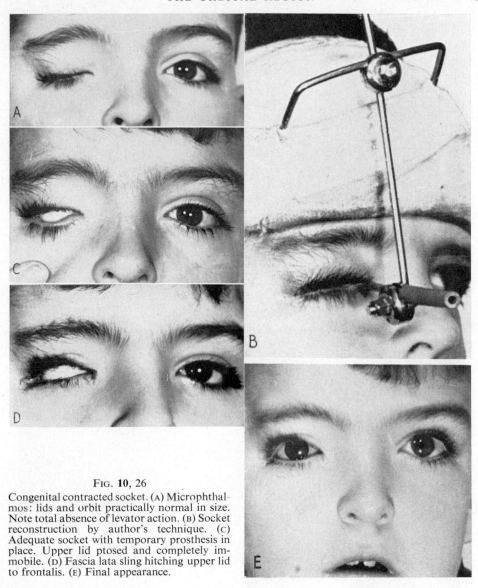

FIG. **10**, 26

Congenital contracted socket. (A) Microphthalmos: lids and orbit practically normal in size. Note total absence of levator action. (B) Socket reconstruction by author's technique. (C) Adequate socket with temporary prosthesis in place. Upper lid ptosed and completely immobile. (D) Fascia lata sling hitching upper lid to frontalis. (E) Final appearance.

muscle has also failed to develop, and if this is the case no fear need exist that the levator will be damaged in this dissection towards the orbital margin. If a levator muscle is present it must, of course, be avoided during the dissection. A suitable plastic mould is inserted, covered by a skin graft, so as to produce a larger socket than will ultimately be required (Fig. **10**, 28); the inevitable contraction of the graft will reduce the socket to a reasonable size. A mould used incorporates a hollow steel tube which emerges at the medial canthal end, and the graft is draped over the mould with the loose ends gathered together on the posterior surface. This ensures a continuous sheet of skin graft behind the area of the union of the lid margins, and

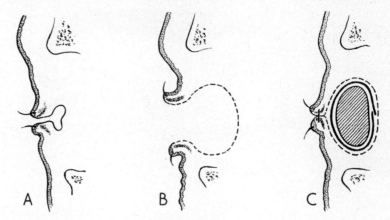

Fig. 10, 27

Author's technique for reconstructing total eye socket. (A) Pre-operative condition. (B) Excision of all conjunctiva, except that on the inner surface of the lids near the margin. (C) Insertion of skin-covered conformer with unbroken skin surface presenting behind a sub-total tarsorrhaphy.

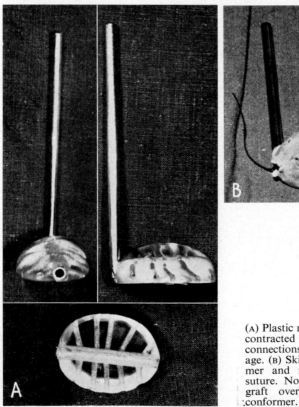

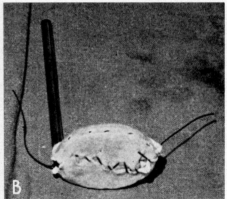

Fig. 10, 28

(A) Plastic mould or conformer for use in contracted sockets. Note steel tube with connections to lateral openings for drainage. (B) Skin graft draped round conformer and retained by continuous silk suture. Note drainage holes stabbed in graft over openings of channels in conformer.

this latter is carried out as a subtotal tarsorrhaphy by everting the lid margins and inserting a continuous pull-out monofilament nylon suture into the exposed tarsal plate on either lid (Fig. **10**, 27C). The skin graft should be of medium thickness to avoid undue contraction, but at the same time it must be thin enough to avoid carrying with it an excessive number of sweat and sebaceous glands which will tend to produce a rather unpleasant odour in the eye socket. The steel tubing is fixed to a plaster head-cap by a system of rods connected by universal joints. This prevents the mould from tilting and at the same time allows irrigation of the socket to be carried out during the six weeks before the tarsorrhaphy is divided.

If levator muscle function is absent the ptosis of the upper lid must be corrected using a fascia lata sling (see Ptosis, page 224).

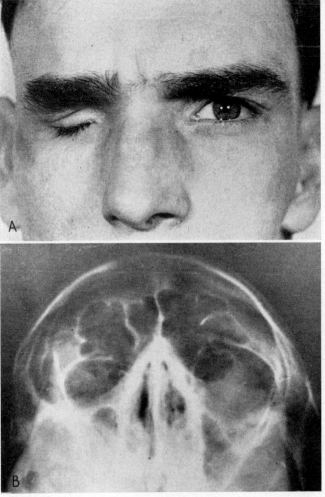

FIG. **10**, 29

Congenital contracted socket. (A) Anophthalmos: tiny palpebral aperture with rudimentary lids. (B) X-ray showing underlying bony orbit markedly underdeveloped.

Anophthalmos

In patients presenting with true anophthalmos the problem is considerably greater than in the majority of those in which even a tiny rudimentary eye is present. The reason for this is two-fold: firstly, the whole of the orbit will be greatly reduced in size and will be at a lower level than the orbit on the normal side: secondly, the palpebral aperture itself will be very small and the lids may only be a half of the

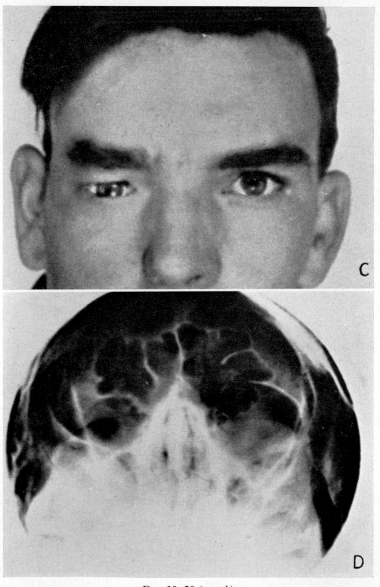

FIG. **10**, 29 (*contd.*)

(c) Socket constructed by author's technique. Upper lid raised by fascia lata sling attached to frontalis. (D) X-ray showing removal of bone of lateral and infero-lateral margin of orbit to enable socket to be reconstructed.

normal length of the eyelids (Fig. **10**, 29A and B). Similar orbital deformities may occasionally be present in patients with microphthalmos.

On the few occasions on which the writer has had to deal with this problem the mucosa has been excised as described above, and the dissection for the new socket has been made *outside* the underdeveloped orbital bones. Additional room for the socket has been obtained by excision of some of the bone forming the orbital margin but this removal of bone has been confined to the lateral and inferior walls. A skin-lined socket is reconstructed using the technique described above, but the lateral canthus is split for a distance which will provide a palpebral aperture approximating to the normal in length so that an adequate sized mould can be inserted. This cantho-tomy is closed when the lids are united by a tarsorrhaphy, and is again re-opened when the tarsorrhaphy is divided. The end result of this procedure leaves much to be desired, both in the positioning of the new socket and in the abnormal appearance of the lateral canthus and the lateral part of each eyelid (Fig. **10**, 29C and D). As there is no eye present it would be perfectly reasonable to graft a line of lashes on the lateral segment of the eyelids, or artificial eyelids could be applied to these areas. Another possibility would be to rotate the existing lash-bearing medial half of the margin of the lower lid and implant it in the lateral half of the upper lid. The pedicle would be divided in two weeks. This would, of course, necessitate reconstructing the lower lid by the technique of rotating the cheek and lining the new sector of the lower lid with cartilage taken from the nasal septum (see Coloboma of the Upper Lid, page 228).

Tessier has recently demonstrated a method of dealing with the orbital problem in these patients in which, by suitably placed incisions, he sections the various walls of the orbit, displaces them outwards to produce a reasonable sized orbit, and fills in the intervening gaps with bone grafts. Even with such a radical approach to the orbital problem there is still the question of reconstruction of a socket, and more particularly, the missing part of the eyelids at the outer canthus has still to be dealt with.

J. C. MUSTARDÉ

REFERENCES

BEARD, C. (1969). *Ptosis*. St. Louis: Mosby.

DUKE-ELDER, Sir STEWART (1952). *Textbook of Ophthalmology*, Vol. 5, pp. 4653–4658. London: Kimpton.

EVERBUSCH, O. (1883). Zur operation der congentalen blepharoptosis. *Klin. Mbl. Augenbeilk*. **21**, 100–107.

ISAKSSON, I. (1962). *Studies of Congenital Genuine Blepharoptosis*. Goteborg: Orstadius.

JONES, L. T. (1964). The anatomy of the upper eyelid and its relation to ptosis surgery. *Am. J. Ophthal*. **57**, 943–959.

MUSTARDÉ, J. C. (1959). The treatment of ptosis and epicanthal folds. *Br. J. plast. Surg*. **12**, 252–258.

MUSTARDÉ, J. C. (1966a). *Repair and Reconstruction in the Orbital Region*, p. 324. Epicanthus and telecanthus. Edinburgh: Livingstone.

MUSTARDÉ, J. C. (1966b). *Repair and Reconstruction of the Orbital Region*, p. 163. Reconstruction of the upper lid. Edinburgh: Livingstone.

MUSTARDÉ, J. C. (1968a). Experiences in ptosis correction. *Trans. Am. Acad. Ophthal. Oto-lar*. **72**, 173.

MUSTARDÉ, J. C. (1968b). Reconstruction of the upper lid and the use of nasal mucosal grafts. *Br. J. plast. Surg*. **21**, 367–377.

CHAPTER XI

HYPERTELORISM

Surgical correction of orbital hypertelorism by swinging the two orbits closer together (Fig. **11**, 1) is made possible by the fact that the optic foramina themselves are in more or less normal position, and thus the optic and oculo-motor nerves need not be interfered with as the orbits are moved. Hypertelorism is usually associated with other defects, particularly clefts and craniostosis.

Clefts. (1) Facial: including clefts of lip, palate or nose, vertical or oblique orbito-maxillary clefts, and lateral proboscis. (2) Cranial: these include meningo-encephalocele, nasal dermoid and glioma, and epignathic tumours.

Craniostosis. This in particular includes the cranio-facial dysostoses of Crouzon and Apert.

Previously, surgery was either limited to correction of the external deformities, e.g. epicanthus, telecanthus, wide eyebrows, etc. (Webster and Denig, 1950), or to attempts to move the eye and orbital contents without moving the whole of the bony orbit (Converse and Smith, 1962). Such techniques are not suitable to any but minor degrees of hypertelorism.

Pre-operative study

Radiological examination is the most important pre-operative study, and the position of the anterior clinoid processes is checked by horizontal tomography. Lateral views revealing the situation of the cribiform plate are also important.

PRINCIPLES OF THE OPERATIVE TECHNIQUE

Protection of the anterior lobes by covering the meninges six months prior to the main operation with dermis or a pericranial graft is no longer advocated (Fig. **11**, 4) and a pericranial graft, sutured in place over weak areas of the dura, is carried out at the time of the operation.

Movement of the whole of the bony orbit towards the midline is achieved by the following technique.

1. Total ethmoidectomy, except for the os planum of the sphenoid.

2. Removal of the whole of the nasal septum to reduce the risk of nasal atresia.

3. Avoidance of damaging the optic nerves by locating the site of the optic canal, and by stripping all the orbital periosteum up to within 10 mm of the posterior pole of the orbit.

4. Preservation of the sphenoidal fissure and its contents.

5. Preservation of the lacrimal passages and all of the orbital contents by sub-periosteal dissection within the bony orbit.

6. Approximation of the orbits by removal of a central block of bone from the floor of the skull, the nose, the ethmoids and the maxillae (producing an interorbital width of 12 to 15 mm).

7. Insertion of bone grafts into the gaps left in the floor of the skull and in the temporal and orbital regions by the medial swinging together of the orbits.

238

8. Restoration of the skeleton of the nose by a bone graft, and fixation of the medial canthi in a new position.

All the above should be carried out in a single operation.

Other deformities may have to be dealt with, e.g. correction of facial clefts, anti-mongoloid slope of the palpebral apertures, inequality of the level of the orbits or deformities of the nose itself (Fig. **11**, 3).

Careful selection of patients must be made to ensure that they are psychologically suitable for such surgery, and it is probable that the operations should be carried out early in life so as to avoid the development of amblyopia by providing the opportunity for making fusion possible.

It should be realised that where there is a wide divergence of the orbits there is almost invariably a lowering of the cribriform plate—by as much as 20 mm—and there may be other less easily detected deformities of the nasal or facial bones such as bifid septum, deformities of the malar or maxillary bones, etc.

In patients with craniostosis, exophoria may be present and is produced by protrusion of the eyeballs, lateral deviation of the optic axes and decrease in size of the orbits themselves. It will be obvious that when gross deviation of the ocular axes is present, fusion of the images is quite impossible (Fig. **11**, 2).

CLASSIFICATION OF HYPERTELORISM

First degree

These are patients with an intercanthal distance of between 30 and 34 mm. More often than not there is really only a telecanthus (Mustardé, 1963) either congenital or post-traumatic, with no true hypertelorism. Various disguising procedures are used in such patients to deal with the telecanthus and epicanthal folds which may be present (p. 207).

Second degree

In these patients the intercanthal distance is above 34 mm but there is no gross orbital deviation or exophoria (Fig. **11**, 6).

Three methods of tackling the problem by osteotomy have been tried.

1. Part of the medial wall of the orbit is removed and a partial ethmoidectomy carried out. This is of no great value in moving the eyes towards the mid-line.

2. The whole of the medial wall, along with the infero-medial angle and medial third of the orbital floor, are removed, but again the results are of little value.

3. Mobilisation of the medial wall (after partial ethmoidectomy), the floor and the lateral wall of the orbit. This extra-cranial operation produces good results, but the writer inclines increasingly towards a more radical cranial approach, especially if the cribriform plate is much lowered.

The details of the extra-cranial technique will be discussed later.

Third degree

Here (Figs. **11**, 1; **11**, 2; **11**, 3; **11**, 4), the inter-orbital distance is very considerably increased but, more important, the orbits are rotated outwards: although the face is no larger the distance between the lateral canthus and the external auditory meatus

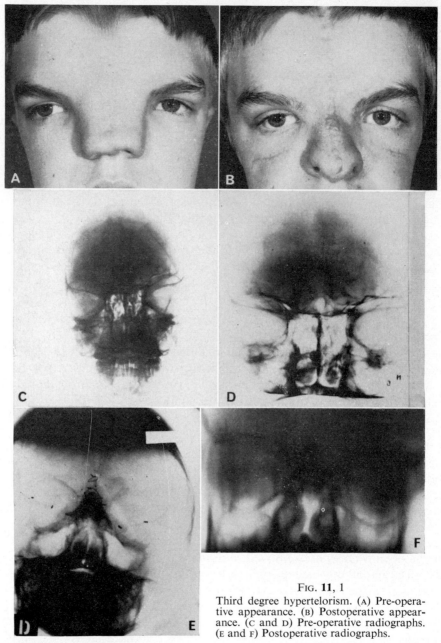

Fig. **11,** 1

Third degree hypertelorism. (A) Pre-opera-tive appearance. (B) Postoperative appear-ance. (C and D) Pre-operative radiographs. (E and F) Postoperative radiographs.

is decreased. In third degree cases the ethmoids may be double the normal width and the medial orbital walls will lie at an oblique angle to each other. The cribriform plate will be situated at a very low level and the eyebrow ridges will be very far apart. A low extracranial osteotomy below the cribriform plate would not permit mobilisation of the roof of the orbits but might damage the cribriform plate and enter the meninges,

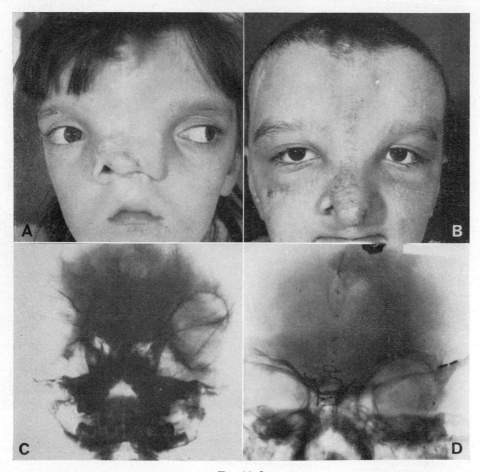

FIG. **11**, 2

Third degree hypertelorism showing deviation of ocular axes. (A) Pre-operative. (B) Postoperative. (C) Pre-operative radiograph. (D) Postoperative radiograph.

and it would not really deal with the wide frontal bone and upper part of the ethmoids, which are the real cause of the hypertelorism.

To bring such divergent orbits together requires total removal of the ethmoids, cribriform plate, crista galli and olfactory nerves. After much trial and error a technique has been finally arrived at which involves the complete mobilisation of all four orbital walls but which preserves intact a small cone at the apex of the bony orbit some 10 mm from the optic foramen, thus avoiding damage to the optic nerve.

OPERATIVE PROCEDURES

1. A frontal craniotomy is carried out, the frontal bone being removed and later replaced as a free graft.

2. The dura with the enclosed frontal lobes is raised up from the floor of the anterior

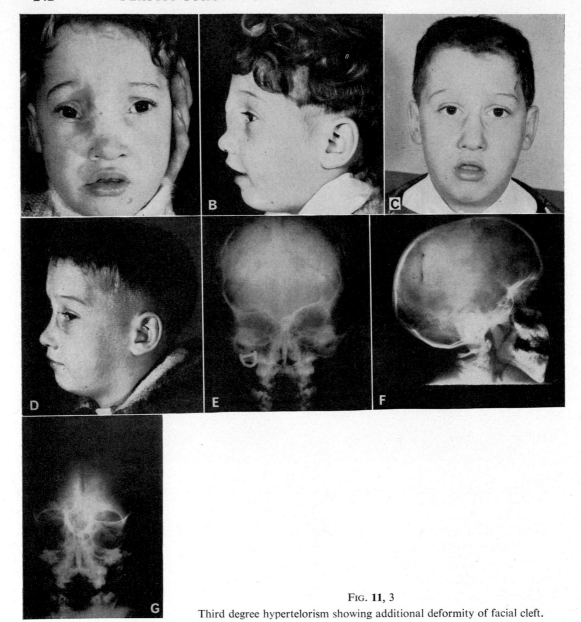

Fig. 11, 3

Third degree hypertelorism showing additional deformity of facial cleft.

fossa of the skull. The olfactory nerves are severed and any tears or leakages in the dural covering are closed by direct suture or, if large, by suturing a graft of pericranium (taken from behind the area of the craniotomy) over the area. The whole of the anterior fossa up to the optic chiasma is exposed.

3. A mid-line incision is made over the nose and through this all of the tissues of the nose and lateral to it can be raised from the underlying facial skeleton.

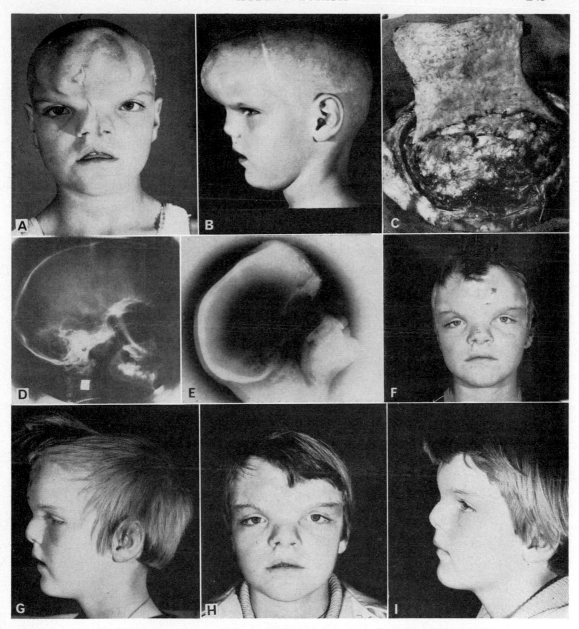

FIG. 11, 4

Third degree hypertelorism; two-stage correction (first stage no longer used: see text). (A and B) Appearance shortly after insertion of dermis graft to cover anterior lobes (first stage). (C) Fixation of dermis graft over dura of frontal lobes. (D and E) Pre- and postoperative radiographs demonstrating dermis graft. (F to I) Postoperative appearance shortly after, and some time after, correction of hypertelorism.

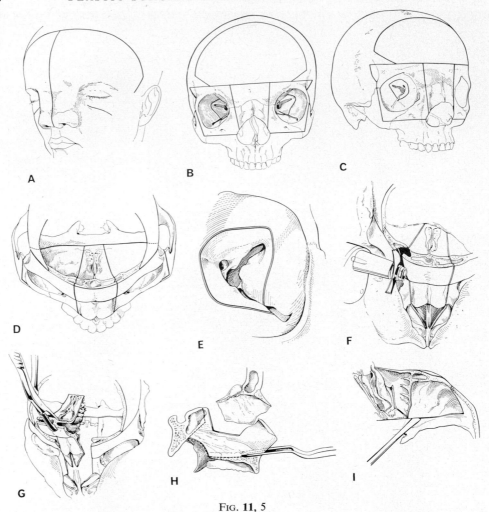

FIG. 11, 5

Surgery of third degree hypertelorism. (A to D) Bone sections to separate orbits from rest of face and skull. (E) Cone of bone left around optic foramen. (F to H) Removal of fronto-ethmoid-nasal bloc. (I) Section across roof of orbit.

4. Incisions are made along the infero-lateral orbital margins to give access to the lateral parts of the orbit, the malar bones, and temporal fossae (Fig. **11**, 1B).

5. Sub-periosteal dissection around all four orbital walls, up to 10 mm from the optic foramen, exposes the whole orbit for subsequent osteotomy and preserves all of the orbital structures intact within the cone of periosteum (the naso-lacrymal duct must be carefully preserved under direct vision).

6. Fronto-naso-ethmoid resection (Fig. **11**, 5A to G). A carefully estimated central block of the floor of the anterior fossa and frontal bone, the whole of the ethmoids, and the nasal septum in its entirety (including the central area of the maxillary process around the cavity of the nose) is removed.

7. Osteotomies are carried out via the various facial incisions to divide the whole

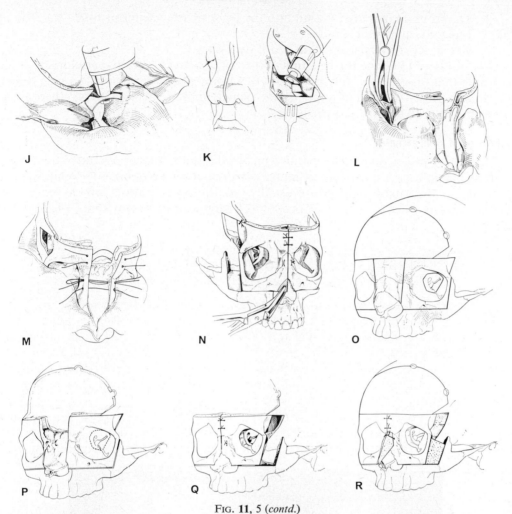

FIG. **11**, 5 (*contd.*)

(J and K) Step section of zygoma. (L to Q) Mobilisation of orbits towards mid-line. (R) Bone grafts to fill defects and retain orbits in new position.

of the bony orbit from the skull and facial bones (Fig. **11**, 5H to K), preserving intact the bony cone around the optic foramen (Fig. **11**, 5E).

8. The bony orbits are now brought towards the mid-line, partly by direct medial displacement and partly by true rotation (Fig. **11**, 5L to Q).

9. Bone grafts are inserted into the floor of the anterior fossae lateral to the displaced orbital roofs, and between the zygomatic processes and the zygomatic bones in the line of section of the fronto-zygomatic region (Fig. **11**, 5R).

10. Bilateral cantho-plexy is carried out to fix the medial canthal ligaments to each other by a deep trans-nasal suture (Fig. **11**, 3C), followed by a bone graft to support the nasal bridge line. The lateral canthi will take up a more or less correct position as the periosteum becomes re-attached to the zygomatic bones.

11. The frontal lobes are lowered into the reconstructed anterior fossa, the frontal bones replaced, and the scalp closed.

12. The nasal cartilages are reshaped if necessary.

It is still hard to define the best time for surgical correction of hypertelorism. If we consider that fusion is the only important functional problem we must operate before the fourth year if we are to hope for the ocular improvement. After 12 there is no other problem than nose growth.

Additional operations

There may still be many deformities which will require further operative treatment, such as hypoplasia of maxilla or zygoma, short upper lip, coloboma of eyelids, ptosis, mandibular deformities, etc. More usually, additional operations on the nose may be required in order to correct deformities of length, or of size or shape of the nasal apertures.

SUB-CRIBRIFORM INTERCRANIO-FACIAL OSTEOTOMY
(*Second degree hypertelorism*)

In less gross cases of hypertelorism (Fig. **11**, 6), where the divergence of the orbits is not so great as to produce extreme obliquity of the vertical axes, a reduced procedure which is confined to the skeleton of the face below the level of the cribriform plate may be carried out. Such an operation, avoiding the need for a cranial approach, is technically easier than the cranio-facial operation but has, nevertheless, many of its risks, particularly of meningeal puncture, due to damage to a very low cribriform plate—a feature of any abnormally wide ethmoid region.

The surgeon operating on these cases by this modified route may have to balance his decision between making a horizontal section in the ethmoid area low enough to avoid damage to the cribriform plate and the meninges, and at the same time making

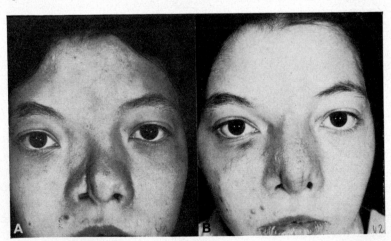

FIG. **11**, 6
Second degree hypertelorism. (A) Pre-operative. (B) Postoperative.

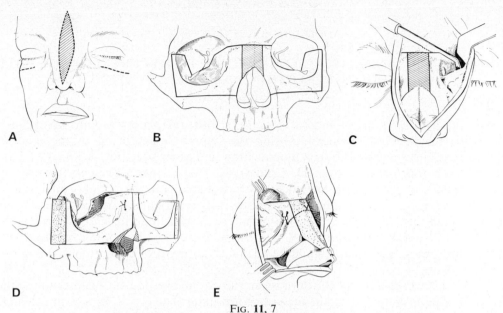

FIG. **11**, 7

Sub-cribriform correction of second degree hypertelorism (see text).

the section sufficiently high to permit partial but effective removal of the ethmoid mass and mobilisation of the medial orbital walls to allow the orbital cones to be moved towards each other. The writer has had three patients in whom there was a c.s.f. leak during this type of approach—although they all subsequently made satisfactory recoveries.

The operative procedure (Fig. **11**, 7) may be either in the nature of a sagittal splitting of the facial bones followed by a horizontal section below the level of the cribriform plate, first anteriorly and then posteriorly, or a Le Fort III procedure situated through the fronto-zygomatic process near the roof of the orbit. The important point is to effect a satisfactory mobilisation of the orbits—apart from the roofs. This is carried out by sub-periosteal dissection of the lining of the orbit which will then permit osteotomies to be carried out to free the orbit from the malar and maxillary bones. These osteotomies must be above and behind the equator of the eyeball if they are going to produce adequate results.

P. TESSIER

ADDENDUM I TO CHAPTER XI

ONE-STAGE CRANIOFACIAL OSTEOTOMY IN HYPERTELORISM WITH PARAMEDIAN RESECTION AND PRESERVATION OF OLFACTORY NERVES

The observation that, in most cases, the cribriform plate was not significantly enlarged (the increase in width causing the hypertelorism being in the anterior ethmoid region) suggested to us a modification of Tessier's technique which we have performed in four patients (Figs. **11**, 8 and **11**, 9). This technique presents two advantages: it can be performed in one stage instead of two, and it preserves olfaction.

A frontal scalp flap extending laterally to the preauricular area, is outlined and incised in the usual manner. The scalp flap is raised subperiosteally down to the level of the supraorbital arches. A segment of frontal bone is then removed (the size of the removed segment should be adequate to provide exposure of the anterior cranial fossa).

Subperiosteal elevation of the dura is carefully done over the entire anterior cranial fossa, to a point as far medial as the cribriform plate. The elevation is then extended backward to the level of a horizontal line extending through the posterior portion of the cribriform plate, medial to the lateral border of the cribriform plate, and lateral to the full extent of the anterior cranial fossa. Intravenous mannitol injections shrink the brain and facilitate the retraction of the frontal lobes.

The periosteum is then raised externally from the lower portion of the frontal bone and the supraorbital arches; this subperiosteal elevation is continued laterally over the temporal fossa, exposing the lateral wall of the orbit. A probe assists in locating the inferior orbital fissure. Exposure of the superior orbital rim is then continued. As the periosteum is elevated, the supraorbital nerves and vessels stay with the orbital contents when they exit through a supra-orbital notch; if they exit through a foramen, removal of the orbital roof and floor of the foramen permits the nerves and vessels to follow the orbital contents and the coronal flap. The pulley of the superior oblique is also detached subperiosteally.

Subperiosteal elevation is continued around over the periorbita of the roof of the orbit. Medially, the lacrimal sac is raised from the lacrimal groove, along with the attachments of the medial palpebral ligament, and the elevation is extended backward over the lamina papyracea. Laterally, the subperiorbital elevation is extended backward along the lateral wall of the orbit until the inferior orbital fissure is exposed. The orbital contents are now separated from the entire periphery of the orbit, with the exception of the apex.

This periorbital elevation should be done with great care. The risk of ocular complications, such as retrobulbar haemorrhage, appears to be minimal, however, if the surgeon's instruments remain outside the periorbita throughout the operation. Traction on the orbital contents during the operative procedure should be carefully avoided, for fear of injury to the optic nerve.

The infraorbital nerve is now located and subperiosteal elevation over the anterior

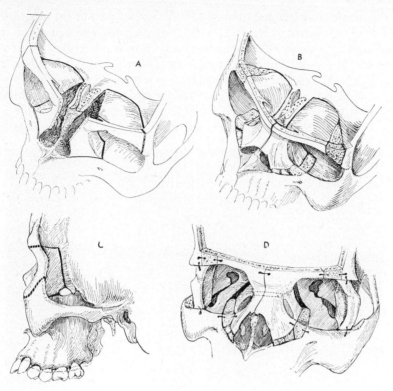

FIG. **11**, 8

One-stage medial orbitotomy, with preservation of the cribriform plate. (A) Outline of the medial orbital oseotomy, the shaded areas represent the areas of bone resection. (B) The extent of the bone resection. (C) After medial displacement. (D) Bone grafts fill the gaps.

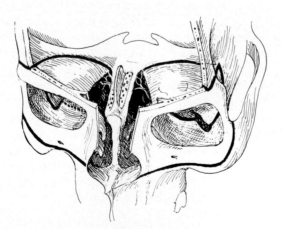

FIG **11**, 9

Outline of the subtotal orbital osteotomy with preservation of the cribriform plate.

surface of the maxilla is extended medially to the lateral wall of the nose and inferiorly to the edge of the pyriform aperture. The root of the nose and bony dorsum are then exposed through a midline skin incision which may be extended downward as far as the tip of the nose, and upward through the entire scalp flap for better exposure.

A medial (Fig. **11**, 8) or a subtotal orbitotomy (Fig. **11**, 9) is then performed. A central segment of bone is removed from the nasofrontal area, the ethmoid sinus is exenterated, and two wedges of bone are resected from the roof of the ethmoid on each side of the cribriform plate, which is preserved (Fig. **11**, 8A and B). Procedures

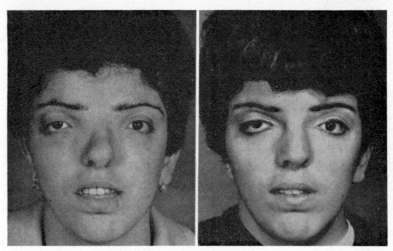

FIG. **11**, 10
Left—pre-operative appearance of patient with true ocular hypertelorism.
Right—after procedure illustrated in Figure **11**, 8.

to narrow the nose and eliminate the bifidity (consisting of resection of bone, septal cartilage and bone, lateral and alar cartilages) complete this procedure. Resection of excess skin is done to approximate the medial ends of the eyebrows.

Bone grafts (costal in children, iliac in adolescents) are wired into the bony gaps; the resected frontal bone is trimmed to fit the modified frontal defect and maintained by wire fixation.

Both the medial orbitotomy and the subtotal orbital osteotomy have been done successfully by this one-stage technique, which preserves the olfactory nerves. In four patients, two underwent a medial orbitotomy, and two a subtotal orbital osteotomy. An additional procedure was added, however, to the medial orbitotomy: the lateral wall of the orbit was severed from its connections and displaced medially for a distance equivalent to the amount of medial displacement of the medial portion of the orbit (Fig. **11**, 8C and D). Thus, enlargement of the orbital cavity was avoided, as well as the resultant risk of enophthalmos (Fig. **11**, 10).

JOHN M. CONVERSE AND JOSEPH RANSOHOFF

ACKNOWLEDGEMENT

Figures **11**, 8, 9 and 10 and text are reproduced by permission of the Editor of *Plastic and Reconstructive Surgery*.

ADDENDUM 2. TO CHAPTER XI

CORRECTION OF MINOR DEGREES OF HYPERTELORISM

In patients who have a minor degree of hypertelorism, in which the eyes are not more than 10 to 12 mm further apart than normal, correction of the divergence of the ocular axes may be carried out by a very modified technique involving a facial approach (Fig. **11**, 11). As Tessier points out, a purely facial approach cannot be attempted unless the level of the cribriform plate is above the line of the centres of the eyeballs, but in these minor degrees of hypertelorism it is most likely that the cribriform plate will be at a high enough level. This should be ascertained by X-ray exmination baefore surgery

The medial wall and medial half of the roof and floor of the orbit are readily

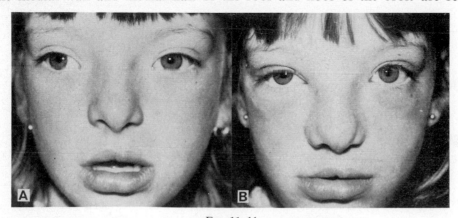

FIG. **11**, 11

Minor degree of hypertelorism. (A) Pre-operative appearance: interpupillary distance 64 mm, intercanthal distance 40 mm. (B) Postoperative appearance: interpupillary distance 56 mm, intercanthal distance 34 mm.

explored by a nasal approach similar to that used by the writer for trans-nasal glioma resection. The incision is carried round both alar bases and across the vault of the anterior nares between the upper and lower alar cartilages (Fig. **11**, 12A). The two incisions are united across the columella and the lower half of the nose can be raised up from the underlying facial skeleton leaving the upper alar cartilages still attached to the nasal bones. It will be found that in a child this allows exposure of the glabellar area (Fig. **11**, 12B) and the supra- and infra-orbital margins as far as the midline (Fig. **11**, 12C). With a chisel both nasal bones are freed and the periosteum is then scraped away from the maxilla at the infra-medial angle so as to expose the bone overlying the naso-lacrimal duct (Fig. **11**, 13A). This bone is carefully removed so that the naso-lacrimal duct and the lacrymal sac above it can be visualised and preserved in the next stage. Stripping of the periosteum at the infra-medial angle is continued into the orbit and, after incising the periosteum along the inferior margin of the orbit, the periosteum is stripped up within the orbit to about a centimetre beyond the equator of the eye and as far laterally as can be reached through this exposure. The periosteum at the supra-medial angle is likewise incised around the orbital margin and is stripped away from the orbital bone, carrying with it the trochlea and the superior oblique muscle. The dissection is continued as far laterally as possible and should reach into the orbit 1 cm behind the equator of the eye. The dissection should not involve the whole of the medial wall of the orbit as it is important that the

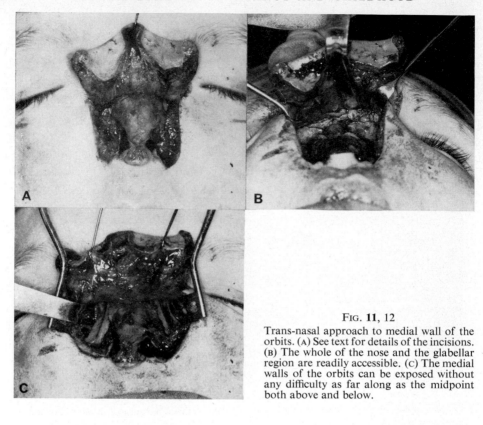

FIG. 11, 12

Trans-nasal approach to medial wall of the orbits. (A) See text for details of the incisions. (B) The whole of the nose and the glabellar region are readily accessible. (C) The medial walls of the orbits can be exposed without any difficulty as far along as the midpoint both above and below.

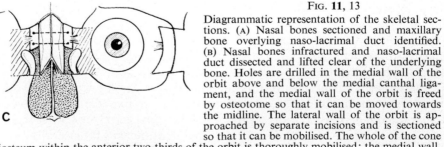

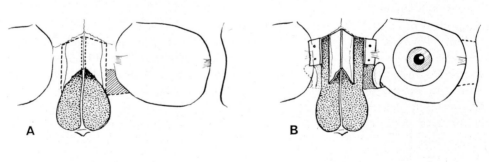

FIG. 11, 13

Diagrammatic representation of the skeletal sections. (A) Nasal bones sectioned and maxillary bone overlying naso-lacrimal duct identified. (B) Nasal bones infractured and naso-lacrimal duct dissected and lifted clear of the underlying bone. Holes are drilled in the medial wall of the orbit above and below the medial canthal ligament, and the medial wall of the orbit is freed by osteotome so that it can be moved towards the midline. The lateral wall of the orbit is approached by separate incisions and is sectioned so that it can be mobilised. The whole of the cone of periosteum within the anterior two-thirds of the orbit is thoroughly mobilised; the medial wall, along with the thin bone overlying the ethmoid air cells, is forced in towards the midline and the medial orbital margin is wired to its fellow on the opposite side.

periosteum should be left intact and attached to the bone along with the medial canthal ligament over the remaining part of the medial wall of the orbit. This area is now cut free with a chisel except along the line joining it to the thin bone overlying the ethmoidal air cells (Fig. **11**, 13B).

Attention is now turned to the lateral part of the orbit, and the periosteum along the orbital margin is divided through incisions based at the junction of the lid and cheek skin and within the lateral extremity of the eyebrow. The periosteum of the orbit is completely stripped up along the floor and roof of the orbit until the lateral wall is reached and, as before, the dissection is carried out to 1 cm beyond the equator of the eyeball. Care must be taken in the region of the infra-orbital nerve to ensure that this structure is not damaged. The lateral wall is now sectioned by a chisel above and below and these two lines of section are united within the orbit in the line to which the periosteum has been stripped up. The lateral wall is now freed and mobilised towards the midline and, having ascertained that the periosteum within the orbit is completely free from the roof and floor in the anterior part of the orbit, the medial wall with the attached medial canthal ligament is now fractured towards the midline along with the thin wall of the ethmoid air cells by the use of the thumb or a suitable instrument.

It should now be possible to shift the cone of the periosteum within the orbit along with the medial and lateral walls so that the eye can be moved bodily towards the midline. The medial orbital wall, carrying with it the medial canthal ligament, is drilled in two places and a soft stainless steel wire having been passed through the drill holes on either side, the wire is tightened to bring the medial walls of the orbits into the desired position. Overcorrection should be carried out as there is a slight tendency for the canthi to drift laterally in the first few postoperative months. The lateral wall need not be fixed and the various skin wounds are closed in layers. A plaster of Paris splint is applied to the nose and should be wide enough to produce pressure on the area of the medial canthi. The plaster of Paris nose splint and 'Roman helmet' side flaps over the lateral orbital margins should be incorporated in a plaster of Paris headcap so that it will continue to exert pressure for three weeks postoperatively.

Considerable oedema of the eyelids is to be expected in the first 10 days postoperatively but sutures may be removed at a week and the oedema will subside within 10 to 14 days.
                                                                J. C. MUSTARDÉ

REFERENCES

CONVERSE, J. M. & SMITH, B. (1962). An operation for congenital and traumatic hypertelorism. In *Plastic and Reconstructive Surgery of the Eye and Adnexa*. Ed. Troutman, R. C., Converse, J. M. & Smith, B. London: Butterworth.

CONVERSE, J. M. *et al.* (1970). Ocular hypertelorism and pseudohypertelorism. *Plastic reconstr. Surg.* **45**, 1–13.

GREIG, D. M. (1924). Hypertelorism: a hitherto undifferentiated congenital craniofacial deformity. *Edinb. med. J.* **31**, 560.

HAGE, J. (1960). Surgical approach to the external and internal nose, with a supplementary report on two cases of nasal glioma. *Br. J. plast. Surg.* **12**, 327–339.

MUSTARDÉ, J. C. (1963). Epicanthal folds and the problem of telecanthus. *Trans. Ophthal. Soc. U.K.* **83**, 397–411.

O'BRIEN, P. (1970). The surgical approach to nasal glioma. *Br. J. plast. Surg.* **23**, 1.

TESSIER, P. (1967). Entretiens sur la chirurgie orbito-cranienne. Paris.

TESSIER, P. L., GUYOT, G. & ROUGERIE, J. (1967). La Greffe dermique—procédé de protection cérébro-méningée et de blindage duremérien. *Annls Chir. plast.* **12**, 94–101.

TESSIER, P. L., GUYOT, G., ROUGERIE, J., DELGET, J. P. & PASTORIZA, J. (1967). Ostéotomies cranio-naso-orbito-faciales. Hypertelorismes. *Annls Chir. plast.* **12**, 103–118.

WEBSTER, J. P. & DENIG, E. G. (1950). Surgical treatment of the bifid nose. *Plastic reconstr. Surg.* **6**, 1.

CHAPTER XII

CRANIO-FACIAL DYSOSTOSIS
(DISEASES OF CROUZON AND APERT)

Premature closure of suture lines in the vault of the skull (cranio-stenosis) produces deformities of the vault and base due to abnormal pressure building up within the cranium itself. When these deformities are accompanied by certain specific facial deformities the name of Crouzon's disease or Apert's disease is applied to the resultant clinical picture. In the writer's view these two conditions are essentially similar but in Apert's disease the deformities tend to produce a more monstrous effect, and the hands are also deformed (syndactylism). An increased intracranial pressure is usually present and in time it may produce neurological symptoms which are only relieved by decompression osteotomy. The deformity of the skull may be mainly due to arrest in transverse development (scaphocephaly) or decrease in both antero-posterior and transverse width (brachycephaly or oxycephaly—tower skull). As far as the base of the skull is concerned the increase in intracranial pressure tends to push the base down behind the face and the cribriform plate and ethmoids in particular are prolapsed downwards. The effect on the orbits is to render these very shallow, with the roofs of the orbits becoming practically vertical. The great wings of the sphenoid are pushed forwards, contributing still more to reducing the depth of the orbit, and the lateral orbital walls fail to project forwards fully. There is in addition a hypoplasia of the maxilla, with underdevelopment of the orbital floors in a forward direction. As a result of the foregoing, the eyeball is pushed forward to such an extent that the equator of the globe may lie wholly outside the orbital rim (Fig. **12**, 1A to D). There is often a moderate degree of hypertelorism, but owing to the frequency of ocular muscle imbalance or even paraplegia, the eyes themselves may turn out in a lateral direction and this exaggerates the appearance of hypertelorism—as well as rendering fusion impossible.

There are in addition deformities of the nose (rhinomegaly), the chin (prognathia), the external canthus (dystopia with anti-mongoloid slant), and the upper lid (ptosis), all of which will require to be dealt with (Fig. **12**, 1E to G).

The aim of surgical intervention should be simultaneous correction of the exophthalmos and the retroposition of the maxilla by bringing forward the whole facial mass. The technique is designed not only to deepen the orbits but to increase the vertical diameter at the same time. (Attempts to deepen the orbit merely by adding bone grafts to the orbital margin do little to improve the condition, as the palpebral and lacrimal structures are not brought forward by this technique which merely disguises the real deformity.) Hypertelorism, if present, is also corrected at the time of the facial osteotomy (Fig. **12**, 2).

The reasons for operating are threefold: (1) improvement in function—ocular, maxillary, nasal, phonetic, (2) improvement in appearance and (3) psychological improvement (obviating the stigma of monster).

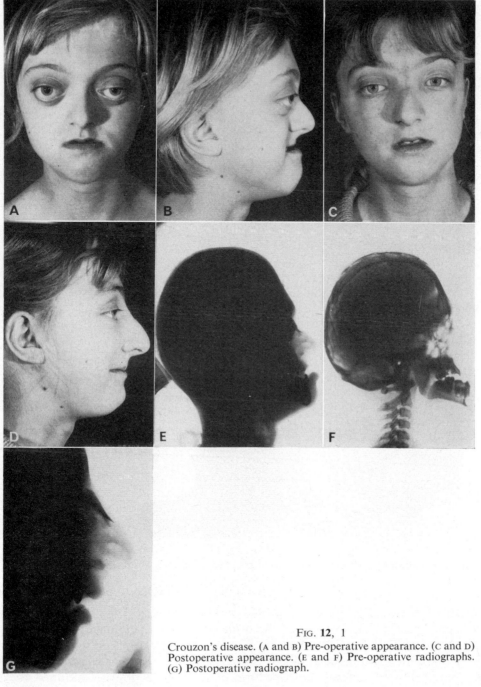

Fig. 12, 1

Crouzon's disease. (A and B) Pre-operative appearance. (C and D) Postoperative appearance. (E and F) Pre-operative radiographs. (G) Postoperative radiograph.

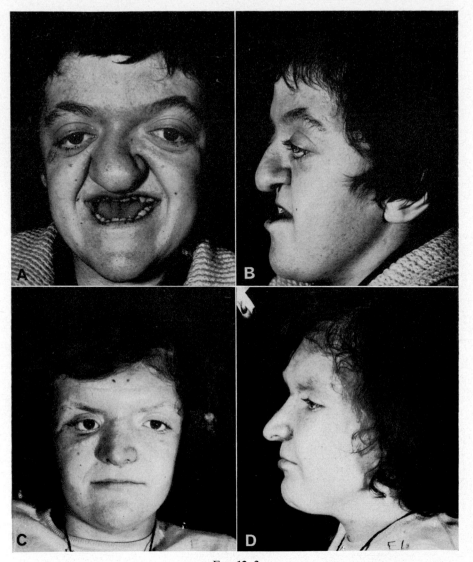

FIG. 12, 2

Apert's disease. (A and B) Pre-operative appearance. (C and D) Postoperative appearance.

PRINCIPLES OF OPERATION

1. Through carefully placed facial and frontal incisions (Fig. 12, 3), the orbit is approached and the periosteum of the orbit stripped systematically from the roof, floor, lateral and medial walls, incising it along the orbital margins.

2. Mobilisation of the facial bloc is commenced by a transverse section across the nasal bloc below the line of the cribriform plate. This section is continued back to within 15 mm of the optic foramen (Fig. 12, 4A). Damage to the cribriform plate at this stage, with c.s.f. leak, is the chief operational risk.

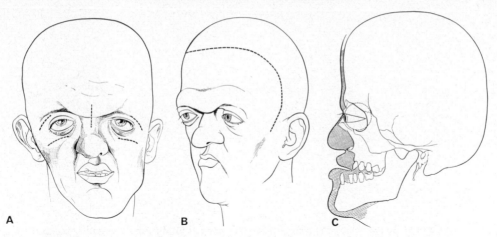

FIG. **12**, 3

Siting of incisions, with reference to skull, to permit complete stripping of periorbita and subsequent bone sections.

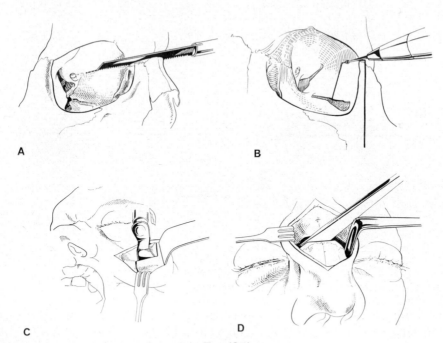

FIG. **12**, 4

Commencement of bone section of orbit. (A) Across root of nose and along medial wall. (B) Vertically on zygoma. (C) Completing zygomatic step. (D) Dividing nasal septum.

PS K

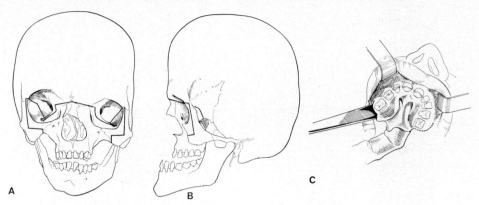

FIG. **12**, 5

(A and B) Bone sections complete. (C) Section between maxilla and pterygoid process.

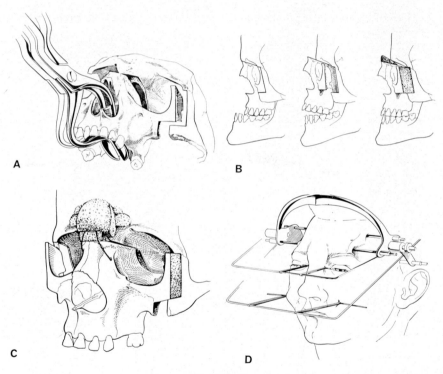

FIG. **12**, 6

Forward traction of facial bloc and insertion or onlay of bone grafts.

3. Section of the lateral walls is now carried out, and the cut is brought vertically down through the fronto-zygomatic region (Fig. **12**, 4B).

4. The bone cuts are now joined across the floor of the orbit.

5. After sagittal splitting of the outer wall of the orbit, the malar bone is cut by a step osteotomy (Figs **12**, 5 and **12**, 6).

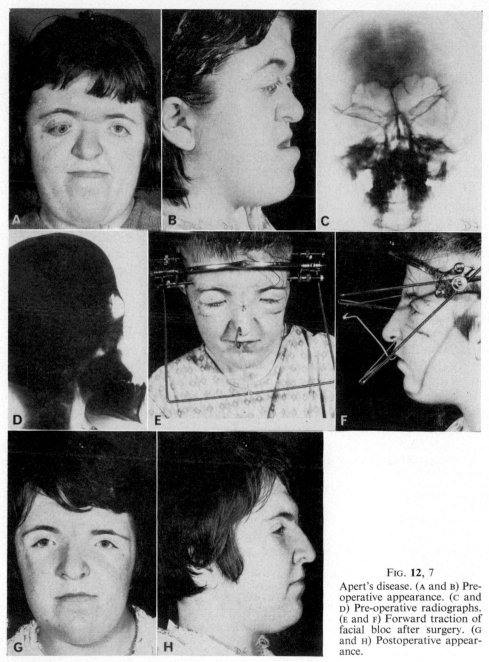

FIG. **12**, 7

Apert's disease. (A and B) Pre-operative appearance. (C and D) Pre-operative radiographs. (E and F) Forward traction of facial bloc after surgery. (G and H) Postoperative appearance.

6. Through the mouth an osteotomy is carried out between the maxilla and pterygoid process (Fig. **12**, 5C).

7. Freeing of the facial bloc is now possible, and using special forceps—and with the aid of forward traction by means of a capstan attached to a diadem which is

fixed to the skull—the whole bone bloc is drawn forward (Fig. **12**, 6). This forward transposition should be exaggerated by up to 10 mm to allow for some tendency to sink back a little postoperatively. The soft palate must be carefully preserved from injury at this stage.

8. Bone grafts are placed in the gap between the nasal bones and the frontal bone, between the separated parts of the zygomatic bones, and between the maxilla and pterygoid processes. The forehead contour is built up by additional bone grafts (Fig. **12**, 6c).

9. Postoperative traction may be exerted on the facial bloc by fixation to the diadem for a better control of the occlusion or when posterior bone grafts seem insufficient (Fig. **12**, 6D and **12**, 7).

10. Complementary surgical procedures are usually required to correct the additional deformities already mentioned, including nasal reduction (particularly in Apert's disease), application of bone grafts to the anterior surface of a very under-developed maxilla, nasal septal resection, mentoplasty, correction of lateral canthal dystopia, shortening of the levator muscle, etc. and these procedures may be carried out in one or two stages, four to six months after the main operation.

Age for operation

It might be considered that an operation such as that described above should not be carried out on the growing facial bones of a child. Neurosurgeons have shown us that age is no limitation as far as operations on the skull are concerned, and it is the writer's belief that growth is not materially affected in the face, particularly as the various suture lines are left practically undisturbed. Relief of compression symptoms and of ocular malfunction are an important argument for early operation. The writer considers that between the ages of 3 to 5 years represent theoretically the most suitable times for operation.

In practice, however, operation has been carried out after 10 years of age because of the greater ability to control the bite after the permanent teeth have erupted (Fig. **12**, 7).

P. Tessier

REFERENCES

Apert, E. (1906). De l'acrocéphalosyndactylie. *Bull. Mém. Hôp. Paris*, **23**, 1310.

Crouzon, O. (1912). Dysostose cranio-faciale héréditaire. *Bull. Mém. Soc. méd. Hôp. Paris*, **33**, 545.

Crouzon, O. (1932). Sur la dysostose cranio-faciale héréditaire et sur les rapports avec l'acrocéphalo-syndactylie. *Bull. Mém. Soc. méd. Hôp. Paris*, **48**, 1568.

Gillies, H. & Harrison, S. H. (1959). Operative correction by osteotomy of recessed malar maxillary compound in a case of oxycephaly. *Br. J. plast. Surg.* 3, 123.

Longacre, J. J., de Stefano, G. A. & Holmstrand, K. (1961). The early versus the late reconstruction of congenital hypoplasias of the facial skeleton and skull. *Plastic reconstr. Surg.* **27**, 489.

Tessier, P. (1967a). Ostéotomies totales de la face. Syndrome de Crouzon. Syndrome d'Apert. Oxycéphalies, scaphocéphalies, turricéphalies. *Annls Chir. plast.* **12**: 4, 1967.

Tessier, P. (1967b). *Entretiens sur la chirurgie orbito-cranienne*, Paris.

CHAPTER XIII

THE NOSE

ATRESIA

Unrecognized posterior choanal atresia is sometimes the cause of asphyxial death in the newborn. The atresia results from the persistence of the buccal pharyngeal and the buccal nasal membranes. In normal embryonic development these membranes perforate. The blocking partition may be membraneous, consisting of soft tissue on either side, or there may be a bony wall between the soft tissue membranes. The condition may be unilateral or bilateral. Bilateral choanal atresia in the newborn may require urgent treatment. However, the unilateral type will be more difficult to recognize since it causes fewer symptoms. In an infant who has difficulty in breathing through the nose, the passage of a flexible catheter through the nose to the nasal pharynx will confirm the diagnosis. X-ray studies using radio-opaque media injected through the nose will be helpful.

The condition may be corrected surgically by either of two approaches, a transpalatine approach or a transnasal approach. The transpalatine approach is considered the method of choice in the older child while the transnasal approach is usually used in the infant. Beinfield (1959) advises, in infants, performing the operation under a topical anaesthesia of the nasal mucous membrane; this is the nasal approach (Fig. **13**, 1).

First, a mechanical airway should be inserted. A special retractor designed by Beinfield for protecting the posterior nasopharyngeal wall should be used to prevent perforating the pharyngeal fascia. A special curette designed by the same author, marked at a distance of $1\frac{1}{4}$ and $1\frac{3}{4}$ in. from the tip serves as a guide to prevent perforation. A finger should be placed in the nasal pharynx to guard the posterior pharyngeal wall. First the curette is inserted to the $1\frac{1}{4}$ in. mark and, beginning at the floor of the nose, the soft tissue lining and the bone are curetted away. After removal of the bone, one may insert the curette an additional $\frac{1}{2}$ in. to make sure there is adequate bony opening. The toughness of the pharyngeal mucous membrane will require an incision to increase the opening. When a sufficiently large opening has been obtained, a No. 12 rubber catheter is passed through the nose and the pharynx into the mouth and grasped there. A transparent plastic tube equivalent to No. 18 French tubing is attached to the oral end of the catheter, which is then carefully withdrawn through the nose with a plastic tube following. They are guided through the nose by the finger held above the soft palate. One should make sure that the posterior end of the nasal tubing protrudes through the newly created opening into the pharynx. The anterior end should protrude slightly from the nostrils and here it can be secured by a suture fastened to an adhesive strip.

In the older child, the transpalatine approach is advised (Fig. **13**, 2). A midline incision can be used in the hard palate and this extended posteriorly or, as recommended by Roopenian and Stemmer (1958), a horse shoe-shaped incision similar to that used in a pushback palate operation can be utilised. A mucoperiosteal flap is

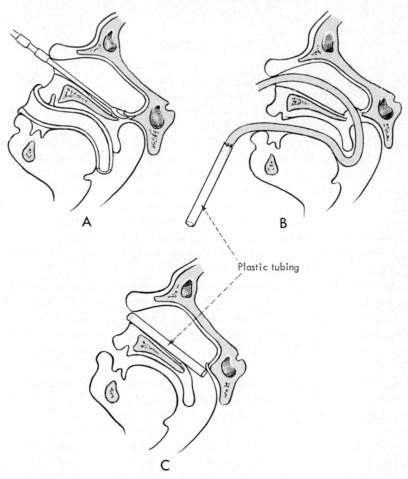

FIG. **13**, 1

(After Beinfield.) Trans-nasal operative approach for posterior choanal atresia in the newborn. (A) An oral airway is in place. Beinfield's special curette is inserted through the nose. The surgeon's index finger should be inserted into the posterior nasal pharynx to guard it while the lining and bone are curetted away. (B) An opening sufficiently large to admit a No. 18 catheter should be made. This is passed through into the mouth where similar-sized plastic tubing is attached. (C) The tubing is then withdrawn through the opening into the nose to the nostril. The tubing is secured as it emerges from the nostril.

elevated, preserving both palatine arteries. The nasal mucous membrane can then be incised posteriorly. The posterior membrane together with its bone can then be resected, possibly taking a portion of the posterior vomer and the posterior margin of the bony palate. Sufficient mucous membrane should be preserved to allow reflecting flaps, as shown in Figure **13**, 2E, to resurface the residual raw areas. If sufficient mucosa cannot be obtained for this purpose, a free skin graft inserted on a postnasal plug should be utilised.

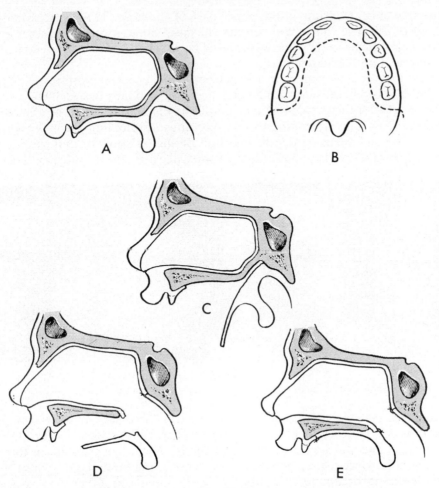

FIG. **13**, 2

For the older child, a transpalatine approach is used in posterior choanal atresia. (A) Vertical section showing the obstruction. (B) The broken line indicates the palate incision. It is similar to that used for a pushback palate operation. (C) The entire mucoperiosteum of the palate is elevated, preserving both palatine arteries. (D) An incision is made in the nasal mucous membrane of the palate. The obstructing bone is ablated but the mucous membrane is preserved. (E) Mucosal flaps are reflected to cover the denuded bone. If necessary, a free skin graft may be inserted on a postnasal plug.

DERMOID CYSTS

These are comparatively rare. In a review of the literature for the last 50 years, Crawford and Webster (1952) collected only 51 cases of nasal dermoid cysts in addition to their own 14 cases.

A dermoid cyst of the nose is a congenital malformation caused by embryonal inclusion of ectodermal remnants within the nasal septum. The usual site is in the midline of the nose and the cysts appear in two locations, either in a lower cartilaginous area (Fig. **13**, 3) or in the upper part of the nose. Those appearing in the upper part of the nose will spread beneath the nasal bone, protruding either into the glabellar region or the lower edges of the nasal bone. They must be differentiated from encephaloceles and haemangiomas.

The cyst may not be evident in the newborn and becomes noticeable only as it grows. The cyst is generally non-tender and increases gradually in size. If the secretions escape through a drainage opening the contour of the nose may still be affected. One occasionally finds hair protruding from a tiny sinus leading into the cyst. This sinus can be probed and varies in depth. Injection of such a sinus or cyst with a radio-opaque material followed by X-ray examination will clarify the diagnosis and delineate

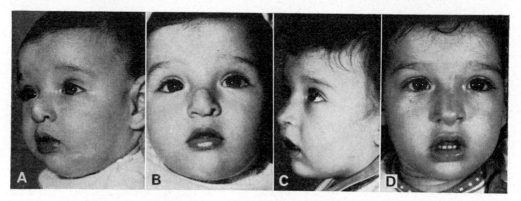

FIG. **13**, 3

Dermoid cyst of the nose. (A and B) Pre-operative. (C and D) Postoperative.

the path of the cyst, thus facilitating the surgery. It is necessary, of course, to dissect out carefully the entire lining of the cyst. Cysts located in the lower part of the nose, in the cartilaginous portion, present less difficulty than when they are in the upper part of the nose. Here it may be necessary to unroof the bony nasal arch or to split the nasal bones to obtain access to the cyst and contents. If a dye such as Bonnie's Blue is injected into the sinus at the time of operation, the dissection is easier.

HAEMANGIOMA

Haemangiomas may be found in any part of the nose. They are bluish or purplish in colour, compressible, and have a rather characteristic doughy feeling. One does not find a draining sinus in the haemangioma nor, of course, the protruding hairs that may occur in the dermoid cyst. Haemangiomas are sometimes present at birth but usually appear shortly after. The usual course is regression although the haemangioma may increase in size and may sometimes ulcerate. Regression may leave no residual disfigurement and hence no treatment may be required. However, after regression even the residual disfigurement may require surgery. In the presence of ulceration or continued growth it is advisable to treat the haemangioma. This is especially true if it constitutes a grotesque disfigurement of such magnitude that it may cause psychological complications. Surgery is indicated if the tumour can be removed in one

operation without endangering the child's life or causing further disfigurement
(Fig. **13**, 4). In larger haemangiomas that do not regress combined radio-therapy and
surgery may be utilised.

Haemangiomas of the tip of the nose may be approached either through a split
columella incision or a columella lift incision that follows the margin of the columella

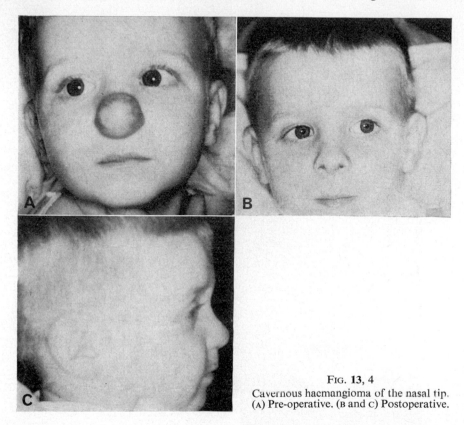

FIG. **13**, 4
Cavernous haemangioma of the nasal tip.
(A) Pre-operative. (B and C) Postoperative.

and the margins of the nasal tip. In either event, the skin flap should be reflected and
the haemangioma dissected away completely and the bone coagulated. The skin may
be preserved if it has not been invaded. If it has been invaded, the closure may be
difficult.

NASAL ENCEPHALOCELE

Nasal encephalocele is a rare congenital defect present and noticeable at birth
(Fig. **13**, 5). It is an ependyma-lined space filled with cerebrospinal fluid communicat-
ing directly with the ventricles of the brain. It may protrude on a stalk through the
foramen caecum into the glabellar area. The encephalocele is compressible and it does
not present the smooth, even swelling of a dermoid cystic mass. The encephalocele
should be completely excised and the dural defect closed. It is important to diagnose

PS K 2

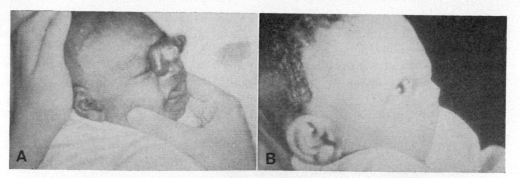

Fig. 13, 5
Nasal encephalocele. (A) Pre-operative. (B) Postoperative.

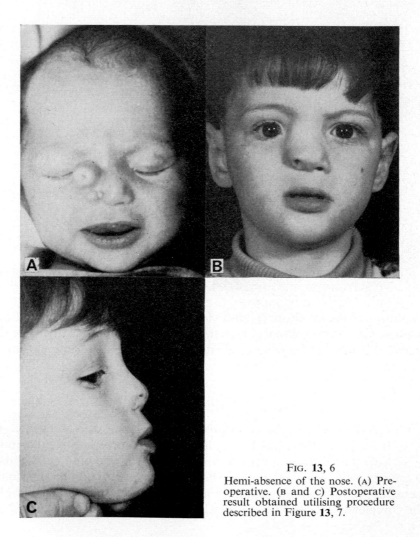

Fig. 13, 6
Hemi-absence of the nose. (A) Pre-operative. (B and C) Postoperative result obtained utilising procedure described in Figure 13, 7.

and operate upon these cases early since they may ulcerate with consequent meningitis.

NASAL GLIOMA

This is a tumour of neurological origin usually present at birth. The usual site is in the midline at the root of the nose, sometimes on one side or the other (Dawson and Muir, 1956). The tumour is firm, rounded, nodular and attached to the bone. The glioma lies beneath the bone but penetrates through it. It will gradually increase in size unless removed and will expand the nasal bone. The proper treatment is complete excision.

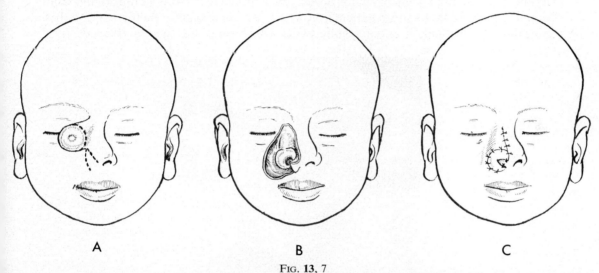

A   B   C

FIG. **13**, 7

Barsky's operation for hemi-absence of the nose. (A) The broken line indicates the incision. This is circumferential at the free end of the snout-like projection. The incision is connected medially to an inverted V on the side of the nose. This V is elevated as a small flap. (B) Wide undermining of the skin covering the projection is carried out. A supplementary incision is made along the medial side of the projection and the V-shaped flap inserted to increase the size of the opening. (C) The closure.

HEMI-ABSENCE OF THE NOSE WITH LATERAL PROBOSCIS

This is an extremely rare congenital malformation. We have had only one of these cases and two have come under our observation elsewhere. In our own case, the left side of the nose was completely normal but on the other side a small snout-like projection arose in the region of the inner canthus of the eye. This projection was tubular and there was a small amount of mucous secretion at the lower end (Fig. **13**, 6). Radiographic examination with injection of radio-opaque material showed a small pouch extending backward for 1 or 2 cm. The operation designed for the correction of this condition in one stage is shown in Figure **13**, 7.

A. J. BARSKY

ADDENDUM TO CHAPTER XIII

BIFID NOSE

(MEDIAN DYSRAPHIA OF THE FACE)

Bifid nose, or cleft nose, is a rare but important congenital deformity and its surgical correction may present quite a problem. Sanvenero-Rosselli (1953) has suggested that the deformity should be included in the malformations resulting from disturbances of fusion of the median anterior raphé.

Embryological pathology

Median dysraphia of the face seems to be related to both genetic and environmental factors, and the family history may reveal other afflicted persons (Francesconi and Gianni, 1963, 1964). In some patients, however, no such genetic factor may be discoverable, for instance in monozygotic twins where only one twin is affected. It is

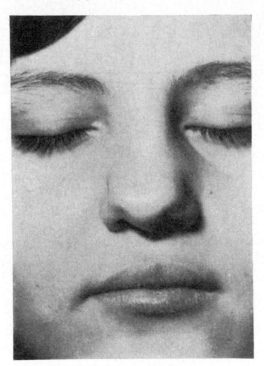

FIG. 13, 8

Mild form of bifid nose. A small groove is present in the tip region.

possible in the latter cases to suggest an interaction between genetic susceptibility to developmental disturbance and exogenous factors in the early stage of embryo growth (Fraser, 1959). It has been postulated that disturbances of fusion of the median anterior raphé may be related to anomalous growth of the primitive arterial network in the embryo (Sanvenero-Rosselli, 1953; Stark et al., 1965), and to temporary hypoxia with local accumulation of toxic products inhibiting normal fusion of symmetrical lateral structures.

Clinical findings

Clinically, bifid nose (rhinoschisis) may present in a number of forms varying from a slight groove in the lower part of the nose (Fig. **13**, 8), to the true bifid nose where the two halves are completely separated (Figs. **13**, 9 and **13**, 10). The nasal

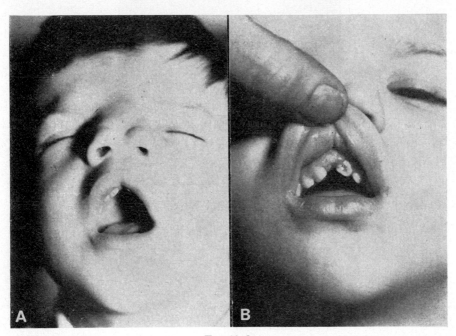

FIG. **13**, 9

(A) Patient with bifid nose. (B) As in (A) showing median cleft of upper lip, which extended into palate.

septum is frequently affected and there may be duplication of the cartilaginous septum with severe disturbance of the airways. In adult life the nasal bones are found to be completely flat, and perhaps separated by a groove. In severe cases hypertelorism is present (Fig. **13**, 10). Median cleft of either of the lips, of the tongue, of the upper or lower jaw, or of the hard and soft palate may be found in addition.

Treatment

While plastic surgery can certainly be called on to repair congenital malformations (Fig. **13**, 11), it must be pointed out that extensive surgical procedures performed in early childhood on delicate structures such as the nose may be dangerous. Although perhaps producing a satisfying result initially, the late result may be disastrous due to interference with normal tissue growth as the result of the trauma of the operation. Nevertheless, small operations as shown in Figure **13**, 11 can be performed in childhood to improve nasal respiration and get rid of some of the deformity, but a full

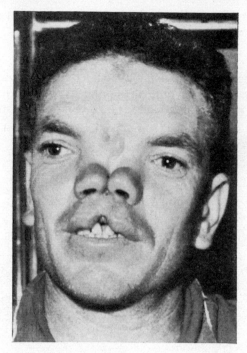

FIG. 13, 10

Adult with bifid nose. Note flattening and separation of nasal bones, and median cleft of upper lip.

plastic repair of the nose—which will involve cartilage and bone—must be deferred until late childhood or early adult life when the nasal structures are more developed.

HEMI-ABSENCE OF THE NOSE

Although hemi-absence of the nose (Fig. **13**, 12) is not a frequent malformation, numerous problems arise not only from a theoretical point of view but also from that of plastic repair.

Berblinger (1928) considers hemi-absence of the nose to be a hyporhinia but, as it can be associated with lateral proboscis (Fig. **13**, 13) (see also p. 267), it is better to consider the former as hypoplastic disrhinia and the latter as dystopia.

Embryological pathology

This anomaly of development of the nose seems to be mostly related to environmental factors, as family histories do not reveal clear hereditary data.

While hemi-absence of the nose probably stems from an arrest of embryonic growth of the lateral nasal process (possibly due to aplasia of its vascular network), lateral proboscis could represent a morphologic deviation under a noxious stimulus from the naso-frontalis process.

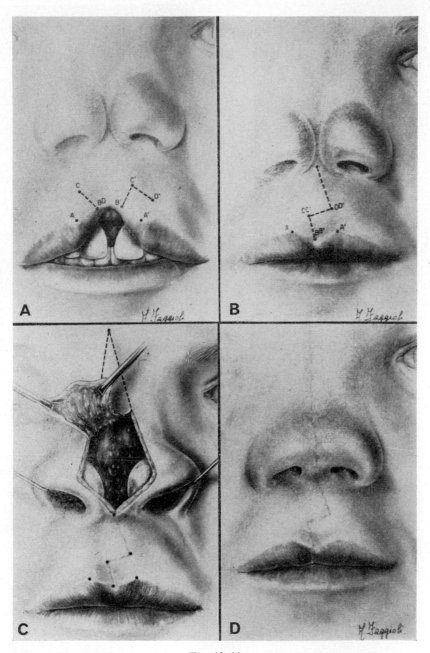

FIG. **13,** 11

(A to D) Technique for repair of bifid nose and median cleft of lip. (Courtesy of *Minerva Chirurgica.*)

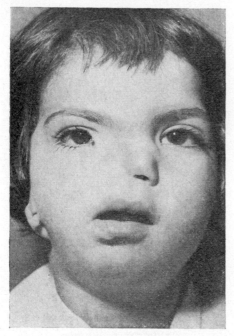

FIG. **13**, 12

True hemi-absence of the nose, with associated severe malformation of ear, lids and oral opening.

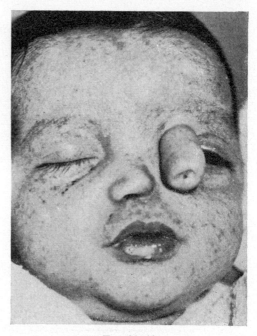

FIG. **31**, 13

Hemi-absence of the nose with lateral proboscis.

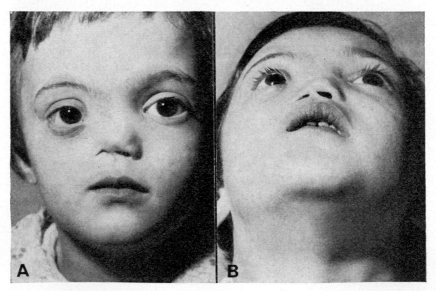

FIG. **13**, 14

The left opening of the nose is reconstructed with a free skin graft.

Clinical findings

The clinical picture of this malformation is very typical. The nose appears perfectly well developed on one side, while the other is completely missing. Only a single nostril is present, almost in a median position, and the piriform opening is narrowed by a soft or a bony membrane of the affected side, resulting in a very poor function of the nasal airways. The bridge of the nose is flat, as the nasal bone and the frontal process of the superior maxillae are missing or underdeveloped.

Treatment

As has been recently stressed, nasal respiratory disturbance has a strong influence on the moulding of the facial bone structures and on the growth of the whole body; it is therefore necessary to restore the nasal openings during childhood (Fig. **13**, 14A and B), although reconstruction of the nose must be deferred until the end of nasal growth. A 'proboscis lateralis', if present, can be opened and sutured in a proper position to restore the alar rim and the lateral wall of the nose but it is important not to sever its pedicle until the end of childhood.

G. FRANCESCONI

ACKNOWLEDGMENTS

Figures **13**, 1; **13**, 2 and **13**, 7 are reproduced from *Principles and Practice of Plastic Surgery*, 2nd edition by A. J. Barsky, S. Kahn and B. E. Simon (1964) by kind permission of the McGraw Hill Book Company.

REFERENCES

BARSKY, A. J., KAHN, S. & SIMON, B. E. (1964). *Principles and Practice of Plastic Surgery*. New York: McGraw Hill.

BEINFIELD, H. H. (1959). Surgery for bilateral bony atresia of the posterior nares in the newborn. *Archs Otolar.* **70**, 1–7.

BERBLINGER, W. (1928). Die Storungen des Formweschsel. Missbildungen der Nase. In Henke and Lubarsch: *Handb. Anat.* III, 1. Berlin.

CRAWFORD, J. K. & WEBSTER, J. P. (1952). Congenital dermoid cysts of the nose. *Plastic reconstr. Surg.* **9**, 235–260.

DAWSON, R. L. G. & MUIR, I. F. K. (1956). The fronto-nasal glioma. *Br. J. plast. Surg.* **8**, 136–143.

FRANCESCONI, G. & GIANNI, E. (1963). La Disrafia Mediana anteriore della faccia. *Minerva stomat* **12**, 447.

FRANCESCONI, G. & GIANNI, E. (1964). Su alcuni casi di rare malformazioni congenite delle cavita nasali. Contributo embriogenetico, tassonomico e bio-dinamico funzionale. *Minerva stomat.* **13**, 592.

FRASER, F. C. (1959). Causes of congenital malformations in human beings. *J. chron. Dis.* **10**, 97.

ROOPENIAN, A. & STEMMER, A. L. (1958). Congenital posterior choanal atresia. *Am. J. Surg.* **96**, 802–806.

SANVENERO-ROSSELLI, G. (1953). Developmental pathology of the face and dysraphic syndrome. An essay of interpretation based on experimentally produced congenital defects. *Plastic reconstr. Surg.* **11**, 26.

STARK, R., WASHIO, H., DE FOREST, M. & BROQUE, S. (1965). The role of vascular deficiency in the production of congenital malformation. *Plastic reconstr. Surg.* **35**, 478.

CHAPTER XIV

CORRECTIVE AND RECONSTRUCTIVE SURGERY IN DEFORMITIES OF THE AURICLE IN CHILDREN

The reconstruction of deformities of the external ear, especially those involving an absence of major portions, presents the reconstructive surgeon with a severe challenge to his technical skill and reconstructive ingenuity. Mimicking the delicate contours, closely applied skin and flexibility of the auricle often presents a well-nigh impossible challenge and in the present state of the reconstructive art a degree of compromise is demanded.

Historically the first attempts at reconstruction of the auricle are documented in the Sushruta Samhita (Bhishagratna, 1907). Cheek flaps were used to replace the loss of a large portion of the external ear. Tagliacozzi (1597) and later Dieffenbach (1845) both advocated the use of local flaps in the repair of defects of the auricle. It remained for Gillies in 1920 to lay the ground work for the modern concepts of reconstruction of large traumatic or congenital defects of the auricle by the use of costal cartilage grafts. Pierce (1930) instituted the use of the retroauricular split-thickness graft to form a postauricular sulcus.

Macrotia first attracted the attention of Cocheril (1894), who reduced the large ears by the excision of wedges of skin and underlying cartilage but it was not until 1910 that Luckett founded the basis for modern-day techniques for the correction of the protruding ear. Many varied methods for the correction of the protruding ear have been described since that time and notable among these are Barsky (1938), Young (1944), Gonzales-Ulloa (1951), McEvitt (1947), Converse et al. (1955), Holmes (1959), Converse and Wood-Smith (1963), Stenstrom (1963) and Mustardé (1964).

Anatomy

The auricle, a delicate structure of cartilage and closely applied skin, lies at an angle of approximately 30° to the adjacent scalp. The skin is closely applied to the underlying delicate, flexible, fibroelastic cartilage from which the perichondrium is peeled with difficulty. The auricle is supplied with blood by the superficial temporal and postauricular arteries and possesses a rich subcutaneous anastomotic vascular supply.

Sensation is provided by the greater auricular nerve which is aided by branches of the lesser occipital and auriculotemporal nerves. Local anaesthesia is obtained in this region by block of these nerves. The auricularis posterior muscle is occasionally well developed in patients who are able to wiggle their ears voluntarily but, apart from this amusing antic, it serves little use to its owner. The intertragus muscles are vestigial and incapable of great activity.

Embryologically the middle ear is derived from the first pharyngeal pouch which develops a dilation of its lateral extent, constricting medially to form the Eustachian tube. The lateral extent comes into contact with the ectoderm of the floor of the first branchial cleft. The ossicles are developed from the first and second branchial arches, the first arch contributing the malleus and incus and the second arch the stapes.

The external ear develops in the region of the first branchial cleft and adjacent first and second branchial arches. The mandibular arch contributes a small amount to the external appendage, the major contribution arising from the hyoid arch. At about 8 weeks of development, the primary meatus forms as a depression coming into contact with the expanding first entodermal pharyngeal pouch. The mesoderm intervening between the enterderm remains as the tympanic membrane.

His first described the external auricle in 1899 and his observations were confirmed by Arey in 1954; six hillocks developed along the first and second arches about the first branchial cleft, at the fifth intra-uterine week. Those hillocks lying on the hyphoid arch contribute the major portion of the external auricle, the first and sixth hillocks remaining relatively stable in position (Wood-Jones and Wen, 1934). Much contention still exists as to the exact relationship between these structures and anatomical defects, but microtia and faulty development of the first and second arches is frequently but not invariably seen.

MICROTIA

Microtia, a word of Greek derivation which signifies 'small ear' is a congenital malformation which varies in its extent from total absence (anotia) or small remnants to a truly miniature auricle (Fig. 14, 1). The external deformity is complicated by the functional disability of deafness, the result of imperforation of the external auditory

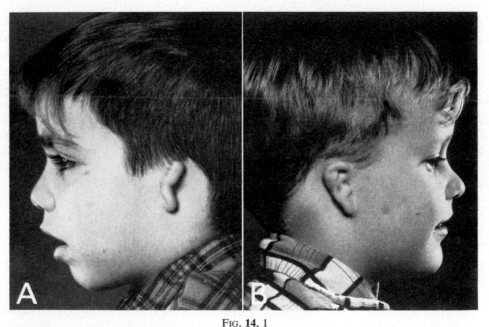

FIG. 14, 1

Variations in microtia. (A) Typical microtia with small remnants. (B) Microtia in 'small ear' with relatively large remnants.

canal, absence of the tympanum and deformity of the middle ear and ossicles.

Microtia is observed once in every 20,000 births (Holmes, 1959) with the unilateral type of microtia occurring approximately six times as frequently as the bilateral deformity (Dupertuis and Musgrave, 1959). Associated with the microtia is a failure of the development of the middle ear and this has prompted many investigators to explore the middle ear region in hopes of producing serviceable hearing.

Ear construction and hearing

It is generally agreed that attempts to improve hearing by opening the middle ear are contraindicated in unilateral microtia (Bellucci and Converse, 1960; Derlacki, 1968). The surgically established external auditory canal impinges upon the tissue and vascular supply of the area and complicates the subsequent reconstructive surgery whilst the hearing improvement does not warrant imposing upon the patient a lifetime of otologic care. When new techniques of otologic surgery make such procedures possible, the surgery should be done after the completion of the auricular reconstruction.

SURGICAL TECHNIQUE

The present concept of auricular construction is based upon the placing, in a first stage, of a meticulously fabricated autogenous cartilage framework into a subcutaneous pocket after a careful predetermination of the position of the transplant. It is emphasized that the implantation of the cartilage framework is done prior to any other surgical procedure in order that the vascularization of the skin and subcutaneous tissue be unimpaired.

The need for an adequate cartilage framework was understood by Gillies (1937), who employed maternal cartilage homografts, by Peer (1948), who prefabricated the cartilage framework by means of diced autogenous cartilage placed in a mould embedded in the abdominal wall, and by Tanzer (1959) who meticulously refined the technique of carving and assembling fragments of autogenous costal cartilage. The history of the development of the various techniques of reconstruction of the auricle was reviewed by Converse in 1958.

Cronin (1966) has introduced the use of a preformed silicone rubber auricular framework but as with all inanimate objects placed in close relationship to the skin surface has experienced problems of exposure and subsequent sepsis around the silastic framework. Although several acceptable auricular reconstructions have been completed we do not at this time favour this method.

The techniques described in this paper (Converse, 1969) are modifications of techniques previously described (Tanzer, 1959; Converse, 1963).

It is advisable, when possible, to provide the child with a new auricle prior to the beginning of his schooling. This plan offers the advantage of averting the psychological trauma which the patient is apt to suffer from the taunts he is subjected to by his schoolmates and the additional advantage of avoiding absences from school during the periods of treatment. Some children, however, have poorly developed costal cartilages at the age of 5 or 6 years, and for this reason the auricular reconstruction must be postponed. Barinka (1966) deliberately postpones the surgery until

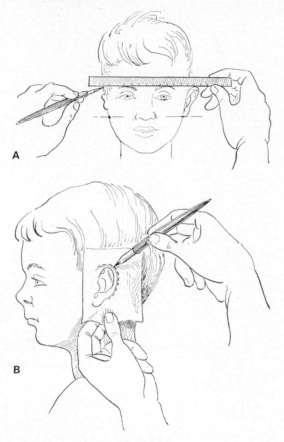

FIG. **14**, 2

Planning the new ear. (A) The position of the proposed new auricle is determined by comparison with the contra-lateral auricle. (B) The contour of the contralateral auricle is traced on transparent pliofilm.

after the age of 10 years in order to obtain sufficient cartilage to provide a carefully carved transplant.

Planning and placing the new auricle

Much of the success of the auricular construction depends upon careful pre-operative planning. The size, shape and position of the proposed new auricle are determined by the size, shape, and position of the unaffected auricle. The size of the auricle has already nearly reached adult proportions (Adamson *et al.*, 1965; Farkas *et al.*, 1966) thus, by making the new one slightly larger, symmetry between the two auricles will be maintained. Tanzer (1968) has observed growth in the reconstructed auricle.

An outline pattern of the unaffected auricle serves as a model (Fig. **14**, 2). This outline is traced in ink on a piece of transparent pliofilm or X-ray film placed over

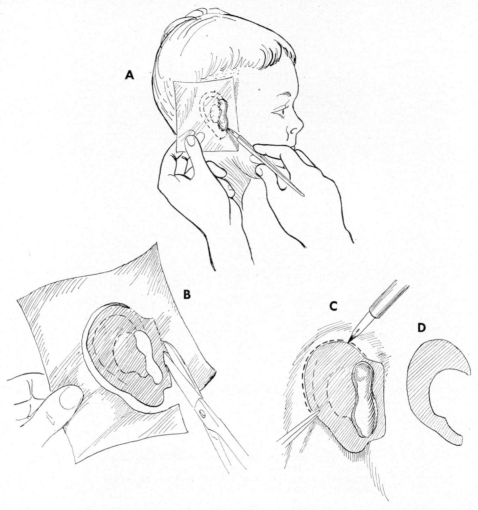

FIG. **14**, 3

Positioning the new ear. (A) The pliofilm pattern is placed in position over the microtic ear. The contour of the auricular remnants is traced. (B) The pattern of the new auricle is cut out of the pliofilm. A cut-out has also been made along the line delimiting the auricular remnants. (C) (Left) Pattern to be placed over the microtic ear at operation. (Right) Pattern of the proposed costal cartilage graft. (D) The pattern is placed over the auricular remnants, the latter fitting into the opening provided in the pattern. The outline of the proposed new ear is traced on the patient's skin.

the auricle. The auricle normally occupies a position below a horizontal line drawn through the upper edge of the eyebrow and behind a vertical line extending upward from the mandibular angle, the patient's teeth being occluded. These landmarks are of assistance when the head is oriented according to the Frankfurt horizontal plane. The angle of the mandible may be in an abnormal position on the defective side; asymmetry of the mandible is frequently associated with congenital microtia, and is a complicating factor in planning the position of the new auricle. The location of the upper border of the new auricle is best determined by comparison with the unaffected ear on full face examination (Fig. **14**, 2).

The pattern is placed in position on the defective side (Fig. **14**, 3A). The auricular remnants furnish invaluable tissue for a new lobule and should be preserved and the contour of these remnants is outlined on the pliofilm pattern. The area outlined over the remnants is cut through and removed (Fig. **14**, 3B) thus permitting the pattern of the auricle (Fig. **14**, 3C) to be placed in the correct position with the auricular remnants protruding through the opening in the pliofilm (Fig. **14**, 3D). The auricular remnants in this way assist in establishing the correct position of the new auricle when the patient is lying on the operating table.

Careful planning of the placement of the new auricle and the use of the centrifugal relaxation technique, which will be explained later in the text (see Fig. **14**, 6B), have resolved the problem of the hairline. It is not longer necessary to raise an area of the scalp as a flap, folding it upon itself and skin grafting the resulting raw area, in a preliminary stage. The centrifugal relaxation technique moves the hairline away from the auricular transplant. A few remaining hair follicles over the reconstructed ear can be successfully eliminated by electrolytic depilation.

At operation, the pattern is placed over the auricular remnants and serves to outline the position of the new auricle (Fig. **14**, 3D). It is later applied over the area of junction of two adjacent costal cartilages over, or in, the vicinity of the common cartilage formed by the union of the eighth, ninth, and tenth costal cartilages (Fig. **14**, 4).

The four principal stages of auricular construction

A new auricle can be constructed in four successive stages spaced at adequate time intervals. These are: (1) the fabrication and placement of the new auricular framework; (2) retroauricular skin grafting and placement of the lobe; (3) the 'valise handle' procedure and the construction of the external auditory canal and the tragus; and, (4) the construction of the concha.

First Stage: Fabrication and Placement of the New Auricular Framework

Removal of costal cartilage. On the operating table prior to the initiation of anaesthesia the area of the common cartilage to the eighth, ninth, and tenth ribs is located by palpation. The child's body is then flexed and a horizontal flexion crease is located and outlined with a marking pencil or pen (Fig. **14**, 4A). If the incision is made within the flexion crease subsequent scarring will be minimized. It is essential to make a sufficiently long incision to provide adequate exposure. Vertical or oblique skin incisions should be avoided as children are prone to develop hypertrophic or keloidal scars in this area. A longer, adequately healed incision line in a natural skin fold is less visible than a short, hypertrophic scar. After incision of the skin, of the fascia covering the musculature, the rectus and superior oblique muscles are cut transversely and the perichondrium covering the cartilage is exposed. Extraperichondrial dissection is then extended downward to the lower rim of the thoracic cage. Extraperichondrial elevation of the tissues is started by sharp dissection and then by blunt gauze dissection. Subperichondrial dissection would be safer, but is

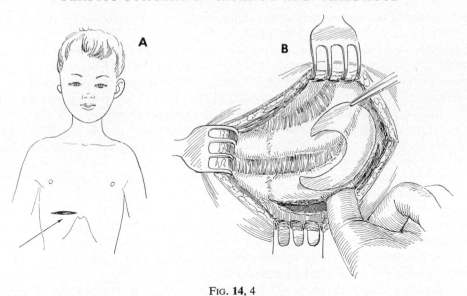

FIG. **14,** 4

First stage: removal of costal cartilage. (A) Line of incision for the exposure of costal cartilages. (B) The pattern of the new auricular framework is placed over the costal cartilages.

not feasible because two adjacent costal cartilages must be removed and the perichondrium is invaginated between the cartilages.

Throughout the years, blunt gauze dissection has proved to be the safest method of separating the pleura from the undersurface of the costal cartilages. In young children, the muscular layer between the cartilage and the pleura is extremely thin and often the pleura is in intimate contact with the perichondrium. Should the pleura be punctured or torn, pneumothorax is prevented by an increase of pressure through the closed system of anaesthesia under intratracheal intubation which maintains the lung in an expanded state. A traumatic pneumothorax is not a serious complication in a patient with good respiratory function of the opposite lung on condition that the patient is anaesthetized in a closed system. Expansion of the lung can be maintained by the anaesthetist in this manner. As soon as the opening in the pleura is discovered, aspiration is employed to suck the blood from the pleural cavity and the tear is closed with silk sutures. If closure of the pleural tear is not feasible, because of the inaccessibility of the tear, closing the muscle layer over it usually suffices. Intrapleural cavity catheter drainage may be required. Re-establishment of lung function occurs within a few days after the pneumothorax.

The cartilage of the auricular framework is removed from the area of the junction of the eighth, ninth and tenth costal cartilages through a transverse incision placed in a natural skin fold (Fig. **14,** 4A). The semirigid plastic pattern is placed over the surface of the costal cartilages and outlined in ink. As the transplant is removed through the entire thickness of the cartilage, the inner surface of the cartilage must be freed in order that the operator's hand may be placed under the cartilage, protecting the pleura (Fig. **14,** 4B).

When the costal cartilage is removed from the same side as the defective ear, it is turned inside-out to reproduce the outward curvature and inclination of the auricle. The perichondrium of the outer surface then becomes the inner surface and serves as a splint, binding the two adjacent costal cartilages together. The perichondrium is removed from the inner surface which becomes the outer surface of the new ear framework and this surface is carved into the characteristic convolutions of the framework of the ear.

An adequate auricular cartilaginous framework can usually be made of four pieces of cartilage. The main fragment provides the major portion of the new scapha with the exception of the anterior portion which requires the addition of a smaller piece. In the older child, the onlay graft for the rim of the helix is obtained from the periphery of the graft from the full thickness of the cartilage. In the younger child, it is usually necessary to employ two separate pieces for the onlay; these pieces are joined in a bevelled fashion.

The thoracic wound is then closed in layers, the skin closure being done by means of a 4/0 continuous interdermal removable suture. Careful haemostasis is necessary to avoid haematoma.

Preparation of the auricular framework. The use of a large, round cutting burr activated by an air turbine has facilitated the carving of the cartilage (Fig. **14**, 5A). The main fragment should be thinned as much as possible and through-and-through perforations may be placed judiciously, while still maintaining sufficient rigidity for its upright position, and the portion of the cartilage situated anterior to the helical rim should be deeply grooved. The lateral surface of the border of the helix is then flattened to receive a cartilage onlay which is also shaped with the air drill. The anterior surface of the onlay is grooved and the rim border should be sharp. The posterior surface of the helical rim onlay is given a rounded convex shape in order to simulate the shape of the normal rim of the helix. After the carving and shaping of the four pieces, they are joined by a fine calibre stainless steel wire (Fig. **14**, 5B and C). The wires are twisted, the ends cut and buried as illustrated in Figure **14**, 5D.

The cartilage framework should be fabricated with great care and patience for upon the quality of its shape and contour will depend the ultimate success of the ear reconstruction.

Implantation of the cartilage framework. The pattern is now placed over the cartilaginous remnants and an ink outline of the contour of the new ear is made upon the skin. The outline of a vertical incision is then made immediately posterior to the auricular remnants (Fig. **14**, 5E). The skin of the area is ballooned out by subcutaneous infiltration of a solution of procaine-adrenalin by means of a Pitkin automatic refilling syringe (Fig. **14**, 5F). This 'hydraulic dissection' elevates the skin and sub-cutaneous tissue from the underlying structures and facilitates subsequent dissection.

By careful subperichondrial dissection, the cartilaginous remnants are removed (Fig. **14**, 6B) and a loose flap of skin is thus obtained which can be extended backward to cover the exposed cartilage (Fig. **14**, 6C).

The principle of centrifugal relaxation. The skin of the area is carefully separated from the underlying structures over, and immediately beyond, the area previously outlined by the pattern (Fig. **14**, 6A).

The cartilage framework is now introduced subcutaneously (Figs. **14**, 6B and C)

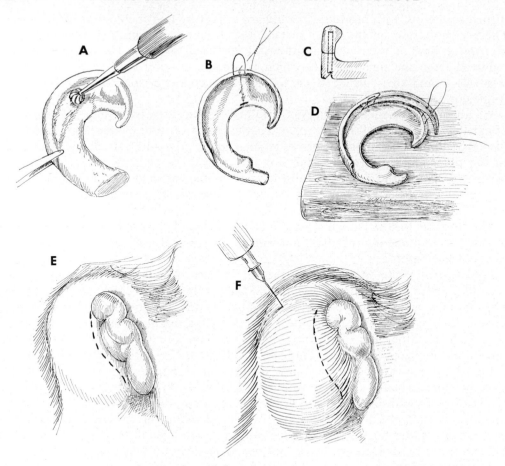

FIG. **14**, 5

First stage: fabrication and implantation of the auricular framework. (A) Carving the auricular framework by means of an air-turbine driven drill. (B) Fine calibred stainless steel wire is employed to assemble the pieces of cartilage. (C) The cartilaginous onlay is being wired into position. (D) The stainless steel wire is buried in the cartilage. A small incision is made with the point of the knife into the cartilage permitting the twisted wires to be buried. (E) Outline of the line of incision for the implantation of the cartilaginous framework. (F) The cutaneous layer is being elevated by subcutaneous injection of a solution of procaine-adrenalin.

The cartilage transplant and the projection of the helical rim raises the skin over the cartilage framework (Fig. **14**, 6B). This centrifugal relaxation usually results in an exposure of a portion of the cartilaginous framework. An additional flap of skin is required to cover the framework and can usually be prepared at the expense of the skin covering the cartilaginous remnants (Fig. **14**, 6C).

Adaptation of the overlying skin to the cartilage framework is the next step. The skin must be brought into intimate contact with the cartilage in the groove situated immediately anterior to the helical rim. It must also be loose enough to adapt itself to the contour of the posterior aspect of the rim of the helix. Mattress sutures are placed through the skin edges then through the cartilage in the antihelical groove

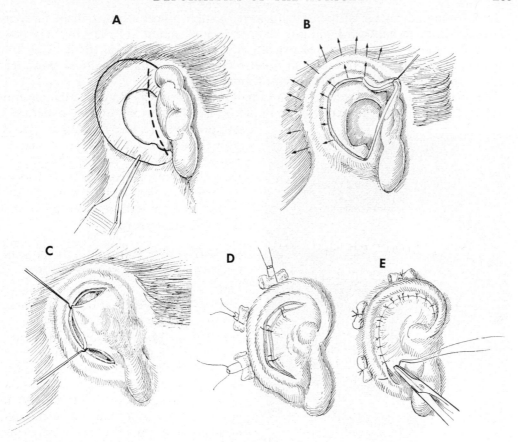

FIG. **14**, 6

First stage: implantation of the auricular framework. The principle of centrifugal relaxation. (A) Outline of the incision and placement of the pattern. (B) After the placing of the auricular framework, the covering skin relaxes in a centrifugal manner establishing a skin defect at the site of the original incision. (C) After removal of the cartilaginous remnants, a skin flap has been developed which encloses the defect produced by the centrifugal relaxation. Mattress sutures are placed through skin and cartilage. (D and E) Illustrate skin suturing and placement of the mattress sutures.

and brought out through the scalp posteriorly to the cartilaginous framework (Fig. **14**, 6D).

Three or four of these mattress sutures are necessary to provide the close adaptation of the skin to the framework. Coaptation of the skin edges is then completed by fine interrupted sutures (Fig. **14**, 6E).

This technique of centrifugal relaxation offers two advantages:

1. The skin with a thin layer of subcutaneous tissue is adequately relaxed over the cartilaginous framework and is able to adapt itself to the framework. Cartilage resorption is caused by pressure exerted by the covering cutaneous layer. The cartilage framework will maintain its original shape if soft tissue pressure is avoided. Blanching of the skin, a sign of excessive tension, does not occur and thus the danger of necrosis of the overlying skin and exposure of the subjacent cartilage is avoided.

2. A second advantage of the centrifugal relaxation procedure is that the hairline moves upward and backward and thus the presence of undesirable hair over the new auricle is avoided. The centrifugal relaxation procedure has obviated the need for preliminary rolling up of the scalp in order to provide a suitably hairless skin area prior to the implantation of the cartilage framework.

The operation is completed by placing small pledgets of teased out Acrilan cotton carefully moulded into the convolutions of the ear framework and a moderately compressive pressure dressing is placed over the area for a few days. A helmet made of plastic material (Fig. **14**, 7) protects the transplanted cartilage framework during sleep and is worn by the patient at night during the entire period of auricular construction.

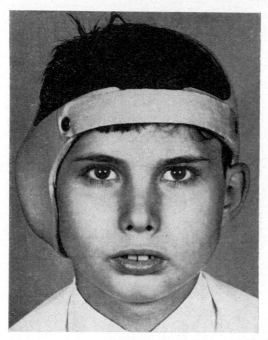

FIG. **14**, 7
Photograph of the patient wearing the helmet which protects the transplanted auricular framework during sleep.

SECOND STAGE: RETROAURICULAR SKIN GRAFTING AND PLACEMENT OF THE LOBE

After a time interval of two or three months, the auricular framework is raised (Fig. **14**, 8A, B and C). It is important that a portion of the upper part of the auricle remain attached to the cranium to ensure fixation of the new auricle and adequate blood supply. It is imperative to deepen the sulcus underneath the cartilage graft until the skin in the conchal area is reached as the skin graft should be placed in contact with the skin anterior to the cartilage framework (Fig. **14**, 8C and D). This precaution is essential to ensure that the depth of the retroauricular sulcus will be maintained during the postoperative healing period. Loss of the depth of the sulcus due to contraction of the skin graft results if the raw surface of the skin graft and of the skin situated anterior to the framework in the conchal area are not in contact. The scalp tends to retract backward, increasing the amount of skin graft required and leaving a recessed hairline. This inconvenience can be avoided by advancing and suturing the scalp to the mastoid periosteum by means of mattress sutures (Fig. **14**, 8E and F; **14**, 9A), prior to skin grafting.

The auricular remnant, now consisting of soft tissue only, is incised along its point of attachment leaving a small pedicle for blood supply (Fig. **14**, 9B and C). The remnant is now rotated posteriorly and its raw edge sutured into an incision made in the lower part of the helix border. The ilne of the former attachment of the remnant is closed by direct approximation.

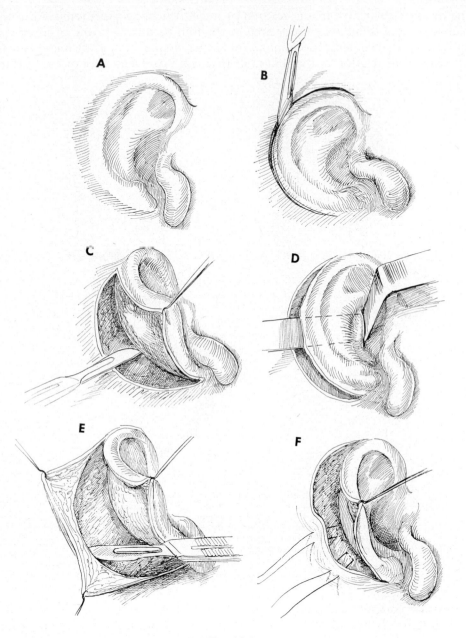

FIG. **14,** 8

Second stage: retroauricular skin grafting. (A and B) An incision is made around the periphery of the implanted auricular framework. (C) The auricular framework is raised. (D) The undermining must extend to a point anterior to the auricular framework as illustrated. (E) The scalp is undermined. (F) Advancement of the scalp is maintained by mattress sutures placed through the mastoid periosteum.

The retroauricular raw area is covered by a split-thickness graft removed from the gluteal area, a most suitable donor area in children because scarring of more visible areas is avoided. The dental compound mould technique (skin graft inlay) is usually employed for the fixation of the skin graft (Fig. **14**, 9D). Dental compound, softened

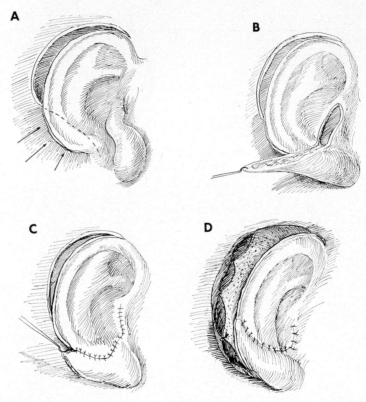

FIG. **14**, 9

(A) The scalp has been advanced, thus diminishing the retroauricular raw area. (B) The auricular remnants are raised. (C) The auricular remnants are sutured to the skin covering the auricular framework. The lower end of the cartilaginous framework penetrates the lobe. (D) A split-thickness skin graft placed over a dental compound mould provides the skin resurfacing of the retroauricular area.

in hot water, takes an impression of the raw area; it is then hardened by a spray of sterile ice water.

The dental compound mould carrying the skin graft inlay is left in position for five or six days. A period of final healing then takes place during which the usual postoperative care of skin grafts is given with careful attention to the area of junction of the skin graft with the covering skin along the helix border.

The new auricle now has a scapha, a helix and a lobe and the anterior border of the cartilaginous framework constitutes an antihelix. The new ear now requires a simulated external auditory canal, a tragus, and a concha which will be provided in subsequent stages.

THIRD STAGE: THE VALISE HANDLE PROCEDURE AND THE CONSTRUCTION OF A TRAGUS AND SIMULATED EXTERNAL AUDITORY CANAL

A suitable time interval must be allowed before undertaking this stage. A period of two months is usually adequate. A through-and-through incision is made through the skin of the retroauricular fold, the knife incising the skin along the anterior border of the cartilage implant (Fig. **14**, 10A). The helix is now raised laterally, remaining attached to the cranium above and below. This procedure is referred to as the 'valise handle' procedure (Tanzer, 1959). The edge of the skin covering the anterior lateral portion of the framework is sutured to the edge of the postauricular skin graft (Fig. **14**, 10B).

All of the skin situated anteriorly to the postauricular skin graft is now raised as a flap with an anterior pedicle. The flap is retracted forward exposing the area of the future concha and simulated external auditory canal. The flap is thinned by excision of subcutaneous tissue from its under surface. All of the subcutaneous tissue of the area is now excised until the periosteum of the mastoid is reached (Fig. **14**, 10C and D). The flap is then replaced, its anterior portion being folded upon itself to provide a tragus, and the posterior portion of the flap being placed against the mastoid periosteum (Fig. **14**, 10E). At this point, it is noted that a defect remains over the mastoid periosteum; this is covered by a full-thickness graft from the postauricular area from the unaffected ear, if available, from the supraclavicular area in male patients or by means of a medium-thickness skin graft from the gluteal area (Fig. **14**, 10F). Both the skin graft and the skin flap should be maintained by means of a pressure dressing against the mastoid periosteum in order that the cul-de-sac of the simulated external auditory canal be situated against the cranial bone. Pressure is maintained by pledgets of acrylan cotton and a compressive dressing.

FOURTH STAGE: CONSTRUCTION OF THE CONCHA

The provision of a concha is an important additional and final procedure to complete the constructed auricle. This is achieved by means of a composite graft of concha taken from the unaffected ear. In the vast majority of cases, the unaffected ear shows a lop-ear deformity. The removal of a composite graft of skin and cartilage from the concha of the unaffected ear assists in correcting the protrusion of the auricle. An operation to correct the protruding ear may also be necessary.

Following the healing of the 'valise handle' procedure, the new auricle may be retracted away from the cranium leaving an opening between the upper and lower attachments of the valise handle to the cranium. It is in this opening that the new concha will be fitted.

An outline is drawn along the site of the future antihelix and an incision made (Fig. **14**, 11A). A turnover hinge-flap is raised by separating the skin from the cartilage transplant, the pedicle of the flap being the skin covering the posterior aspect of the cartilage framework (Fig. **14**, 11B). Excess cartilage is now excised from the anterior border of the cartilage framework in order to permit making a concha of adequate size. The turnover hinge-flap is folded back, raw surface forward, and its free border is sutured into an incision made in the skin covering the mastoid process (Fig. **14**, 11C, D and E). The shape and size of the concha is now obtained. A piece of soft metal

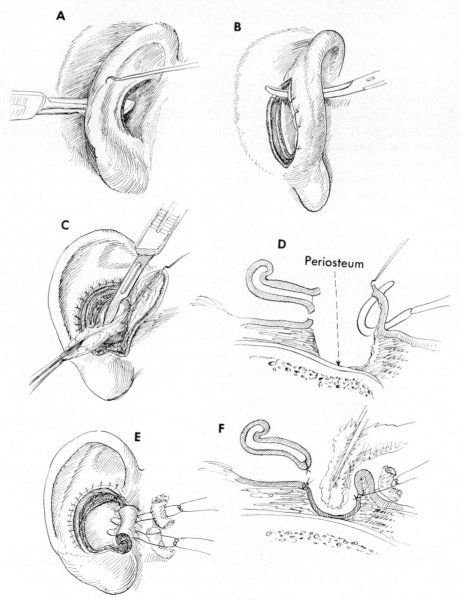

Fig. **14**, 10

Third stage: the 'valise handle' procedure and construction of a tragus and simulated auditory canal. (A) A through-and-through incision is made through the depth of the new retroauricular fold incising the skin along the anterior border of the cartilaginous implant. (B) The edge of the skin covering the anterolateral aspect of the cartilaginous framework has been sutured to the edge of the skin covering the posteromedial aspect. (C) The skin covering the future conchal area is raised as a flap with its pedicle situated anteriorly. The subcutaneous tissues are resected down to the mastoid periosteum. (D) Diagrammatic representation illustrating the resection of the subcutaneous tissues down to the mastoid periosteum. (E) Formation of the tragus by the folded flap. (F) A full-thickness graft is placed over the mastoid periosteum and maintained by a pressure dressing. Diagram illustrating the skin graft in position and the placing of the pressure dressing.

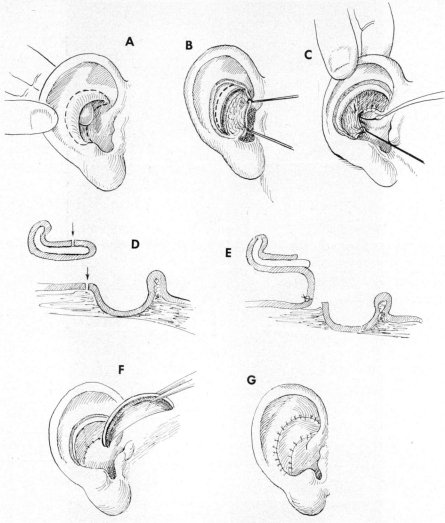

Fig. **14**, 11

Fourth stage: construction of the concha. (A) Outline of the flap to be raised from the skin covering the auricular framework. An outline of the incision to be made through the skin grafted area is also indicated. (B) The flap is raised. The dotted line indicates the amount of cartilage to be resected to enlarge the concha. (C) The free edge of the flap is sutured into the incision made in the skin grafted area. (D and E) Diagrams demonstrating the use of the flap to form the posterior skin of the new concha. (F) The composite graft of conchal skin and cartilage from the contralateral concha is ready for transplantation. (G) The composite graft is sutured into position.

(Asche, 28 gauge) is cut out as a pattern and fitted over the raw area. The soft metal pattern is placed over the raw area and tested for size. The pattern is then applied to the concha of the unaffected ear and serves to outline a composite graft of skin and cartilage. When the composite graft is removed from the donor ear and transferred to the defective ear, the medial edge of the graft becomes lateral and vice versa. It is

PS L

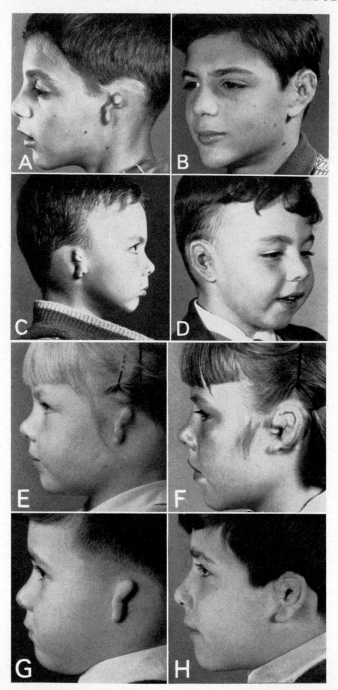

FIG. **14**, 12

Examples of patients with microtia who have undergone auricular reconstruction. The pre-operative appearance of the patient is shown in A, C, E and G; the postoperative appearance in B, D, F and H.

necessary, therefore, to place the metal pattern in an upside down position on the donor ear in order that the graft, after transfer, will fit the defect as planned. The donor area of the composite graft is covered by a retroauricular full-thickness skin graft. The graft (Fig. **14**, 11F) is now inserted into the defect and is closely adapted to the edges of the defect by sutures with close approximation of the skin edges of the graft defect (Fig. **14**, 11G). The outer edge of the cartilage of the conchal composite graft is fitted into a groove made along the under surface of the auricular cartilaginous framework. This procedure ensures the maintenance of an adequate degree of protrusion of the newly constructed auricle while the donor ear is brought closer to the side of the head. The two auricles thus tend to show the same amount of protrusion from the side of the head.

Examples of reconstructed auricles in patients with unilateral congenital microtia are shown in Figure **14**, 12.

BILATERAL MICROTIA

Bilateral microtia requires bilateral reconstructive procedures similar to those employed for unilateral microtia. As conchal cartilage is not available, the construction of the ears is terminated after the valise handle procedure. A concha can also be provided by placing a suitably shaped costal cartilage graft subcutaneously after raising the new auricle from the cranium.

Microtia in the first and second arch syndrome

A type of mandibulofacial dysostosis often referred to as the first and second arch syndrome has, as one of its frequent accompaniments, microtia. Hypoplasia of the mandible, maxilla, occasionally the orbit and facial paralysis are characteristic features of this syndrome in which there may be an underdevelopment of the entire one half of the skull. Construction of the missing auricle is one of a multitude of procedures required (see pp. 35 and 75).

Accessory auricles

Small protuberances, usually situated anteriorly to the microtic ear, often referred to as accessory auricles may be present. They should be resected, a simple procedure. Occasionally, they may connect through epithelized tunnels with the microtic ear or the middle ear. Sebaceous material may exude from these epithelized tracts which also require resection.

Prosthetic implants and prosthetic auricles

Cronin (1966) has employed a silicone implant to simulate the cartilaginous framework of the auricle. This implant is placed subcutaneously in a fashion similar to the cartilaginous transplant. The authors have had no personal experience with this technique.

Artificial ears, external prosthetic replacements for the auricle, are made to simulate the external ear and are maintained in position by means of an adhesive glue. An artificial ear is employed when surgical reconstruction is not feasible or contraindicated. The simulation is excellent when the prosthesis is made by an expert. Disadvantages of the artificial ear are that it can be avulsed readily and the colour matching is disrupted when the patient acquires a sun-tan. Most patients prefer a surgically reconstructed ear.

PROTRUDING OR LOP EAR DEFORMITY

A frequent congenital malformation, the protruding or lop ear deformity (Fig. **14**, 13) has attached to it a certain element of ridicule which can result in psychologic trauma in the affected child. For this reason operative correction at the age of 5 or 6 years, prior to schooling, is desirable.

A number of techniques are available for the surgical correction of the protruding ear. We have routinely employed the technique of Converse *et al.* (1955) and modified by Converse and Wood-Smith (1963), and with it have produced results satisfactory to both ourselves and the patient.

The first techniques for the correction of the lop ear deformity were described by Dieffenbach in 1845 and involved the removal of a segment of skin from the post-auricular sulcus followed by a direct closure thus using the skin as a form of dynamic support of the auricle in its corrected position. Morestin (1903), further modified this by excising an underlying portion of conchal cartilage to reposition the auricle closer to the patient's head; both surgeons, however, failed to appreciate the importance of the unfurled antihelix and it remained for Luckett in 1910 to appreciate the significance of this abnormality and evolve a method for its correction.

The Luckett technique

Luckett's procedure involved the excision of a strip of skin and cartilage on the scalp aspect of the antihelix followed by approximation of the cut edges of the auricular cartilage by means of exerting sutures. The problem with this technique is the production of a very sharp antihelical border thus failing completely to mimic the soft rounded contour of the normal antihelix.

Many variations of Luckett's technique exist, all attempting to soften the sharpness of the newly produced antihelix and some attempting to combine the correction with a removal of excess of conchal cartilage by direct excision of concha.

The McEvitt technique

McEvitt published a modification of the Luckett technique in 1947. He made parallel incisions along the lines of the body of the antihelix and its crura without excision of cartilage; the weakening of the cartilage in this region allowed a relatively smooth moulding of the antihelix to a more normal contour. In the excessively prominent ears, his technique was modified by the removal of a strip of cartilage and emphasis is placed on the need to remove a portion of the base of the antitragus in order to prevent excessive protrusion in this region.

A variation of this weakening and moulding method of correction of the antihelical deformity is that proposed by Holmes (1959) whereby careful incisions in the form of fish scales are produced on the postauricular aspect of the ear thus allowing for backward forming a new antihelix fold. The operation is completed by the resection of a strip of skin leaving intact the subcutaneous tissues, from the posteromedial aspect of the auricle. Ju *et al.* (1963) incised along the line of the antihelix on the anterolateral aspect of the auricle modifying the tragus and the conchal rim under direct vision. This procedure, we feel, offers the distinct disadvantages of making a scar in a prominent site albeit one barely visible, and of running the risk of haematoma formation between skin and cartilage on the anterolateral aspect of the auricle.

Mustardé (1964) produces an antihelix fold by means of buried non-absorbable mattress sutures without incising the cartilage (p. 306).

Evaluation of the deformity

The lop ear deformity requires careful preoperative analysis of its component parts in order to adapt the variations of the technique to the variations of the deformity.

The main characteristics of the lop ear are a poorly developed antihelix, an overdeveloped conchal cartilage and an increased angle between the lobule and the scalp. The following outline illustrates the various elements in the analysis of the lop ear deformity.

Analysis of the component parts

1. The antihelix is unfurled in:
   a. The body of the antihelix;
   b. The posterior-superior crus;
   c. The body and posterior-superior crus.
2. The concha shows excess cartilage:
   a. As uniform excess;
   b. In the upper third to upper half;
   c. In the lower third to lower half;
   d. In both upper and lower thirds.
3. The helix rim and conchal rim show size disparity (the cup or shell ear deformity).
4. The lobule shows:
   a. An increased angle of protrusion;
   b. An excess lobule size.
5. The machiavelian ear shows:
   a. Poor definition of the helix rim;
   b. Usually an excessive ear size;
   c. An excess conchal cartilage;
   d. A weak auricular cartilaginous framework.
6. The auricle shows a left side to right side size disparity.
7. Associated anomalies are:
   a. Darwin's tubercle;
   b. Preauricular tubercle;
   c. Miscellaneous anomalies.

The antihelix is commonly unfurled. The superior crus is poorly defined and passes imperceptibly into both the scapha and the triangular fossa which appear as a flattened area, in contrast to the inferior crus which is usually well developed. The

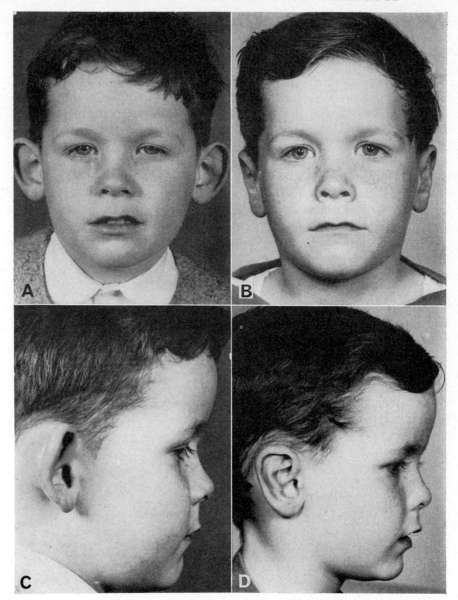

FIG. 14, 13

(A and C) Typical apearance of patient with lop ear deformity. (B and D) Postoperative views of the patient.

formation of the new contour. Converse *et al.* (1955) weakened the spring of the antihelix by the use of an electrically driven wire brush passed along the line of the antihelix. Stenström (1963) undermines the skin over the anterolateral aspect of the new antihelix and then, with a special instrument, scratches the anterior surface of the cartilage along the undermined channel. According to the author, the cartilage curls body of the antihelix is also flattened. Correction requires a partial tubing (the tube being wider superiorly) of both the body and the superior crus to form a smooth convexity between the helix and the conchal rim. Figure **14**, 13 shows a patient with flattening of the superior crus and body of the antihelix.

Excess of conchal cartilage is found throughout (Fig. **14**, 14A), or the excess may be confined only to the upper third or half (Fig. **14**, B), or to the lower third (Fig. **14**, 14C); cartilage may also be in excess above and below, being apparently of normal size in the intermediary portion (Fig. **14**, 14D). This variable component must be

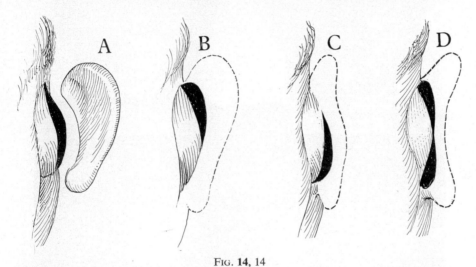

FIG. **14**, 14

Variations in the shape of the concha. (A) Uniform conchal cartilage excess. (B) Upper third to upper half conchal cartilage excess. (C) Lower third to lower half conchal cartilage excess. (D) Upper and lower third conchal cartilage excess.

evaluated before surgical removal of conchal rim as it governs the concho-scaphal angle and the vertical angle made by the ear with the skull. The importance of adequate removal of conchal rim in the upper and lower thirds cannot be over-emphasized in order to prevent the relatively common postoperative 'telephone' deformity noted in Figure **14**, 14D.

Occasionally there is a relative disparity of conchal rim size to helix rim giving an excessive 'cup' like or 'shell' appearance. The cause of this disparity may be either an excessive size of conchal rim or a relative shortage of helix. In its fully developed state, this deformity is that of a microtic ear.

The lobule may meet the mastoid process at an excessive angle. Correction is achieved by removal of both lobule tissue and mastoid skin and not by an excision of lobule skin alone which results in a deformity of the lobule.

The machiavelian ear represents a total distortion of the auricular anatomy and shows failure of definition of the helix rim, unfurling of the crura and the body of the antihelix, excess of conchal cartilage, and a general weakness of the whole auricular cartilage (Fig. **14**, 15).

Disparity in size may exist between the ears of the left and the right sides. If marked,

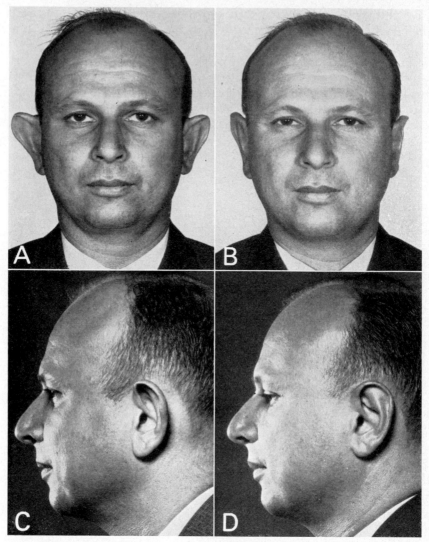

Fig. **14**, 15

(A and C) The machiavelian ear, pre-operative appearance. (B and D) The machiavelian ear, postoperative appearance.

this may be corrected by wedge excision of auricular skin and cartilage in the region of the scapha (Tanzer, 1962).

Embryonic vestiges, such as an excessively large Darwin's tubercle or preauricular tags may be removed at the time of correction of the lop ear deformity.

TECHNIQUE

The auricle is examined and the deformity analysed. This analysis is aided by pressure in the scaphal region to form an antihelix and bring into evidence the scaphal region to form an antihelix and bring into evidence the scaphal depression and the posterior border of the superior crus of the antihelix (Fig. **14**, 16A and B). It also allows evaluation of the conchal component and of the amount of skin to be removed posteriorly (Fig. **14**, 16C and D).

The operative field is prepared and draped and the procedure outlined above repeated. The patient's hair is neither clipped nor shaved. The ear is folded back by gentle pressure in the region of the scapha to produce a tubing of the body of the antihelix and the superior crus of the antihelix. The posterior border of the antihelix

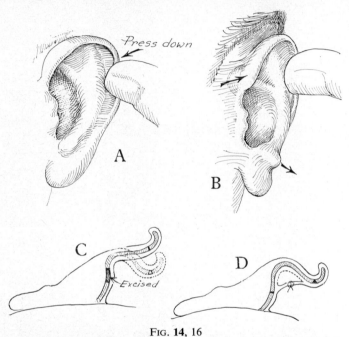

FIG. **14**, 16

Planning the corrective operation. (A) Pressure in the scaphal region forms an antihelix body and superior crus. (B) Further scaphal pressure brings into prominence the conchal rim. (C) Diagrammatic representation of the conchal and skin excess. (D) Diagrammatic representation of the corrected ear.

and the superior crus of the antihelix are outlined in ink on the anterolateral aspect of the auricle together with the anterior border of the superior crus, which is thrown into prominence by gentle pressure between the finger and thumb in the region of the junction between the superior and inferior crura (Fig. **14**, 17A and B). A third line is marked, it is parallel and immediately adjacent to the superior helical rim between the two previously marked lines but joining neither. The conchal rim is marked on the anterolateral aspect of the auricle extending superiorly into the region of the cymba conchae and inferiorly to the external auditory meatus (Fig. **14**, 17C and D).

An ellipse of postauricular skin is removed. The excision of this excess skin exposes the perichondrium. The centre line of this ellipse is determined by the passage of needles from the anterolateral aspect of the auricle through the centre line of the body of the antihelix and the superior crus (Fig. **14**, 18B and C).

Haemostasis is secured by electrocoagulation of the bleeding vessels. Skin and sub-

PS L 2

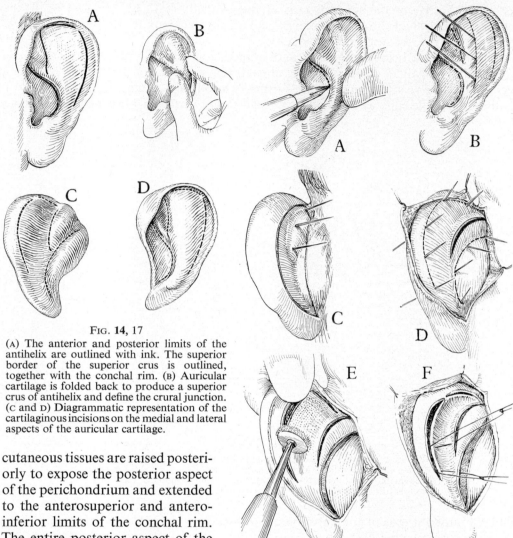

FIG. **14**, 17

(A) The anterior and posterior limits of the antihelix are outlined with ink. The superior border of the superior crus is outlined, together with the conchal rim. (B) Auricular cartilage is folded back to produce a superior crus of antihelix and define the crural junction. (C and D) Diagrammatic representation of the cartilaginous incisions on the medial and lateral aspects of the auricular cartilage.

cutaneous tissues are raised posteriorly to expose the posterior aspect of the perichondrium and extended to the anterosuperior and anteroinferior limits of the conchal rim. The entire posterior aspect of the concha is exposed down to its junction with the mastoid process (Fig. **14**, 18D).

By means of straight cutting needles, passed from the lateral aspect of the auricle to its postauricular aspect, the posterior border of the antihelix and the superior crus, the superior border of the superior crus, the anterior border of the superior crus, and the

FIG. **14**, 18

(A) The conchal rim definition is aided by pressure in the scaphal region. (B) Centre line of the superior crus and body of the antihelix is marked by needles. (C) The ellipse of skin and subcutaneous tissues is removed. (D) The skin edges are undermined, cartilage segments are outlined, and incisions are made through the cartilage to outline the marked segments. Note that the incisions do not join one another. (E) In some cases the auricular cartilage is thick and must be thinned to accomplish the tubing. This is accomplished by means of a wire brush electrically driven. (F) Sutures are placed in order to form the antihelix body and superior crus.

conchal rim are outlined. The needles may be left in place and the incisions join them or small ink spots may be made where the needle points perforate the auricular cartilage. Incisions are made through the cartilage up to, but not including, the perichondrium over the anterolateral aspect of the auricular cartilage (Fig. **14**, 18D). It will be noted that none of the incisions join one another, there being a gap of a few millimetres between the ends of each. Often the cartilage of the body of the antihelix and the superior crus requires thinning to facilitate its folding; an electrically driven wire brush or high speed nitrogen driven burr is employed for this purpose (Fig. **14**, 18E). The brush removes perichondrium and a layer of cartilage allowing for its

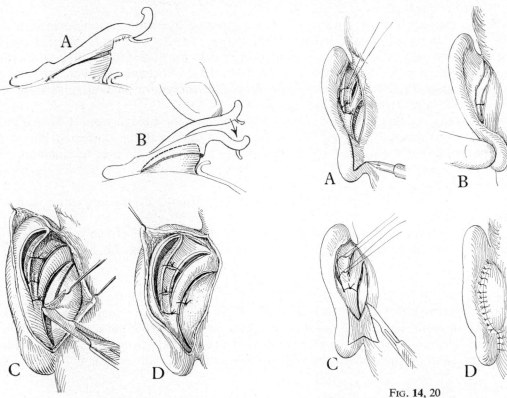

FIG. **14**, 19

(A and B) Conchal rim excess is evaluated by pressure in the region of the scapha. (C) The previously determined strip of conchal rim is excised. (D) Conchal rim and antihelix are joined by a single suture.

FIG. **14**, 20

(A) When the lobule protrudes, an ink line in the form of a 'V' is made on its medial aspect. (B) Freshly marked lobule is pressed against the mastoid process. (C) The segment of skin so outlined is excised. (D) Retroauricular defect is closed by interrupted sutures.

folding into a tube. The use of the wire brush is not always necessary as the cartilage is often sufficiently resilient to permit tubing without pretreatment.

Tubing of the cartilage is maintained by the use of 4/0 white nylon or chromic catgut sutures. The first of these sutures is placed immediately below the junction of the crura of the antihelix with the body of the antihelix, and the second, in the superior crus of the antihelix immediately above the crural junction (Fig. **14**, 18F). The sutures are tied with sufficient tension to produce the desired contour of the antihelix (see Fig. **14**, 13D).

At this stage, we have achieved the restoration of the antihelix and by means of pressure exerted in the scaphal region the amount of conchal rim resection, required to set the auricle back in a satisfactory position, is determined (Fig. **14**, 19). An ellipse of conchal cartilage is removed from the appropriate portion of the conchal rim medial to the previous conchal rim incision. Skin lying on the anterolateral aspect of the concha is undermined for a distance of 3 to 4 mm from the edges of the new conchal rim. The edges of the conchal and antihelix cartilage are approximated by means of a single suture (see Fig. **14**, 13D).

When the lobule of the ear protrudes, we continue the skin incision downward to the lobule along a line in the shape of a 'V' (Fig. **14**, 20A). Pressure of the freshly marked lobe skin against the mastoid skin makes an imprint outlining a mirror image of the skin to be resected (Fig. **14**, 20B). This 'W'-shaped segment of skin is removed (Fig. **14**, 20C), haemostasis secured, and the entire postauricular incision closed with interrupted 5/0 nylon sutures (Fig. **14**, 20D).

A pressure dressing is applied; we use small pledgets of Acrilan wool (Chemstrand Corporation) carefully packed within the convolutions of the corrected ear and covered with fluffed out gauze and cotton pads applied with mild pressure maintained by use of a cotton bandage. The pressure dressing remains undisturbed for a period of five days.

A small fold of excess skin in the conchal fossa usually disappears within two to three months.

This technique avoids sharp ridges resulting from folding of the cartilage, and produces a natural appearing concha, antihelix lobule (see Fig. **14**, 13B and D).

CRYPTOCIA

Cryptocia was first described by Kubo in 1930 and is a rare anomaly in which the upper pole of the auricle has failed to separate completely from the scalp. Correction of this deformity involves the freeing of the buried auricle from the adjacent scalp and provision of a new sulcus by shifting of skin flaps or skin grafting.

'SHELL' OR 'CUP' EARS

Caused by a deficiency in the length of the helix rim and scapha in the upper part of the auricle, this deformity is intermediary between a microtic and a protruding ear. Increase in the length of the helix rim by the addition of tissue (a local flap or a composite graft from the contralateral auricle in unilateral deformities) or by the release of the antero-superior attachment of the helix rim, combined with a procedure similar to the operation for protruding ears, will remedy the deformity (Figs. **14**, 21; **14**, 22 and **14**, 23).

When the tissue deficiency is more extensive, the surgical treatment becomes similar to that of the microtic ear: the missing cartilage framework must be provided.

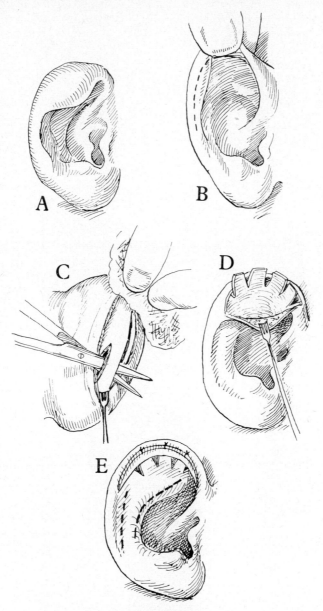

FIG. **14**, 21

The cup ear deformity: a technique application in moderate deformities (after Musgrave). (A) Illustrates the deformity. (B) Correction of the deformity by straightening the cartilage. (C) Incisions through the scaphal cartilage to correct the protrusion of the auricle. (D) Incisions through the helix permitting straightening the cartilage. (E) The corrective procedures on the auricular cartilage are completed.

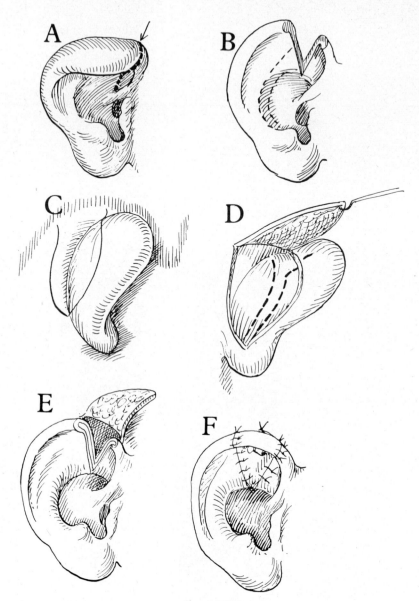

FIG. **14**, 22

The cup ear deformity: a technique to remedy tissue deficiency. (A) Outline of incisions through the anterosuperior portion of the auricle. (B) The auricle assumes a corrected position. A defect appears. (C) Outline of skin flap from retroauricular area. (D) The skin flap is raised. Incisions are outlined to correct the protrusion of the auricular cartilage. (E) A cartilage graft may be placed in the defect. (F) The skin flap covers the cartilage; the operation is completed. A simplified version of this operation is the insertion at stage B of a composite graft from the contralateral ear.

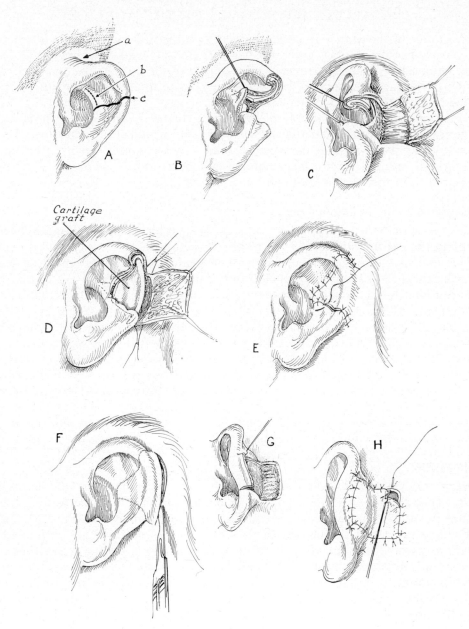

FIG. **14**, 23

The cup ear deformity: another technique to remedy tissue deficiency. (A and B) The auricle is incised through its mid-portion. The upper portion of the auricle assumes a corrected position. (C) A retroauricular flap is raised. (D) Costal cartilage is carved and transplanted into the defect. (E) The cartilage is covered by the skin flap. (F, G and H) In a second stage, the auricle is raised and a skin graft covers the retroauricular defect.

TRAUMATIC DEFORMITIES OF THE AURICLE

Deformities of the auricle in children result from various types of accidents and from burns. The deformities seen vary from irregularity and notching of the helix border, from faulty primary suture of a laceration of the auricle, to total traumatic avulsion of the ear (an extremely rare occurrence) or to total loss of the auricle from burning, a more frequent occurrence.

Because of the rich blood supply of the auricle, tissue is rarely lost in lacerations as a lacerated flap of auricular tissue even when pedunculated on a narrow strip of tissue, will survive. Adjustments must be made, in secondary repair, particularly along the helix border where a tongue and groove or Z-plasty type of procedure may be required to restore the smooth continuity of the helix.

Otohaematoma: the cauliflower ear

This type of deformity is caused by a direct blow on the ear or by traction exerted by pulling the ear forward and is the result of haemorrhage between the auricular cartilage and its covering perichondrium. If untreated, the fibrosis which develops in a haematomatous area produces a deformity commonly referred to as a cauliflower ear, and similar to the deformity frequently seen in pugilists. Preventive treatment is early evacuation of the haematoma and obliteration of the dead space after evacuation of the blood. In order to prevent recurrence of the haematoma, the soft tissue must be collapsed against the cartilage. Dental compound, softened in warm water and moulded over the area and maintained by a pressure dressing, is one method; another technique is the placing of through-and-through mattress sutures tied over bolsters of cotton or gauze, care being taken to avoid excessive pressure which would result in necrosis of the auricle.

Late treatment consists in surgical exposure of the area and carving down the fibrotic tissue in order to restore adequate contour.

Perichondritis

Loss of auricular skin usually results from burns of the external ear and an under-lying perichondritis is an all too frequent sequel. Recent studies at the Brooke Army Hospital Burns Unit have recommended the early removal of cartilage when perichondritis is evident in the burned ear in order to preserve as much non-affected cartilage as possible and the integrity of the covering skin (Dowling *et al.*, 1968).

If the decision is made to utilize this method of therapy, it is essential that it be carried out under adequate antibiotic cover early in the course of the burn and as soon as possible after evidence of cartilaginous involvement is found. Reconstruction is best attempted by a modified tunnel technique but not prior to complete softening of the auricular skin and completion of coverage of other burn sites.

Loss of auricular skin

Traumatic avulsion of the skin may occur but a more frequent cause of loss of skin is a burn. This is always a serious event as the exposed auricular cartilage undergoes necrosis complicated by perichondritis and possible loss of the entire auricular framework. Small areas of skin loss over the anterolateral aspect of the auricle may be repaired by skin grafting. More extensive uncovering of the auricular framework requires coverage by a scalp flap in order to preserve the cartilage. At a later date, the scalp flap is removed and replaced by a skin graft. Deformities resulting from loss of skin may cause the auricle to be bent forward in a protruding ear deformity when skin is lost over the anterolateral aspect of the ear. When skin is lost in the retro-auricular area, the retroauricular sulcus is obliterated and the auricle is collapsed against the cranium.

The remedy to these deformities is the replacement of the missing skin and an operation for the correction of the lop ear deformity, as previously described, may be necessary.

Lacerations and loss of skin in the external auditory canal results in stenosis and interference with audition. The treatment of stenosis of the external auditory canal is resection of the scar tissue, the fabrication of a mould of dental compound which is then covered by a split-thickness graft. An important precaution is to fabricate an acrylic tube which must be worn for a period of many months after the operation in order to prevent secondary contraction and recurrence of the stenosis.

Loss of skin along the helix border is a frequent occurrence particularly following burns. The deformity may be corrected by mobilizing the retroauricular skin forming a new helical rim and repairing the secondary defect left by the advancement of the retroauricular skin by means of a fine calibred tube pedicle flap taken along a horizontal line parallel to the skin folds of the neck, from the mastoid area, the pre-auricular area or from the inner aspect of the arm.

Loss of auricular cartilage

The technique of replacement of the missing auricular cartilage which, in traumatic deformities, varies from the loss of the helical portion of the scapha to total loss of the auricular cartilage is similar to the technique employed in congenital microtia.

The presence of well-vascularized skin and the release of skin tension over the transplanted cartilage are, as in the case of auricular construction and congenital absence, essential for the success of the reconstruction. Various techniques are available for the reconstruction of partial traumatic defects of the auricle.

J. M. CONVERSE AND D. WOOD-SMITH

ADDENDUM TO CHAPTER XIV

CORRECTION OF PROMINENT EARS USING BURIED MATTRESS SUTURES

The basis for using permanently buried mattress sutures to form or reform an antihelix fold is the fact that the auricular cartilage, stripped completely of all the connective tissue which tends to hold it in a pre-determined shape, is much more pliable than is generally appreciated. Because of this, and provided the cartilage is completely cleared of all connective tissue, it can readily be bent into a new shape and held in position by mattress sutures, with very little tension on the latter—and without any need for scoring or thinning or otherwise interfering with the cartilage itself. Where no antihelix fold exists at all (Fig. **14**, 26A) the technique is very simple and merely consists of insertion of three or four silk mattress sutures in such a position that they create an antihelix fold; but in ears where an antihelix fold is already formed (Fig. **14**, 27A) and the ear is prominent because of an excessively deep concha or excessively large upper pinna, the existing fold must be completely eradicated and a

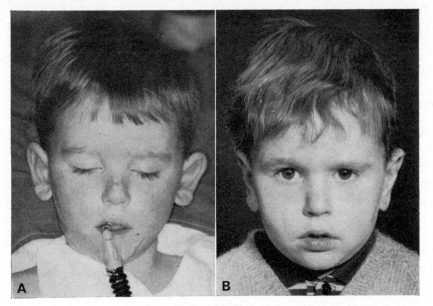

FIG. **14**, 24

Patient with bilateral prominent ears. (A) Pre-operative appearance. On the patient's left there is no antihelix fold: on the patient's right there is a well-formed antihelix fold and a deep concha. (B) Postoperative appearance.

new fold created closer to or further from the auricular-cephalic angle. Patients with ears in this latter category thus provide additional problems due to the pre-existing fold, and we have accordingly two basic types of prominent ears depending on whether or not a well-formed antihelix fold already exists (see Figs. **14**, 24 and 25).

Prominent ears with no existing antihelix fold

This technique is illustrated in Figure **14**, 26, series A to P. An antihelix fold is

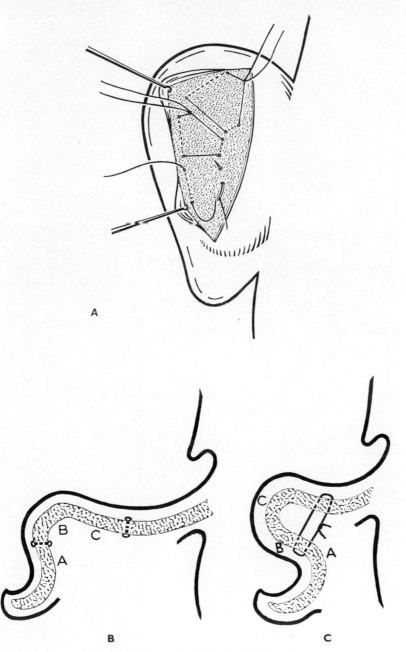

FIG. **14**, 25

Principles of the technique. (A) Insertion of non-absorbable mattress sutures in cartilage to produce antihelix fold (technique to be used on left ear). (B and C) Rolling of antihelix to create new fold closer to the scalp and making use of excess concha (technique to be used on right ear) (ref. Fig. **14**, 24).

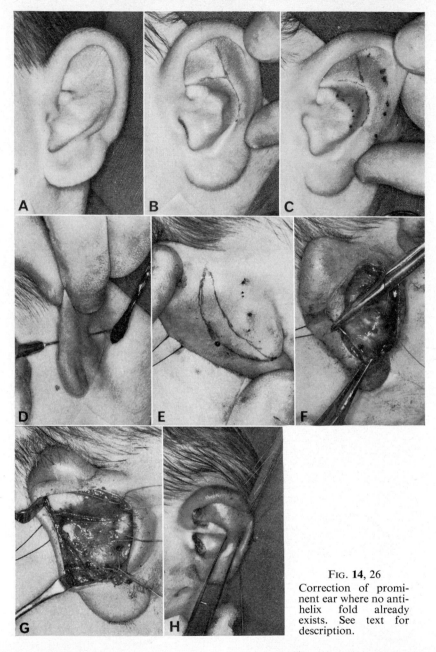

Fig. 14, 26
Correction of prominent ear where no antihelix fold already exists. See text for description.

created in a suitable position by manipulation with the fingers and the summit of this fold is marked in ink on the anterior skin surface (B). The position of three (or four in large ears) mattress sutures is marked out so that each 'bite' of the lower sutures lies 8 to 10 mm from the summit of the fold (C), or a line lying midway between the crura. The suture marks are carried through the auricular cartilage

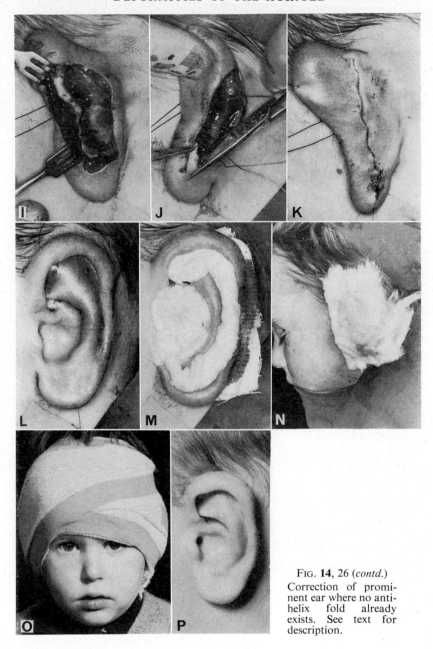

FIG. **14**, 26 (*contd.*) Correction of prominent ear where no antihelix fold already exists. See text for description.

using an ink-loaded hollow hypodermic needle (D). An ellipse of skin, 1 cm wide and about 4 cm in length, is excised from the posterior surface of the ear. This ellipse should be so sited and be large enough to allow adequate exposure of the ink marks in the cartilage (E). All excess fat and subcutaneous tissue is removed from the posterior surface of the auricular cartilage and, using curved blunt-pointed scissors, the posterior surface of the cartilage is completely exposed, from the cephalo-auricular angle to the periphery at the rim of the ear (G). This adequate exposure is essential to permit the final skin wound to lie well away from the buried mattress sutures and their knots.

The mattress sutures are now inserted (F) into the pre-determined marks in the cartilage, and it will help in pulling the cartilage into the correct shape if the knots in the lower two sutures are on the inferior component of the stitch whilst the knot on the upper suture is on the superior component (G). The material used for the buried mattress sutures should be white or colourless to avoid the possibility of the sutures being seen underneath the anterior skin and 3/0 white silk has been found to be perfectly satisfactory. The sutures must be inserted through the full thickness of the auricular cartilage, including the perichondrium on the anterior surface, but must not include the skin or dermis (a small quantity of saline injected subdermally beneath the anterior skin of the ear at the site of the ink marks can be of help here). The sutures are not drawn tight until all are inserted, and it is of importance that the tightening should be carried out whilst the anterior surface of the ear is kept under observation so that the surgeon can determine exactly how tight the suture should be to produce the desired fold. As soon as the correct degree of folding has been produced an assistant places the jaws of a pair of plain forceps across the fold to hold it in position (H) whilst the surgeon completes the knot in the suture. It is best to start with the lowest suture and work upwards. When all three sutures have been tied and a satisfactory fold has been produced (if the fold is *not* satisfactory any particular suture can be untied or removed and replaced and the fold adjusted accordingly), the loose ends of the sutures are cut off as close to the knot as possible (I). If the lobule is still projecting forward, a wedge of skin and fat can be raised from the lower end of the wound directly behind the lobule (J). Once the skin edges are sutured together, using a running intradermal stitch of 3/0 monofilament nylon (K and L), the latter is tied lightly over a small pack placed behind the ear. Such a stitch can be drawn out at the time of the first dressing with no difficulty even in the youngest child and saves pulling the ear forward to expose the suture line.

The various contours of the ear are now packed (M) with damp cotton wool which, on drying, will form an ideal cast for the ear and will, by smoothing out small kinks, help to produce the perfect shape of the various hollows of the normal ear (N). An elastic bandage is applied over the dressing and is not disturbed for 12 days (O). At this time all dressings are removed and the patient or his parents are advised that some form of protection such as a football scrum cap should be worn over the ears at night for a further two weeks (P).

Prominent ears with an existing antihelix fold

This technique is illustrated in Figure **14**, 27, series A to H. Where a fold in the auricular cartilage already exists it must be eradicated before a new fold can be created at the desired site. The technique of the operation is basically similar to that already described—with one or two important points of difference. The summit of the existing fold is marked (A). The summit of the new fold is now marked (B) and this entails rolling the cartilage either closer to or further away from the scalp, and the site of the

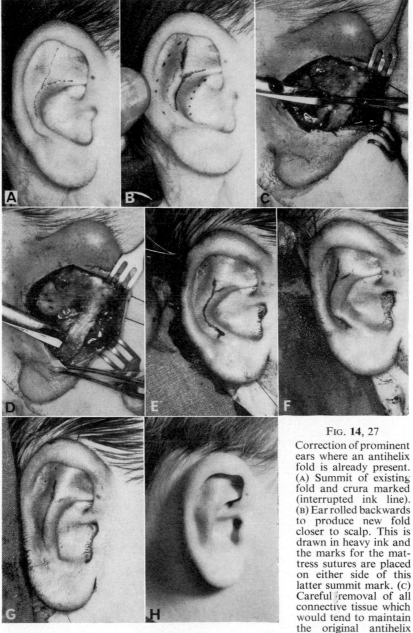

Fig. 14, 27

Correction of prominent ears where an antihelix fold is already present. (A) Summit of existing fold and crura marked (interrupted ink line). (B) Ear rolled backwards to produce new fold closer to scalp. This is drawn in heavy ink and the marks for the mattress sutures are placed on either side of this latter summit mark. (C) Careful removal of all connective tissue which would tend to maintain the original antihelix fold. (D) Freeing of the cartilage of the tail of the helix from the cartilage at the antitragus to help in the obliteration of the original fold. (E) Mattress sutures have been inserted but not tightened. Original fold still visible. (F) Mattress sutures tightened. New fold using part of the concha now created. (G) Excision of triangle of skin from posterior aspect of lobule and closure of the skin defect produce normal position of ear. (H) Postoperative appearance.

proposed sutures is indicated on either side of the new fold line. The cartilage is marked as before and the posterior surface of the cartilage exposed after removal of an ellipse of skin. Eradication of all connective tissue from the posterior surface of the cartilage must be carried out with great thoroughness (C) especially at the site of the existing antihelix fold where a considerable amount of fibrous tissue will be found in the depth of the fold. This fibrous tissue will retain the pre-existing fold unless it is thoroughly removed, and time should be spent on this, even to the extent of leaving bare cartilage, as it is the crux of the whole operation. At the lower end of the antihelix fold where it is becoming acute the sides of the fold separate into two distinct structures, the tail of the helix and the cartilage of the antitragus, and these two structures should now be completely separated from one another using scissors (D). This will permit the lower end of the antihelix fold to be moved more readily, as the two cartilages will slide, one on the other.

The silk sutures are now inserted and, beginning with the lower one they are tightened as described above. It will be found that the fold will roll into its new position (E and F), provided that all fibrous tissue has been thoroughly removed from the posterior surface of the cartilage. The subsequent steps of the operation are carried out as already described.

As already stated, to correct a horizontally shelving lobule, a wedge of skin and fat from the posterior surface of the lobule is removed in continuity with the existing skin defect. Once the continuous nylon suture has been inserted to close the skin wound it will be found that this pulls the soft lobule back into a normal position (G and H).

J. C. MUSTARDÉ

REFERENCES

ADAMSON, J. E., HORTON, C. E. & CRAWFORD, H. H. (1965). The growth pattern of the external ear. *Plastic reconstr. Surg.* **4**, 466.

AREY, L. B. (1954). *Developmental Anatomy. A Textbook and Laboratory Manual of Embryology.* 6th ed. Philadelphia: Saunders.

BARINKA, L. (1966). Congenital malformations of the auricle and their reconstruction by a new method. *Acta Chir. plast.* **8**, 53.

BARSKY, G. (1938). *Plastic Surgery.* Philadelphia: Saunders.

BELLUCCI, R. J. & CONVERSE, J. M. (1960). The problem of congenital auricular malformation. Part I Construction of the external auditory canal. Part II Construction of the auricle in congenital microtia. *Trans. Am. Acad. Ophthal. Oto-lar.* **64**, 840.

BHISHAGRATNA, K. K. L. (1907). *An English Translation of the Susruta Samhita.* Calcutta: Wilkins Press.

COCHERIL, R. (1894). Essai sur la restauration du pavillon de l'oreille. *Paris Thesis. Lille.*

CONVERSE, J. M. (1958). Reconstruction of the auricle. Part I *Plastic reconstr. Surg.* **22**, 150; Part II *Plastic reconstr. Surg.* **22**, 230.

CONVERSE, J. M. (1963). Construction of the auricle in congenital microtia. *Plastic reconstr. Surg.* **32**, 425.

CONVERSE, J. M. (1969). Construction of the auricle in unilateral congenital microtia. *Fourth International Congress in Plastic Surgery*, p. 619. Amsterdam: Exerpta Medica.

CONVERSE, J. M., NIGRO, A., WILSON, F. A. & JOHNSON, N. (1955). A technique for surgical correction of lop ears. *Plastic reconstr. Surg.* **15**, 411.

CONVERSE, J. M. & WOOD-SMITH, D. (1963). Technical details in the surgical correction of the lop ear deformity. *Plastic reconstr. Surg.* **31**, 118.

CRONIN, T. D. (1966). Use of a silastic frame for total and subtotal reconstruction of the external ear: preliminary report. *Plastic reconstr. Surg.* **37**, 399.

DERLACKI, E. L. (1968). The role of the otologist in the management of microtia and related malformation of the hearing apparatus. *Trans. Am. Acad. Ophthal. Oto-lar.* **72**, 980.

DIEFFENBACH, J. E. (1845). *Die Operative Chururgie.* Leipzig: Brockhaus.

DOWLING, J. A., FOLEY, F. D. & MONCRIEF, J. A. (1968). Chondritis in the burned ear. *Plastic reconstr. Surg.* **42**, 115.

DUPERTUIS, S. M. & MUSGRAVE, R. H.: Experience with the reconstruction of the congenital deformed ear. *Plastic reconstr. Surg.* **23**, 361.

FARKAS, I. G., DOBISIKOVA, M. & HAJNIS, K. (1966). An anthropometric contribution to the determination of reconstruction timing for hypoplastic and aplastic auricles. *Antropologie*, **4**, 1.

GILLIES, H. (1920). *Plastic Surgery of the Face*. London: Hodder and Stoughton.

GILLIES, H. (1937). Reconstruction of the external ear with special reference to the use of maternal ear cartilage as the supporting structure. *Revue Chir. struct.* **7**, 169.

GONZALEZ-ULLOA, M. (1951). An easy method to correct prominent ears. *Br. J. plast. Surg.* **4**, 207.

HIS, W. (1899). Zur entwixkelung des Acusticofacialisgebiets beim Menschen. *Arch. Anat. Phys. Anat.* Abth. Suppl.

HOLMES, E. M. (1959). A new procedure for correcting outstanding ears. *Archs Otolar.* **69**, 409.

JU, D. M. C., LI, Ch. & CRIKELAIR, G. F. (1963). The surgical correction of protruding ears. *Plastic reconstr. Surg.* **32**, 283.

KUBO, I. (1930). Beltrag zur Kenntnis der amniogenen Misskldung mit besonderer Berucksichtigung der Entstehung der Amniotischen Verwachsungen. *Virchows Arch. path. Anat. Physiol.* **276**, 241.

LUCKETT, W. H. (1910). A new operation for prominent ears based on the anatomy of the deformity. *Surgery, Gynec. Obstet.* **10**, 635.

McEVITT, W. F. (1947). The problem of the protruding ear. *Plastic reconstr. Surg.* **2**, 481.

MORESTIN, H. (1903). De la reposition et du plissement cosmetiques du pavillon de l'oreille. *Revue Orthop. Chir. Appar. mot.* **4**, 289.

MUSTARDÉ, J. C. (1964). The correction of prominent ears with buried mattress sutures. In *Modern Irends in Plastic Surgery*, ed. Gibson, T. London: Butterworths.

PEER, L. A. (1948). Reconstruction of the auricle with diced cartilage grafts in vitallium ear mould. *Plastic reconstr. Surg.* **3**, 653.

PIERCE, W. P. (1930). Reconstruction of the external ear. *Surgery, Gynec. Obstet.* **50**, 601.

STENSTRÖM, S. J. (1963). A 'natural' technique for correction of congenitally prominent ears. *Plastic reconstr. Surg.* **32**, 509.

TAGLIACOZZI, G. (1597). *De Curtorum Chirurgia per Institionem*. Bindoni.

TANZER, R. C. (1959). Total reconstruction of the external ear. *Plastic reconstr. Surg.* **23**, 1.

TANZER, R. C. (1962). The correction of prominent ears. *Plastic reconstr. Surg.* **30**, 236.

TANZER, R. C. (1968). Personal communication.

WOOD-JONES, F. W. & WEN, I. C. (1934). The development of the external ear. *J. Anat., Lond.* **68**, 525.

YOUNG, F. (1944). Casts and pre-casts cartilage grafts. *Surgery, St. Louis*, **15**, 735.

CHAPTER XV

CONGENITAL FACIAL PARALYSIS (PALSY): UNILATERAL AND BILATERAL

Congenital facial paralysis occurs in both unilateral and bilateral types. The unilateral palsy may be associated with other cranial nerve involvement and is most commonly observed in the first and second branchial arch syndrome (Rogers, 1964; Grabb, 1965). This syndrome (p. 291) consists of a spectrum of congenitally malformed facial structures which develop embryologically in the first and second branchial arches, and in their associated intervening first branchial cleft, first pharyngeal pouch, and in the primordia of the temporal bone (Grabb, 1965). When unilateral palsy is present in this syndrome, it is usually found in combination with a unilateral microtia, and an underdeveloped maxilla and mandible on the same involved side.

Surgical treatment of a child affected by *unilateral* congenital palsy has been described by Champion (1958) and by Freeman (1964). In congenital cases, in which neural repair is no longer possible, Champion advocates surgical correction, i.e., fascial lata sling suspension, before school age is reached. To prevent overcorrection in a child, the repair should be done in stages, which also helps to avoid the damaging effects of suspensory tension on the child's diminutive and delicate facial structures.

To reanimate the paralyzed corner of the mouth, Freeman prefers using an external approach for a masseter transplant to the orbicularis oris muscle, the transplant reinforced by a circumoral fascial strip usually placed as a preliminary at least five weeks prior to the masseter transfer. Others perform the masseter transfer by an oral approach to avoid placing scars on the skin of the cheek.

For correction of paralyzed eyelids, Freeman prefers to use an overlapping tarsorrhaphy, and usually reserves the temporalis muscle for a reanimation muscle transfer procedure only if the tarsorrhaphy is inadequate. Champion recommends a lateral tarsorrhaphy of an edge as an alternative procedure. Removal of a small ellipse of skin from above the eyebrow region may also give a much improved appearance to the whole upper part of the paralyzed face.

It should be emphasized, however, that there is a sad lack, to date, of any significant series of cases or comparative studies in which paediatric and adult patients are evaluated for both the similarities and differences in the aetiology of their paralyses, the type and number of different surgical procedures employed to correct their paralyses, and the length of the postoperative follow-up evaluation period. Thus, it is still very difficult for the surgeon to recommend, as yet, one specific surgical procedure in preference to another.

The first historical reference to *bilateral* congenital facial paralysis was apparently made by von Graefe in 1880 although the syndrome has been attributed to Möbius who in 1888 described several cases of the disorder and in 1892 reported on six cases of bilateral abducens and facial nerve palsy; it is to this group that Möbius's name has been assigned by medical historians.

The most comprehensive reviews of this rare syndrome are those of Henderson (1939), Danis (1945), Reed and Grant (1957), Harrison and Parker (1960) and Dalloz

314

and Nocton (1964). Although some cases of the syndrome demonstrate no hereditary history (Reed and Grant, 1957), and thus represent nongenetic forms of the disorder, Van der Weil (1957) described the syndrome in 46 persons in 6 generations, suggesting an autosomal dominant form of inheritance. In three other reports where parental consanguinity existed, recessive inheritance was suggested. From the limited information currently available, it is possible to explain the inconsistency in the familial incidence of this syndrome by the action of an irregular dominant gene.

Clinical course and physical characteristics

The Möbius syndrome is relatively uncommon (Fig. **15**, 1 and **15**, 2) and only about 125 cases have been reported to date (Gorlin, 1964). Because of the association of other congenital defects, the affected child is very rarely taken to a plastic surgeon, and more often is initially seen by the paediatrician, ophthalmologist, orthopaedic

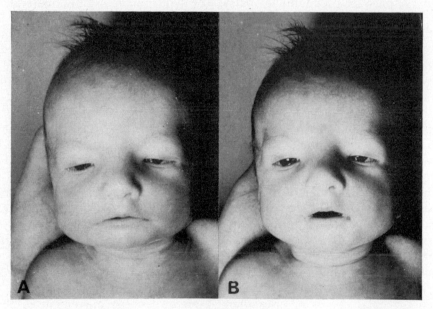

FIG. **15**, 1

Typical masklike facies in Möbius syndrome, with drooping of corners of mouth, wide nasal bridge and epicanthic folds. (*From Nisenson et al., 1955.*)

surgeon or child psychiatrist. The basic features of the Möbius syndrome—which is essentially a bilateral facial paralysis seen at birth combined with ocular muscle paralysis (and often with congenital anomalies of the extremities)—include the following:

1. Bilateral or unilateral loss of abduction of the eyes.
2. Bilateral or unilateral, complete or incomplete facial weakness.
3. Primary or secondary congenital deformities of the extremities.
4. Possible other involvement of the brachial musculature.
5. Possible other cranial nerve palsies.

Diagnosis in infants

Although the physical characteristics of the Möbius syndrome are present in the infant at birth, their detection and evaluation quite often present a difficult problem in differential diagnosis. It is here that the familiarity of a paediatrician with the physical characteristics of 'normal facial expression' in a newborn or young infant becomes of prime importance. One of the most commonly observed diagnostic signs in the infant's first few days of life is a masklike facial expression (Fig. 15, 1B) which becomes particularly evident when the infant is crying (Rubin, 1967) combined with an incomplete closure of the eyelids during sleep, and a difficulty in sucking because of the defects of the motor mechanisms of the lips. When they cry, these infants produce a type of whining noise and their laughter is a series of short 'pleasant' phonations (Nisenson *et al.*, 1955). When the infant winks, the winking movement is feeble and slow. The syndrome is frequently mistaken soon after birth for bilateral traumatic facial nerve palsy or pseudobulbar palsy. The syndrome is usually bilateral.

Diagnosis in children

The faces of children with this syndrome are also masklike, motionless and devoid of any expression. Not uncommonly, their speech is imperfect because of a pronounced inability to use the lips in forming words. There is almost always a drooping of the corners or angles of the mouth, and not infrequently a constant drooling of saliva. Food tends to lodge in the cheeks when the child eats and frequently it must be pushed out by the child's fingers (Reed and Grant, 1957). The palpebral fissures never completely close, and when the child attempts to close the lids there is quite often an involuntary movement of the eyes in an upward direction—Bell's phenomenon (Rubin, 1969). The pupils usually react to light and accommodation, and the head moves in the direction of the desired visual field owing to absence of abducting eye muscle movements beyond the midline, and paralysis of horizontal gaze. Convergence is usually present but defective, and the pupils constrict normally during convergence. Convergent strabismus is sometimes present. Owing to defective orbicularis oculi muscles and incomplete lid closure, some children have tearing, infrequent blinking and a tendency to develop recurrent, low grade keratoconjunctivitis due to exposure (Reed and Grant, 1957).

When the child laughs or cries there is no discernible movement of the facial muscles. In some children, the epicanthal folds are quite prominent, giving them the appearance of mongolism, and, unfortunately, some of these children have actually been mistaken for Mongolian idiots.

Unlike acquired facial nerve palsies, there is usually no sagging of the facial tissues. Involuntary contraction of the facial muscles, such as that seen in cases of Bell's palsy, is not generally observed. When the cheek flesh is palpated between the thumb and finger, it feels especially thin (Reed and Grant, 1957). If the bilateral palsy is not complete, the lower portions of the face are frequently less affected than the upper. In a third of the cases reported by Henderson (1939) the facial palsy was complete, but when it was incomplete, it had a characteristic distribution, with the muscles in the perioral region being the least affected and the only muscles which were capable of any movement.

Other associated anomalies

In Henderson's review of 61 cases he observed that not every case of facial diplegia was associated with abducens palsy or other ocular palsies, but most of the cases showed other congenital deformities, chiefly clubfoot, syndactylism, or absence of fingers and toes. In addition, hypoplasia of the pectoral muscles and brachial deformities were also detected. In these 61 cases, 45 had abducens palsy, 15 had ophthalmoplegia externa, 18 had lingual palsy, 6 had ptosis, 4 had trigeminal palsy, 19 had clubfoot, 23 had convergent strabismus, 13 had brachial malformations and 8 had pectoral muscle defects.

It is not uncommon for cases of Möbius syndrome to be accompanied by other cranial nerve defects including those of the motor trigeminal, oculomotor, glosso-pharyngeal and hypoglossal nerves.

Most patients with the syndrome are of normal intelligence, despite the retarding influence of congenital palsy in their formative years (Rubin, 1969). Gorlin and Pindborg (1954) report that mental retardation, in most cases not severe, occurs in approximately 10 per cent. of affected persons.

Aetiology

In his original review, Möbius suspected that the underlying aetiological factor in this syndrome was a degeneration of the central nervous system nuclei of the sixth and seventh cranial nerves. Subsequently, Lennon (1910), Richards (1953) and Dalloz and Nocton (1964) suggested that the cause might actually be a primary defect in the mesoderm with a primary agenesis or aplasia of the facial and ocular muscles and a secondary degeneration of the nerves supplying those muscles. They suggest, there-fore, that the Möbius syndrome is actually a defect in, or absence of, ocular and facial muscles with a secondary failure of development of the nerve supplying those muscles, and ultimately a degeneration of their central nervous system nuclei as a result of disuse.

Circumstantial evidence to support their hypothesis was provided by Bedrossian and Lachman (1956). They made a surgical exploration, using forced duction tests, in which they observed that adhesions and cheek ligaments, although seeming to bind down the medial and lateral rectus muscles, when freed, still did not permit the patient to abduct or adduct either eye, despite some improvement in the patient's near point of convergence. This suggested to them that, as in previous cases, the actual pathological process was peripheral in the ocular muscles themselves and in their attachments, and probably not in the nuclei of the brain stem. The controversy of a central nervous system hypoplasia versus a primary peripheral muscle defect or absence with secondary nerve degeneration has not yet, however, been conclusively settled by neuropathologists interested in this problem, although most contemporary authors seem to favour the latter concept rather than the former.

Treatment

Since most of these children are mentally normal, despite the fact that they appear dull and have verbal difficulties, they should be treated at as early a stage as possible to restore a fairly normal facial appearance, thus avoiding the stigmata and the

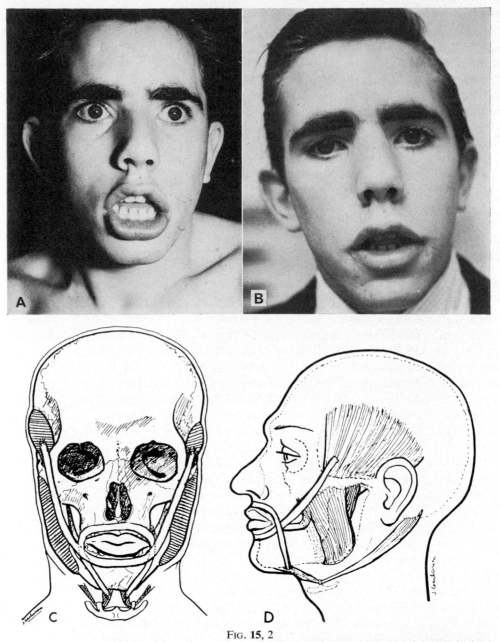

FIG. 15, 2

(A) Möbius syndrome with inability to occlude the lip borders and almost complete immobility of the face. (B) Postoperative view: the lower lip is no longer pendulous and an improvement in facial mobility is made possible by masseteric contraction. (C) Two bands of fascia lata circumscribe the buccal orifice. One of them passes under and between the muscle fibres of the lower lip and is fixed to the temporalis muscles. The other passes under and through the anterior belly of the digastric muscles. The latter is passed through the fibres of the upper lip, the former through the lower lip. (D) A flap of masseter is detached and fixed into a new position at the buccal commissure. (*From Pierre et al., 1960.*)

psychological cruelties that usually ensue when they are placed among other unaffected 'normal' children. Very little, however, has been done surgically or is reported in the reconstructive surgical correction of the Möbius syndrome. One of the few papers dealing specifically with the syndrome from the standpoint of surgical correction was written by Pierre *et al.* (1960). They described a ptsosis of the lower lip and labial inclination of the lower anterior teeth, which gave the patient (Fig. **15**, 2A) a rather ridiculous and stupid appearance; this was only one part of his total facial immobility, which they corrected by a reanimation procedure with two bands of fascia lata which circumscribed the buccal orifice. One band of fascia lata was placed like a chin strap, running from one temporal muscle to the other, passing through the lower lip in a suspensory fashion to help overcome and reduce the lip ptosis.

In addition, a myoplasty was performed, using an anterior band of masseter muscle, which was fastened at the level of the commissure itself (Fig. **15**, 2C and D). The second band of fascia lata was passed under the anterior branch of the digastric muscle and the action of the forward pull of this muscle was transmitted to the commissure by means of the fascia lata band. The aesthetic result in this single case was very satisfactory (Fig. **15**, 2B). The entire appearance of the face was markedly modified and from the static or motionless standpoint it looked much more normal; from a dynamic or functional standpoint, a slight mobility of the oral commissures was achieved.

In the surgical approach to this problem, in addition to correcting the drooping of

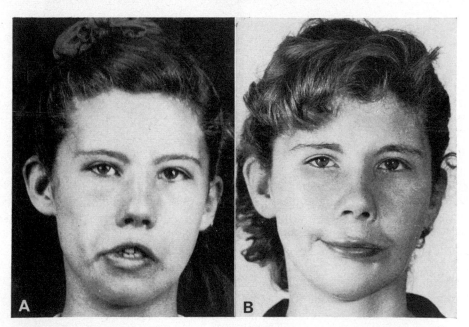

FIG. **15**, 3

(A) Patient attempting to smile before operation. Note the slight muscular action to the right of the mouth, and short upper lip. (B) Condition after bilateral masseter transplantation and lengthening of the upper lip by bilateral perialar cheek excision and a modified V-Y procedure. (*From Webster, 1956.*)

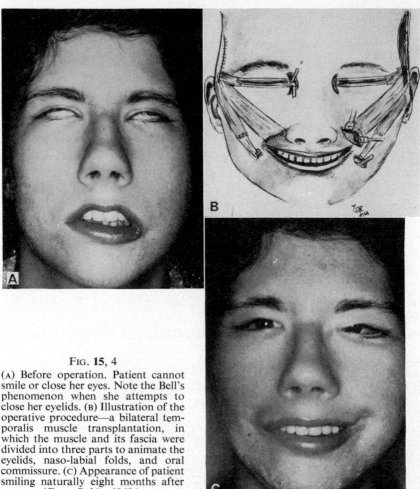

Fig. **15**, 4

(A) Before operation. Patient cannot smile or close her eyes. Note the Bell's phenomenon when she attempts to close her eyelids. (B) Illustration of the operative procedure—a bilateral temporalis muscle transplantation, in which the muscle and its fascia were divided into three parts to animate the eyelids, naso-labial folds, and oral commissure. (C) Appearance of patient smiling naturally eight months after surgery. (*From Rubin, 1969.*)

the corners of the mouth, some of the displeasing facial appearance might also be corrected by repairing the wide nasal bridge, reducing the 'bird-like' profile, and correcting the epicanthal folds that are common in some of these patients. Webster (1956) described such surgery in one patient, who was treated by a bilateral masseter transplantation, and lengthening of the short upper lip by a bilateral perialar cheek excision and a modified V-Y procedure (Fig. **15**, 3A and B).

Recently, Rubin (1969) reported successful animation of an expressionless face in a 21-year-old girl of more than average intelligence suffering from Möbius syndrome. He divided the temporalis musculature into three parts, using each part respectively to animate the eyelids, the nasolabial folds and the corners of the mouth (Figs. **15**, 4A to C), thus permitting the patient to smile and close her eyelids in a much greater approximation of normal expression than she had ever been able to accomplish before.

BLAIR O. ROGERS

REFERENCES

BEDROSSIAN, E. H. & LACHMAN, B. E. (1956). Congenital paralysis of sixth and seventh nerves: Congenita facial diplegia, congenital oculofacial palsy, Möbius syndrome. *Am. J. Ophthal.* **41**, 304.

CHAMPION, R. (1958). Re-animation of facial paresis in children. *Plastic reconstr. Surg.* **22**, 188.

DALLOZ, J. C. & NOCTON, F. (1964). Le syndrome de Moebius: à propos de deux observations nouvelles. *Archs Fr. Pédiat.* **21**, 1025.

DANIS, P. (1945). Les paralysies oculo-faciales congénitales: à propos de trois observations nouvelles. *Ophthalmologica,* **110**, 113.

FREEMAN, B. S. (1964). Facial palsy. In *Reconstructive Plastic Surgery,* ed. by Converse, J. M., Vol. III, 1124. Philadelphia: W. B. Saunders Co.

GORLIN, R. J. & PINDBORG, J. J. (1964). *Syndromes of the Head and Neck,* pp. 370–377. New York: McGraw-Hill.

GRABB, W. C. (1965). The first and second branchial arch syndrome. *Plastic reconstr. Surg.* **36**, 485.

GRAEFE, A. VON & SAEMISCH, T. (1880). *Handbuch der Gesamten Augenheilkunde.* Vol. 6. Leipzig: Wilhelm Engelmann.

HARRISON, M. & PARKER, N. (1960). Congenital facial diplegia. *Med. J. Aust.* **47**, 650.

HENDERSON, J. L. (1939). The congenital facial diplegia syndrome: Clinical features, pathology and aetiology: A review of sixty-one cases. *Brain,* **62**, 381.

KAKAR, P. K., SAWHNEY, K. L. & SAHARIA, P. S. (1966). Familial Bell's palsy: case report. *J. Lar. Otol.* **80**, 628.

LENNON, M. B. (1910). Congenital defects of the muscles of the face and eyes (Infantiler Kernschwund of Moebius): Report of three cases. *Calif. St. J. Med.* **8**, 115.

MÖBIUS, P. J. (1888). Ueber angeborene doppelseitige Abducens-Facialis-Lähmung. *Münch. med. Wschr.* **35**, 91 and 108.

MÖBIUS, P. J. (1892). Ueber infantilen Kernschwund. *Münch. med. Wschr.* **39**, 17, 41 and 55.

NISENSON, A., ISAACSON, A. & GRANT, S. (1955). Masklike facies with associated congenital anomalies (Möbius syndrome). *J. Pediat.* **46**, 255.

PIERRE, M., BUREAU, H. & GARBARINO, J. (1960). Diplégie faciale congénitale: syndrome de Moebius: correction chirurgicale. *Annls Chir. plast.* **5**, 181.

REED, H. & GRANT, W. (1957). Möbius' syndrome. *Br. J. Ophthal.* **41**, 731.

RICHARDS, R. N. (1953). The Möbius syndrome. *J. Bone J. Surg.* **35**-A, 437.

ROGERS, B. O. (1964). Rare craniofacial deformities. In *Reconstructive Plastic Surgery,* ed. Converse, J. M. Vol. 3, 1213. Philadelphia: Saunders.

RUBIN, A. (1967). *Handbook of Congenital Malformations,* p. 128. Philadelphia: Saunders.

RUBIN, L. (1969). Congenital bilateral facial paralysis—Moebius syndrome: surgical animation of the face. In *Transactions of the Fourth International Congress of Plastic Surgery.* Amsterdam: Excerpta Medica.

VAN DER WEIL, H. J. (1957). Hereditary congenital facial paralysis. *Acta Genet.* **7**, 348.

WEBSTER, J. P. (1956). The surgical treatment of bilateral congenital facial paralysis. *Fortschr. Kiefer-u. Gesichts-Chir.* **2**, 159.

CHAPTER XVI

SPECIAL PROBLEMS OF FACIAL PARALYSIS IN CHILDHOOD: THE USE OF THE STERNOCLEIDOMASTOID MUSCLE

The usual treatment of facial paralysis in childhood is described elsewhere (Chap. XV) but occasionally special problems will be encountered which will require measures to be taken for their solution.

Problem 1: Lack of growth of denervated side of face

When facial paralysis occurs in the rapidly developing and enlarging face, the muscles do not grow on the paralysed side, and a discrepancy in the size of the two sides of the face may become obvious. Supporting the face with static small facial slings will assist in restoring symmetry to the sagging mouth and cheek, but will not provide tissue to reconstruct the deficit of facial tissues on the paralysed side. A method which has been performed successfully by us consists of utilizing the sternocleidomastoid muscle on the paralysed side, as an innervated muscle transplant, and to transfer the muscle belly subcutaneously to the cheek where the ends of the muscle are attached to the labial commissure and to the upper and lower lip.

PROCEDURE

A transverse incision is made above the clavicle, and the clavicular and sternal ends of the sternocleidomastoid muscle are divided as far distally as possible. The incision is undermined superiorly and the sternocleidomastoid muscle is dissected free to the level of the ninth nerve which innervates the muscle. The blood supply to this muscle enters high on the belly and should be preserved.

A second incision is made in front of the ear and below the angle of the mandible to expose the superior portion of the sternocleidomastoid muscle. The muscle is dissected further, the vessels and nerves stretched cautiously, and the entire belly of the muscle can then be brought upward to the limit of the length of the muscle and its vessels and nerves.

The cheek is then undermined to the appropriate level (similar to a facelift) and small incisions are made in the lower lip at the mucocutaneous junction, the upper lid at the mucocutaneous junction, and at the commissure. The sternocleidomastoid muscle is brought forward into this subcutaneous pocket and is sutured to the labial musculature using 5/0 mersilene sutures (Fig. 16, 1A). The sternocleidomastoid scarcely

FIG. 16, 1

Sternocleido-mastoid muscle. (A) Transferred to the lip and left attached to mastoid bone. (B) Transferred to the zygomatic arch to provide vertical pull in facial paralysis.

322

has sufficient vertical pull to mobilise the cheek adequately if it is left attached
in the original mastoid area and, if desired, the superior attachment of the muscle
at the mastoid process can be divided, and the entire muscle transposed on its neuro-
vascular stalk. The mastoid end of the sternocleidomastoid muscle can be sutured to
the tough periostium of the zygomatic arch (Fig. 16, 1B). We prefer, however, to
delay the division of the mastoid end of the muscle for three to six weeks until
adequate attachment of the distal end has been assured.

Two objectives are accomplished by the transfer of this muscle. First, the muscle
provides dynamic animation of the previously paralysed face, and tissue excursion of
1·0 to 2·5 cm ($\frac{1}{2}$ to 1 in) is usually obtained. Secondly, the bulk of the muscle adds

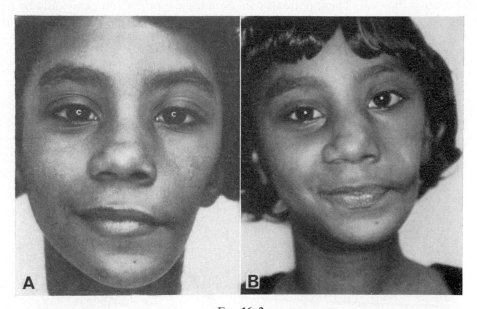

FIG. 16, 2

(A) Congenital facial paralysis in 10-year-old female. (Note lack of growth of left face and
asymmetry of lips.) (B) Postoperative view after transfer of s.c.m. muscle to upper and lower lip.
(Note animation of lips and fullness of cheek.)

substance to the deficient cheek area, and aids in restoring contour and symmetry
(Fig. 16, 2). Normal growth of the face and transferred muscle has been noted postoperatively in our small series, and these patients have not required static facial slings
for further correction.

Problem 2: Multiple cranial nerve paralysis

Infrequently following encephalitis and other serious infantile diseases, various
combinations of cranial nerve dysfunctions will exist in the same patient. Bilateral
seventh nerve paralysis in combination with bilateral fifth nerve paralysis may occur
to produce almost intolerable conditions. When such bilateral facial paralysis exists,
the lips are flaccid and the lower lip will evert: the mouth hangs permanently open
(Fig. 16, 3A), and continuous drooling will be a severe problem. Frequently the

nerves to the tongue and pharynx are involved, and swallowing and tongue motion are impaired to further complicate the problem.

If both the seventh and fifth nerve functions are absent bilaterally, a static facial sling can be positioned from attachments made bilaterally on each zygomatic arch, extending subcutaneously through the top of the lower lip to provide lip height and a lip sulcus for saliva pooling.

Such patients will have additional problems if the hyoid-mandibular musculature is functioning. Since all biting mechanisms are absent because of temporalis, ptergoid and masseteric paralysis, the mandible has no counter-acting pull to the constant traction of the anterior inframandibular musculature, and the mandible soon becomes 'bowed'. These patients can close their mouths and chew only by using manual pressure on the anterior inferior portion of the mandible, or by moving their

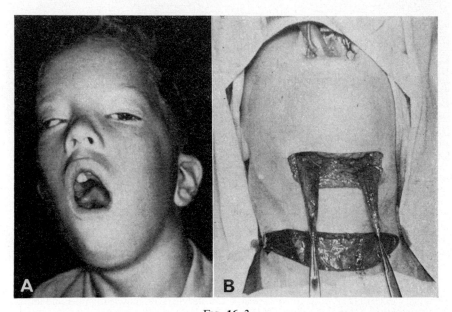

FIG. 16, 3

(A) Pre-operative view of bilateral facial and bilateral trigeminal nerve paralysis. Patient is unable to close mouth. The mandible is bowed. (B) At operation for transfer of the s.c.m. muscle to the mandible to produce closure of the mouth. The two s.c.m. muscles are crossed under the symphysis to provide a vertical pull.

head to one side and using shoulder elevation under the mandible. Usually the posterior molar teeth occlude, and the remaining ramus of the mandible curves to produce a severe open bite anteriorly.

The correction of this problem is difficult, if not impossible. Elastic chin straps have been worn by our patients; however, young children do not tolerate these. Orthodontic banding and elastic traction will not provide adequate force without disrupting the teeth.

We have again resorted to the sternocleidomastoid muscle in this unusual problem, and the patients have gained much relief, but not total correction.

PROCEDURE

Bilateral incisions (or a single long incision) are made above the clavicle on each side of the neck above the sternocleidomastoid muscle. The muscles are detached from their sternal and clavicular attachments and are freed to the vascular and nerve stalk. An incision is made under the chin, the bodies of the right and left sternocleido-mastoid muscle are brought forward under the chin, where they are crossed and each sutured to the opposite side of the mandibular periostium and to each other (Fig. **16**, 3B). The mastoid attachment of each muscle is higher than the chin and therefore provides some vertical traction. If necessary, the mastoid ends of the muscle can be transferred at a second stage to the zygomatic arch area, for a more direct pull.

When mandibular growth has been established, the mandible can be sectioned, an appropriate area removed, and occlusion restored with surgery. In our series, these patients do not regain enough motor power to provide normal mastication, and they must remain on a semi-soft non-chewing diet, or use external pressure for chewing. This muscle transfer does, however, provide adequate traction to allow continuous mouth closure, and is a source of great comfort to the patient.

C. E. HORTON, J. E. ADAMSON AND R. A. MLADICK

CHAPTER XVII

FACIAL HEMIATROPHY IN CHILDHOOD

Of all the disfiguring diseases that may occur in childhood, progressive facial hemiatrophy is one of the most frustrating. From the surgeon's point of view, treatment results have been disappointing until very recently. This is an equally disheartening situation for parent and child—there are not only the cosmetic defects but also the psychological and financial problems inherent in the long and often unrewarding treatment. The disease is about as illusive as it was when defined by Romberg in 1846.

Many causes have been suggested, but none are clearly causative (Rogers, 1963). Infection, trauma, sympathetic malfunction, and trigeminal peripheral neuritis, are some of the aetiological suggestions. Hereditary factors through an autosomal dominant gene with poor genetic penetrance is supported by some investigators (Gorlin and Pindborg, 1964). Moss and Crikelair (1960) provided some laboratory evidence for the theory of sympathetic origin by producing similar clinical signs in rats who had a sympathectomy. None of this evidence is conclusive. The theory of trauma or infection does not provide a satisfactory answer, and is likely to be coincidence rather than causation. Although there is no proof of genetic origin, the early onset and tendency to occur in more than one member of certain families may merit further study.

Of importance for our present purposes is recognition at onset, the treatments that have been used, and the treatment which seems to have provided the most promising results up to the present.

Diagnosis

The frequency of true unilateral progressive facial hemiatrophy may be under-estimated. Rogers (1963) reported 1,035 cases from the world literature from mid-nineteenth century to 1963. Of the 670 clearly identified cases, 73 had occurred in children under 2 years old. Hemiatrophy often is more severe and rapidly destructive at this early age.

Diagnosis is made more difficult by the fact that there are a number of other unilateral and bilateral facial atrophies. Romberg's disease is not congenital, but it often starts during the first two years of life and almost always starts before the end of the first decade. The maximum atrophy is usually complete within the first two to ten years of the disease's onset.

An obvious wasting of subcutaneous tissue—in fact, of all of the soft tissues on the affected side of the face—is diagnostic. The entire side may be affected or atrophy may follow the three main divisional branches of the trigeminal nerve (Fig. **17**, 1). Focal or spotty increased pigmentation often occurs, usually beginning on the cheek, lip, or forehead, and it may remain at a plateau or progress until a tanned appearance results. *Coup de sabre*, a line like a saber cut going directly down the midline of the face, is characteristic.

Muscle, bone, and cartilage may become involved in the process of atrophy. Even the tongue and ipsilateral salivary gland may be affected. Generalised neurological disorders, Horner's syndrome, exophthalmos, and perspiration defects have been reported with this disease. Contralateral jacksonian epilepsy and trigeminal neuralgia have sometimes accompanied the facial atrophy in the experience of Gorlin and Pindborg (1964).

Microscopic study shows inflammatory changes followed by excess formation of collagen. Both dermis and epidermis are atrophied as may be the adnexal structures. Flattening or absence of the rete pegs also is seen.

The differential diagnosis includes the progressive atrophy seen in linear scleroderma, lypodystrophy (usually a bilateral phenomenon), advanced degrees of facial asymmetry, and sometimes congenital deformities associated with the first and second branchial arch syndrome.

The differences between scleroderma and hemiatrophy are hazy. Indeed, hemiatrophy may result from scleroderma (p. 567). The two may be one and the same process. Typically, however, scleroderma begins with a small 'white spot' on the cheek of a young child which then progresses to low grade inflammatory changes in the skin, subcutis, later resulting in a picture similar to hemiatrophy. The typical *coup de sabre*, however, is most often a feature of Romberg's disease, and rarely seen in scleroderma.

The disease may be slowly or rapidly progressive. Also, it may quickly 'burn out' after a severe beginning in childhood. Ominously, it may appear to have been halted only to begin again as though the evident cessation was only a period of remission.

Treatment

Severity of the deformity and its potential for causing psychic disability in the youngster have led paediatricians and others who treat children to refer these patients to the plastic surgeon. Since it is very difficult to predict the progression of Romberg's disease in children, treatment should not wait until the ailment has run its course.

Traditional methods of reconstruction have proved to be disappointing, and new modalities need to be considered. Grafts of fat, dermis and fat, fascia, as well as bone and cartilage have been used. Alloplastic materials also have been tried. Implants of polyethylene, polyvinyl, and polyurethane were later used. Of course, reconstruction of soft tissue with pedicle flaps was necessary in cases of severe atrophy.

The autogenous materials were frequently absorbed, and it was inconvenient to transfer these in children because of the limited amount of tissue and the risk of a second wound. Synthetic implants were frequently no better because of insufficient soft tissue covering and the high incidence of extrusion. Paraffin injections were abandoned early because of the frequency of granuloma formation.

The method of treatment most recently evaluated is injection of dimethylpolysiloxane (liquid silicone). This material has been under intensive investigation for the past 15 years. It should be said at the outset that dimethylpolysiloxane fluid is viewed as an experimental substance even in experienced hands. Its use in the United States has been permitted pending further study and approval by the Food and Drug Administration. Both laboratory and clinical results to date have been promising.

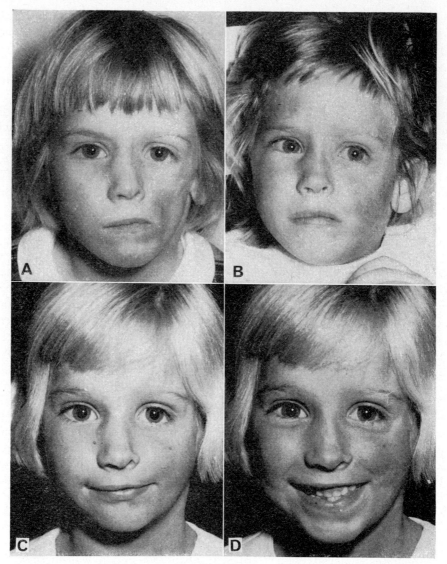

Fig. 17, 1

(A) Pretreatment appearance of typical idiopathic hemiatrophy of the left face in a 4-year-old girl. Progressive duration of about 2½ years. (B) The results after 1 year of dimethyl-polysiloxane fluid injections. A total dose of 15 ml was given at this time. (C) The result four years after beginning therapy. A total dose of 30 ml. The face is slightly firm to palpation, and the increased pigmentation persists. The contour restoration is quite adequate. (D) The patient smiling to show the absence of limitation of mobility.

The belief that the use of dimethylpolysiloxane is warranted when employed in this severe disease which has not been amenable to traditional reconstruction, and personal successful experience with it to date (Ashley *et al.*, 1965; Rees and Ashley, 1966, 1967) leads to the conclusion that this discussion is timely. The author has used liquid silicone injection in the treatment of 20 children, under the age of 15, with

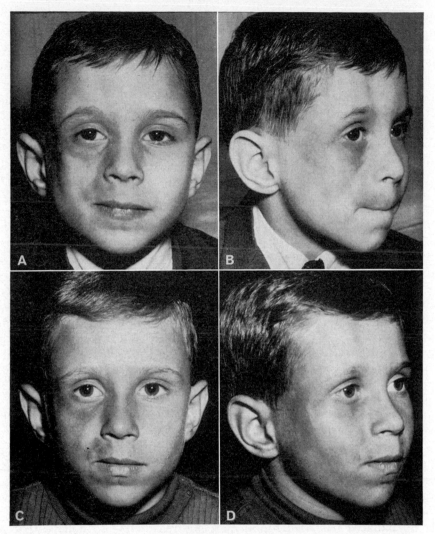

FIG. **17**, 2

(A and B) Pretreatment photographs of a 6-year-old Caucasian boy with hemiatrophy of the right face. Note the patchy increased pigmentation and the coup de sabre of the forehead. No pertinent aetiology was established. The onset was age 2½ years. (C and D) The result 1½ years after beginning silicone fluid injections. 20 ml were given in divided doses of a maximum of 2 ml per injection. As in Figure **17**, 1, the pigmentation changes persist even though the contour is markedly improved.

highly satisfactory results. The longest follow-up is nine years and the shortest is six months as of this writing.

In all cases, the injected area has been near normal to palpation and facial animation uninhibited. No evidence of lymphatic or systemic absorption in children has appeared. The illustrations (Figs. **17**, 1 and **17**, 2) show appearance before and after treatment in two of these children.

PS M 2

Technique

Tranquilization and heavy sedation are used before the procedure. The child's face is washed with hexachloraphene and then with benzalkonium chloride. A small quantity of a local anaesthetic, such as 1 per cent. lidocaine is given to anaesthetise the injection site. Then the dimethylpolysiloxane fluid is injected subcutaneously.

The liquid silicone* used by this author has a viscosity of 360 ccntistrokes (viscosity of water is 1 centistroke) which required modified equipment. A finger-and-thumb adapter from a standard 3 ml syringe is attached to a 1 ml tuberculin syringe, and the narrow column of pressure allows injection through a 26-gauge needle.

The quantity of liquid silicone given is from 0·5 ml to a maximum of 2·0 ml at a treatment. A single injection is given every week or every other week usually for a total of 8 to 12 treatments. The injected quantity must be small especially early in the treatment series to reduce the chance of 'drifting' or overcorrection.

The method of injection is by a 'fanning' technique like that sometimes used in local anaesthesia. Frequent aspiration is important to see that the needle is not in a small vessel. The material is injected slowly, and one begins at the cephalic portion of the defect to compensate for potential 'drifting'.

There have been no side effects in our patients. Post-injection pain and 'drifting' have not occurred. Mild ecchymosis of the area may occur after injection but has usually disappeared within two or three days. Although a longer period of follow-up is necessary, there is at present no reason to believe that true granuloma formation is likely when pure silicone fluid is used, or that there will be spread through tissue planes or lymphatic spread when small volumes are injected as described. Mild subcutaneous fibroplasia is stimulated to produce loculation in a fine reticular fibrous frame.

Conclusions

Facial hemiatrophy in children is indeed a challenge to the reconstructive surgeon and, as always, *primum non nocere* must be the first rule of practice. Previous treatment failures necessarily caused us to look for something which gives reason to hope that these children may have relief of their severe defect and subsequent prevention or alleviation of ensuing psychological problems.

While no panacea has been found, it seems reasonable to believe that present research in the clinical use of dimethylpolysiloxane fluid is the most promising avenue of treatment up to the present time. This statement is based on the author's personal series of 10 cases in childhood and some 20 cases of various forms of facial atrophy as well as pooled data of a longer number of patients treated by other surgeons. It is mandatory, of course, that the parents of the child clearly understand what the surgeon plans to do—that it is experimental and that the long term results will not be certainly known for some years to come. When this is understood and when the treatment is in experienced hands, the results at this time can be said to be rewarding and promising.

THOMAS D. REES

* Dow Corning pure medical grade dimethylpolysiloxane 360 fluid.

REFERENCES

ASHLEY, F. L., REES, T. D., BALLANTYNE, D. L., GALLOWAY, D., MACHIDA, R., GRAZER, F., McCONNELL, O. V., EDGINGTON, M. T. & KISKADDEN, W. (1965). An injection technique for the treatment of facial hemiatrophy. *Plastic reconstr. Surg.* **35**, 640.

GORLIN, R. J. & PINDBORG, J. J. (1964). *Syndromes of the Head and Neck*, pp. 475–479. New York: McGraw-Hill.

MOSS, H. L. & CRIKELAIR, G. (1960). Progressive facial hemiatrophy following cervical sympathectomy in the rat. *Archs oral Biol.* **1**, 254.

REES, T. D. & ASHLEY, F. (1966). The treatment of facial atrophy with liquid silicone. *Am. J. Surg.* **111**, 531.

REES, T. D. & ASHLEY, F. L. (1967). A New Treatment for Facial Hemiatrophy in Children by Injections of Dimethylpolysiloxane Fluid. *J. Pediat. Surg.* **2**, 347.

ROGERS, B. O. (1963). Progressive facial hemiatrophy: Romberg's disease, a review of 772 cases. *Proceedings of the Third International Congress of Plastic Surgeons*, p. 681. Amsterdam: Exerpta Medica.

ROMBERG, M. H. (1946). *Klinische Ergebrusse*. Berlin: Forstner.

CHAPTER XVIII

FACIAL HEMIATROPHY
(THE USE OF AUTOGENOUS MATERIALS)

A deforming disease of obscure origin, facial hemiatrophy seldom affects the power of facial expression or the sensitivity of the skin. It can basically be classified as congenital or progressive.

The congenital form of this disease is characterised by a hypoplasia of the affected side, involving the subcutaneous fatty and connective tissue as well as bone and muscle.

The progressive form generally begins at puberty, without preference for sex or race, with symptoms of a progressive disease which slowly involves the same tissues as in the congenital condition. The scalp itself may eventually be affected and in advanced stages even the tongue, trunk or limbs may be involved. It is usually a unilateral entity and its origin is still not understood.

In the evaluation of 772 cases, Rogers (1964) did not find statistical evidence of hereditary characteristics and feels that there might be a relation with the sympathetic nervous system—as was evidenced by Moss and Crikelair (1959), who reproduced the syndrome in rats after a unilateral cervical sympathectomy.

Facial hemiatrophy with various aetiologies were studied in 14 cases by us. Four of the cases presented Romberg's syndrome and one of these suffered from tocotraumatism. The ages ranged between 7 and 29 years. Four other patients presented facial hemiatrophy since birth: two of them with aplasia auricularis. The other six patients were treated by the same type of surgery but in three the aetiology was traumatic, and in the remaining three the disease was due to X-ray therapy in infancy for treatment of benign skin diseases.

Treatment

The treatment of facial hemiatrophy aims at restoring facial balance without hampering muscular movement and expression. Various kinds of materials have been employed, ranging from grafts of fat, bone, or cartilage, to tubed pedicle flaps and aloplastic substances.

The use of decorticated tubed pedicle flaps was first reported by Newmann in 1953, the advantage being that these flaps are not absorbed, as happens with other living materials which are employed. Patients with facial hemiatrophy generally present a good quality of facial skin, needing only a filling material for restoration of the contour, and in our series preference has been given to the use of decorticated abdominal tube flaps; but it is important to realise that these should only be used once the disease is no longer progressing (Fig. **18**, 1). This rule must be adhered to if absorbtion of the implanted flap is to be avoided, for the aetiological factors for the disease will undoubtedly continue to act in the area if the implant is inserted in the acute phase. This is of basic importance in young patients who must not be operated on too early, and for this reason the illustrations of necessity show operations on older age-groups (Fig. **18**, 2).

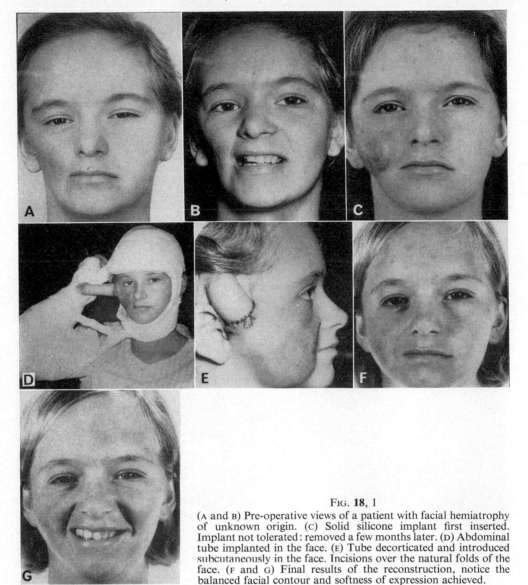

FIG. **18**, 1

(A and B) Pre-operative views of a patient with facial hemiatrophy of unknown origin. (C) Solid silicone implant first inserted. Implant not tolerated: removed a few months later. (D) Abdominal tube implanted in the face. (E) Tube decorticated and introduced subcutaneously in the face. Incisions over the natural folds of the face. (F and G) Final results of the reconstruction, notice the balanced facial contour and softness of expression achieved.

Free dermo-fat grafts have been used with some success where the atrophy has been of a limited nature, but in more extensive cases no advantages have been found with this type of treatment due to the tendency for absorption of the graft, and also due to hardening of the graft with loss of the softness which is so important in the cheek.

In the infrequent cases where the skin itself is involved, a tubed pedicle flap may still be used, but should not be decorticated (Fig. **18**, 3), and unless a large amount of skin and underlying padding is required the flap should not be taken from the

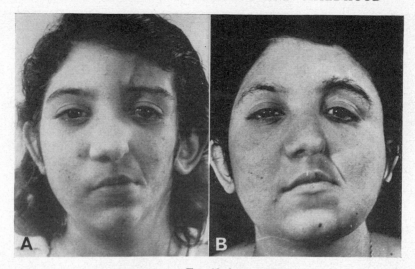

FIG. 18, 2

(A) Pre-operative view of patient with progressive facial hemiatrophy. (B) Final result: the re-established facial contour can be seen.

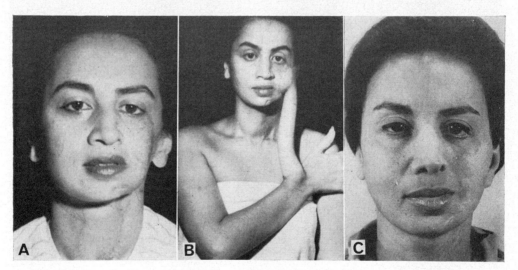

FIG. 18, 3

(A) Pre-operative view of a patient with serious left hemifacial atrophy consequent on X-ray treatment for haemangioma in infancy. Radio-dermatitis involved the skin in this patient, thus requiring skin substitution during the facial reconstruction. (B) Thoraco-abdominal tube which was used in the reconstruction. (C) Final result showing the re-established facial contour and softness of expression obtained.

abdomen, but from a region with better quality skin, such as the thorax, as the whole of the affected area must be resurfaced by means of the flap.

Decorticated tube flaps can easily be adapted to irregularities of various types of deformities (Fig. 18, 4), and in addition they furnish a fresh circulation to the region which improves the local condition of the skin. We consider this therapy as the ideal

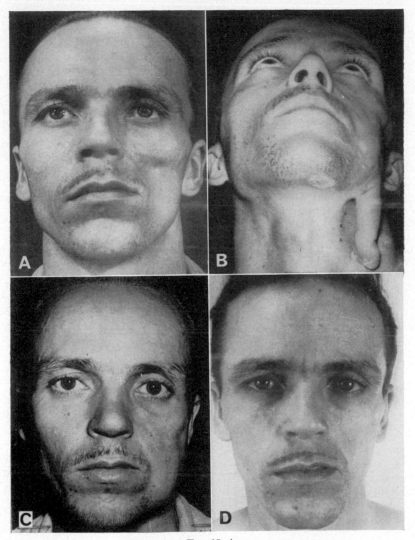

FIG. **18**, 4

(A) Pre-operative view of a patient with Romberg's syndrome. (B) Tubular flap already implanted in the face. (C) Immediate result after disappearance of oedema and partial absorption of the adepose tissue, a constant occurrence in these cases. (D) Final late result.

selective treatment, at least until such time as liquid silicone proves itself to be as good as early experiments would appear to indicate.

In an evaluation of a larger series, the use of solid silicone has not been found to be of great value for the treatment of this specific condition, where large areas have often to be reconstructed (Fig. **18**, 1C). Nevertheless, some excellent results were obtained in smaller areas where a good fixation was provided for the implant—one of the basic conditions for its satisfactory tolerance in any site.

IVO PITANGUY

REFERENCES

ASHLEY, F. L., REES, T. D., BALLANTYNE, D. L., GALLOWAY, O., MACHIDA, R., GRAZER, F., MCCONNELL, D. V., EDGINGTON, T. & KISKADDEN, W. (1965). An injection technique for the treatment of facial hemiatrophy. *Plastic reconstr. Surg.* **35**, 640–48.

BARSKY, A. J., KHAN, S. & SIMON, B. E. (1967). *Princípios y Pratica de la Cirugia Plastica y Reconstructiva.* Buenos Aires: Ed. Méd. Panamericana Sarandi.

BEER, M. (1968). Beitrag zur kenntnis Der Hemiatrophia Facialis progressiva. Inaug. Dissert. Knigsberg i br., L. Krause and Emerlein, 1968.

CRIKELAIR, G. F., MOSS, M. L. & KIIURI, A. (1962). Facial hemiatrophy. *Plastic reconstr. Surg.* **29**, 5–13.

DAVIS, W. B. (1968). Reconstruction of hemiatrophy of face. Case report. *Plastic reconstr. Surg.* **42**, 489–91.

GRABB, W. C. (1968). *Plastic Surgery—a Consise Guide to Clinica Practice.* Ed. Grabb, W. C. & Smith, J. W. Boston: Little Brown.

GORLIN, R. J. & PINDBORG, J. J. (1964). *Syndromes of the Head and Neck.* New York: McGraw-Hill.

KISKADDEN, W. & MCGREGOR, M. W. (1946). Report of a case of progressive facial hemiatrophy with pathological changes and surgical treatment. *Plastic reconstr. Surg.* **1**, 187–92.

LONGACRE, J. J. & DE STEFANO, G. A. (1954). Reconstruction of extensive defects of the skull with split rib grafts. *Plastic reconstr. Surg.* **19**, 186–99.

MOSS, M. L. & CRIKELAIR, G. F. (1959). Progressive facial hemiatrophy following cervical sympathectomy in the rat. *Archs oral Biol.* **1**, 254.

PESKOVA, H. & STOCKAR, B. (1961). Hemiatrophia faciei progressiva: Romberg's disease. *Acta Chir. plast.* **3**, 276.

PITANGUY, I. & BISAGGIO, S. (1967). Radiodermatites como sequela de tratamento de entidades benignas. *Revta bras. Cirug.* **53**, 9–31.

NEWMANN, C. G. (1953). The use of large buried pedicled flaps of dermis and fat. Clinical and pathological evaluation in the treatment of progressive facial hemiatrophy. *Plastic reconstr. Surg.* **11**, 315–332.

PITANGUY, I. & BISAGGIO, S. (1967). Atrofia facial pós-irradiaçao de hemangiomas na infância. *Hospital, Rio de Janeiro* **72**, 715–28.

ROGERS, B. (1964). Rare craniofacial deformities. In *Reconstructive Plastic Surgery.* Ed. Converse, J. M. Philadelphia: Saunders W. B.

WARTEMBERG, R. (1945). Progressive facial hemiatrophy. *Archs Neurol. Psychiat. Chicago* **54**, 75.

CHAPTER XIX

ACQUIRED FACIAL HEMI-HYPERTROPHY (HEMI-GIGANTISM)

Facial giantism, either unilateral or bilateral, may occur as a result of skeletal hypertrophy or may be due to underlying osseous tumours, but on rare occasions the cause of the facial enlargement may be a pathological state arising primarily in the soft tissue. Such lesions are notably: haemangioma, lymphangioma and neurofibroma, and giantism resulting from these conditions is almost invariably unilateral. Although overgrowth or deformity of the facial bones may be present this is a secondary deformity—as distinct from the primary skeletal enlargement of true congenital hemi-hypertrophy (Statne and Lovestedt, 1962; Furnas *et al.*, 1970)— and is responsible for only a minor part of the gigantic size of the face. Despite the difference in pathology and the wide difference in prognosis the three conditions present many clinical features in common and it would seem reasonable to consider them together under the title of this brief note.

Haemangioma

Massive facial haemangioma (Fig. **19**, 1A, B and C) generally runs a course not unlike mixed haemangioma in other parts of the body (Chap. XXXV) in that it may present initially as a very superficial, comparatively flat tumour at birth but rapidly develops a deeper cavernous element until the whole face becomes involved and the distended tissues bulge out in the eyelids and around the mouth so that the eye is completely hidden and the mouth may be partially obstructed. The skin and musculature of the face is greatly stretched and feeding may become very difficult indeed. The treatment of these very large facial haemangiomas presents a grave problem, for the proximity of the cavernous sinus may render injection techniques— if these are favoured—dangerous, whilst the radiotherapist may hesitate to use dosages which may, in order to be effective, produce harmful results on the development of the face or on the underlying eye. Surgery has almost no place, for the unwary surgeon tempted to dissection finds himself looking into open trabeculated blood spaces if he is foolhardy enough to attempt surgical reduction of the gigantic face. In most instances a combination of moderate, superficial doses of radiotherapy and, most important of all, a capacity to be patient, will be in the child's best interests whilst at the same time producing a feeling that 'something is being done', and with the passage of time a very considerable involution of the condition will take place (Fig. **19**, 1D and E).

Whilst it is usually held to be of prime importance to permit the patient to see out of the affected eye in order to avoid the development of amblyopia it is by no means a certainty that this latter will happen even if the eye is covered for some considerable time, and the eyelids may be enlarged to such an extent that surgery to reduce them cannot effectively be carried out without gross destruction of the musculature of the lid itself. Even then it is likely that the patient's ability to see will still be impaired by an immobile, drooping upper lid. Apart from this the whole orbit may be displaced downwards and the orbital bone may be considerably deformed (Fig. **19**, 1G). The downward displacement of the orbit and the considerable likelihood of inability to move the eye freely (because of tumour in the orbit itself) may produce a diplopia

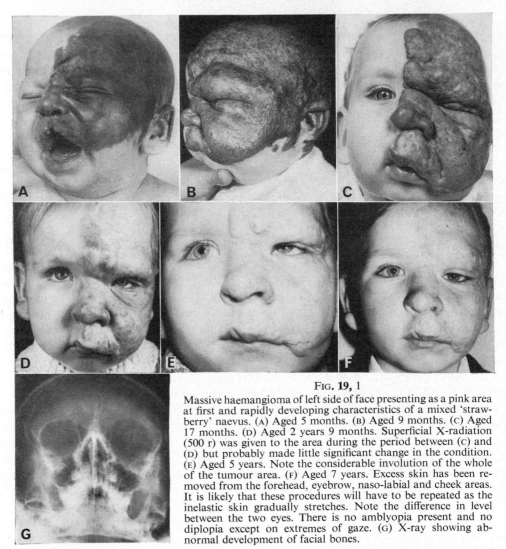

Fig. **19**, 1

Massive haemangioma of left side of face presenting as a pink area at first and rapidly developing characteristics of a mixed 'strawberry' naevus. (A) Aged 5 months. (B) Aged 9 months. (C) Aged 17 months. (D) Aged 2 years 9 months. Superficial X-radiation (500 r) was given to the area during the period between (C) and (D) but probably made little significant change in the condition. (E) Aged 5 years. Note the considerable involution of the whole of the tumour area. (F) Aged 7 years. Excess skin has been removed from the forehead, eyebrow, naso-labial and cheek areas. It is likely that these procedures will have to be repeated as the inelastic skin gradually stretches. Note the difference in level between the two eyes. There is no amblyopia present and no diplopia except on extremes of gaze. (G) X-ray showing abnormal development of facial bones.

which would be difficult to correct, and in gross cases a degree of amblyopia may at least avoid such a troublesome diplopia.

Angiography is only of academic interest, for ligation of facial vessels short of both main arterial trunks to the head and neck is of no practical value in influencing the life history of the condition or reducing the size of the tumour. What should be borne in mind is that although the tissues have been so considerably stretched the facial nerve remains undamaged, unless by interfering surgery, and its function is still retained—a matter of great importance in helping to restore a reasonable appearance to the face in later years once involution has taken place.

When it is evident that no further involution is to be expected, judicious excisions of baggy areas and modified facelifting procedures based in the hairline and around the ears can be employed to reduce the residual drooping of forehead, cheek and eyelids (Fig. **19**, 1F), but the basic alterations in the facial skeleton and the downward displacement of the eye are probably best left alone.

Lymphangioma

Lymphangioma, producing giantism of the face (Fig. **19**, 2A and B), is of the cavernous type and is sometimes referred to as cystic hygroma (Chap. XXXVI). Like the cavernous haemangioma it may present comparatively little deformity originally but rapidly increases in growth until the affected side of the face presents a grotesque gigantic appearance with complete obscuration of the eye and a gross distortion of the mouth. A certain degree of hypertrophy of the maxilla and mandible may develop, but not to any marked extent. Unlike the haemangioma, however, this condition shows no tendency towards spontaneous resolution and must be regarded as permanent. Radiotherapy is of no value here and recourse must be had to surgery.

From the very start the surgical approach must be radical and the massive quantities of tumour tissues should be resected in stages from the forehead, cheeks and inside of the mouth without regard for preservation of the facial nerve. It is the writer's experience that not only is it extremely difficult to dissect out the functioning branches of the facial nerve through such a huge mass of tumour tissue, but, much more important, the facial muscles are so grossly stretched and in themselves impossible to dissect out that it is not feasible to preserve a significant amount of them for any practical use to be made of them.

A series of planned resections should be carried out (Fig. **19**, 2C and D) and, as blood loss can be severe, no attempt should be made to deal with too much of the tumour at any one time. A preliminary ligation of the external carotid artery may be carried out but is likely to make little significant difference in controlling bleeding subsequently. As indicated above it is the writer's opinion that in facial giantism due to this condition, or to neurofibroma (see below), it is unrealistic to attempt to preserve any of the facial nerve or of the facial musculature and, having carried out a radical resection of the tumour, the paralysed side of the mouth or the eyelids should be hitched up at a subsequent stage by any of the standard available techniques such as the use of a fascia lata sling, or the 'motivating' operations involving the temporalis or masseter muscles. These techniques are to be found in standard works on plastic surgery and have no specific points of difference in child patients. It may be possible to achieve a satisfactory hitch of the affected side of the mouth simply by suturing the undersurface of the dermis close to the corner of the mouth on to the edge of the malar prominence, or to the muscle and connective tissue close to this point (Fig. **19**, 3H).

As far as the eyelids are concerned exploration and judicious reduction of tumour tissue should be carried out both on the outside and the inside of the orbital septum,

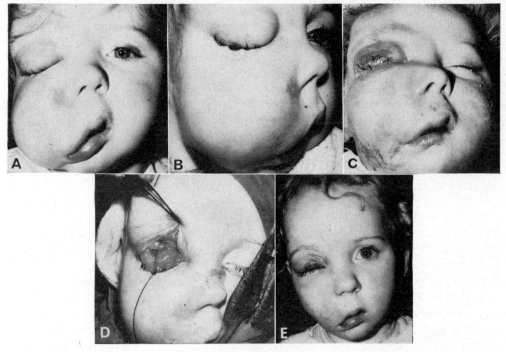

FIG. **19**, 2

Enlargement of right side of face due to massive lymphangioma. (A and B) Pre-operative appearance. No function could be detected in any part of the facial musculature on the affected side of the face. (C) Post-operative appearance after primary resection of tumour tissue *en bloc* from temporal area, eyelid, cheek and neck (via a facelift type of incision). (D) Detail of resection of tumour tissue from upper lid showing attempt to preserve levator muscle. (E) Appearance $3\frac{1}{2}$ years after primary operation. Two intermediate operations have been carried out to resect tissue at the medial canthus and to attempt to raise the right angle of the mouth. Full-thickness wedges of the eyelids have been resected at the outer aspect to reduce the length of the palpebral opening. Note that some levator action has still been preserved. Further work will be required at a later date to improve appearance and lift up the left angle of the mouth.

but these resections should not be done at one and the same time (Fig. **19**, 2D). Shortening of the greatly elongated palpebral fissure may be carried out by resection of full-thickness blocks of the lateral part of each lid. This will produce a temporary increase in oedema of the eyelids but will allow the lateral canthus to be re-established and will reduce the length of the lids to reasonable proportions. Resection of a large block of the upper lid in any site other than the lateral sector is liable to destroy any likelihood of making use of the action of the levator muscle at a later date. If it has been possible to preserve some of this latter muscle it is likely that a resection of a part of it will be required to produce any significant elevation of the upper lid, but no attempt should be made to do this until the size of the lids has been reduced to reasonable proportions (Fig. **19**, 2E). It must be remembered that it is unlikely that any reliance can be placed on utilising frontalis muscle to help in raising the eyelid: in the absence of any means of motivation of the upper lid, it is best to leave the length of the lid long enough to ensure cover of the cornea and make use of crutch spectacles, which have a small soft arm attached to the frame in order to raise the eyelid during waking hours. If it has been possible to reduce the eyelid to reasonable proportions and some elevation of the eyelid has been preserved but the ability to close has been lost because of paralysis of the orbicularis muscle, a small stainless steel spring, as advocated by Morel-Fatio and Lalardrie (1964), may be used to produce closure of the upper lid during sleep.

Neurofibroma

Von Recklinghausen's disease—neurofibromatosis—may, on rare occasions, give rise to a gigantic overgrowth of one side of the face (Duke-Elder, 1952) which starts in infancy deep to a pigmented area of facial skin (Fig. **19**, 3A, B and C). The condition is progressive and is not subject to spontaneous resolution; the pathology is that of a plexiform neurofibroma and macroscopically the tumour tissue resembles large collections of pale worms, up to 1 cm in diameter, all intertwining and fixed together by connective tissue (Fig. **19**, 3E). Both the fifth and seventh cranial nerves are involved and the number of individual nerve fibres which are affected may run into hundreds, so that it is impossible to trace individual nerve branches through the mass of interlacing 'worms' even if it was worthwhile attempting to preserve any of them. The facial bones, particularly the maxilla and the mandible, may also show considerable hypertrophy and deformity (Fig. **19**, 3K). As with cystic hygroma the skin is grossly expanded and may hang down in great tumour-filled folds over the eye or the cheek: the lids may be three times or more the normal length but the orbit itself is not so displaced as in massive facial haemangioma.

As with cystic hygroma of the face, treatment is again directed to serial resection of the whole of the tumour tissue as far as is possible, leaving the underlying bony skeleton with the muscles of mastication practically bare. The approach must be carried out at whatever sites would seem to offer the best advantage and an incision running down the hairline in the temporal region to follow the anterior limit of the ear and thence down beneath the angle of the mandible offers the greatest possibility, with secondary incisions in the naso-labial folds and along the margins of the eyelids (Fig. **19**, 3G). No attempt should be made to preserve any neurological function and excess skin should be excised as in hygroma surgery. Preliminary external carotid ligation may be tried but again seems to make little improvement in control of the bleeding due probably to anastomosis with the vessels of the opposite side of the face and with the deeper parts of the head and neck. The greatest difficulty may be experienced with the enormously expanded mouth and lids and as far as the latter are concerned, despite radical thinning, they may always impede vision. No hesitation should be felt regarding radical resection of tumour in the lids and fornices for unless this is done the eye will certainly never be of any practical value to the patient, and considerable risks can be taken in resection of full-thickness blocks of the lids or in thinning them out (Fig. **19**, 3H). If this is not done the eye itself will be useless, so there is nothing to lose by attempted adequate resection, and if the eye is proptosed by masses of tumour in the orbit it will have to be removed eventually in any case and a prosthesis (probably combining eyelids and an artificial eye) may be the eventual solution to the problem.

One of the striking features of these patients is the abnormally low situation of the

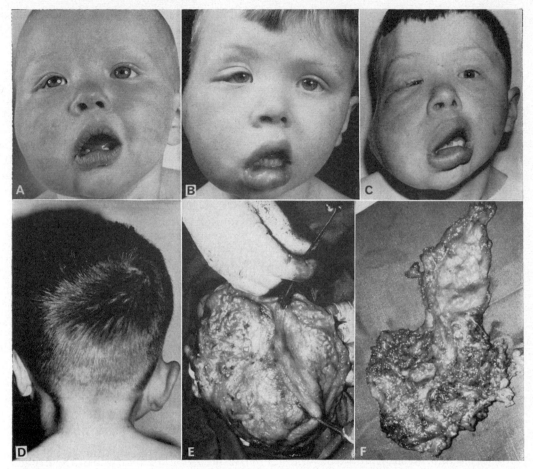

FIG. **19**, 3

Massive enlargement of the right side of the face from neurofibromatosis affecting motor and sensory nerves. (A) Appearance at 9 months. (B) Appearance aged 3 years 4 months. (C) Appearance aged 8 years. No treatment carried out so far. (D) As in (C), showing displacement downwards of the ear on the affected side. (E) Exposure of the face on the affected side at operation. The ear can be seen on the left side of the photograph: the large wormlike masses of involved nerve tissue can be seen particularly clearly above and in front of the ear. Stimulation of the grossly thickened nerve fibres on occasion produced some facial movement but it was not possible to trace any particular nerve for any distance in the mass of intertwining structures which were present over the whole of the side of the face. (F) Resection *en bloc* of the neurofibromatous tissue, including small sections of apparently normal nerve which lead only to areas of pathological involvement.

ear (Fig. **19**, 3D), and this should be corrected early in the programme. Hitching up of the various parts of the face may require one or two operative sessions and should be carried out as described under lymphangioma. There is not the same likelihood that the levator muscle will be preserved as in the latter condition and the probability is that the upper lid should be left covering the cornea, to be raised during the day by the use of a crutch spectacle with a lifting bar in the upper palpebral furrow. Late operations may involve resection of part of the thickened hypertrophic maxilla and mandible.

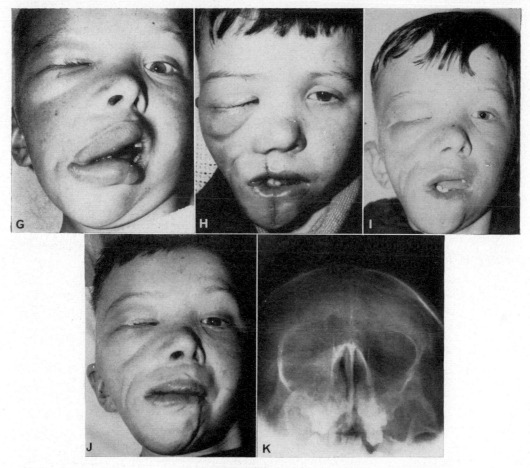

FIG. **19**, 3 (*contd.*)

(G) Appearance shortly after primary resection of neurofibromatous mass. (H) Appearance one year later, following wedge resection of upper and lower lips and further attempt to reduce tumour mass in lower lid by transconjunctival approach. The right angle of the mouth has been hitched to the malar using some of the fibrous tissue present in the cheek following operation one year ago. (I and J) Appearance 6 months after operation described in (H). The oedema of the eyelids is still preventing opening of the latter. Note, there is now considerable hypertrophy of the maxillary alveolus and palate, and of the mandible—particularly in the alveolar region—and this underlying bony deformity adds considerably to the abnormal appearance of the face. This bone change has become more obvious in the past two years and reduction of the excess bone will have to be considered along with other procedures to improve the facial appearance in the future. Note that the displaced ear has again sunk down despite considerable elevation at the earlier operations. (K) X-ray showing deformity of facial bones, particularly of the maxilla and floor of the orbit.

La Ruffa (1967) described a patient with facial hemi-giantism suffering from neuro-fibromatosis in whom 10 separate operations, including ligation of the supposed feeding vessels, were carried out over a period of six years, and who in the end was fitted with an over-all ocular prosthesis with lids attached. This exemplifies the tediousness of the treatment of these patients and the need for gradual controlled resection and restoration over a very long period.

The ultimate prognosis in patients with this condition is poor for, apart from the likelihood of re-appearance of tumour from small nerve fibres hitherto apparently unaffected, the probability of eventual sarcomatous change must always be borne in mind.

J. C. MUSTARDÉ

ACKNOWLEDGMENT

Figures 19, 1A, B, C and D; Figures 19, 3A and B are reproduced by courtesy of Mr Wallace M. Dennison, F.R.C.S.

REFERENCES

DUKE-ELDER, S. (1952). The Ocular Adnexae. In *Textbook of Ophthalmology*, vol. V. p. 5104. London: Kimpton.

FURNAS, D. W. *et al.* (1970). Congenital hemi-hypertrophy of the face: Impersonator of childhood facial tumours. *J. Pediat. Surg.* 5, 344.

LA RUFFA, H. (1967). Facial reconstruction in gigantic neurofibromatosis. *Semana méd. B. Aires*, 74, 981.

MOREL-FATIO, D. & LALARDRIE, J. P. (1964). Palliative surgical treatment of facial paralysis. The palpebral spring. *Plastic reconstr. Surg.* 33, 446.

STATNE, E. C. & LOVESTEDT, S. A. (1962). Congenital hemi-hypertrophy of the face (facial giantism). *Oral Surg.* 15, 184.

CHAPTER XX

CONGENITAL SCALP DEFECTS

The classic congenital scalp defect presents as a depressed area covered by a thin, parchment-like epithelial membrane or as a raw wound with a serosanguinous exudate. It is centred around the midline vertex as a circular, linear or stellate lesion that may or may not have an underlying bone defect. (Ingalls, 1933; Farmer and Maximen, 1960; Walker *et al.*, 1960; Hodgeman *et al.*, 1965; Cutlip *et al.*, 1967.) Although single defects predominate, double lesions are reported in 20 per cent. of the cases and triple lesions in 8 per cent. (Ingalls, 1933; O'Brien and Drake, 1960; Cutlip *et al.*, 1967.) In rare cases they appear in the occipital and postauricular areas (Cutlip *et al.*, 1967).

Although the diameter ranges from a few millimeters up to 10 cm, the most common defect is the circular, 'punched-out', 1 to 2 cm wound (Fig. 20, 1). Linear lesions tend to lie along the saggital suture and are usually related to an underlying bone defect frequently believed to be merely a widened suture. The stellate lesions (often very large) are generally located between the fontanels, rarely on the posterior scalp. The frequency of an underlying bone defect is directly proportional to the size of the ulceration; the small circular lesions are usually not accompanied by a bone defect, while a majority of the large stellate lesions are.

Biopsies of the involved area will reveal a lack of inflammation and necrosis,

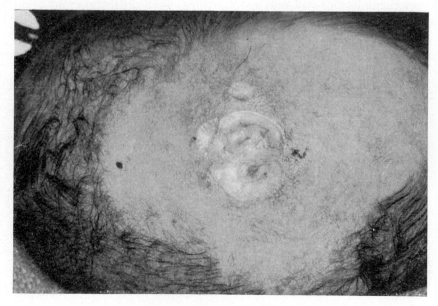

FIG. 20, 1

This view looking towards the vertex of the scalp shows a classic congenital scalp defect. This infant was born with a thin epithelial membrane overlying this depressed defect. There was no underlying bone defect in this case. (Photograph courtesy of Dr L. Ware.)

absence of deep dermis, dermal structures, fat and muscles and a sparcity of elastic fibres in the surrounding skin (Walker *et al.*, 1960; Hodgeman *et al.*, 1965; Cutlip *et al.*, 1967).

Incidence and aetiology

By 1965, approximately 250 cases were reported in the literature (Resnik *et al.*, 1965). Firstborn female infants have been slightly in the majority (Peer and Van Duyn, 1948). Although there have been a significant number of reports of familial cases, and even in identical twins, the mode of inheritance is not clear, with some suggesting a dominant and others a recessive pattern (Farmer and Maximen, 1960; Hodgeman *et al.*, 1965; Resnik *et al.*, 1965; Cutlip *et al.*, 1967). A significant number of babies with this defect are born prematurely, and there is a frequent history of stillborn siblings (Farmer and Maximen, 1960). Some congenital anomalies reported with this lesion include hydrocephalus, haemangiomas, polycystic kidneys, meningoceles, cleft lip, cleft palate, microphthalmia, limb deformity, spastic paralysis and verrucous nevi.

Grieg's embryologic explanation is presently the most accepted and relates the defect to arrested midline development. Since the dorsal midline region of the embryo undergoes so many changes and structural re-arrangements, it is surprising that these defects are not more numerous (O'Brien and Drake, 1960; Hodgeman *et al.*, 1965).

Treatment

Small superficial lesions will heal spontaneously with protection and good wound hygiene, but larger lesions with underlying bone defects expose the meninges and/or

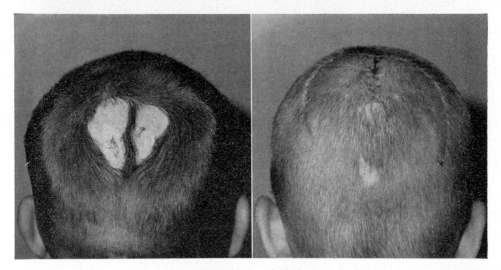

FIGS. **20**, 2 and **20**, 3

An 8-year-old boy with a healed congenital scalp defect present since birth. The bone had regenerated under this thin, atrophic, epithelial membrane. Closure was carried out by sliding two rotation flaps towards the midline. (Photographs courtesy of Dr B. Defiebre.)

vascular sinuses and must be operated on early. These larger, more serious defects can result in death due to meningitis or haemorrhage. Depending on their size, these lesions can be closed by direct approximation, by local flaps, or by split-thickness skin grafts. Although in Ingalls' paper (1933) the mortality was reported as 20 per cent, the prognosis is now generally good, except in large lesions overlying the saggital sinus. Neurosurgical consultation may be necessary in these difficult cases which occasionally require ligating this sinus.

In those lesions which heal spontaneously, a depressed, hairless, atrophic scar results which later can be staged out or closed with local flaps (Figs. **20**, 2 and **20**, 3). Bone defects do not usually require bone grafting, as once good soft tissue coverage is established, the bone will regenerate.

R. A. MLADICK, C. E. HORTON and J. E. ADAMSON

REFERENCES

CAMPBELL, W. (1826). Case of congenital ulcer on the cranium of a fetus, terminating in fatal haemorrhage on the 18th day after birth. *Edinb. J. med. Sci.* **5**, 82.

CUTLIP, B. C., CRYAN, D. M. & VINEYARD, W. R. (1967). Congenital scalp defects in mother and child. *Am. J. Dis. Child.* **113**, 597.

DINGMAN, R. D. (1958). Surgical treatment of defects of the scalp. *J. Int. Coll. Surg.* **30**, 148.

FARMER, A. W. & MAXIMEN, M. D. (1960). Congenital absence of skin. *Plastic reconstr. Surg.* **25**, 291.

HODGEMAN, J. E., MATHIES, A. W. & LEVAN, N. E. (1965). Congenital scalp defects in twin sisters. *Am. J. Dis. Child.* **110**, 293.

INGALLS, N. W. (1933). Congenital defects of the scalp (studies in the pathology of development). *Am. J. Obstet. Gynec.* **25**, 861.

JOHNSON, J. B. (1954). Congenital skin defects; report of 3 cases. *J. Int. Coll. Surg.* **21**, 599.

KAHN, E. A. & LEMMEN, L. J. (1950). Unusual congenital anomalies of neurosurgical interest in infants and children. *J. Neurosurg.* **7**, 544.

O'BRIEN, B. McC. & DRAKE, J. E. (1960). Congenital defects of the skull and scalp. *Br. J. plastic Surg.* **13** 102.

ORMSBY, O. S. & MONTGOMERY, H. (1954). *Diseases of the Skin*, p. 698. Philadelphia: Lea & Febiger.

PEER, L. A. & VAN DUYN, J. (1948). Congenital defect of the scalp. *Plastic reconstr. Surg.* **3**, 722.

RESNIK, S. S., KOBLENZER, P. J. & PITTS, F. W. (1965). Congenital absence of the scalp with associated vascular anomaly. *Clin. Pediat.* **4**, 322.

SAVAGE, D. (1957). Localized congenital defects of the scalp. *Archs Derm.* **75**, 266.

WALKER, J. C., KOENIG, J. A., IRWIN, L. & MEYER, R. (1960). Congenital absence of skin. *Plastic reconstr. Surg.* **26**, 209.

CHAPTER XXI

CRANIUM BIFIDUM

PATHOLOGY

The term cranium bifidum means a protrusion of the meninges through a gap in the cranium. If the sac contains c.s.f. and brain tissue it is called an encephalocele; if it contains no neurological elements it is known as a cerebral meningocele (Ingraham and Matson, 1954). The sac may be covered by intact skin and subcutaneous tissue but more frequently the meninges are exposed. In the latter variety there is considerable danger of injury to the meninges causing rupture any time after birth and rupture of the sac of very large encephaloceles during labour is not unknown. It is usually stated that the opening in the skull is always situated in the midline, but this is not invariably the case, and we have seen encephaloceles in which the opening was in the parietal bone at some distance lateral to the sagittal suture. In the vast majority of cases the opening is in the occipital bone, but anterior encephaloceles protruding above the bridge of the nose or protruding into the naso- or oropharynx have been described (Ingraham and Swan, 1943). In the commoner occipital encephalocele the brain tissue found in the sac is usually either part of the cerebellum or the posterior part of the cerebral occipital lobes.

INCIDENCE

This malformation is relatively rare, having an incidence of approximately 10 per cent., or less, of the incidence of myelomeningocele (Lorber, 1961; Eckstein and Macnab, 1966). During the last 16 years 837 newborn infants with myelomeningocele have been admitted to the Liverpool Regional Neonatal Surgical Centre; during the same period only 67 infants with encephalocele have been admitted.

CLINICAL PICTURE

In occipital encephaloceles the protrusion of the meninges is obvious on inspection. The sac may be small (Fig. **21**, 1) or enormous in size, sometimes considerably larger than the infant's head (Fig. **21**, 2). About a quarter of the cases have an obvious microcephalus. These are usually the cases with large encephaloceles and air ventriculograms performed in these infants often show gross associated malformations of the brain. Hydrocephalus develops in over 50 per cent of infants with encephalocele, but is often of only moderate degree (Lorber, 1967).

In children with anterior encephalocele, especially in those where the encephalocele protrudes into the naso- or oro-pharynx, the diagnosis may not be immediately obvious and the malformation is not infrequently discovered at a later date. Severe associated malformations are common with encephaloceles.

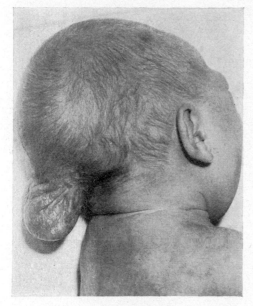

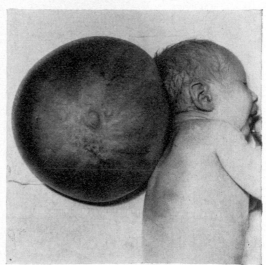

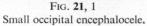

FIG. **21**, 1
Small occipital encephalocele.

FIG. **21**, 2
Giant occipital encephalocele.

TREATMENT

Indication for operation

Whilst encephaloceles which are not covered by skin should be operated upon as soon as possible, to prevent trauma and infection of the sac, skin covered encephaloceles do not need urgent operation. Most surgeons would not favour operation in infants with obvious microcephaly. Fortunately some of the most severe cases with large amounts of brain tissue in the encephalocele sac die either shortly after birth, or as the result of operation. Facilitation of nursing is a frequent indication for surgery. If surgery is withheld it is impossible to foretell whether the infant will die quickly or will continue to live for many months or years. The size of the encephalocele is not of itself a guide to prognosis; the ultimate result depends on the amount of brain tissue in the sac or, more accurately, on how much normal brain tissue will be left inside the skull after operation. Surgical amputation of the cerebellum during the neonatal period does not leave the patient with any gross physical handicap, but ablation of the occipital lobes will invariably cause blindness.

Technique

The skin surrounding the neck of the encephalocele is incised. In most encephaloceles the skin of the scalp extends some distance up the neck of the sac and there is usually no difficulty in preserving enough skin for adequate closure without tension. The incision is deepened and extended subcutaneously towards the margin of the occipital bony defect. If possible the dissection should not be carried out in the plane of cleavage between the dura mater and the subcutaneous tissues, as the dura, which is frequently very delicate, can easily be injured. An attempt should therefore

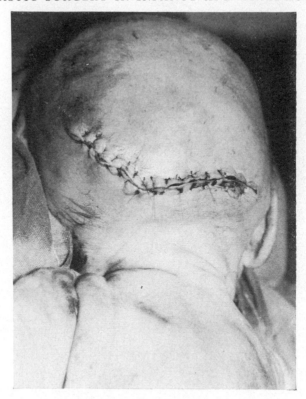

FIG. **21**, 3
After amputation of the encephalocele sac and closure of its
neck, the skin defect is closed in a transverse direction.

be made to leave as much subcutaneous tissue as possible around the neck of the
encephalocele. Great care must be exercised when approaching the rim of the defect
in the occipital bone as not infrequently large veins run from the extra-dural veins
to the neck of the sac. These will bleed profusely if injured and will retract within the
cranial cavity if accidentally severed (Rickham and Johnston, 1969).

Once the neck of the encephalocele has been clearly defined the sac is opened and
the interior inspected. Anything in excess of a minimal amount of nervous tissue
within the sac will have to be ablated, as reduction of nervous tissue into the cranial
cavity under pressure will invariably cause death. Resection of parts of the brain is
often a very haemorrhagic procedure; all bleeding vessels must be meticulously
ligated or coagulated with diathermy. The neck of the sac is then repaired using
continuous non-absorbable sutures and if possible the repair is reinforced by suturing
subcutaneous tissue and flaps of galea over the defect. The skin is then sutured using
vertical mattress sutures. It is usually easiest to suture the skin defect in a transverse
direction (Fig. **21**, 3). Drainage is not employed, but a compression bandage should
be used.

Postoperative management

Provided no infection occurs and provided the brain damage has not been too excessive, children stand the excision of even large encephaloceles quite well. If hydrocephalus develops this will have to be dealt with once the incision has healed (Chap. XXII).

PROGNOSIS

The prognosis for children who have been operated upon for encephalocele depends on the quantity and quality of the remaining brain. If this is adequate the prognosis will be good. Microcephalic children and children in whom large quantities of brain tissue have been removed at operation will be retarded or will have severe neurological sequelae (Barrow and Simpson, 1966; Lorber, 1967). Associated hydrocephalus, on the other hand, is not associated with a bad prognosis provided it is speedily and efficiently corrected.

P. P. RICKHAM

REFERENCES

BARROW, N. & SIMPSON, D. A. (1966). Cranium bifidum. *Aust. Paediat. J.* **2**, 20.
ECKSTEIN, H. B. & MACNAB, G. H. (1966). Myelomeningocele and hydrocephalus. *Lancet* **1**, 842.
INGRAHAM, F. D. & MATSON, D. D. (1954). *Neurosurgery of Infancy and Childhood*. Springfield, Illinois: Thomas.
INGRAHAM, F. D. & SWAN, H. (1943). Spina bifida or cranium bifidum. *Proc. Staff Meet. Mayo Clin.* **27**, 33.
LORBER, J. (1961). Systematic ventriculographic studies in infants born with meningomyelocele and encephalocele. *Archs Dis. Child.* **36**, 381.
LORBER, J. (1967). The prognosis of occipital encephalocele. *Devl. Med. Child. Neurol.* Suppl. **13**, 75.
RICKHAM, P. P. & JOHNSTON, J. H. (1969). *Neonatal Surgery*. London: Butterworths.

CHAPTER XXII

HYDROCEPHALUS IN CHILDHOOD

Definition

By hydrocephalus we understand a condition in which the volume of cerebral portion of the c.s.f. is becoming progressively too large for the cerebral volume (Lange, 1966). Theoretically hydrocephalus can be caused by excessive secretion of c.s.f., a block in the pathway of the fluid, or a failure of absorption. In childhood the second possibility is the only one of practical importance (Rickham and Johnstone, 1969).

Historical notes

Although the condition must have been known to physicians since the dawn of medical science, it was first accurately described at the beginning of the seventeenth century (Vesalius, 1725). During the last 150 years (Hemmer, 1969) many attempts have been made to cure this condition but most of the successes were only limited and temporary. It was not until 1956, when the engineer, J. Holter, modified the valve originally designed by Nulsen and Spitz (1952), that it became a practical proposition to drain the excessive c.s.f. from the lateral ventricle into the heart with the aid of a silicon rubber system containing a no-return valve.

Pathological notes

In a short chapter on hydrocephalus a detailed discussion of the very complicated physiology and pathology of c.s.f. formation and absorption is out of place. Dandy and Blackfan's classical work (1914) seemed to indicate that the choroid plexus in the lateral cerebral ventricles was the sole producer of c.s.f. It is now known, however, that only 60 per cent of the fluid is thus formed and that the remaining 40 per cent is produced in the subarachnoid space (Bering, 1965). In 1933 it was shown that the fluid was absorbed by the arachnoid villi (Weed, 1914), but subsequent studies have revealed that the villi account for only 10 per cent of the total absorption and that the perineural spaces and the ependyma appear to be the main site of absorption (Howarth and Coope, 1955; Bowsher, 1957).

The most common cause of hydrocephalus in childhood is a congenital block in the c.s.f. pathway. In about 20 per cent of these cases the site of the obstruction is one of the narrow parts of the pathway, i.e., the aqueduct or one of the foramina (Forrest et al., 1966). In 80 per cent it occurs in conjunction with spina bifida cystica as a result of the associated Arnold Chiari malformation, a herniation of the tongue-like process of the cerebellum and the lower part of the medulla oblongata through the foramen magnum, causing crowding of the structures in the posterior fossa. Infection is second to congenital malformation as a cause of hydrocephalus in childhood. Any type of meningitis may cause hydrocephalus by producing adhesions in the sub-arachnoid spaces; infections due to Staphylococci, E. Coli and Klebsiella, Meningo-cocci, etc., may all be responsible.

352

Incidence

Of all the children born with myelomeningocele (the incidence of which in this country is roughly 2 per 1,000 births), 80 per cent also suffer from congenital hydrocephalus. In addition, hydrocephalus without myelomeningocele occurs in about 0·3 to 0·4 infants per 1,000 births (Rickham and Johnstone, 1969).

Clinical picture

In a minority of cases the child has an abnormally large head at birth; in most cases, however, congenital hydrocephalus only gradually becomes obvious after birth. Hydrocephalus following meningitis usually only develops when the meningitis is abating or has been completely cured.

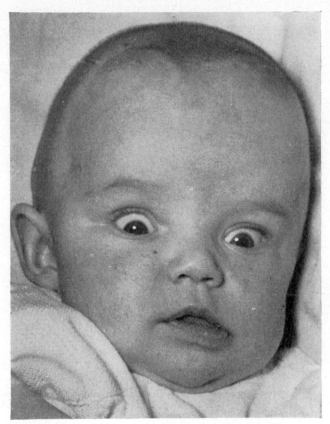

FIG. 22, 1
Infant with hydrocephalus showing 'setting sun sign'.

PRESENTING SIGNS AND SYMPTOMS

1. An abnormally rapid increase in the size of the head.
2. The 'setting sun sign' due to downwards rotation of the eyeballs (Fig. **22**, 1).
3. A bulging fontanelle, which though often present is not an invariable sign.
4. McEwen's sign (the cracked pot sound on percussion).

PS N

5. Progressive spasticity due to the destruction of the cerebral white matter; and

6. Signs of cranial nerve paralysis, especially a converging squint and abductor palsy of the vocal cords (Rickham, 1965). On the other hand, papilloedema rarely, if ever, occurs in congenital hydrocephalus (Macnab, 1966).

SPECIAL INVESTIGATIONS

If hydrocephalus is suspected the diagnosis can be confirmed by measurement of the intraventricular pressure via a brain needle inserted through the lateral angle of the fontanelle into one lateral cerebral ventricle. In cases of progressive hydrocephalus the pressure is usually, although not invariably, increased above the normal.

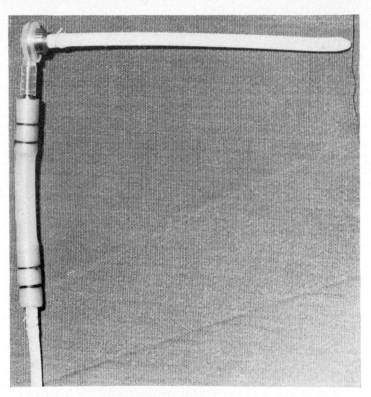

FIG. 22, 2

Holter valve connected proximally to ventriculostomy reservoir with silicon cap and side-arm connecting it to the ventricular catheter. The lower end of the valve is connected to the atrial catheter.

Cerebrospinal fluid is then aspirated through the needle and replaced by injected air, which will outline the ventricular system on radiography. An air ventriculogram which shows dilated cerebral ventricles confirms the diagnosis.

Treatment

Once the diagnosis of hydrocephalus has been made, operation should be proceeded with as soon as possible so as to halt the progressive destruction of brain tissue.

As has been stated above, drainage of c.s.f. from the lateral ventricle into the blood stream by means of a system containing a no-return valve has become the method of choice; only the Holter valve system (Rickham and Johnstone, 1969) will be described briefly here (Fig. **22**, 2).

TECHNIQUE

A semicircular scalp incision is made behind and above the right ear and scalp and pericranium are reflected. A burr hole is drilled through the skull at a point lying at the junction of the upper and middle third of a line between the tip of the right mastoid process and the vertex. A gutter 2 cm long is cut through the skull, running downwards from the burr hole (Fig. **22**, 3). A brain needle is now inserted through the dura and cerebral cortex into the right ventricle. Having ascertained the distance

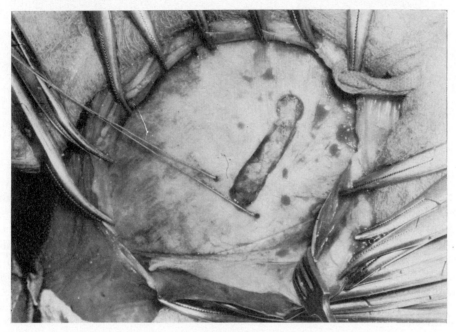

FIG. **22**, 3

After reflecting the scalp and pericranium a 5 mm wide hole has been drilled through the skull and a 2 cm long gutter has been cut through the bone running from the drill hole in a downwards direction. The first pair of small holes has been drilled near the lower end of the gutter and a nylon suture which will subsequently fix the valve to the bone, has been passed through it.

of the lateral ventricle from the surface, a suitably long silastic rubber ventricular catheter is inserted into the ventricle with the aid of a stilette and connected to a small circular cup, the ventriculostomy reservoir (Rickham and Penn, 1965). The right internal jugular vein is now exposed in the neck through a short tansverse incision and a silver impregnated, radio-opaque silicon rubber atrial catheter is pushed down the vein under radiographic control, so that its fine tip comes to lie in the right atrium (Rickham, 1968). The upper end of this catheter is connected

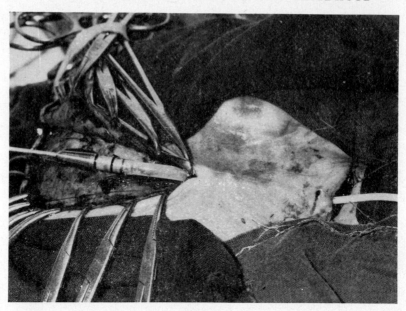

FIG. **22**, 4

The valve and its introducer are pulled from the neck incision subcutaneously to the scalp incision.

to the lower nozzle of the Holter valve, and the catheter is fixed in the vein by a ligature. With the aid of a long, curved haemostat a subcutaneous tunnel is made between the upper scalp incision and the incision in the neck and the Holter valve, with the upper end attached to a guide and the atrial catheter attached to its lower end, is pulled through the subcutaneous tunnel until its upper nozzle emerges from the scalp wound (Fig. **22**, 4). The upper nozzle is then connected to the ventriculostomy reservoir with the aid of a silicon cap with side-arm and is fixed to the skull with ligatures which have been passed through small burr holes drilled at the sides of the gutter in the bone (Fig. **22**, 5). The incisions are then closed (Fig. **22**, 6).

Complications

The two main complications of this operation are infection and blockage of the drainage system.

INFECTION

This can occur soon after the operation or may be delayed for many months or years. Primary infection may be due to faulty technique but more commonly bacteria from a distal focus of infection, such as a skin or urinary tract, travel via the blood stream into the c.s.f., and then settle in the valve. The operation of insertion of a valve must, therefore, only be performed when there is no focus of infection anywhere in the body. Delayed infection, mainly due to the staphylococcus albus, usually follows a bacteraemia.

Whatever the cause of the infection, the bacteria tend to settle in the valve and the

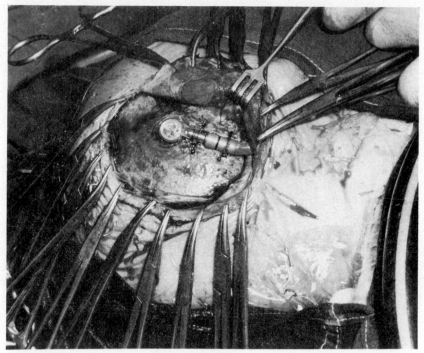

Fig. **22**, 5

The upper end of the valve has been connected to the ventriculostomy reservoir and has been fixed to the skull by two nylon sutures passed through two pairs of small burr holes placed laterally to the gutter in the bone.

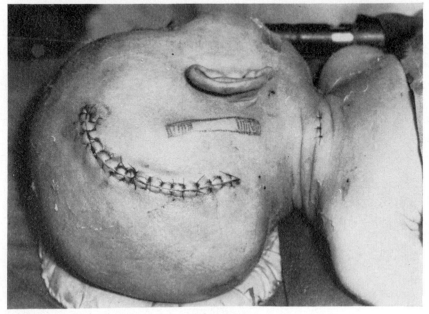

Fig. **22**, 6

The incisions in scalp and neck have been closed. The position of the valve has been outlined on the skin.

infected c.s.f. passing through the valve into the heart will cause a septicaemia. This can rarely be cleared up with antibiotic treatment alone, and in many cases the whole infected drainage system will have to be removed.

BLOCKAGE OF THE DRAINING SYSTEM

The most common site of blockage in the first few months after operation is in the ventricular catheter (Sayers, 1965). Usually small blood or fibrin clots are the blocking agents. This complication is particularly common in small infants, who have a relatively high concentration of fibrinogen in their c.s.f.

Blockage of the atrial catheter is usually a late complication, caused mainly by the patient's growth. In the growing child the atrial catheter is slowly pulled out of the atrium and once its end comes to lie in the superior vena cava the segment of the vein containing the catheter frequently thromboses and drainage stops (Nulsen and Becker, 1965).

The use of the ventriculostomy reservoir has made unblocking of the ventricular catheter a relatively minor procedure in the majority of cases and only a small percentage of these children need replacement of the catheter (Rickham and Penn, 1965). If the atrial catheter blocks it will have to be replaced and if it is impossible to pass a new catheter through the thrombosed right internal jugular vein it may be

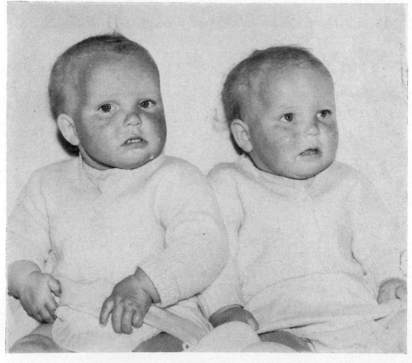

FIG. 22, 7

One of these 12-month-old twins had a gross hydrocephalus at birth and had a Holter valve operation when 2 weeks old.

necessary to use the right external jugular, the left internal or external jugular vein or even the vena azygos for insertion of the catheter into the right atrium.

PULMONARY EMBOLI

This complication used to be reported frequently (Erdohazi *et al.*, 1966) but it has become a rarity since the introduction of an atrial catheter with a thin flexible end, the so called type C catheter (Sayers, 1965).

Prognosis

In spite of complications necessitating revision of the drainage system in some cases, the majority of the results have so far been very satisfactory. Provided the children are operated upon early, before the progressive hydrocephalus has caused too much damage to the brain, the head will be of normal size (Fig. **22**, 7) and in nearly 90 per cent. the intelligence will not differ markedly from that of normal children (Mawdsley *et al.*, 1967).

P. P. RICKHAM

REFERENCES

BERING, E. A. (1965). Pathophysiology of Hydrocephalus. In *Workshop in Hydrocephalus*. Ed. Shulman, K. Philadelphia: Children's Hospital.

BOWSHER, D. (1957). Pathways of absorption of proteins from cerebrospinal fluid. *Anat. Rec.* **128**, 25.

DANDY, W. E. & BLACKFAN, K. D. (1914). Internal hydrocephalus. *Am. J. Dis. Child.* **8**, 406.

ERDOHAZI, M., ECKSTEIN, H. B. & CROME, L. (1966). Pulmonary embolisation as a complication of ventriculo-atrial shunts inserted for hydrocephalus. *Devl. Med. Child. Neurol.*, Suppl. **11**, 36.

FORREST, D. M., HOLE, R. & WYNNE, J. M. (1966). Treatment of infantile hydrocephalus using the holter valve. *Devl. Med. Child. Neurol.* Suppl. **11**, 27.

HEMMER, R. (1969). *Dringliche chirurgische Eingriffe an Gehirn, Rückenmark und Schädel im frühen Säuglingsalter*. Stuttgart: Ferdinand Enke.

HOWARTH, F. & COOPE, E. R. (1955). The fate of certain foreign colloids and crystalloids after subarachnoid injection. *Acta anat.* **25**, 112.

LANGE, S. A. (1966). *Surgical Treatment of Progressive Hydrocephalus*. Amsterdam: North Holland Publishing.

MACNAB, G. H. (1966). The development of knowledge and treatment of hydrocephalus. *Devl. Med. Child. Neurol.* Suppl. **11**, 1.

MAWDSLEY, T., RICKHAM, P. P. & ROBERTS, J. R. (1967). The long term results of early operation on open myelomeningoceles and encephaloceles. *Br. med. J.* **1**, 663.

NULSEN, F. E. & BECKER, D. P. (1965). The control of progressive hydrocephalus in infancy by valve-regulated venous shunt. In *Workshop in Hydrocephalus*, ed. Shulman, K. Philadelphia: Children's Hospital.

NULSEN, F. E. & SPITZ, E. B. (1952). Treatment of hydrocephalus by direct shunt from ventricle to jugular vein. *Surg. Forum*, **2**, 399.

RICKHAM, P. P. (1965). The management of hydrocephalus. In *Proceedings of a Symposium on Spina Bifida*. London: National Foundation for Research into Poliomyelitis and Other Crippling Diseases.

RICKHAM, P. P. (1968). The use of silver impregnated silastic catheters in the holter valve operation. *Devl. Med. Child Neurol.* Suppl. **15**, 14.

RICKHAM, P. P. & JOHNSTON, J. H. (1969). *Neonatal Surgery*. London: Butterworths.

RICKHAM, P. P. & PENN, I. A. (1965). The place of the ventriculostomy reservoir in the treatment of myelomeningoceles and hydrocephalus. *Devl. Med. Child Neurol.* **7**, 296.

SAYERS, M. P. (1965). In *Workshop in Hydrocephalus*, ed. Shulman, K. Philadelphia: Children's Hospital.

VESALIUS, A. (1725). *Opera Omnia Anatomica et Chirurgica*. Batavorum: J. du Vivie and J. and H. Verbeek.

WEED, L. H. (1914). Studies on cerebro-spinal fluid. *J. med. Res.* **26**, 31.

CHAPTER XXIII

THE NECK

CONGENITAL DEFECTS

Pterygium Colli (Webbed Neck)

Pterygium colli or webbed neck is a congenital defect in which there are thick folds of skin and subcutaneous tissue on the lateral aspect of the neck extending from the mastoid region to the acromion. They are usually bilateral, but may be unilateral. The neck appears short, thick and broad, but may not be absolutely short once the deformity is corrected. The postero-lateral hairline may be placed lower and more anterior than normal. There is frequently an excess of skin in the horizontal circumference of the neck (Fig. **23**, 1).

The cause of this condition is not known. No familial tendencies have been

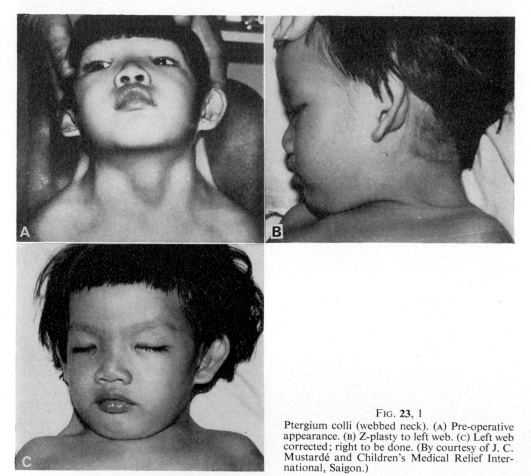

Fig. **23**, 1
Ptergium colli (webbed neck). (A) Pre-operative appearance. (B) Z-plasty to left web. (C) Left web corrected; right to be done. (By courtesy of J. C. Mustardé and Children's Medical Relief International, Saigon.)

reported. The deformity may occur as an isolated entity or may be associated with regional or generalized deformities. The commonest regional associated deformity is that of the Klipped Feil Syndrome or of the other cervical spine abnormalities. Unilateral neck webbing may occur with variants of Sprengles shoulder anomaly. The usual generalised anomaly associated with pterygium colli is Turner's syndrome.

Treatment is by Z-plasty at 1 to 6 years of age. Paired flaps give the best correction. Multiple smaller Z-plasty flaps in continuity may be necessary to avoid further displacement of abnormal hairlines to a more conspicuous region. Large excesses of neck skin may require vertical posterior midline elliptical skin excisions to give maximum improvement. Results are best when the neck is not absolutely short, there is no associated gross regional deformity, the hairline is not displaced and the central arm of the rotated flaps can be designed to be close to a normal neck fold. If hair must be transposed to an undesirable region to effect adequate lengthening of the web it can be excised and replaced by a free skin graft at a later date.

TORTICOLLIS (WRY NECK)

Torticollis is a condition produced principally by shortening of the sternomastoid muscle, although in long-standing cases the deep fascia will be involved as well as the adjacent deep muscles of the neck. The condition may be primary in the sterno-mastoid muscle or secondary to conditions outside that muscle. It may be present at or shortly after birth or appear later in childhood.

The head and neck are held relatively immobile and the head is canted or drawn

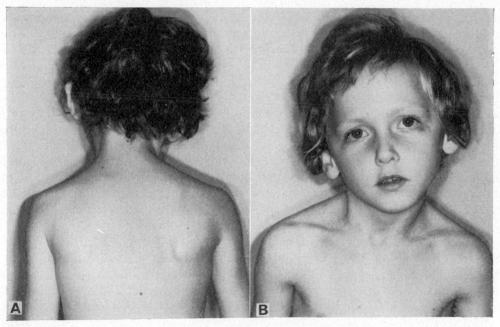

FIG. 23, 2

Torticollis (wry neck). Shortening of the right sternocleidomastoid muscle has canted the head towards the right shoulder and has rotated the chin point to the left of the midline.

PS N 2

toward the shoulder of the affected side (Fig. **23**, 2). The face or head is turned or rotated to the opposite side. In longer standing cases there will be flatness of the lower face on the involved side and even of the whole face and head on that side. The distance between the outer canthus and the corner of the mouth will eventually be less on the involved side, the arch of the eyebrow flatter and a secondary scoliosis may develop to help keep the eyes level.

Congenital torticollis

This is the commonest form. Immediately or shortly after birth the neonate will be noticed to have a relatively immobile head and to hold his head canted toward one shoulder and rotated to the opposite shoulder. Attempts to move the head and touch the neck on the involved side may produce crying. Palpation of the sternomastoid muscle of the involved side will show shortening and a round or fusiform mass, usually in the central third of the muscle, which may be tender and warm. This so-called sternomastoid tumour was originally thought to be due to haemorrhage from birth trauma, perhaps due to tearing of an end artery. It is now considered by many to be a neonatal angiofibromatous overgrowth similar to haemangioma.

Secondary torticollis

This may be present at birth or appear later in life. Cervical spine congenital abnormalities are a common cause and should be ruled out by X-ray whenever there is any doubt, particularly in the more advanced or long-standing cases. Strabismus may produce what has been called *ocular torticollis*. Even hysteria may produce the deformity. Spasm of the sternomastoid muscle secondary to lymphadenitis may produce transient torticollis. It is important to rule out all the secondary forms because only congenital torticollis benefits from local treatment.

Many cases of neonatal torticollis will resolve spontaneously in three to nine months, while others respond favourably to intensive physiotherapy. Active physiotherapy should be initiated as soon as the diagnosis has been made. It is difficult to carry out effective physiotherapy after 9 months of age. An assistant holds the trunk, arms and shoulders while the therapist manipulates the head, canting it to the normal side and rotating it toward the involved side. Massage of the stretched muscle and tumour reduces spasm. Positioning baby and crib so that it must turn to the side of the lesion to satisfy its developing interests will aid spontaneous regression. If the sternomastoid tumour does not resolve in three to nine months, the muscle will be replaced by shortened fibrous tissue and the deformity become chronic. Such cases will require sternomastoid tenotomy.

Sternomastoid tenotomy should be done at 12 to 18 months of age for all cases of primary torticollis in which the condition is still present at that age. An incision including platysma is made $\frac{1}{2}$ to 1 in. above the clavicle, parallel to a neck crease or its continuation, down to sternomastoid muscle. The sternal and clavicular heads are cut under direct vision and allowed to retract fully. Excision of muscle is rarely indicated. The posterior fascia or pseudosheath is palpated with a finger. This structure almost always contains shortened fibres and should be transected under direct vision, protecting the deeper vital structures. The regional deeper muscles, splenius capitus, trapezius and scaleni are examined. Involvement of these is rare, but if present must be transected. Only platysma and skin are closed. A subcuticular suture will decrease needle marks.

Young cases require no immobilisation because of their spontaneous activity. Older patients, or recurrent cases, require immobilisation either by an eccentric soft padded neck collar, or, a plaster cast holding the head in the over-corrected position. Active physiotherapy and posture instruction in front of a full-length mirror is started one week postoperatively.

MIDLINE FISSURE AND SINUS

The midline of the neck is the site of a relatively rare congenital defect (Fig. 23, 3) representing defects in midline fusion as the paired lateral arches are developing. The

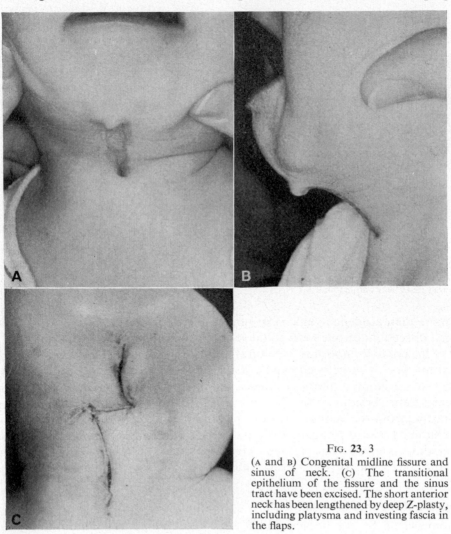

FIG. 23, 3
(A and B) Congenital midline fissure and sinus of neck. (C) The transitional epithelium of the fissure and the sinus tract have been excised. The short anterior neck has been lengthened by deep Z-plasty, including platysma and investing fascia in the flaps.

distance between mentum and manubrium is shorter than normal. The midline skin will be the site of a fissure or groove the base of which may contain transitional epithelium (Fig. **23**, 4). Skin excrescences or tags may be present together with epidermal sinuses. The sinuses rarely pass deep into the neck but may extend up or down toward the manubrium for varying distances.

Treatment may be carried out as early as 3 months of age. It consists of excision of the abnormal skin in fissures and tags and sinus tracts. Midline lengthening is usually necessary by single or multiple pairs of Z-plasties which include skin, platysma and investing fascia.

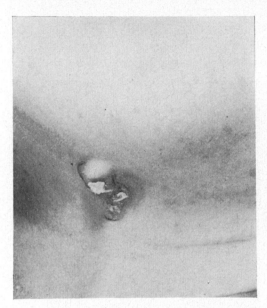

Fig. **23**, 4

Congenital midline sinus of neck. There was a subcutaneous extension superiorly to the mentum and inferiorly to the manubrium. Microscopically the excised tissue was hamartomatous.

Branchiogenic Anomalies

Most congenital deformities of the neck can be related to the differentiation of the primitive branchial system, and attempts have been made to classify accordingly. This differentiation is a complex incompletely understood process. It is common for clinicians to classify or think of these lesions in ways which may be more practical from a clinical point of view. Some clinicians classify these conditions as *lateral lesions* and *midline lesions*. Others think of these lesions as lesions of the facial nerve (first branchial cleft anomalies) and lesions of the hypoglossal nerve (second branchial cleft anomalies). Both systems have practical merits.

Embryology

An understanding of the embryology is of more than academic value. The surgery of congenital neck lesions is usually a regional dissection, or one local to the lesion, rather than a block dissection. Knowledge of the possible important structures usually related to each congenital condition makes this type of surgery safe and possible.

The neck develops as a series of ridges and furrows known as branchial arches and branchial clefts. Lesions of the first branchial cleft may present anywhere along the line starting from the auditory meatus, passing immediately behind the angle of the mandible and forward along, or immediately below, the inferior border of the body of the mandible. Lesions of the second cleft may occur anywhere along the line running from the lower end of the sternocleidomastoid muscle upwards to the tonsillar pillar.

Anomalies of the first branchial cleft

Anomalies of the first branchial cleft are considerably less common than those of the second branchial cleft, and they tend to present in more varied ways. For this reason they are more commonly misdiagnosed and mistreated.

These lesions may be present at birth or develop later—usually in infancy or childhood (Fig. **23**, 5). It is common for them to present as recurring areas of inflammation and chronic draining sinuses behind or immediately beneath the mandible (Fig. **23**, 6). There may be a sinus or fistula in the earlobe or a connection to the external auditory canal.

The very common *preauricular sinus* is tempting to consider as a variant of the first branchial cleft anomaly because of its proximity to that embryological region. The fact that this lesion is so much more common, has such a constant opening just above and in front of the tragus, almost always ends blind against the cartilage of the most anterior portion of the superior conchal fossa and almost never is related to the facial nerve, is against it being considered a variant of the first branchial cleft lesion.

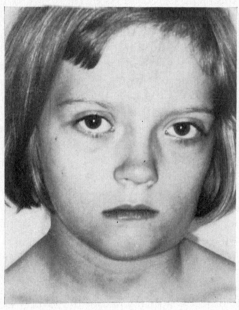

FIG. **23**, 5

First branchial cleft cyst. Excision had been carried out in infancy only to recur at 5 years of age. Excision at that time was much easier because the cyst wall was formed better.

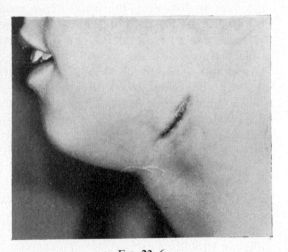

FIG. **23**, 6

First branchial cleft cyst and sinus. There had been recurring episodes of swelling beneath the mandible which had been drained several times. At operation a tract extended up and communicated with the outer inferior part of the auditory canal and was adherent to the facial nerve.

The preauricular sinus is frequently bilateral. It is not uncommon for one parent to have a similar lesion. They frequently exist throughout life as a pin-point dimple or opening which produces no symptoms but may occasionally extrude a small amount of sebaceous material. An occasional sinus becomes red and tender. The swelling is frequently 0·5 to 1·0 cm anterior to the sinus opening. It may discharge spontaneously through the sinus opening. The more anterior swelling may ulcerate through the skin and discharge there.

An asymptomatic preauricular sinus requires no treatment other than a prophylactic warning to parents to keep the area clean. If there has been an episode of inflammation in the sinus or anterior to it one should treat this conservatively with compresses. Once the acute episode is resolving the lesion should be excised. The opening is included in an elliptical skin excision. A fine probe is placed in the tract and the tract excised. This almost always goes down to conchal cartilage. The cases with anterior inflammation may have attenuations of the tract extending out that way or there may be no obvious extension. Careful excision of the tract usually cures such cases. Occasionally it is necessary to excise skin and deeper granulation tissue over the anterior area and rotate in surrounding skin for a direct closure.

The treatment of a *true first branchial cleft sinus or fistula* involves a decision whether or not a classical exposure of the facial nerve will be necessary or advisable. This lesion is always approached with the knowledge that a main stem or branch of the facial nerve will be in close proximity to some portion of the lesion. If the facial nerve is approached directly and followed through the lesion, parts of the lesion will frequently be left unexcised and the lesion will recur. The author prefers to identify the lesion and stay in a plane very close to it, carefully dissecting along the tract as one does in following the facial nerve itself, watching for the first signs of facial movement. In this way it is possible to avoid injury of the facial nerve. A well-functioning nerve stimulator will be of value to some operators, as an adjunct to other methods of nerve preservation.

Infections have usually been present in first branchial cleft lesions. If present they must first be treated by incision and drainage with careful placement of the incision to accommodate its inclusion in formal excisions later. Three to six weeks should be allowed for early resolution. If one can choose the stage when there is a soft, well-formed wall around the tract rather than friable granulation tissue or dense fibrous tissue, excision will be easier and safer.

An elliptical incision to include the sinus opening is made. A fine probe similar to a No. 2 lacrimal duct probe is passed gently into the sinus tract to identify its general direction and the incision is extended, usually posteriorly to the region of the earlobe. Careful dissection is continued along the tract. An occasional tract will be fistulous, ending in the auditory canal close to the external auditory meatus. The internal opening should be excised but in a manner that will not narrow the ear canal.

If the first branchial cleft lesion is a cyst, the lesion is approached in the same way with a direct incision over the cyst. It is helpful to identify the mandibular branch of the facial nerve as the posterior facial vein crosses it in some of these lesions. Once one has recognised the surface of the cyst, general dissection is carried out directly on its surface, again watching for facial nerve activity and not cutting a strand of tissue until one is certain it is not a nerve filament.

Recurrences are common when previous infection has been present and parents should be warned of this possibility in a judicious manner.

Anomalies of the second branchial cleft

More common than anomalies of the first branchial cleft, these fall into four categories: (1) ectopic ear tissue, (2) branchial sinus, (3) branchial fistula and (4) branchial cyst.

Ectopic ear tissue. This may appear at any point along the sternomastoid line (Fig. **23**, 7). It may take the form of skin or skin-cartilage excrescences or of cartilage embedded superficially in the sternomastoid muscle. Simple surgical excision is indicated.

Branchial sinus and fistula. These are the commonest lesions of branchial origin seen in the neck. They are frequently present at birth but may not be noticed until later childhood because they are minute. Mucous discharge draws attention to them.

They may occur anywhere along the anterior border of the lower two-thirds of the sternomastoid muscle, most commonly at a point just below

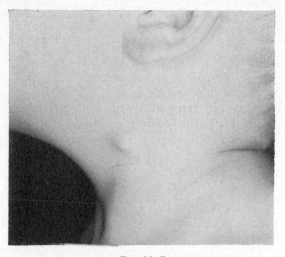

Fig. **23**, 7

Ectopic ear tissue in the neck.

the junction of the distal and middle thirds of that muscle (Figs. **23**, 8 and 9). Half of the lesions will turn out to be fistulous at operation. The internal opening is difficult to see pre-operatively without dye injection because it is hidden in the vicinity of the tonsillar fauces. Efforts to identify it pre-operatively are not necessary. Dye injections at the time of operation can be as troublesome as helpful. It is not uncommon for the dye to exude into surrounding tissues and obscure the operative field rather than delineate the tract.

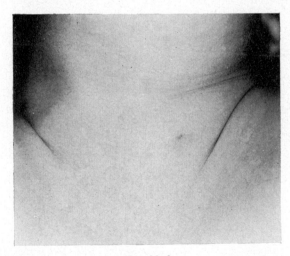

Fig. **23**, 8

Branchial sinus. The small sinus opening is just visible on the left neck. The drop of clear fluid contralaterally could be mucous from another sinus, but happens to be a tear!

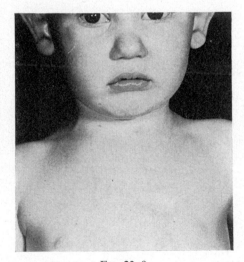

Fig. **23**, 9

Bilateral branchial sinus opening. There was a fistulous tract on both sides extending to the posterior tonsillar pillar areas.

Second branchial cleft cysts. These are not common, especially in infancy. They tend to appear later in childhood or in adult life.

Operation

The patient is positioned with the neck extended and the head rotated to the opposite side, and the head and chest slightly elevated. After preparation and draping the assistant temporarily turns the head anteriorly and flexes the neck to allow accurate identification of the neck creases. With the head in this position a short transverse ellipse, parallel to skin crease, is drawn to include the sinus opening. A second incision

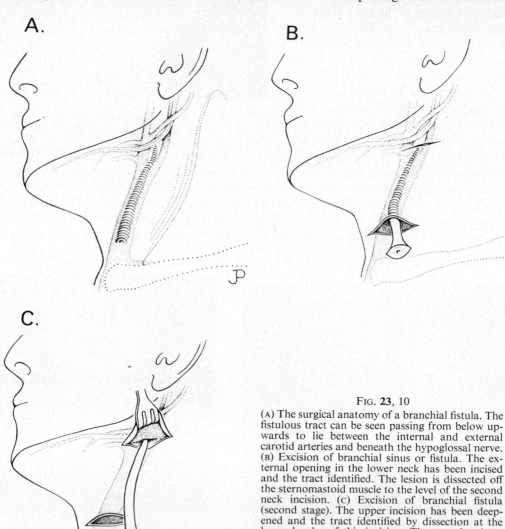

Fig. 23, 10

(A) The surgical anatomy of a branchial fistula. The fistulous tract can be seen passing from below upwards to lie between the internal and external carotid arteries and beneath the hypoglossal nerve. (B) Excision of branchial sinus or fistula. The external opening in the lower neck has been incised and the tract identified. The lesion is dissected off the sternomastoid muscle to the level of the second neck incision. (C) Excision of branchial fistula (second stage). The upper incision has been deepened and the tract identified by dissection at the lower border of this incision. The tract has been delivered into the second incision. Dissection is continued proximally beneath the upper border of the second incision using gentle traction and dissection on the lesion.

line is marked parallel to a neck fold at the junction of the middle and upper third of the sternomastoid muscle. The head is returned to its rotated and extended position (Fig. **23**, 10A, B and C).

The sinus is excised with its ellipse of skin. The fine probe is passed into it gently, to avoid fabrication of false tracts in areolar tissue planes. Dissection is carried out proximally on the anterior border of the sternomastoid muscle. As one approaches the upper incision site the tract commences to pass deeper. The second incision is made and the dissected tract identified below, and passed up into the second incision. From here, dissection is continued along the wall of the tract. Many sinuses end at this level or even closer to the skin.

From this point on the lesion usually lies between the internal and external carotid arteries below and the hypoglossal nerve above. The dissection is carried as high as possible. The tract may end anywhere along the line and will be totally excised. If it persists as a fistula it can be transected when the dissection has gone beyond the vessels and nerve. It does not require ligation, although some surgeons prefer to ligate. It is not necessary to identify the internal opening. The skin incisions are closed without drainage.

Pathology

Superficial sinuses will be lined with squamous epithelium. Deeper sinuses and fistulae are lined with collumnar, often ciliated collumnar, epithelium reminiscent of the respiratory tract. The walls contain lymphoid tissue.

Results

Elusive deep portions of sinus or fistula are the cause of recurrence. Perforation of the tract by forceful probing or confusing a narrowing of the fistulous tract with the end of a sinus tract are the usual causes. Recurrences are commoner after cyst excision than after sinus or fistulae excision. Parents should be warned of this possibility.

THYROGLOSSAL DUCT CYST

The commonest midline lesion of the neck in infancy is the thyroglossal duct cyst. These are usually not noticed at birth, but appear between 3 months and 13 years of age. Parents notice a round swelling in the region of the hyoid bone, but often consider it an enlarged Adam's apple. The swelling is often not noticed until it becomes red and sore. It may recede, with or without discharge, only to return. This lesion presents as a dermal sinus only occasionally. Less frequently the swelling may present near the foramen caecum of the tongue. A fistula may be present between the foramen caecum and anterior neck, although the author has never seen one.

The swelling is usually at the lower border of the hyoid bone and almost always moves with the hyoid bone on swallowing (Fig. **23**, 11). Occasionally it may be above the hyoid, or lower in the neck over the thyroid cartilages. It may be slightly off the midline. Older children may complain of dysphagia, a fullness in the throat or a tight collar.

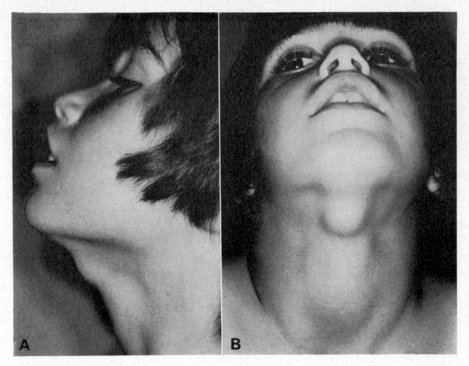

FIG. 23, 11

Thyroglossal duct cyst. The lesion moves briskly and synchronously with the hyoid bone.

Embryology

The development of the neck is closely related to that of the tongue. As the neck elongates the tuberculum impar divides the primitive tongue into two parts. One part descends in the neck and differentiates to become the thyroid gland. The line of descent may persist totally, or in part, as a thyroglossal duct tract.

Treatment

The lesion should be excised once it is noticed unless acutely inflamed. With the assistance of a paediatric anaesthetist, the operation is frequently done at 3 months of age. It was formerly customary to wait until infants were older. If a lesion becomes inflamed during the waiting period its management is more difficult.

Lesions which are inflamed may resolve spontaneously or fluctuate and point. The latter lesions will require incision and drainage. This should be done with a short transverse incision in the location of the future formal excision site. When the inflammatory reaction has subsided, usually in three to six weeks, formal excision should be undertaken.

The surgeon should approach this lesion with a plan to carry out the radical operation of Sistrunk (Fig. 23, 12A to F). A conservative excision is followed by a higher recurrence rate because it is difficult to identify tract remnants macroscopically at operation.

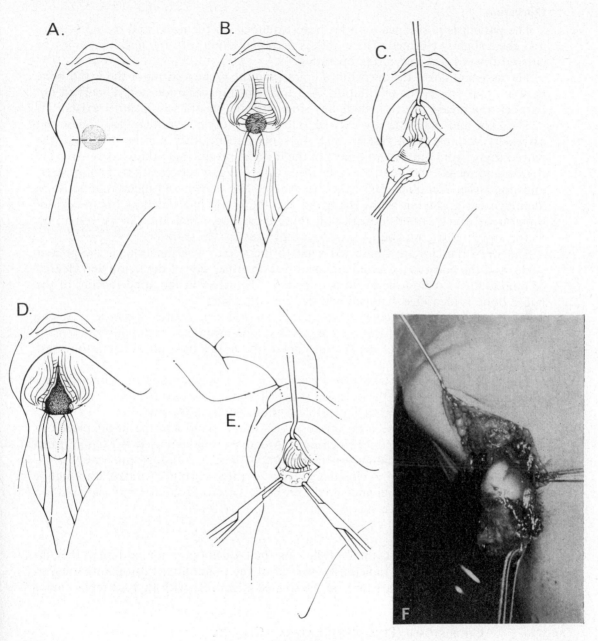

Fig. **23**, 12

Thyroglossal duct cyst operation. (A) The incision in or parallel to that crease over or beneath the lesion. (B) To show the surgical anatomy. The strap muscles are transected beneath the hyoid bone and thyrohyoid membrane identified. (C) Enough dissection is carried out above the lesion to allow identification of the hyoid bone on either side of the lesion. (D) The hyoid bone has been transected on either side of the lesion, leaving the lesion attached to the body of the hyoid (not shown in this diagram). (E) With a double gloved finger in the mouth and traction on the specimen, a core of tongue muscle is excised up to the foramen caecum in continuity with the specimen. (F) The final stage of the operation.

Operation

The patient is positioned with his head extended on the neck, and the neck, head and chest slightly elevated. The mouth is prepared along with the neck, so it may be entered towards the end of the operation.

The assistant flexes the draped head, grasping the greater cornu of the hyoid bone between two fingers for orientation. A 3 to 6 cm transverse incision is marked out parallel to a crease line to include any sinus opening or old scar if either exists.

The skin and platysma are excised. The strap muscles are identified. These are extremely variable from case to case. In some patients they will be thick and the paired thyrohyoid muscles will meet in the midline producing a thick cover over the thyrohyoid membrane. In other cases there will be a gap between these two muscles, allowing easier identification of the membrane. The thyrohyoid membrane must be identified early, staying below the hyoid and the lesion but watching for the exceptional tract which extends down to the thyroid cartilage, instead of, or as well as, up to the region of the tongue.

The strap muscles are transected beneath the hyoid. The junction of the greater cornu and the body of the hyoid are identified on either side of the lesion and cleared of muscle in the region the hyoid is to be cut. The artery at the upper border of the hyoid bone is identified clamped and tied on either side.

At this stage it may become obvious that the lesion is entirely separate from the hyoid. If one is certain of this the conservative operation may justifiably be resorted to. If there is doubt about the discreteness of the lesion the radical operation must be proceeded with.

The hyoid bone is cut with heavy scissors or fine bone-cutting instruments. The freed body of the hyoid with the lesion attached to it is dissected from the pharyngeal wall, as far from the hyoid as is possible without entering the pharynx.

The second glove is placed on the surgeon's minor hand and the finger placed in the mouth resting on the foramen caecum. A core of tongue muscle is excised up to the foramen caecum, including the tract if one is present, although one rarely is.

The tongue muscle gap is closed with two or three chromic sutures, although a tight closure is not essential and should probably be avoided. Platysma and skin are closed. A drain is not necessary.

Results

Recurrences are not as common following the radical operation, although they do occur. Parents should be judiciously warned of the possibility. Postoperative hypothyroidism is extremely rare and can be treated effectively with thyroid replacement therapy.

CHORISTOMA (PERSISTANT LATERAL CERVICAL CYSTIC THYMUS)

It is of both practical and academic value to distinguish the lesion known by these names from the branchial cyst. It may occur spontaneously, after trauma or after infection as a mass in the line of the lower two-thirds of the sternomastoid muscle (Fig. 23, 13A and B). Deviation of the trachea to the opposite side is common.

Treatment is by surgical excision through a transverse skin crease incision. Step-

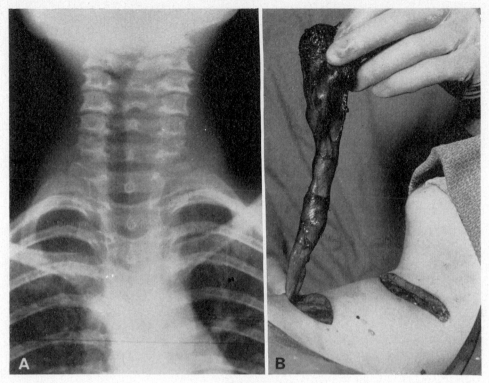

Fig. **23**, 13

(A) Choristoma (persistent lateral cervical cystic thymus). The lesion in the left neck is displacing the trachea to the right. (B) To demonstrate the lesion and the operative procedure. Stepladder incisions are used and the excision starts above at about the level of the bifurcation of the carotid artery and proceeds inferiorly, usually to a point beneath the manubrium sterni. (Courtesy, The Editors, *Canadian Journal of Surgery*, **6**, 178–86, 1963.)

ladder incisions may be necessary with the second incision lower than the first. The lesion will be alongside the carotid sheath from the bifurcation of the carotid above to varying levels in the region of the manubrium sterni below. Its lower limits have always been able to be defined from the lower neck incision in our experience.

The lesion will contain thymic tissue in varying degrees of differentiation and cystic degeneration, together with variable amounts of ciliated or columnar epithelium derived from the third pharyngeal outpouching. Lymphoid tissue is not a constant feature.

TUMOURS

BENIGN

Lymphangioma (cystic hygroma)

This topic is also discussed in Chapter XXXVI.

Cystic hygroma is a term used to name one clinical type of lymphangioma, namely

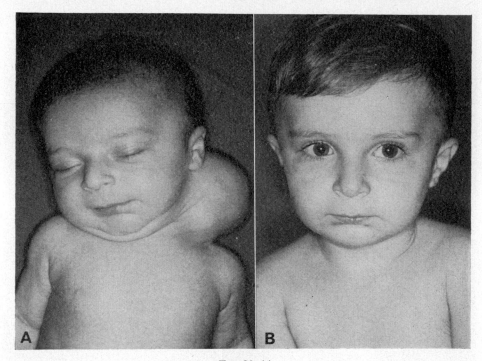

Fig. **23**, 14

(A) Lymphangioma. The lesion was excised at 3 months of age. (B) Excision has been planned so that scars will lie in or parallel to skin creases.

a cystic lymphangioma. The term is non-specific pathologically, but will be difficult to supplant clinically. Lymphangioma is commonest in the neck, about 60 per cent of all cases occur there and so will be described in detail in this section (Fig. **23**, 14A and B).

PATHOLOGY

Controversy exists as to whether the lesion is a true neoplasm, a hamartoma or a result of congenital dysplasia of lymphatics. It is likely that misplaced displastic lymphatic tissue is sequestrated in the developing foetus. If lymphatic channels or spaces between areas of lymphatic tissue become filled with lymph or blood or inflammatory products they may enlarge, even becoming cystic. Macroscopically the lesions are multilobular and multiloculated. They may be relatively discrete or diffuse with tongues and sheets of tissue extending out along fascial planes, between nerves and vessels and actually 'invading' muscle and other tissue. The lesion may contain dilated channels, small and large cysts. Opening an apparently unilocular cyst will usually show it to be haphazardly honeycombed or trabeculated resembling the bladder. The contained fluid may be clear, amber, cloudy, blood-tinged or frankly bloody. Microscopically the lesion consists of flattened epithelial cell walls or linings forming cystic spaces. It will be difficult to tell from many haemangiomata, and pathologists rely on the clinical diagnosis to a considerable extent.

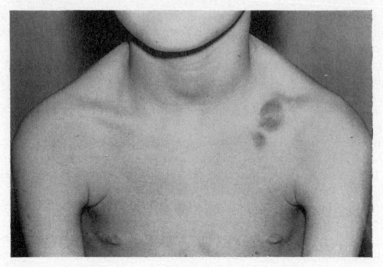

Fig. 23, 15

Lymphangioma simplex. There was involvement of the skin and the subcutaneous tissues only.

CLASSIFICATION

Lymphangioma simplex: superficial, primarily cutaneous or mucous membrane involvement manifested by red papular or vesicular lesions (Fig. 23, 15).

Lymphangioma cavernosa: deep usually diffuse involvement without large cyst formation. The limits of this type are often impossible to define at operation or on histological examination.

Lymphangioma cystica (cystic hygroma): large cysts which may be relatively well circumscribed.

Lymphangioma complex: when multiple areas are involved such as the neck and the axilla, or the neck and the floor of the mouth.

DIFFERENTIAL DIAGNOSIS

The lesion is frequently difficult to distinguish from the haemangioma. Both may give a bluish hue to overlying skin. Both may be associated with regional dilated veins. Indeed the two lesions may occur together. Congenital lymphoedema is difficult to distinguish and both may occur together, particularly in the extremities.

Branchial cleft cyst is difficult to distinguish but this lesion is usually confined to the line of the sternocleidomastoid muscle, while lymphangioma is usually more extensive. Lipoma, or lipomatosis can be a problem when the lesion occurs in an extremity.

NATURAL LIFE HISTORY

The lesion is usually present at birth or appears in the first few months of life. Both this lesion and the branchial cleft cyst may appear later in life throughout childhood and even in adult life. They may be small, only to enlarge with alarming speed and magnitude. The enlargement may be associated with trauma, a respiratory infection, skin scratches or episodes of spontaneous lymphangitis. Each new enlargement may decrease spontaneously or persist.

There has been no true reported case of lymphangioma undergoing malignant change. The fear of this need not enter into the consideration of a patient with this condition.

The role of the phenomenon of spontaneous regression is not as well documented for lymphangiomata as for haemangiomata. It has been the author's observation that lymphangioma left in at the time of operation will never enlarge in some cases, while in others this residual tissue will undergo marked cystic enlargement and channel dilatation. This is in all probability due to alterations within residual tissue, rather than new growth. Peripheral growth has been described.

To study spontaneous regression, the cases of lymphangioma at The Hospital for Sick Children, Toronto were studied. They were divided into two groups—those in whom tissue was left in, usually around the carotid sheath contents, and those in whom all lymphangiomatous tissue was considered to be excised. There was a recurrence of a mass in about 25 per cent of both groups. This suggests that residual lymphangioma tissue can be dormant, or regress. It also suggests that as complete an excision as possible should be done.

TREATMENT

It is unreasonable to wait too long for a cervical lymphangioma to resolve spontaneously. Also, ulcerating and weeping lesions tend to develop severe infections. Surgical excision is the treatment of choice. This can be carried out on the very young child when good anaesthesia and supportive treatment is available. Radiation therapy, radon seat insertion and sclerosing solutions have all been described as treatment measures. The lesions are usually widespread and are relatively radio resistant, requiring large fields of and tumour doses of radiation. The long-term radiation effects may be as problematic as the original lesion.

The patient is prepared for a blood transfusion and is positioned with the neck extended, the head and chest slightly elevated. Whenever possible the incision or excision sites are designed to lie parallel to skin creases. An elipse of skin may be excised as part of the initial dissection. The dissection is carried on down to the cyst wall where the visible margin of the lesion is. The longer one can keep cysts intact, the more satisfactory the excision will be. When cysts are opened, the tumour mass collapses and becomes difficult to delineate from the normal tissue. Normal tissue should not be sacrificed to gain exposure or accomplish modified block dissections. Vital structures should not be sacrificed. Surgically produced deformities can be as deforming as the original lesion. On the other hand, the more complete the excision the less likely the recurrence.

Haemangioma

The neck is a common site for haemangiomata. The management of the pure haemangioma of the neck is the same as for other regions of the body (Chap. XXXV). It is worthy of note that many cervical haemangiomas are mixed haemangioma-lymphangiomata and as such do not undergo spontaneous regression as promptly as pure haemangiomata do.

Dermoid cyst

Dermoid cysts may present anywhere in the neck but are seen most commonly in the upper half of the neck just off the midline where they may be difficult to tell pre-operatively from a thyroglossal duct cyst (Fig. 23, 16A and B). Add to this the syndrome of the multiple epidermal cyst.

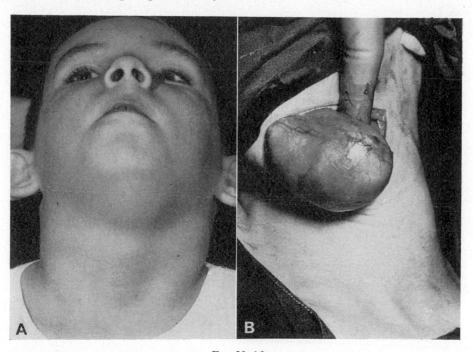

FIG. **23**, 16
(A) Dermoid cyst of neck. The lesion is in the mylohyoid triangle. (B) Appearance at operation.

Calcifying epithelioma of Maherbe

This interesting lesion of childhood and adolescence presents as intra- or sub-cutaneous lumps, which are somewhat mobile and have a firm edge on palpation. They are treated by surgical excision and will be found to have a thin wall enclosing calcified material. Both should be removed.

MALIGNANT

Malignant cervical tumours are very rare in children, with the exception of lymphomas, and they must be distinguished from specific and non-specific lyphanden-itis. It is not proposed to discuss their management in a volume of this specialised nature, however, and surgical works devoted to general plastic or paediatric surgery should be consulted for such information.

W. K. LINDSAY

REFERENCES

FARMER, A. W. (1950). *Essays in Surgery*, pp. 131–144. Toronto: University of Toronto Press.

FIELDING, J. F., FARMER, A. W., LINDSAY, W. K. & CONEN, P. E. (1963). Cystic degeneration in persistent cervical flamus: a report of four cases in children. *Can. J. Surg.* **6**, 178–186.

GOTTLIEB, E. & LEWIN, M. L. (1966). Congenital midline cervical clefts of neck. *N. Y. Jl Med.* **66**, 712–718.

McPHAIL, N. & MUSTARD, R. A. (1966). Branchial cleft anomalies: a review of 87 cases treated at The Toronto General Hospital. *Can. med. Ass. J.* **94**, 174–179.

MONROE, C. W. (1966). Midline cleft of the lower lip, mandible and tongue. *Plastic reconstr. Surg.* **38**, 312–319.

PALETTA, F. X. (1966). Lymphangioma. *Plastic reconstr. Surg.* **37**, 269.

POLLOCK, W. F. & STEVENSON, E. O. (1966). Cysts and sinuses of a thyroglossal duct. *Am. J. Surg.* **112**, 225.

WILLIAMS, D. W. (1952–53). Congenital midline cervical cleft and web. *Br. J. plast. Surg.* **5**, 87–93.

SISTRUNK, W. E. (1920). The surgical treatment of cysts of the thyroglossal tract. *Ann. Surg.* **71**, 121.

SECTION 2

TRUNK

CHAPTER XXIV

SPINA BIFIDA

There are few malformations in which the lesion may involve so many systems in the body as spina bifida cystica. The term 'spina bifida' is applied to a developmental gap in the vertebral column through which the contents of the spinal canal may protrude. Except in its simplest form (spina bifida occulta), it is usually a very grave anomaly and is commonly associated with anomalies of the spinal cord and paralysis of the lower limbs—both motor and sensory—with trophic and vasomotor changes in the skin and paralysis of the sphincters. There may be multiple developmental errors and many patients die at or soon after birth.

The incidence in the general population is said to be 1 in 800 births. Having had one child with overt spina bifida, parents should be warned that the chance of the malformation appearing in any later child is approximately 1 in 25. After the birth of a second child with spina bifida, the risk of recurrence increases to 1 in 10.

Embryology

Early in intra-uterine life the neural groove appears as a longitudinal furrow in the ectoderm on the dorsal surface of the embryo. The edges of the furrow unite to form a tube from which the nervous system is developed. The tube becomes separated from the surface by mesoderm, and on the ventral side the vertebral bodies develop round the notochord. The developing vertebral arches fuse, first in the thoracic region, and fusion then extends up and down. Failure of fusion gives rise to spina bifida which is frequently associated with maldevelopment of the spinal cord and membranes.

Spina bifida occulta

This is a common anomaly which is usually of no significance and is often discovered accidentally by radiography. Frequently only one vertebra (lumbar or sacral) is affected and there is no protrusion of cord or membranes. A local patch of hair, a naevus, a lipoma or a small circular or ovoid area of atrophic or parchment-like skin in the lumbosacral region are suggestive of an underlying bone deficiency (Fig. **24**, 1). The condition rarely gives rise to symptoms in childhood. Minor anomalies in spinal fusion seldom if ever have any causal relation to enuresis. In later childhood and adolescence neurological signs may appear, due to increasing tension produced at the site of the defect by disproportionate growth of vertebral column and spinal cord. Local skin lesions may have to be removed for cosmetic reasons.

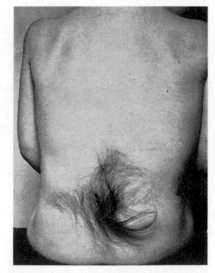

FIG. **24**, 1
Spina bifida occulta. Pre-operative condition, showing tuft of hair (see Fig. **25**, 1).

381

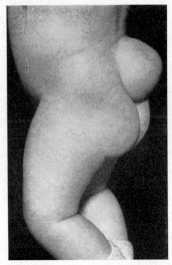
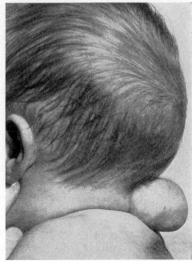

A   B

FIG. **24**, 2

Meningocele. (A) Lumbo-sacral. (B) Cervical.

Spina bifida cystica

While we have used the terms 'meningocele', 'myelo-meningocele' (meningomyelo-cele), 'syringomyelocele', and 'myelocele', it is convenient to group all these lesions under the broad term of 'spina bifida cystica'. In the rather uncommon meningocele there is no nerve involvement: in all the other lesions there is myelodysplasia in varying degrees with associated paralysis.

Meningocele. There is a herniation of the meningeal coverings through a gap in the vertebral arches and this presents as a midline swelling in the back, most commonly in the lumbo-sacral region (Fig. **24**, 2A), but occasionally in the cervical or thoracic region (Fig. **24**, 2B). Rarely the defect presents to one or other side of the midline. The meningocele is usually covered completely by normal skin or the covering may consist of a thin and translucent layer which readily ulcerates and ruptures. No individual meningeal layers can be distinguished in this covering. The swelling is cystic and may become more tense when the child cries. A meningocele may be translucent or it may be associated with an excess of lipomatous or angiomatous tissue.

Although the pathologist may report ectopic nerve elements in the excision specimen, there is no myelodysplasia and no paralysis. Meningoceles constitute about 14 per cent of all cases of spina bifida cystica.

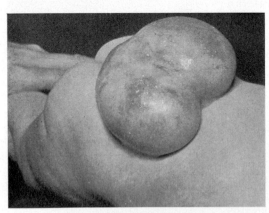

FIG. **24**, 3

Lumbo-sacral myelomeningocele.

Meningomyelocele. To outward appearances the swelling may resemble the less common pure meningocele, but in this anomaly there are always nerve elements in the sac (Fig. **24**, 3). These elements vary from normal or ectopic nerves, ectopic spinal cord, to the cauda equina or the cord itself. The swelling may be entirely cystic or there may be solid elements. If cerebrospinal fluid is aspirated and replaced by air, a lateral radiograph may show the nerve elements coursing across the sac. Lumbosacral meningomyelocele is usually associated with motor and sensory paralysis of the lower limbs as well as paralysis of the bladder and rectum; trophic ulcers develop readily. There may be associated club foot—usually talipes equino-varus. Evident hydrocephalus may be present at birth or it may develop later. This form of hydrocephalus is commonly associated with the Arnold Chiari malformation, in which a cone of medulla and cerebellum is prolonged downwards through the foramen magnum.

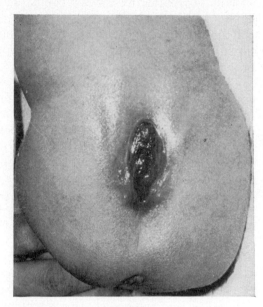

Fig. **24**, 4
Myelocele.

Syringomyelocele. In this rare anomaly the presenting features are similar to those of meningomyelocele, but the central canal of the cord is greatly dilated. The condition is only of embryological interest.

Myelocele. Arrest of development has occurred before closure of neural groove (Fig. **24**, 4) and the infant presents with a raw elliptical area from which the open cord discharges cerebrospinal fluid. At one time this condition was rarely compatible with life. Many babies were stillborn; others died within a few days from infection of the cord and meninges. Since the introduction of chemotherapy, many lesions start to epithelialise and, after a few days, present with a cystic swelling resembling meningomyelocele.

Differential diagnosis

The only conditions which may give rise to difficulty in differential diagnosis are posterior enteric remnants and sacrococcygeal teratoma (Chap. XXX). Lipomata are rare tumours in infancy and childhood but they do occur in the lumbosacral region— usually to one side of the midline. Such lipomata are almost invariably associated with spina bifida.

Management

In 1957 in the Royal Hospital for Sick Children, Glasgow, we estimated that 90 per cent of babies born with spina bifida cystica died of meningitis, of progressive hydrocephalus, or of the complications of paraplegia. About 4 per cent lived as permanent invalids in wheelchairs and 2 per cent were able to lead an independent life after multiple orthopaedic procedures. Only 1 baby in 50 grew up to lead a normal life! Today ventriculo-peritoneal drainage has been replaced by ventriculo-atrial drainage, *q.v.*, and the prognosis in hydrocephalus is greatly improved. Advances in chemotherapy have allowed us to control meningeal infection. We have been compelled to reassess our orthopaedic procedures for dealing with paralysis and deformity and have made considerable progress in making incontinent children both healthy and socially acceptable by various forms of urinary deviation and regulation of bowel habit.

Before undertaking treatment an attempt is made to explain to the parents what surgery has to offer to their child. Except in patients with spina bifida occulta the prognosis is always guarded.

There is an early mortality of almost 40 per cent. In a simple meningocele with good skin covering, operation is not performed until after the infant is 3 months old. In 86 per cent of patients with spina bifida cystica (meningomyelocele, syringomyelocele and myelocele) operation is performed within the first 24 hours of life— not only to save life but to prevent deterioration in function. Many of these infants (more than 60 per cent) now survive, and by early operation we can lessen their disability. It is often possible to close the spinal defect in layers. Haemangiomatous staining of the skin is common in all types of spina bifida and after operation the haemangiomatous area may temporarily become more extensive. Over a period of years we have found that the incidence of progressive hydrocephalus is about 50 per cent, both in patients subjected to early operation and in those on whom operation is delayed (Chap. XXII).

Occasionally, babies with a serious spinal defect (e.g. myelocele) are born with active lower limbs and yet within a few hours after birth there is complete paralysis of the legs and sphincters. This terrifyingly rapid deterioration is due to drying of the cord rather than to infection or the formation of granulation tissue. As soon as possible after birth, the exposed cord is protected and kept moist with sterile isotonic saline solution or cast vinyl film while awaiting transport to a neurological or surgical paediatric unit. Even during operation, the spinal cord is kept moist with saline as it can be subjected to further drying from the heat of the operating room and from the overhead operating light.

When the back is closed the patient is reviewed in consultation with paediatric orthopaedic colleagues. The common limb deformities are paralytic club foot and paralytic dislocation of the hips. By manipulation, by the use of callipers and by stabilising operations, every effort is made to render the child ambulant as early as possible.

It is important to find out early if the neuropathic bladder can empty freely; this is done by excretory urography and micturating cystography. Operation on a meningocele or meningomyelocele will never improve bladder function and may even make the situation worse.

Urinary infection is controlled by chemotherapy, and excessive leakage may be avoided by keeping the volume of urine in the bladder as small as possible. The mother, and later the child, is taught to empty the bladder at regular intervals by manual pressure. By school age a boy can usually manage a portable urinal, but this apparatus is rarely successful in the female. In the female it may be justifiable to deviate the urine using a free ileal or colonic loop. This type of surgery is not without risk. Postoperatively blood-urea tests should be supplemented by estimations of serum chlorides, plasma bicarbonate and phosphates. On a few occasions we have known girls to gain reasonable urinary control when they reach puberty, but often at the expense of increased residual urine.

Important as it is to achieve urinary continence, preservation of renal function is of even greater importance. Patients with spina bifida who survive the early hazards of meningitis and hydrocephalus commonly die of renal failure. Recurrent infection may be suppressed by continuous chemotherapy.

Colostomy is seldom required for bowel incontinence. By the intelligent use of laxitives and suppositories, if necessary supported by a fairly short period of hospital or other suitable institutional treatment, bowel habits are usually rendered socially acceptable. Despite early closure of the spinal defect and the success of ventriculo-atrial drainage there is still a relatively high mortality from meningitis and infection of the urinary tract. All but 14 per cent of the children are paraplegic and many require repeated readmission to hospital.

WALLACE M. DENNISON

REFERENCES

BENTLEY, J. F. R. (1968). A scheme for the management of urinary dysfunction associated with spina bifida. *Z. Kinderchir.* **3**, 365.

MUSTARDÉ, J. C. (1966). Meningomyelocele: the problem of skin cover. *Br. J. Surg.* **53**, 36.

SMITH, J. S. & BENTLEY, J. F. R. (1969). Pre-operative protection of myeloceles with cast vinyl film. Studies on hydrocephalus and spina bifida. *Develop. Med. and Child. Neur.* **20**, 57.

PS O

CHAPTER XXV

THE SURGICAL TREATMENT OF SPINA BIFIDA

Spina bifida occulta

No treatment is required for the bifid spine or spines, but the overlying triangle of hair-bearing skin is an embarrassment and should be removed. This can be done by excision and direct closure in a few patients, but in the majority will necessitate the use of a moderately thick skin graft (Fig. **25**, 1) to provide cover. Late signs of neurological involvement in the lower limbs or urinary bladder may indicate the need for exploration of the spinal cord and release of restricting bands or a short ligamentum dentatum.

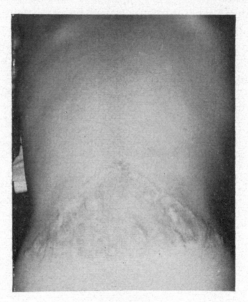

FIG. **25**, 1

Spina bifida occulta: hair-bearing area replaced by split skin graft (see Fig. **24**, 1).

Meningocele

True meningoceles containing no neural tissue are comparatively rare (Fig. **25**, 2A) and generally involve only one, or at most, two, bifid spines: they may occasionally arise from the occipital region of the skull. Treatment is comparatively simple and, whilst not an emergency procedure, should be carried out as soon as is possible in the thin-walled variety to avoid the risk of rupture of the covering layers. It consists of dissection of the neck of the meningocele (Fig. **25**, 2B) to allow the skin-covered meningeal sac to be removed and the spinal defect to be covered by plicating flaps of lumbo-dorsal fascia from either side. No difficulty should be experienced in closing the skin wounds by direct approximation (Fig. **25**, 2C).

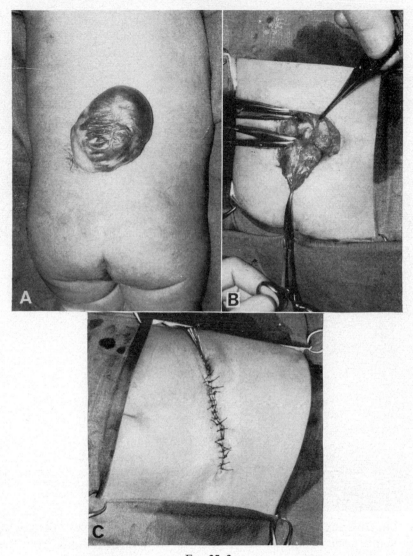

FIG. **25**, 2

Meningocele. (A) Pre-operative condition. (B) Single spine only affected: note narrow pedicle of meninges. (C) Skin closure easily effected.

Meningomyelocele

Most cystic spinal swellings are not true meningoceles but contain a varying amount of neural tissue, and despite the large size they may present on the surface (Fig. **25**, 3A) they generally arise, like the true meningoceles, from a single bifid spine —rarely two or more. Sometimes they are found to be ruptured at birth with c.s.f. leaking freely from them, and they must be closed as rapidly as possible to prevent the onset of meningeal infection. The risk of rupture is always present in the early stages in thin-walled cysts and they should be dealt with as semi-emergency cases

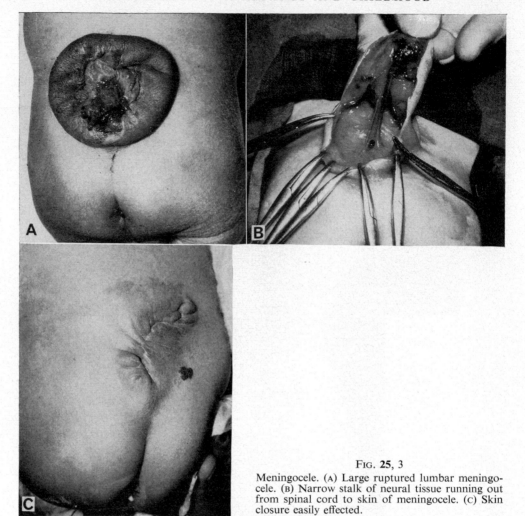

FIG. 25, 3
Meningocele. (A) Large ruptured lumbar meningocele. (B) Narrow stalk of neural tissue running out
from spinal cord to skin of meningocele. (C) Skin
closure easily effected.

unless the skin covering is obviously adequate. Operation involves opening the sac of
the cyst to identify the neural tissue, which will be found emerging from the gap in
the spinal canal and running out towards the surface layers (Fig. 25, 3B). As in simple
meningoceles the neck of the meningeal sac is carefully dissected by incising all round
the meningocele and carrying the incision into the fatty layer which surrounds the
neck of the sac. In very large meningomyeloceles some of the true skin around the
base of the swelling may be preserved, but this makes dissection of the neck of the
sac more difficult. As much of the neural tissue as possible should be saved—it is
quite probable that a large proportion of it is non-functional, undifferentiated tissue,
but this is difficult to determine. The neural tissue should be securely covered by a
layer of meninges and, if need be, a laminectomy is carried out on the vertebral arch
immediately above in order to accommodate the bulk of the neural tissue and meningeal covering. The remainder of the meninges and skin is discarded.

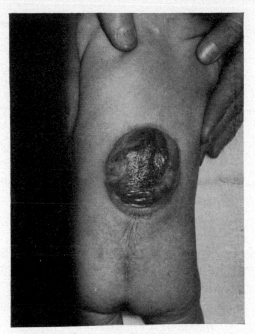

FIG. 25, 4
Severe spina bifida with neural tissue exposed on surface.

Flaps of lumbo-dorsal fascia are brought across from each side to provide strong cover and the skin is closed direct. Even where a relatively enormous meningo-myelocele is present there is usually no difficulty in obtaining skin closure (Fig. 25, 3C) although a rotation flap may occasionally have to be used.

Myelocele

Strictly speaking, myeloceles are flat and non-cystic with bifid spines lying opened out at 180° (Fig. 24, 4), but cystic swellings may exist on either side of the plaque of exposed neural tissue even at birth (Fig. 25, 4), and such lesions are sometimes referred to as meningomyeloceles. The exposed neural tissue is extremely sensitive for the first few hours after birth, and if touched in any way gives rise to a massive reflex reaction in the lower limbs with increase in spasm of the muscles. This reflex is quickly lost, and the limbs lose any power of movement they may have had in a matter of a few hours, so that operation on these babies is one of the most pressing of all neonatal emergencies. (The following account of the technique evolved by the writer, and the accompanying photographs are taken from *Plastic and Reconstructive Surgery*, Vol. 42, No. 2, by permission of the publishers, Williams and Wilkins.)

In cases of extensive and severe spina bifida (Fig. 25, 4), where the cord is grossly involved and neural tissue is presenting on the surface as a red, raw area, the problem of repairing the actual neural tube and its immediate coverings usually presents little technical difficulty (Fig. 25, 5A and B). The abundance of meningeal lining from the cystic tumour around the cord tissue provides adequate material which can be

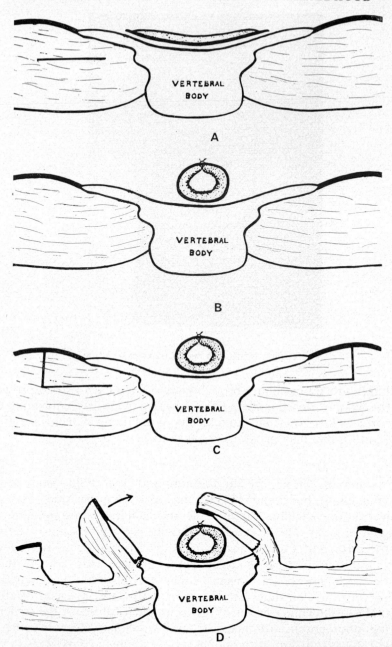

Fig. 25, 5

Schematic representation of steps in repair of severe spina bifida. (A) Neural tissue opened out as a flat plaque. (B) Neural tissue tubed and covered by meningeal layer. (C) Lateral muscle mass incised along lines indicated. (D) Bifid spinous processes fractured and osteo-muscular flaps brought over to form new spinal canal over reformed spinal cord.

brought up as a flap on each side to cover over the neural tissue. The real difficulty is to produce a strong covering layer for the reconstructed cord and meninges, which will be adequate for practical purposes, and yet be simple and safe to obtain.

In this severe type of case, the spines are not only bifid but the bifid processes are turned outward to lie horizontally. For all practical purposes the lumbodorsal fascia

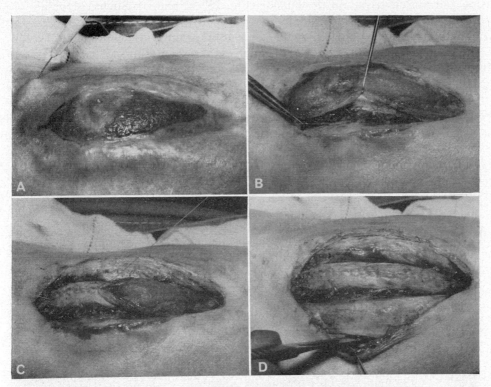

FIG. 25, 6

Photographs of steps in repair. (A) Injection of dilute adrenalin solution into skin around defect. (B) Separation of neural tissue and meninges from skin by sharp dissection. (C) Suturing meningeal layer to form water-tight covering over tubed neural tissue. (D) Vertical incision into lateral muscle mass.

is restricted to two comparatively narrow strips on the lateral side of the tips of the widely separated processes; when mobilized, these narrow strips of fascia are completely inadequate to stretch across the defect in the spine to form a protective covering.

The further problem of provision of skin-cover over the neural tube and its meningeal coverings is sometimes almost insurmountable in these cases, where seven or eight spines may be affected. Widespread undermining and flap rotation (Paterson, 1959), although it may sometimes permit skin and subcutaneous tissue to be brought over the area, is often followed by wound break-down and necrosis of tissue, due to tightness of the suture line and to interference with the vascular supply of the skin.

In addition to this, even if one is able to obtain a sound covering layer of skin for the neural tissues, the reformed cord is left vulnerable and ill-protected; in most cases, it is lying on the summit of an abnormally convex spine (Nash, 1963).

Some time ago it became apparent to the writer that all of the problems enumerated above might be overcome if the whole of the lateral mass of spinous processes and spinal muscles could be turned in to form a new spinal canal, with a bony skeleton inside and muscle tissue on the outside (Fig. **25**, 5c and D). Such a structure would not only provide adequate protection for the cord, but the muscle on the outside would form a suitable bed on which to place free skin grafts (Mustardé, 1966).

The operative technique which has evolved has the additional merit of requiring almost no undermining of the skin; hence, apart from the elimination of necrosis of the skin, there is considerably less blood loss than it was previously possible to achieve. Indeed, by injecting local anaesthetic with Adrenalin around the junction of the meningomyelocele and under the skin of the back (Fig. **25**, 6A), the blood loss has been cut down to minimal proportions and no intravenous therapy is necessary.

The technique, which is carried out in the first few hours of life to prevent irrecoverable paraplegia (Sharrard, 1963; Maudsley *et al.*, 1967), involves excision of the thin, transparent epithelium on the surface but careful preservation of all true skin on

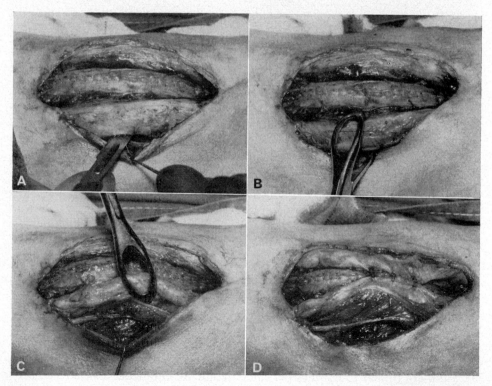

FIG. 25, 7

(A) Muscle dissection carried horizontally toward tips of bifid spines. (B) Each bifid spine is grasped by Lane's tissue forceps at its narrowest point near lamina. (c) The bone is fractured and the osteo-muscular flap turned medially. (D) Osteo-muscular flaps brought across spinal cord to meet in midline.

the meningomyelocele, whether discoloured or not. The meningeal layer, overlying the outwardly displaced spinous processes and lumbodorsal fascia, is incised around the periphery (Fig. **25**, 6B) and turned in as a flap on each side so that it can be sutured in a water-tight junction over the inverted neural tissue (Fig. **25**, 6C). If the exposed neural tissue is very large in area, it can be tubed and then covered by the meninges.

An incision is made vertically into the mass of the spinal muscles on either side, about 2 cm lateral to the tips of the bifid spines (Fig. **25**, 6D). At first, this incision is carried in vertically to a depth of 1·5 cm, and then the knife is turned horizontally so that the muscle mass is undermined to within about 3 mm of the horizontally lying tips of the bifid spines (Fig. **25**, 7A).

Each of the bifid spines is carefully located and fractured inward (Fig. **25**, 7C), using a suitable instrument such as Lane's tissue forceps; the muscle mass at each side, along with the fractured spinous processes, is brought across to meet its counterpart to form a musculo-osseous covering for the reconstructed cord (Fig. **25**, 7D). The suturing together of these lateral masses is best done in two planes: a deep lumbo-dorsal fascial layer (Fig. **25**, 8A), and then a superficial muscular layer (Fig. **25**, 8B). This prevents any later tendency for the reconstructed spinal canal to gape open. If

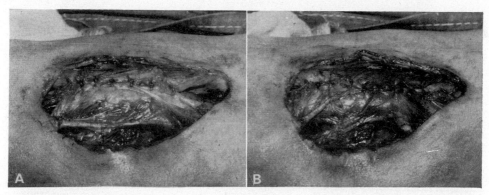

FIG. **25**, 8

(A) Lumbo-dorsal fascia is sutured. (B) Spinal muscle mass sutured over the lumbo-dorsal fascia layer.

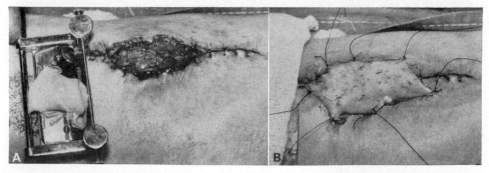

FIG. **25**, 9

(A) Skin sutured to underlying muscle mass *without tension*. (B) Skin graft applied to any remaining exposed muscle.

PS O 2

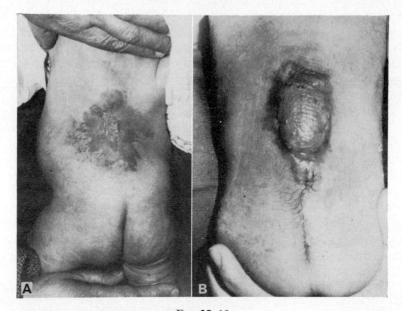

FIG. 25, 10

(A) Postoperative result in case shown in Figures **25**, 6 to **25**, 9. (B) Final result in case shown in Figure **25**, 4.

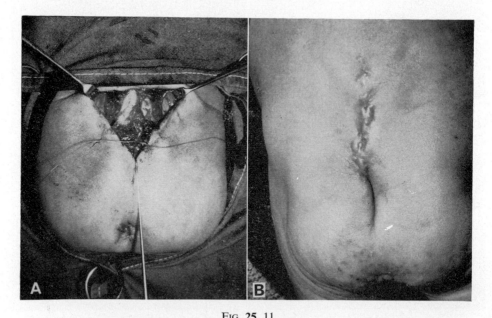

FIG. 25, 11

Lumbo-sacral myelocele (similar case to Fig. **24**, 4). The lower cord and cauda equina are protected by turning over a thin slice of cartilage of the iliac crest along with the detached lumbo-dorsal fascia.

the sacrum is involved, the lumbo-dorsal fascia attached to the iliac crest is turned in, along with a thin slice of the cartilage of the crest, to provide a covering layer (Fig. **25**, 11).

The skin of the back, and any skin which has been preserved from the lateral walls of the meningocele, is now sutured to the underlying muscle *without any tension* (Fig. **25**, 9A). It may be better to leave an area of muscle exposed in the centre if there is the slightest tightness on the skin edges when an attempt is made to close the defect. When the skin can be easily approximated, the edges are sutured together and a light pressure dressing is applied. If the defect cannot be completely closed without tension, a split-skin graft is cut from one of the buttocks and is sutured to the edges of the defect (Fig. **25**, 9B). The ends of the sutures are left long, tied over a pad of cotton wool or plastic sponge, and a top dressing is applied overall, using adhesive plaster for fixation. One week later, the dressings over the skin graft are removed; the dressings over the donor site are left untouched for one more week.

As would be expected, the exposed muscle layer readily accepts a skin graft (Fig. **25**, 10A). The end result, whether the skin has been closed directly or a graft applied, is to produce a soundly healed spine with protective bony arches, and with a substantial layer of soft tissue on top of this (Fig. **25**, 10B).

Early closure of severe spina bifida may tend to accelerate the appearance of hydrocephalus, and some indication of the likelihood of the onset of this condition may be obtained from the presence or absence of greatly enlarged fontanelles at birth. This subject is dealt with in detail in the succeeding section.

J. C. MUSTARDÉ

REFERENCES

COOPER, D. G. W., HOWARD, D. R. & PIKE, J. (1966). *The cause of death in children with myelomeningocele or hydrocephalus.* Read at the Annual Meeting of the Association for Research into Hydrocephalus and Spina Bifida, Bristol.

MAUDSLEY, T., RICKHAM, P. P. & ROBERTS, J. R. (1967). Long-term results of early operation on open myelomeningoceles and encephaloceles. *Br. med. J.* **1**, 663.

MUSTARDÉ, J. C. (1966). Meningomyelocele: the problems of skin cover. *Br. J. Surg.* **53**, 36.

MUSTARDÉ, J. C. (1968). Reconstruction of the spinal canal in severe spina bifida. *Plastic reconstr. Surg.* **42**, 109.

NASH, D. F. E. (1963). Meningomyelocele. *Proc. R. Soc. Med.* **56**, 506.

PATERSON, T. J. (1959). The use of rotation flaps for excision of lumbar meningomyelocele. *Br. J. Surg.* **46**, 606.

SHARRARD, W. J. (1963). Meningomyelocele: prognosis of immediate operative closure of sac. *Proc. R. Soc. Med.* **56**, 501.

CHAPTER XXVI

HYPOSPADIAS

DEFINITION AND HISTORY

Hypospadias is a congenital defect in which the urethral meatus is located in an abnormal position on the ventral surface of the penis or in the scrotum or perineum. (Hypospadias: Greek *hypo*—'under' and *spadizo*—'to tear off'.) The prepuce usually forms a hood over the dorsal portion of the glans penis. The glans is flattened, tipped ventrally, and grooved on the ventral surface. The tissues of the penis, within a triangle formed by the urethral meatus and the lateral edges of the hooded prepuce, are abnormal. The skin is thin and friable. A broad band of subcutaneous fibrous tissue extends from the existing meatus to the glans causing a ventral curvature of the penis called 'chordee'. (Latin *chorda*—'string'.) Hypospadias is often associated with other congenital abnormalities. In severe cases and when the testes are undescended, sex determination is difficult.

Galen has been credited with first describing this anomaly some time in the second century. Paulus of Aegineta (625–690 A.D.) suggested amputation of the deformed penis distal to the hypospadiac urethra. Dieffenbach in 1837 attempted unsuccessfully

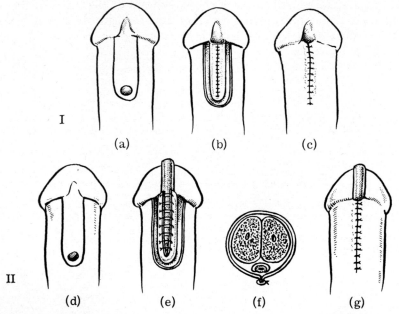

FIG. 26, 1

The two techniques of Duplay. The first (I) is a modification of that of Thiersch. The chordee having been relieved at a previous stage, a flap of skin is outlined (a), formed into a tube (b), and covered by the penile skin (c). The second technique (II) is similar but the flap of skin was not made large enough to be brought around the catheter. Epithelial growth of the buried skin allowed a complete tube to form (d, e, f, g).

to repair hypospadias. The first successful hypospadias repair was reported in 1842 by Mettauer, a pioneer surgeon from the backwoods of Virginia. Dr Mettauer also suggested for the first time the correction of the chordee by the use of 'subcutaneous incisions in succession until the organ is liberated'. Three famous French surgeons, Duplay (1880), Ombredanne (1923) and Nove-Josserand (1919) made the first modern contributions to hypospadias repair. Duplay was the first to recommend opening the skin of the penis to excise completely the tissues causing chordee as a preliminary operation. To repair the urethra he made parallel incisions on the ventral penile skin extending from the urethra to the glans. In his first description, he modified the procedure of Thiersch and made a tube of the skin so outlined by partially undermining and sewing it over a catheter. Later he found that a smaller median strip of skin could be used if the lateral edges of this median strip were undermined, partially elevated, and sutured around a catheter. He stated, 'Although the catheter is not really covered (by the skin strip) there are no ill effects upon the new canal.' Coverage was obtained by mobilizing the lateral skin flaps so that they could be brought together over the midline. Without stating so, he demonstrated the principle that a strip of buried skin would continue to grow until a canal had been formed by growth of the lateral skin edges (Fig. **26**, 1).

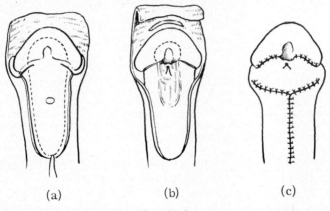

(a) (b) (c)

FIG. **26**, 2

The technique of Ombredanne. A large flap of skin is incised and elevated. A purse string suture is sewn around the edges of the flap and into the glans (a). Pulling on the purse string suture causes this skin to form a baggy tube to connect the meatus to the distal end of the penis (b). This was covered with a perforated perputial hood (c). The results of this operation left much to be desired.

In 1923, Ombredanne recommended a distally based flap at the urethral meatus, brought forward with a purse-string suture to the tip of the penis (Fig. **26**, 2). He also recommended a buttonhole type of preputial hood flap to transfer the prepuce to the ventral penile surface. This preputial flap was later modified and popularized by Nesbit.

The use of free split-thickness skin grafts to reconstruct the urethra was proposed by Nove-Josserand in 1919. Because split-thickness skin grafts contract, many strictures resulted from this surgery and therefore many other urethral substitutes were tried. Bladder mucosa, vein grafts and the appendix have all been advocated at one time or another for urethral reconstruction and have fallen into disrepute. Isografts and homografts of urethra have also been tried and discarded. McIndoe in 1937 recommended multi-staged repair of hypospadias and advocated the use of split-thickness skin grafts to reconstruct the urethra; however, he felt that splinting

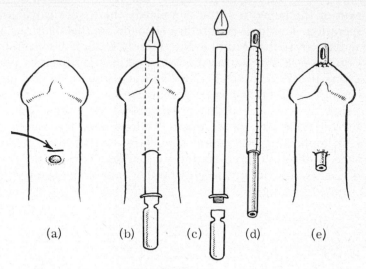

(a)   (b)   (c)   (d)   (e)

FIG. 26, 3

The technique of McIndoe. An incision is made distal to the urethral meatus (a). A special trocar is then passed the length of the shaft of the penis and out through the glans (b). The trocar comes apart (c) allowing introduction of a catheter to which has been fixed a split-thickness skin graft tube (d). The graft is attached at the distal and proximal ends, and the tube is left in place 6 months (e).

for a minimum time of six months after surgery was necessary prior to the final stage of anastomosing the proximal urethra to the newly constructed 'skin graft' distal urethra (Fig. 26, 3).

Numerous other types of hypospadias repair have been described in the literature. Many of these repairs have merit, many others have been discarded long ago. Backus in 1960 found over 150 techniques of hypospadias surgery in the literature. More have been added since that time. Modern techniques for repair of hypospadias usually stem from modifications of older operations. These techniques can be classified as either multi-staged or one-stage procedures, and these can be divided into those using only penile skin, those using penile and scrotal skin and those using free grafts in the repairs.

Multi-stage repairs include that of Sir Denis Browne who, in 1949, noting that a buried strip of skin would automatically form a tube, devised an operation quite similar to the method of Duplay. This operation is very popular at the present time and gives excellent results in capable hands. Byars in 1955 modified an operation described by Thiersch and Duplay and recommended multiple layers of sutures to aid the skin closure in the reconstruction of the urethra. His technique advocates surgical construction of the urethral tube and immediate coverage with lateral skin flaps.

The procedure of Bucknall (1907) utilizing the scrotum in the repair of hypospadias has been modified in two directions and each is quite popular and successful today. Cecil (1932) and Culp (1951) form the urethra from penile skin and bury it in the scrotum. At a later procedure the scrotal skin is excised and used to cover the ventral surface of the penis. Wehrbein (1943) and Smith (1955) utilize a previously formed tube of scrotal skin to cover the newly formed urethra.

One-stage procedures utilize either a tubed free graft of hairless skin or skin from the local area formed into a tube and covered with local skin. All reconstruction is accomplished at the time of the release of the chordee. We began the development of our one-stage procedure in 1955, as an extension of the work of Young and Benjamin (1949) and McCormack (1954). Humby in 1941 reported 12 cases of one-stage repair also using a full thickness free graft. Broadbent *et al.* (1961), Des Prez *et al.* (1961), Mays (1951), Aronoff (1963) and Mustardé (1965) have also reported one-stage repairs using penile skin in continuity for urethroplasties.

At the present time no magic solution has been found for the problem of hypospadias. Complications in healing frequently follow all types of operations. As with most surgical problems, there are many paths leading to successful correction. In certain hands, one path may be easier to travel than another. We feel, however, that any physician interested in this problem must keep abreast of new advances in this field and should take advantage of improving techniques when available.

INCIDENCE AND CLASSIFICATION

Culp states that approximately 8,000 hypospadiac children are born each year in the United States. This is an approximate incidence of one in every 313 live male births. In Denmark, Sorenson found a similar incidence of one hypospadias patient per 300 live male births. Crawford (1963) in England and Campbell (1951) in the United States found a somewhat lesser incidence. Ross noted that 14 per cent of all patients gave the history of more than one hypospadias problem occurring in the same family. In our series of approximately 135 cases, we have had two father-son combinations, one family with two hypospadiac sons but three other normal boys and another with three hypospadiac brothers. There is no evidence that maternal disease during pregnancy has contributed to the formation of this condition. Sorenson feels that hypospadias is transmitted by a recessive gene. Modern chromosomal studies have shown no defect characteristic of genital anomalies, but techniques now available show only gross abnormalities in the chromosomes.

We classify hypospadias according to the position of the urethral meatus: glandar, distal penile, midpenile, penoscrotal junction, scrotal or perineal hyposapdias (Fig. **26**, 4). Approximately two-thirds of our cases have been distal penile. Sorenson reported that three-fourths of his cases were glandar or distal penile. Culp has found that 'once the associated chordee is corrected' about 28 per cent of his cases have been penile, 45 per cent penoscrotal, 16 per cent scrotal and 10 per cent perineal.

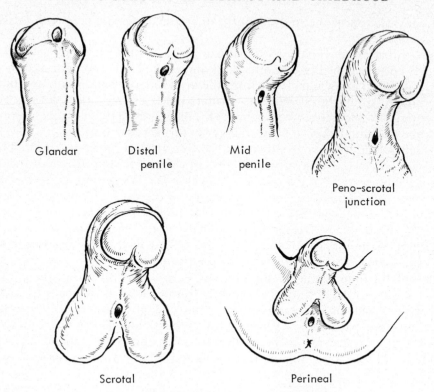

Glandar   Distal penile   Mid penile   Peno-scrotal junction

Scrotal   Perineal

FIG. 26, 4
Classification of degrees of hypospadias.

Embryology

At the end of the second week of embryonic development, a mesodermal cell layer begins to form at the primitive streak near the dorsal end of the embryo. The mesodermal cells move peripherally as they proliferate. Dorsal to the primitive streak the mesodermal cells pile up to form a ridge where the ectoderm and entoderm have fused. These become the cloacal ridge and membrane. After the tail fold forms, these structures come to lie on the ventral wall of the embryo, at the termination of the hindgut. Proliferating mesoderm continues to grow anterior to the cloacal membrane, forming the genital tubercle. Further development of this tubercle occurs by growth and extension of its caudal aspect. The cloacal folds extend along the ventral surface of the genital tubercle producing urethral folds which extend to the tip. As the cloaca is separated into bladder and rectum, the urogenital membrane (anterior half of the cloacal membrane) opens.

This growth is the same for both sexes and has occurred prior to the development of the gonads. As the primitive germ cells move into the gonadal ridge, gonadal development begins. The 'Y' chromosome of the male karyotype causes development of testes. The testes secrete a substance which causes the external genitalia to develop a male configuration from the indifferent stage. In the absence of this determiner, development will be female.

The genital tubercle elongates to become the phallus with the glans at the end. The urethral groove deepens. The edges of this groove become prominent and fuse to form a tube. A prominent median raphe marks the line of fusion which progresses from the urogenital opening distally. The glans becomes deeply grooved but does not close to form the glandar urethra until later as the formation of the prepuce occurs.

A defect in the quantity or quality of the male evocator, or premature cessation of its production will cause varying degrees of feminization of the external genitalia. The resultant deformity is hypospadias.

PATHOLOGICAL ANATOMY

In the usual case of hypospadias, the penis of the newborn is of normal size and is curved ventrally by a dense band of fibrous tissue which extends from the abnormally situated meatus of the urethra distally to the glans. We feel this fibrous tissue to be the result of anomalous development of the structures which would have surrounded the normal urethra—the corpus spongiosum, Buck's fascia and dartos fascia. This

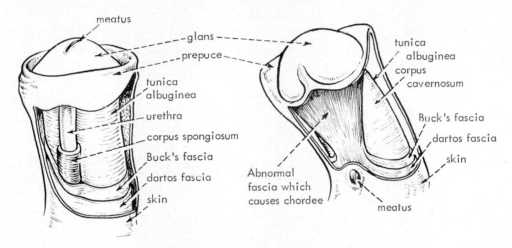

FIG. 26, 5

Anatomy of normal penis, and penis with hypospadias. In hypospadias the normal structures—urethra, corpus spongiosum, Buck's fascia, and dartos fascia—are replaced by a fan shaped band of fibrous tissue which holds the penis in chordee.

fibrous tissue extends forward from the end of the normal corpus spongiosum, surrounds the urethra, and inserts distally into the base of the glans in the sulcus between the glans and corpora cavernosa (Fig. 26, 5). Occasionally there may be hypoplasia of the penis. The meatus may be small and dilatation or meatotomy soon after birth may be necessary to allow normal micturition.

In some instances the urethra will end in the midshaft of the penis, yet a small mucosal tract may extend distally and end in a blind pouch. Occasionally the penis may be twisted and the raphe which is normally situated in the ventral midline may

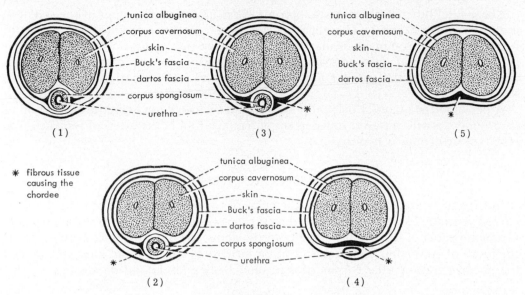

FIG. **26**, 6A

Cross-section of penis. Normal (1). Type III chordee without hypospadias (2). Type II chordee without hypospadias (3). Type I chordee without hypospadias (4). Hypospadias (5). These conditions differ only in the layers of tissue on the ventral surface of the penis which are abnormal and replaced by fibrous connective tissue (*). It is this tissue which must be resected to straighten the penis. When the urethra is present, it need not be sacrificed to accomplish this.

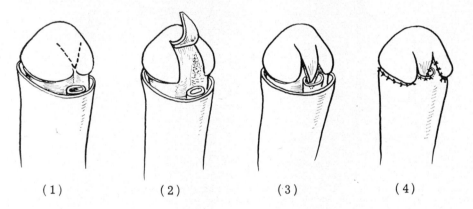

FIG. **26**, 6B

When the urethral meatus is at the frenulum of the glans and there is Type I defect proximal to that, repair is accomplished by making a circumcising incision leaving the urethra attached to the skin (1). After release of the chordee a 'V' shaped flap is raised on the glans (2). This is set into an incision made in the urethra (3), and the skin is reapproximated to the corona of the glans (4). Excess perputial skin is excised at that time.

be extended to one side or the other of the shaft. The scrotum may extend superiorly around the base of the penis (anterior scrotum), or in the case of scrotal or perineal hypospadias will be cleft in the midline. The glans will usually be indented at the fossa navicularis, simulating a normal urethral opening at the tip. Rarely a congenital

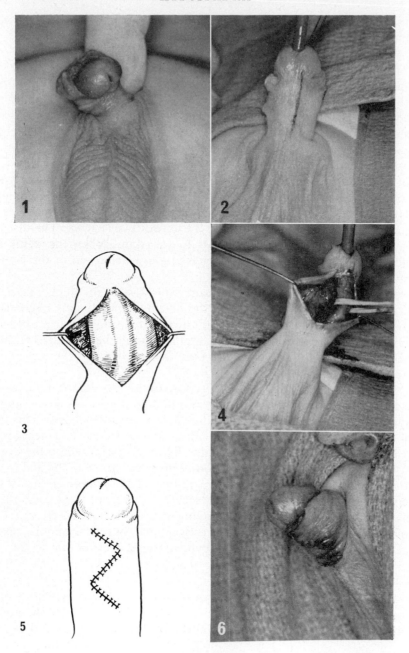

FIG. 26, 6c

Release of chordee without hypospadias. (1) Pre-operative—chordee without hypospadias. (2) A longitudinal incision is made lateral to the midline. (3) Exposure of the fibrous tissue and the urethra. (4) Resection of tissue causing chordee. When the fibrous tissue has been resected, the penis will straighten without cutting the urethra. (5) Z-plasty is used to close. (6) Note that the penile shaft is straight (lateral view).

urethral fistula may be present in association with hypospadias. In 10 per cent of all cases of hypospadias, cryptorchidism is present and must be treated.

Chordee without hypospadias (congenital short urethra)

Hypospadias will rarely occur without chordee, but about 10 per cent of our series of primarily operated cases have had 'chordee without hypospadias'. This condition has previously been termed by some 'congenital short urethra' and it has been recommended by many authors that the urethra must be divided to straighten the penis, creating a large urethral fistula which can later be reconstructed at a second stage. A one-stage repair of this deformity can be accomplished, however, without division of the urethra. We have found three types of chordee without hypospadias (Fig. 26, 6). In the first, the urethra is present as a thin tube of mucous membrane lying directly beneath the skin. The fibrous tissue causing the chordee lies between this structure and the tunica albuginea of the corpora cavernosa. This tissue can be resected leaving the thin urethra attached to the skin. When the penis has been straightened the skin and urethra will stretch to allow extension of the penis and no urethroplasty will be necessary.

In the second type, the corpus spongiosum will be present. Buck's fascia and the dartos fascia will be abnormal and form the fibrous band. In this circumstance the tissue to be resected will lie lateral to the urethra with a small central extension deep to the urethra. To release this chordee the urethra should be separated from the skin and the abnormal tissue removed by stripping the urethra and the tunica albuginea of the corpora cavernosa.

In the third type of chordee without hypospadias, the defect involves only the dartos fascia. The abnormal tissue in this situation seems always to be lateral to the urethra and in two of our cases involved only a segment of the shaft. It is important in each of the first two types of chordee without hypospadias to remember that dissection at the glans must be carried out laterally to the point where the dorsal hood of prepuce originates. If necessary, the hood of prepuce can be mobilized to cover the ventral surface of the penis. The urethra will extend the length of the straightened penis when all the fibrous tissue has been resected. In many of these cases the prepuce completely surrounds the penis and circumcision can be carried out when the straightening has been accomplished. It is conceivable that there may be cases of true congenital short urethra, but we have not encountered such in our series.

Female hypospadias

Hypospadias can occur in the female; however, it usually requires no surgery since the urethral opening is still within the vaginal vault. In severe cases, the urethra may be short enough to compromise urinary control and surgical repair will be necessary.

Hypospadias 'cripples'

The repair of hypospadias is a difficult and delicate procedure and all methods of repair are accompanied by complications and failures. Once postoperative scar tissue has formed on the ventral surface of the penis, it becomes more difficult with each unsuccessful stage to create an unscarred, unrestricted penis and to reconstruct the urethra. Some unfortunate patients may have undergone many stages of surgery and become what we term 'hypospadias cripples'. To repair this condition we recommend the relentless resection of all scar tissue on the penis. All ventral segments of the previously unsuccessfully reconstructed urethra should be sacrificed, leaving only the dorsal roof to form the outer skin surface of the penis. When the scar tissue causing chordee has been resected, it is usually possible at the same stage of surgery to use a graft of full-thickness skin (taken from a hairless area) and to burrow through the shaft from the normal proximal urethra to the tip of the glans to complete the reconstruction. A 'V'-shaped flap of glandar mucosa should be used to form an elliptical anastomosis at the tip of the glans. A wide elliptical anastomosis between the tube graft and the urethra should also be performed proximally. A scrotal flap is

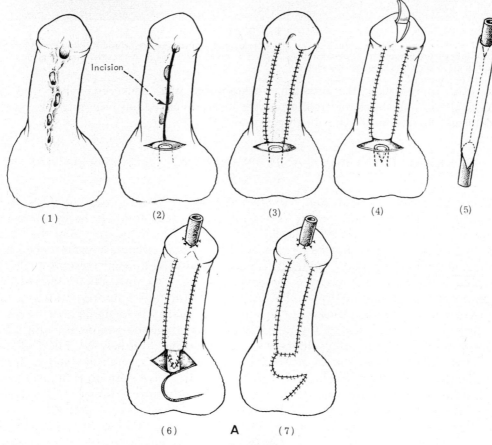

Fig. 26, 7a

Repair of hypospadias cripples. Repair of the multiple fistulas in this patient would not be feasible (1). An incision is made opening the repaired urethra back to the pre-existing normal urethra (2). The repaired urethra is excised leaving its roof as the ventral skin of the penis. The normal urethra is dissected free and incised (3). A 'V' flap is elevated from the glans and the skin of the shaft is undermined (4). A skin graft tube (5) is inserted beneath the skin to replace the urethra. This is facilitated by making the distal anastomosis to the 'V' flap, then pulling the catheter and the graft through before inserting the catheter into the urethra and making the proximal anastomosis (6). The skin is then closed (7).

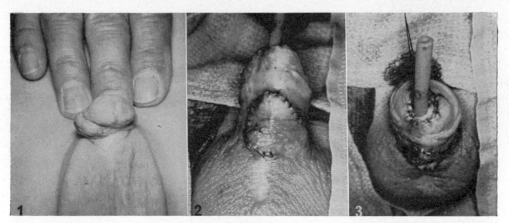

FIG. **26**, 7B

Hypospadias cripple (6 operations elsewhere) (1). Release of ventral scar tissue and full thickness graft for urethral reconstruction (2). Anastomosis of graft at tip of penis, using 'V' shaped midline glandar flap to allow an elliptical anastomosis (3).

then used to resurface the proximal anastomosis area. This repair has worked successfully in nine cases referred to us with severe hypospadias crippling. One such patient had undergone 14 previous operations (Fig. **26**, 7).

GENERAL PRINCIPLES AND TREATMENT OF HYPOSPADIAS REPAIR

When a newborn is first seen with hypospadias, it is important to assess the adequacy of the urethral opening. Occasionally a meatotomy is necessary as a preliminary step to the proposed surgical procedures. It is mandatory that the child with hypospadias should not be circumcised. If a ritual circumcision must be performed, special dispensation should be obtained and only a small incision made in the child to allow all the prepuce to remain for later reconstruction. Jewish law requires only that blood be drawn. This is probably the most important advice that the paediatrician and obstetrician can give the parents and will facilitate later successful surgery. A careful search for other associated congenital anomalies must be performed. An intravenous pyelogram should be done routinely on all cases of hypospadias. Cystoscopy should be carried out in the more severe cases and in those in which the true sex is in doubt. Sex chromatin studies have been done in all of our cases since the procedure was described, and recently chromosome studies have proved the maleness of one of our patients with very ambiguous genitalia.

The growth of the child and particularly of the penis should be evaluated at intervals until the organ is large enough to undergo the delicate surgery required to correct the condition. In our opinion, surgery is best performed somewhere between 18 and 24 months of age. We do not set an arbitrary time for this surgery but prefer to wait until the penis is large enough to allow adequate dissection and reconstruction. Rarely have we had to wait until 3 or 4 years of age. As the child gets older, the fascial layers of the penis become more fibrotic and dissection is more difficult. Therapy with anterior pituitary-like hormone has not caused satisfactory growth in our patients in whom it has been used and fibrosis of the fascia has seemed to increase, making the procedure more difficult. We have not used testosterone.

There are five criteria of successful hypospadias repair: (1) the chordee should be completely relieved so that the penis is unrestricted in motion; (2) the urethra should be brought to the tip of the penis; (3) a solid stream of urine should flow from the urethra on micturition with no splattering, splashing or backflow; (4) the external surface of the penis should be symmetrical and no abnormal tissue tags or fistulas should be present; and (5) normal sexual functions of the penis should be possible.

For many years competent surgeons have said that chordee release and urethroplasty should not be performed at one operation. The fear was expressed that if chordee recurred after the urethra had been reconstructed, secondary surgery would be more difficult. In the past, two or more stages for resection of the bands causing chordee frequently have been necessary because of inadequate surgery. Urethral reconstruction was often complicated by multiple fistulas, strictures and diverticula. Because of these possible complications, it was felt desirable to stage most hypospadias repairs. Our experience has demonstrated that these fears are no longer as appropriate as they have been in the past. In our repair wide unhindered exposure of the ventral surface of the penis has allowed complete resection of the tissues causing chordee. We have not had a case of recurrent chordee in any of our one-stage hypospadias cases. If chordee should recur following surgical resection, it would indicate to us that our surgery had been inadequate. Simultaneous chordee release and urethroplasty using local flaps is difficult, because adequate exposure of the tissues causing the chordee cannot be accomplished with facility if blood supply to the local flaps is to be maintained. As a result, flaps taken at some distance from the chordee area, or full thickness skin grafts (which do not contract) have been recommended by various authors. These techniques have been well established over a period of time, and it is no longer correct to say that it is improper to do a one-stage repair of hypospadias. Conversely, now it is proper for the patient to ask, 'Why cannot I have a one-stage repair of hypospadias?'

Reconstruction of the urethra

Following adequate resection of the tissues causing chordee, the urethra may be reconstructed with skin from various areas. If it is formed from local tissues, the flaps must be designed in such a way (1) to preserve blood supply, and (2) to extend to the tip of the penis. Many operations have been performed in the past in which the urethra was left at the base of the glans, with the idea that normal function of the urethra in micturition and in the deposition of sperm in the vagina would occur. If, however, the urethra can be taken to the tip of the penis, the patient is restored to a condition of normalcy. If a circular anastomosis is performed with the epithelium of the glans when the urethra is brought through the tip of the penis, contracture will produce a stricture at the meatus. A circular anastomosis in this position as in any other area of the body will contract. An important contribution to successful hypospadias repair which was originated by the authors is the construction of a glandar 'V'-shaped flap to fit into the anastomosis of the urethra in this area. In this way, distal penile strictures can be avoided. This procedure can be applied to many different techniques of hypospadias repair.

Distant flaps from the scrotum and abdomen have been used for the reconstruction of the urethra for hypospadias because of the lack of skin on the penis even after the transfer of the dorsal hood of prepuce to the ventral surface of the penis. These repairs usually are not desirable because of the formation of hairs within the urethra. If hair is allowed to grow within the urethra, concretions, infection and obstruction can result. Normal hair growth will occur on full-thickness skin grafts, so full-thickness skin grafts used to reconstruct the urethra must be procured from a hairless area such as the prepuce (Horton and Devine, 1963), the inner aspect of the upper arm, the postauricular area or occasionally from the dorsum of the foot. If split-thickness skin grafts are used, contracture will certainly occur and prolonged splinting is necessary.

FIVE POPULAR TECHNIQUES OF HYPOSPADIAS REPAIR

1. The Denis Browne operation (multi-staged)

The first stage of surgery is done at about 18 months of age. A preliminary meatotomy (to make certain the opening of the urethra is adequate) plus resection of the tissue causing the chordee and the transfer of dorsal penile skin to the ventral surface are the three important elements of the first stage of the repair. A transverse incision is made and the ventral penile skin is undermined from the urethral opening to the glans; the prepuce and a portion of the skin of the shaft are shifted to the ventral side to provide excess skin for later urethral reconstruction. Browne felt that early release of the chordee was essential to allow the penis to develop normally without growth restraint.

The second stage of surgery is completed at about 4 or 5 years of age. At this time a perineal urethrostomy is performed and a peripheral incision is made around a midline strip of skin on the ventral shaft of the penis, extending from the urethral meatus to the inferior portion of the glans. A small triangle of glans is denuded on each side of the midline. By combining wide undermining and a dorsal relaxing incision, lateral skin flaps can then be approximated over the midline longitudinal strip of skin, which remains attached to the ventral surface of the penis. No catheter is placed over the buried strip of skin on the penis. The perineal catheter is usually removed on the tenth postoperative day, thus allowing the perineal fistula to heal spontaneously (Fig. **26**, 8).

Several points of surgical technique are important in this operation. First, an adequate urethral opening must be provided and the first stage meatotomy is essential in most cases. Second, the dorsal longitudinal relaxing incision on the shaft of the penis must not extend past the base of the penis onto the abdominal wall. Incisions on the shaft of the penis heal with a wide, flat, pliable scar unless they encroach upon the abdominal wall. At this point, a hypertrophied, keloid-like scar will commonly occur and may cause a disappointing result. Third, the longitudinal strip of skin which is buried must be wide enough to allow circumferential growth of an adequate, new urethra. This may vary with the size of the patient, but should never be less than

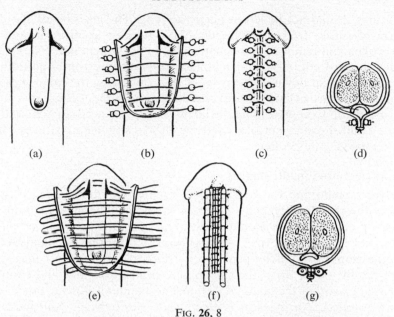

FIG. **26**, 8

Technique of Denis Browne. The chordee having been released, an incision is made outlining a strip of skin from around the urethral meatus to the glans penis (a). The lateral margins of skin are elevated and with the help of an incision on the dorsum of the penis are mobilised so that they can be closed easily over the skin strip. Wire sutures are used to take tension off the suture line (b). These sutures are secured with glass beads (c), backed by a crushed metal sleeve allowing adequate room for oedema which will develop (d). Culp has modified this by placing mattress sutures tied over rubber bolsters (e, f, g). Mustardé has developed an ingenious plastic clamp which has much to recommend it.

1 cm in width, even in a child. In an adult, this should measure 1·5 cm or more. Fourth, to prevent stenosis at this site during healing, the incision should extend well around the distal end of the normal urethra leaving a circumferential cuff of normal skin measuring 4 to 6 mm in all directions. Fifth, the incisions made on the glans penis should extend distally as far as possible to elongate the urethra. This entire technique is simplified by bringing as much tissue as possible to the distal ventral surface of the penis and glans during the first stage of repair. Sixth, tension-relieving sutures should be used when the lateral flaps are brought over the buried strip of skin. Browne secured these sutures with glass beads and crimped metal sleeves so that if necessary the sutures could be loosened from time to time as oedema occurred. The Denis Browne operation, while probably the most popular method to correct hypospadias, is not perfect. Culp (1959) reports a series of complications requiring re-operation in from 22 to 44 per cent of all cases when the Denis Browne technique has been followed. Most authors report a 10 to 30 per cent incidence of fistula formation. The usual complications of this operation consist of fistula formation, retrogression of the urethral meatus from the tip and occasionally stricture formation. This technique is constructed on sound principles and will produce consistent results when meticulous technique is utilised. Sir Denis Browne considered any modification of his original procedure to be the cause of fistulas and failure. It is important that the

relaxing sutures should not be left in place too long. The glass beads should allow at least 0·5 cm of suture free on each side at the time of application and the beads should be broken and removed if oedema begins to bury them in the skin. Culp (1959) has modified this procedure by tying nylon mattress sutures over longitudinal bolsters of rubber tubing to cut down on necrosis of skin caused by the small pressure points of the sutures. Mustardé (1954) endeavoured to avoid such necrosis by using a transparent plastic clamp to approximate the lateral flaps over a broad area and dispensed with through-and-through sutures fixed by beads and metal sleeves. All sutures should be removed in seven days.

2. The Byars operation (multi-staged)

In the Byars technique for hypospadias repair, the first stage consists of the correction of the chordee. Byars also stresses the point that the maximum surface of the available preputial tissue should be utilized by transferring all of the preputial skin to the ventral side of the organ. At surgery a traction suture is first placed through the tip of the glans to hold the penis in a stretched position. An incision is made extending from the distal tip of the existing urethra to the glans and from this point circumferentially around the glans. All abnormal bands of fibrous tissue causing the chordee are resected. An incision is then made through the full-thickness of the unfolded prepuce from the midline to the coronal sulcus. These flaps of prepuce are transferred ventrally to resurface the area between the retracted urethral meatus and the glans. Since the preputial tissue will be used to construct a new urethra, it must be brought to all areas where the new urethra will be formed. This means that the undersurface of the glans must be denuded and that an excess of the preputial flap should be brought forward onto the tip of the penis. A catheter is placed in the existing distal urethra for diversion of the urine to allow the first repair to heal. This initial surgery is usually carried out at 3 years of age.

The second stage of surgery is done at 4 or 5 years of age, thus allowing adequate time for resolution of the scarring and reaction to the first operation. Incisions similar to that of the Denis Browne procedure are made; however, the longitudinal strip of skin is wider, corresponding in millimetres to the size of the catheter which would normally fit the existing urethra. For a 4- or 5-year-old boy, the strip of skin will be somewhat wider than 14 mm to allow a tube to be constructed around a no. 14 French catheter. This median strip should extend forward on the undersurface of the glans as close to the tip of the penis as possible. Following minimal lateral undermining, the longitudinal strip of skin is sutured to form a urethra using 5/0 chromic gut. The lateral flaps are then widely undermined and closed 'in depth' over the reconstructed urethra. Silk sutures have been recommended for the skin repair by Byars (1955). If the procedure is to be completed in two stages, a perineal urethrostomy is performed prior to the urethroplasty. If a three-stage operation is to be performed, the reconstructed urethra is not anastomosed to the distal portion of the existing urethra and a fistula is left to be repaired at a later stage. Byars reports that in the last few years most of his operations have been completed in two stages, although if any question exists as to the desirability of repair he does not hesitate to make this a three-staged operation. No catheter is used to traverse the newly constructed urethra. An elastic bandage to prevent oedema and haematoma formation should be left in place for 5 or 6 days following the surgery. Byars in 1955 reported a series of 52 cases with 12 fistulas. In 1964, he reported 140 hypospadias repairs with only 4 cases of fistula formation in the last 77 patients of the series. Total hospitalization time for the two operations was reported as averaging 14 days (Fig. **26**, 9).

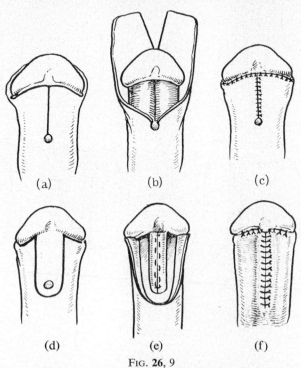

(a)   (b)   (c)

(d)   (e)   (f)

Fig. **26**, 9

Byars technique. An incision is made in the midline from the meatus to the corona, then around the penis proximal to the glans (a). The tissue causing the chordee is resected. The prepuce is unfolded and an incision made in its midline (b). Preputial flaps which are brought to the ventrum of the penis (c). At a later stage a central flap is incised to form the new urethra (d). After the new tube is formed, the lateral skin edges are undermined (e) and closed over the new urethra in a multiple layer closure (f).

3. The Cecil operation as modified by Dr Ormond Culp (multi-staged)

Dr Culp uses his modification of the Denis Browne operation when the urethral meatus is located proximal to the penoscrotal junction. He uses two modifications of the Cecil operation for more distal lesions. The chordee is released by making a transverse incision distal to the urethral meatus. This is extended laterally into the hooded prepuce. The urethra is mobilised and all the constricting tissue is excised. After wide undermining of the skin of the penis and prepuce, the skin incision is closed longitudinally with fine wire or mersilene sutures. The first operation is performed at 18 months of age. The second operation is deferred until the age of 4 or 5 years. At that time a 'U'-shaped incision is made in the ventral skin similar to

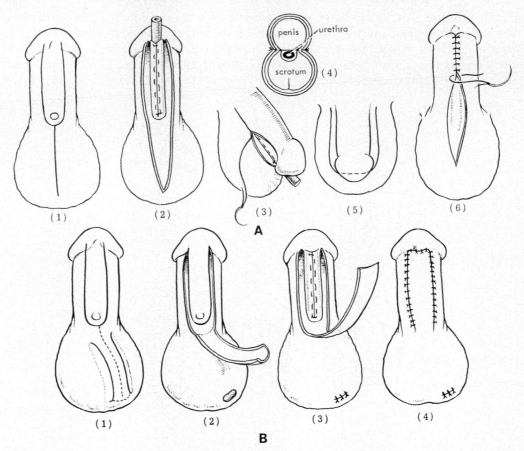

Fig. 26, 10A

Cecil-Culp technique. After preliminary straightening of the penis, a 'U'-shaped incision is made around the meatus on to the glans. A proximal continuation of this incision is carried on to the scrotum for a distance equal to the length of the penis (1). The penile skin flap is formed into a tube with a running suture and the edges of the skin of the penis and scrotum are undermined (2). The penis is sutured to the scrotum in two layers, attaching the subcutaneous tissue of the scrotum to the tunica albuginea of the corpora cavernosa and the skin of the scrotum to the skin of the penis (3, 4). Two to three months later the skin of the scrotum is incised and the penis freed up (5), the defect being closed with silk sutures (6).

Fig. 26, 10B

Wherbein-Smith. At the time of release of the chordee, a tube pedicle is formed with its base at the peno-scrotal junction. The incision for the urethroplasty is carried proximally to open this tube (1). The distal tube end is cut loose and the edges of the skin are undermined (2). The urethra is tubed (3) and covered with the opened scrotal skin tube (4).

the procedures of Browne and Byars. The width of the median strip is determined by the tissue available at the site of the new meatus: 10 to 12 mm (no. 10–12 French catheter) in children and 16 to 18 mm (no. 16–18 French catheter) in older patients. A catheter is inserted into the bladder through the old meatus and the median skin is closed over it as a tube, using chromic gut sutures. A longitudinal midline incision is then made in the scrotum and the penis is buried in the scrotum. Subcutaneous scrotal tissue is sewn to the corpora of the penis and the skin edges of the scrotum are attached to the skin edges of the penis. Reinforcing sutures at the site of the new meatus help to prevent retraction. The catheter is left *in situ* for one week.

The penis and scrotum are divided after an interval of at least two months. An ample strip of scrotal skin is left on each side to be trimmed if redundant. A drain is left in the scrotum for two or three days after closure. Silk skin sutures are left in position for one week.

In more distal lesions the incision in the scrotum is not made in continuity with the penile incision for the original anastomosis. The area to be repaired and at least 1 cm of the normal urethra are buried, and the release stage is similar to the above procedure. About 20 per cent of these cases require further surgical procedures for repair of complications (Fig. **26**, 10). Dr Culp is quite critical of his results, and situations which might be acceptable to others are considered by him to be failures requiring further surgical repair. Also, many of his cases have been 'hypospadias cripples'—the result of previous injudicious surgical procedures (Fig. **26**, 10A).

In the Wehrbein-Smith repair, a tube of scrotal skin, based at the penoscrotal junction, is constructed at the time of the release of the chordee. The tube is made as long as the length of the penis and as wide as half the circumference. At the second stage, the urethra is formed as in the Cecil repair and the penis is immediately resurfaced by the opened anterior tube of scrotal skin (Fig. **26**, 10B).

4. The Horton-Devine operation (one stage)

In 1955 the authors started a combined repair for hypospadias, cooperating and utilising techniques from both plastic surgery and urology. A one-stage repair of hypospadias has evolved and has now been completed in approximately 135 cases of all degrees of hypospadias. In this technique, a perineal urethrostomy is performed initially and an appropriately sized red rubber catheter is sutured into position. (When the urethral meatus is in the perineum, this type of urinary diversion may not be feasible and a suprapubic cystostomy will be necessary.) The red rubber catheter is passed into the urethra until a free flow of urine is obtained. The catheter is manipulated by withdrawing it a slight distance and reinserting it so that only the tip lies in the bladder. The catheter at the penile meatus is then marked with brilliant green marking solution. A catheter guide is passed down the catheter, and the tip of the guide is used to push the catheter against the perineum about midway between the scrotum and the anus. The area is injected with approximately 1 ml of 1:100,000 epinepherine solution to facilitate a bloodless field. An incision is made with a knife through the layers of the perineum until the colour of the catheter can be seen through the urethra. The urethra is then incised with delicate strokes to prevent cutting the catheter. The catheter is drawn out of the urethra so that the distal portion can be grasped. The bell of the catheter is cut off, and the well lubricated distal portion is drawn out through the perineum and secured with sutures of 4/0 black silk. The proper length of catheter in the urethra is ascertained by measuring the distal end so that the previously made mark just reaches the urethral meatus. If too much of the catheter is left in the bladder, bladder spasm and difficulties with drainage will ensue.

A 4/0 black silk suture is taken through the glans, in an area just dorsal to the apex, to provide traction. The assistant's finger is held behind the shaft of the penis

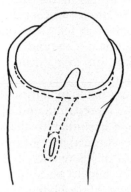

FIG. 26, 11

Incisions are made circumscribing the urethral meatus and extending out to the corona of the glans penis. They are then carried completely around the penis.

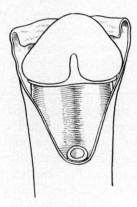

FIG. 26, 12

All abnormal fibrous tissue is removed, cleaning the tunica albuginea of the corpora cavernosa and freeing up the urethra. The prepuce is unfolded.

and pressure is applied to the shaft during all of the operation to reduce bleeding and facilitate dissection. Epinepherine solution (1–2 ml of 1:100,000) is injected into the area of operation to aid in haemostasis. After skin markings are made, incisions are carried around the existing urethral opening and are extended distally on each side of the midline (to remove the thin abnormal ventral skin) to the coronal sulcus from which point they are continued on each side completely around the glans (Fig. **26**, 11). The lateral skin flaps are elevated from the shaft, and all fibrous tissue causing the chordee is removed. The fibrous tissue bands extend around the urethra at the meatus and for a short distance proximally. Dissection should not be carried too far proximally or the normal corpus spongiosum will be entered and bleeding will occur.

The venae profundae of the penis lie between Buck's fascia and the tunica albuginea of the corpora cavernosa, and bleeding from these should not be confused with inadvertent entry into the corpora. The tissue containing these veins and all surrounding fibrous tissues should be excised so that the tunica albuginea of the paired corpora is glistening and clean over the entire field (Fig. **26**, 12). We feel that Buck's fascia and all the tissue superficial to it must be removed from a triangular area extending from around the urethra at the meatus to the glans with the lateral margins of the dissection extending to the base of the prepuce. All bleeding points are easily controlled with coagulation current or 6/0 chromic gut sutures. Atraumatic ophthalmic suture, dyed blue, is used throughout this procedure except for an occasional tension-relieving suture when 5/0 gut is used. The dye helps in

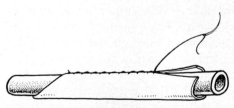

FIG. 26, 13

The distal end of the prepuce is excised in the shape of the desired graft. All the subcutaneous tissue is removed and the full-thickness skin graft tube constructed. A tongue is left at the proximal end opposite the seam and the seam is not carried out to the distal end, leaving a 'V'-shaped end to the skin graft.

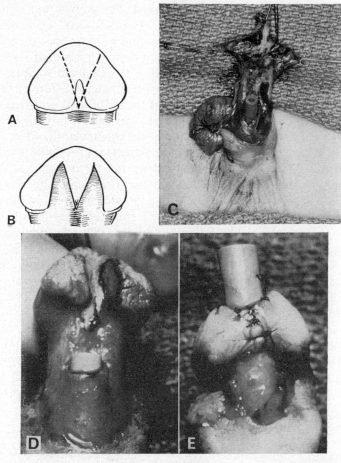

FIG. 26, 14

Diagrams of glandar flaps (A, B). Midline glandar flap elevated and lateral
wings mobilised (C). Midline glandar flap sutured at tip to form dorsal
wall of distal urethra (D). Lateral glandar flaps closed over midline to re-
shape glans and bring urethra to tip of penis (E).

visualising the very thin suture material and the needles developed for ophthalmological surgery are excellent in allowing atraumatic suturing.

The prepuce is then freed and unfolded to its full length. The hypospadiac urethral
opening will now have retracted proximally beneath the intact skin of the penis: an
incision is made along its ventral aspect to provide a large 'V'-shaped groove for an
elliptical anastomosis with the future skin graft urethra. The distance between the
hypospadiac meatus and the extreme tip of the glans is measured with a ruler and
noted. The calibre of the normal urethra has previously been ascertained by gentle
sounding. Ordinarily in the 2-year-old child a no. 10, no. 12, or no. 14 catheter is
appropriate. The number of the French size of catheter corresponds to the circumference of the catheter in millimetres; therefore, if a no. 14 French catheter fits and if
the distance between the proximal hypospadiac meatus and the tip of the glans is

3 cm, a graft measuring 14 mm by 3 cm is desired. The graft is then cut from the distal portion of the prepuce which has previously been unfolded. All subcutaneous tissue is removed from the graft which is sutured around a red rubber catheter. In order to provide an elliptical anastomosis at each end of this skin graft tube, special shaping is necessary (Fig. **26**, 13). At the proximal end, a 0·5 to 1 cm tongue of tissue is left opposite the suture line to fit into the previously made incision in the urethra. The suture line is carried to within 0·5 to 1 cm of the distal end and tied, thus leaving a 'V'-shaped triangular defect to fit a flap to be constructed in the glans.

Attention is then directed to the glans and to the construction of this flap. Dissection is carried out with the scissors separating the glans from the underlying corpora. It is important that this dissection should not extend too far laterally as it will endanger the blood supply of the glans. A 'V'-shaped flap is cut into the glans leaving a triangular wide base at the tip of the glans with a 'V'-shaped point at the coronal sulcus. The flap is elevated and thinned, leaving only a small amount of subcutaneous tissue present on the undersurface. The lateral glandar tissues are then undermined, producing lateral glandar wings of much greater thickness than the triangular flap (Fig. **26**, 14). During this dissection, it will be noted that bands of fibrous tissue extend into the space between the corpora and the glans. Removal of this tissue in the course of dissection allows further straightening of the penis. The 'V'-shaped flap is then sewn down to the shaft of the penis by a 6/0 chromic suture and the penis is ready for the construction of the urethra.

The red rubber catheter holding the skin graft tube is inserted into the proximal urethra, and the anastomosis between the graft and the urethra is performed using 6/0 chromic gut interrupted sutures (Fig. **26**, 15). The 'V'-shaped flap of glandar mucosa is sutured into the defect in the distal portion of the skin graft urethral tube,

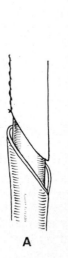
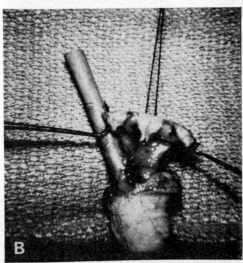

FIG. **26**, 15

Anastomosis of the skin graft tube to the urethra (A). Note how the tongue of graft fits the incision made in the urethra forming a long elliptical anastomosis. Photograph at this stage (B).

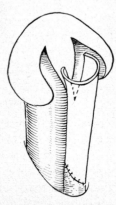

FIG. **26**, 16
Anastomosis of the skin graft tube to the 'V'-shaped flap in the glans. The wings of glans are then rotated to surround the graft and locate the meatus at the tip in the glans.

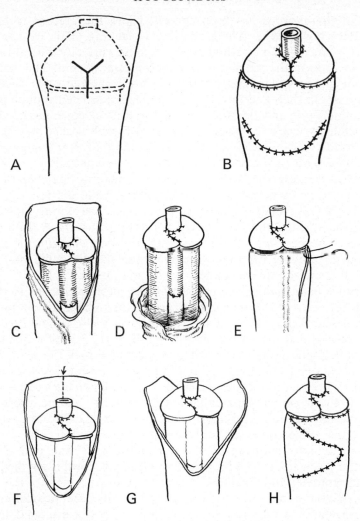

FIG. **26**, 17

'Y'-shaped incision in the preputial flap (A). Completion of the procedure (B). When there is torsion of the penis, the raphe will not be in the midline (C). Completely freeing the skin from the penis will allow the raphe to be brought to the midline (D). This will shift skin from the dorsum to the ventrum of the penis affording good coverage and correcting the twist (E). If the preputial skin is too short for transposition of a hood, an incision is made in the midline of the prepuce (F). The flaps are swung to the ventrum (G), and closed in a Z-plasty fashion to prevent superimposition of the suture line and the graft (H).

again using 6/0 chromic gut with the knots inside the lumen. The lateral glandar wings are elevated and advanced medially around the skin graft and catheter to form a new distal penile urethral meatus (Fig. **26**, 16). This changes the spatulate flat shape of the hypospadiac glans to a normal conical shape and allows the urethral meatus to emerge at the exact tip.

PS P

At this point the chordee has been corrected and the urethra reconstructed. A vascularised covering for the skin graft tube is lacking. This can be obtained in several ways (Fig. **26**, 17). The method most frequently used by the authors is to make a 'Y'-shaped incision in the remaining extended preputial skin. The glans is inserted through the opening and the prepuce is transferred to the ventral surface of the penis in a manner similar to that described by Nesbit. There has been enough preputial skin to obtain the skin graft and provide a hood for ventral coverage in all of our uncircumcised penile hypospadias cases. In the event that the prepuce is inadequate, we take hairless skin from other body areas in the form of a full-thickness graft to make the skin graft tube. This tube must be adequate in length and, if necessary, two pieces of skin can be sutured together with an elliptical anastomosis for extra length.

If torsion of the penis is present pre-operatively, wide dissection is carried out between the skin and the shaft of the penis to the base. The skin of the penis can thus be shifted and the dorsal skin turned to cover the ventral surface of the penis. It will usually be noticed in these cases that pre-operatively the median raphe did not follow the midline but in moving the tissue it can be replaced into the normal position. Abnormal torsion should not be created by this manoeuvre.

Occasionally we have divided the prepuce in the midline, similar to the technique of Byars, and have covered the ventral surface of the penis with the prepuce in this manner. This produces imposition of suture lines over the graft and does not provide as secure a coverage as does the Nesbit type hood or the rotation of the skin of the penis on the shaft. Z-plasties of the preputial skin or the skin of the penile body usually are not desirable in our technique because of impaired vascularity of the sharp angles and flap tips. The prepuce in most cases will be adequate in length to cover to the base of the penis. If the hypospadiac meatus lies proximal to the penoscrotal junction, a scrotal flap should be mobilized to join with the preputial flap to cover the scrotal area. Scrotal flaps carried onto the penis tend to cause torsion.

Following meticulous suturing of the subcutaneous tissue and skin with 6/0 chromic gut, the black silk suture previously used for traction is stitched through the distal end of the catheter and tied loosely to prevent dislodgement of the tube holding the skin graft. We have found the use of silk, nylon, steel and heavier catgut sutures to be unnecessary and to require removal of the sutures at a later date. Sutures of 6/0 chromic gut dissolve in 10 to 12 days, and we do not have to struggle with or hurt the patient with suture removal. Fine mesh nitrofurazone covered gauze is placed over the suture line, multiple bandages are applied, and a fitted elastoplast outer dressing is utilized to hold pressure on the repair (Fig. **26**, 18). With this technique, we can usually finish the entire one-stage hypospadias operation in $1\frac{1}{2}$ hours without undue haste.

The outer bandage is removed on the third day, and the entire penile area is soaked in a sterile saline bath three times a day to remove the remaining bandages. The nitrofurazone gauze must not be pulled forcefully from the area for even slight traction on the repair line may cause a dehiscence and fistula formation. The perineal urethrostomy catheter is connected to straight drainage and irrigated only as necessary. On the seventh postoperative day the red rubber tube is removed from the penis. The perineal urethrostomy catheter remains until the tenth postoperative day at which time it is removed and the patient is allowed to void spontaneously. We urge the patients to void frequently in order to avoid extreme pressures in the urethra during micturition. An antibiotic ointment is placed into the meatus to soften any crusts or clots which form. By using an ophthalmic tipped tube, the tip of the tube can be inserted into the meatus and the meatus kept free of all plugs. Frequent soaking in a warm bath is encouraged up to the fifteenth or sixteenth postoperative day.

With this technique, the total hospital stay varies from 10 to 12 days in the usual one-stage repair. There is only one anaesthesia and one operation. Complications

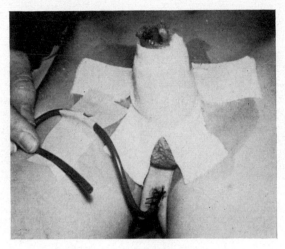

FIG. **26**, 18

Photograph of the dressing. Fine mesh gauze impregnated with Furacin is placed next to the repair. This is covered with a massive layer of gauze sponges, none going completely around the penis. Then pressure is applied with the elastic adhesive material. The perineal urethrostomy can be seen.

have been mild with fistula formation being the problem most frequently encountered. Most fistulas have been small, some having closed spontaneously and others having responded to local treatment with silver nitrate or simple suture. Larger fistulas and those not responding to local treatment have been closed with excision and closure of the urethra and mobilization of a local flap of skin. One haematoma resulted in prolonged postoperative healing with diverticulum formation due to partial loss of the skin graft tube. This was corrected by an inlay graft at a second procedure. Following the use of our 'V'-shaped glandar flap we have had no strictures or retraction of the urethral meatus. Three strictures have occurred at the graft urethral anastomosis. Two responded to dilatation under anaesthesia; one required re-operation. None have occurred since using the tongue and groove anastomosis described herein.

We have followed many of our cases through puberty. The skin graft tube used for urethral reconstruction has grown at an adequate rate and has not caused difficulty. Approximately 78 per cent of our cases have been cured with one operation. When a Nesbit hood is used to resurface the ventral surface of the penis, lateral projections of excess skin occur on the shaft of the penis. This extra ventral skin irregularity ordinarily diminishes in size as the penis lengthens. We have not found it necessary to bring a patient into the hospital for a secondary procedure for cosmetic appearances alone. The lateral tabs of tissue have occasionally been utilized to aid in fistula repair when such repair is necessary postoperatively.

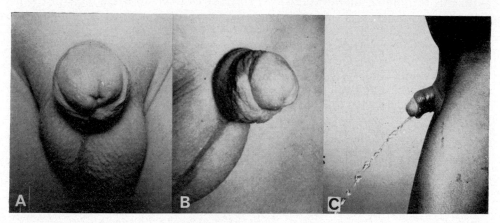

FIG. **26,** 19

Postoperative photographs. Glans penis showing the location of the meatus (A). Shaft of the penis showing the preputial hood moved to the ventral side. Also the meatus in the glans (B). Voiding picture (C).

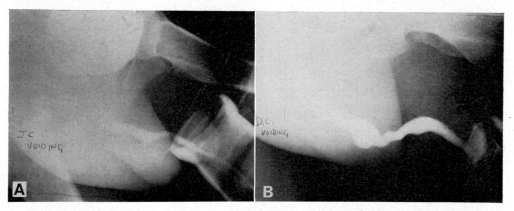

FIG. **26,** 20

Postoperative voiding urethrogram. Perineal hypospadias 9 years postoperative (A). Perineal hypospadias 11 years postoperative (B).

This technique does not offer an easy way to repair hypospadias. It requires meticulous surgical technique and attention to detail. With fewer stages, there is a lesser risk of anaesthesia. Hospitalization with its cost in time and money is minimised and the psychic trauma associated with multiple hospitalization and operative procedures is decreased.

5. The Mustardé operation (one stage)—*Contributed by J. C. Mustardé.*

Minor degrees of hypospadias involving the coronal area or the distal third of the penis comprise by far the greatest number of patients seen in surgical practice. Although the opening of the urethra may not be far removed from the normal opening on the tip of the glans, the hooded prepuce forms a considerable deformity, and the majority of these children have a degree of chordee of the terminal portion of the penis. Circumcision, whilst removing the obvious deformity should never be performed in such children as, should they or their parents decide on operation at a later date the main source of reconstructive material will have been destroyed. The

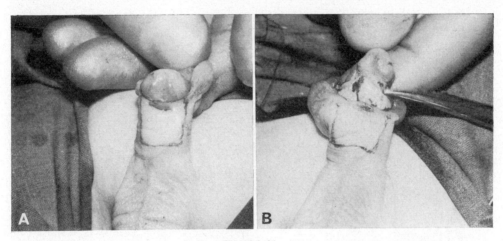

FIG. **26**, 21

Sub-coronal hypospadias. (A) Outline of flap on ventral surface. (B) A coronal incision allows complete correction of chordee with excision of all fibrous bands. (In this particular patient the chordee was corrected before incising around the flap, as is usually done.)

operative technique first published by the writer, in 1965 is designed to correct all three deformities in a moderately simple operation which takes about an hour to perform; it is based on a combination of earlier techniques, notably that of Bevan (1917), but introduces the new concept that by using a completely isolated flap to produce the new urethra, the chordee can be readily corrected at the initial operation. With the addition of a few minor but important improvements the technique is substantially the same as originally described.

Operative technique. A preliminary perineal urethrostomy is carried out (see description under Horton and Devine technique), and a traction suture is inserted into the glans a little on the dorsal side of the tip to avoid interfering with the construction of the opening on the glans which will be made later. A rectangular flap is drawn on the ventral surface of the penis to include the opening of the urethra and extending proximally along the shaft of the penis far enough to allow this flap to connect the opening of the urethra with the tip of the glans once the chordee has been completely overcome (Fig. **26**, 21A). The flap should be about 14 mm in width so that it can be tubed to form a urethra of adequate dimension. It is no longer felt advisable or necessary to cut a fish-tail on the proximal end. The flap is completely undermined except for a strip comprising the distal one-quarter, which is left attached around the urethra: a probe may be inserted into the urethra at this stage to ensure visualization of the latter so that it will not be punctured when dissecting up the flap. The skin of the shaft of the penis lateral to the flap is now widely undermined and an incision is carried out around the corona so that the whole of the prepuce can be lifted away and opened up as in the Ombredanne and Nesbit techniques. The area between the distal edge of the flap and the glans is now carefully dissected and all fibrous tissue is removed, so that the chordee will be completely overcome (Fig. **26,** 21B). The writer does not consider it necessary in these minor degrees of hypospadias

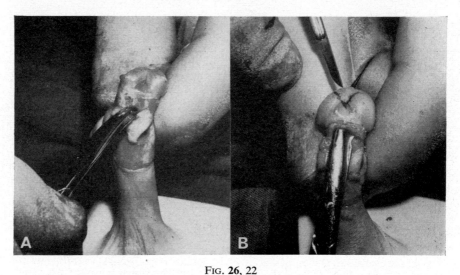

Fig. **26,** 22

(A) Commencement of tunnel immediately distal to base of flap. (B) Tunnel carried up into glans where 'V' incision is made to open it.

to remove the rudimentary corpus spongiosum which may be present between the urethral opening and the glans and considers that the chordee can be completely corrected whilst still preserving this mid-line structure. It must, however, be removed if there appears to be any retention of chordee, or likelihood of retention of chordee, due to this structure, which may be quite substantial in some cases and forms a part of the trifoliate cross section of the penis. (The writer disagrees with Horton and Devine with regard to the morbid anatomy of a number of these hypospadias patients (Fig. **26,** 25).) It is essential that all *fascia* be removed right down to the comparatively thin sheath of this rudimentary corpus spongiosum if it is present, and particularly, the fascia must be removed in the groove between this structure and the corpora cavernosa on each side.

The urethral opening having been displaced proximately as far as it will reasonably go, an incision is made transversely into the substance of the rudimentary corpus spongiosum or into the cavernosa, and, using blunt-pointed scissors a dissection is made up through this structure into the glans (Fig. **26,** 22A). The dissection so made must be wide enough to take the urethral tube without tightness, and once the tip of the glans has been reached the scissors are spread and a 'V' cut made in the glans (Fig. **26**, 22B) in the manner described by Horton and Devine, so that the scissors can be pushed completely through. This method of creating a 'V' opening on the glans in order to avoid a ring scar at the termination of the reconstructed urethra is a point of technique for which the writer is indebted to Horton and Devine and which he considers to be of the utmost importance. The tongue of the 'V' on the glans should be thinned as described by the above named authors and sutured down into the opening in the glans, the ends of the suture being left lying to be used at a later date.

A length of rubber catheter (this is generally 6/8 French) is introduced into the

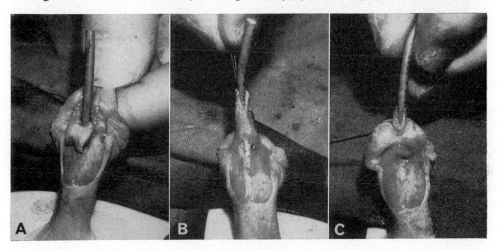

FIG. **26**, 23

(A) 10 cm section of catheter inserted into urethra. The flap has been undermined in its proximal two-thirds. (B) The flap is lifted up and tubed around length of catheter. (C) Catheter and covering brought through tunnel onto surface of glans.

urethral opening and passed proximally until it touches the perineal catheter (Fig. **26**, 23A). The rectangular flap is tubed over the catheter so inserted, except for the last 5 mm at the free end of the flap: the two corners are, however, fixed to the tubing with a temporary suture (Fig. **26**, 23B) to prevent the rubber tube being pulled out as it and its surrounding flap are threaded through the tunnel already dissected (Fig. **26**, 23C). Once this has been done the temporary suture used to fix the corners of the flap to the rubber tube is released and the corners of the flap are sutured into the appropriate corners of the arrow-head opening in the glans. The suture originally holding the tip of the 'V' flap in the glans is used to fix the seam of the urethral tube in position, and the rest of the terminal end of the urethral tube is very carefully married up to the wound in the glans. All the sutures should be of 6/0 chromic gut. Attention is now turned to the site of the opening in the shaft into which the urethral tube was carried. If any loose tissue can be brought across this site without encroaching on the vascular supply to the base of the rectangular flap it should be sutures with 6/0 gut to provide a more secure covering over the entrance to the tunnel.

The prepuce is now opened out, buttonholed after the manner of Ombredanne, and brought across the ventral surface of the penis so that it can be sutured over the

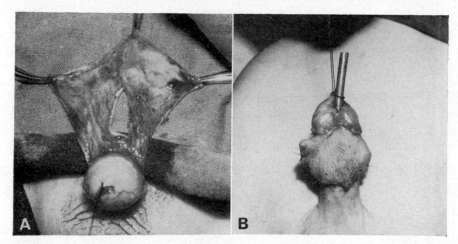

FIG. 26, 24

(A) Prepuce opened out to form Ombredanne type flap with button-hole. (This example is in a different patient from rest of illustrations.) (B) Ombredanne flap brought over to cover ventral surface. Urethral flap sutured to 'V' opening on glans.

whole of the raw area (Fig. 26, 24). If the degree of chordee has been minimal, there will be only a short distance between the opening of the tunnel in the corpus spongiosum and the skin of the glans: in order to provide as large a raw area as possible between these two points, and hence to minimise the risk of fistula formation some of the skin of the glans should be cut away so that the entrance to the tunnel is not underlying the junction of the skin of the glans and the prepucial flap.

Pressure is obtained on the penis and the loose skin of the prepucial flap without any risk of strangulation by means of a small corselet of two-way stretch material which is wound loosely round the penis. The traction suture in the glans is passed through the rubber tube in order to anchor it.

The dressing of the penis, and the rubber tube in the urethra, are removed on the seventh day, with the child in a warm bath, and the perineal catheter is withdrawn on the tenth day.

McComb has recently described what seems to be a sound modification of the writer's technique in which he removes a rosette of mucosa from the tip of the glans and everts the urethral flap over this denuded area, thus totally avoiding stenosis of the new meatus.

Penile hypospadias. The writer has adapted the one-stage technique described above to more severe degrees of hypospadias where the urethral opening is too far proximal to permit a distally-based flap to be used without raising hair-bearing skin. In these patients a Broadbent flap (Broadbent *et al.*, 1961) running from the urethral opening along the shaft and onto the prepuce has been used. This flap, after adequate correction of the chordee, is tunnelled through the distal half of the penis to emerge on the glans as in the writer's one-stage technique and the skin defect on the shaft is covered by swinging over the remainder of the penile and prepucial skin.

A number of these operations have been performed over the past four years, but in a number of cases fistula formation at the proximal end of the reconstructed urethra

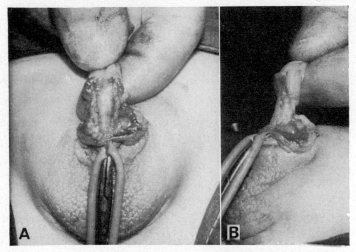

Fig. **26**, 25
Penile hypospadias after correction of chordee. Corpus spongiosum
readily identified distal to urethral opening.

has been a complication which necessitated a secondary operation, and it is felt that
in severe hypospadias a two-stage approach may be the method of choice.

CONCLUSION

For centuries physicians have been looking for the ideal solution to the problem
of hypospadias. Great progress has been made from the time when Paulus of
Aegineta recommended amputation to the present. Although much knowledge has
been gained of the embryology and of the surgical treatment of this malformation,
little has been discovered to help prevent the anomaly. Congenital penile anomalies
seem to represent gradation of one embryological growth continuum. Hypospadias
without chordee and hypospadias cripples respond well to individualized surgical
treatment. Whether the repair is performed in one stage or in multiple stages, all
surgical procedures have become more refined and good results can now be anticipated in all cases. It behooves each surgeon to become cognizant of the latest techniques in this field and choose a technique which will consistently give better results
with less mental and physical trauma to the patient.

C. E. HORTON

REFERENCES

ARONOFF, M. (1963). A one-stage operative technique for the treatment of subglandar hypospadias in
    children. *Br. J. plast. Surg.* **16**, 59–62.
BACKUS, L. H. & DE FELICE, C. A. (1960). Hypospadias—then and now. *Plastic reconstr. Surg.* **25**, 146–
    160.
BEVAN, A. D. (1917). A new operation for hypospadias. *J. Am. med. Ass.* **68**, 1032.
BROADBENT, T. R., WOOLF, R. M. & TOKSU, E. (1961). Hypospadias: one-stage repair. *Plastic reconstr.
    Surg.* **27**, 154–159.
BROWNE, D. (1949). Hypospadias. *Post-grad. med. J.* **25**, 367–372.

BUCKNALL, R. T. H. (1907). A new operation for penile hypospadias. *Lancet*, **2**, 887–890.

BYARS, L. T. (1950). Surgical repair of hypospadias. *Surg. Clins N. Am.* **30**, 1371–1378.

BYARS, L. T. (1955). A technique for consistently satisfactory repair of hypospadias. *Surgery Gynec. Obstet.* **11**, 184–190.

CAMPBELL, M. F. (1951). Undescended testicle and hypospadias. *Am. J. Surg.* **82**, 8–17.

CECIL, A. B. (1932). Surgery of hypospadias and epispadias in the male. *J. Urol.* **27**, 507–537.

CECIL, A. B. (1952). Modern treatment of hypospadias. *J. Urol.* **67**, 1006–1011.

CECIL, A. B. (1955). Symposium on pediatric urology. Hypospadias and epispadias: diagnosis and treatment. *Pediat. Clins N. Am.* **2**, 711–728.

CRAWFORD, B. S. (1963). The management of hypospadias. *Br. J. clin. Pract.* **17**, 273–280.

CULP, O. S. (1951). Early correction of congenital chordee and hypospadias. *J. Urol.* **65**, 264–274.

CULP, O. S. (1959). Experiences with 200 hypospadias: evolution of a therapeutic plan. *Surg. Clins N. Am.* **39**, 1007–1023.

DES PREZ, J. D., PERSKY, L. & KIEHN, C. L. (1961). One-stage repair of hypospadias by island flap technique. *Plastic reconstr. Surg.* **28**, 405–411.

DEVINE, C. J. & HORTON, C. E. (1961). One-stage hypospadias repair. *J. Urol.* **85**, 166–172.

DIFFENBACH, J. F. (1837). Guerison des fentes congenitales de la verge de l'hypospadias. *Gaz. hebd. Méd. Chir.* **5**, 156.

DUPLAY, S. (1880). De l'hypospadias perinio-scrotal et de son traitment chirurgical *Archs gén. Méd.* **23**, 513–530.

FOGH-ANDERSON, P. (1953). Hypospadias: 34 completed cases operated on according to Denis Browne. *Acta Chir. scand.* **105**, 414–423.

HORTON, C. E. & DEVINE, C., Jr. (1963). A one-stage hypospadias repair. In *Transactions of the Third International Congress of Plastic Surgery*.

HORTON, C. E. & DEVINE, C., Jr. (1966). Hypospadias. In *Modern Trends in Plastic Surgery* 2. Section IV. London: Butterworth.

HUMBY, G. (1941). A one-stage operation for hypospadias. *Br. J. Surg.* **29**, 113.

McCOMB, H. (1970). Construction of distal urethra in hypospadias. In *Transactions of the Asian Pacific Congress of Plastic Surgeons*, pp. 214–216. Part I. New Delhi.

McCORMACK, R. M. (1954). Simultaneous chordee repair and urethral reconstruction for hypospadias. *Plastic reconstr. Surg.* **13**, 257–274.

McINDOE, A. H. (1937). The treatment of hypospadias. *Am. J. Surg.* **38**, 176–185.

MAYS, H. B. (1951). Hypospadias—a concept of treatment. *J. Urol.* **65**, 279.

MEULEN, J. C. H. M. van der (1964). *Hypospadias.* Springfield, Illinois: Thomas.

MUSTARDÉ, J. C. (1954). Reconstruction of anterior urethra in hypospadias by buried skin strip method. A simplified and improved technique. *Br. J. plast. Surg.* **7**, 166.

MUSTARDÉ, J. C. (1965). One-stage correction of distal hypospadias: and other people's fistulae. *Br. J. plast. Surg* **18**, 413.

NESBIT, R. M. (1941). Plastic procedure for correction of hypospadias; *J. Urol.* **45**, 699–702.

NESBIT, R. M. (1954). The surgical treatment of congenital chordee without hypospadias. *J. Urol.* **72**, 1178–1180.

NOVE-JOSSERAND, G. (1919). Nouvelle technique pour la restauration en une seance des hypospadias étendus par la tunnelisation avec greffe dermo-epidermique. *J. Urol.* **8**, 449–456.

OMBREDANNE, L. (1923). *Precis Clinique et Operatoire de Chirugie Infantile.* Paris: Masson.

RICKETSON, G. (1958). A method of repair for hypospadias. *Am. J. Surg.* **95**, 279.

SMITH, D. R. (1955). Hypospadias: its anatomic and therapeutic considerations. *J. Int. Coll. Surg.* **24**, 64.

SORENSON, R. Quoted by J. C. H. M. van der Meulen.

THIERSCH, C. (1869). On the origin and operative treatment of epispadias. *Arch. Heilk.* **10**, 20.

WEHRBEIN, H. L. (1943). Hypospadias. *J. Urol.* **50**, 335–340.

YOUNG, F. & BENJAMIN, J. A. (1949). Preschool age repair of hypospadias with free inlay skin graft. *Surgery, St. Louis*, **26**, 384–404.

CHAPTER XXVII

EPISPADIAS AND EXSTROPHY

INTRODUCTION

Epispadias and exstrophy are the two most commonly encountered examples of a group of congenital abnormalities of the lower abdominal wall and urinary tract, in which there is a failure of midline fusion of the ventral wall of the urogenital sinus and associated structures. In all members of the group there is a gap between the pubic bones, which are joined only by a fibrous bar, and a shortening of the vertical distance between the umbilicus and the anus. In exstrophy, the bladder is laid open on the surface, with a low-placed umbilical hernia at its apex and a shortened, open urethral strip below (Fig. 27, 1). In epispadias the bladder is closed over but the urethra is short and the bladder neck is incomplete anteriorly. The corpora cavernosa are loosely connected to one another behind the urethra in the male to form a short upturned penis; in the female the two halves of the clitoris are entirely separate, lying lateral to, and a little behind, the urethral opening (Fig. 27, 2). The anus is brought forward in the perineum and the vaginal orifice faces anteriorly. In the most minor examples of the group, only the glans penis is abnormal, in the most severe (vesico-intestinal fissure) the exstrophied bladder is separated into two halves by a section of the exstrophied bowel representing the opened out ileo-caecal region and associated with imperforate anus. In certain other variants, the bladder is closed and the distal urethra relatively normal, but the pubes are wide apart and the bladder neck is incompetent. There are thus many possible variations upon this theme and treatment has to be adapted to the particular circumstances, but it is important to bear in mind

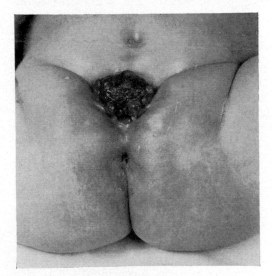

FIG. 27, 1
Exstrophy in the male child.

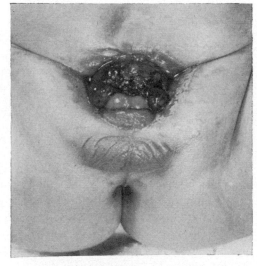

FIG. 27, 2
Exstrophy in the female child.

427

the nature of the handicaps involved and the possible dangers attached in greater or lesser extent to all cases. These handicaps may be listed under six headings, as follows:

The external deformity

In the female epispadias cases this is negligible, so that the abnormality is often overlooked in infancy: in the male epispadias it is relatively slight and concerns chiefly the genital function. The exstrophy of the bladder is obvious and hideous, the bulging inflamed bladder is horrifying to the young parents who are apt to demand urgent surgery. In fact, however, the exposed mucosa can be managed without much difficulty during the first year of life, and operations are better postponed: once the child begins to crawl and walk, the irritation of the coverings becomes more of a problem and if exposure continues into adolescence or adult life there are severe metaplastic changes with the possibility of malignancy. Neoplasms have often been recorded but are of a relatively low grade adenocarcinoma form and seldom metastasise; they are only likely to occur in untreated cases during the third and fourth decades of life, so that they do not present a problem in countries with a high standard of medical care.

The defect of the abdominal wall and pelvic floor

The wide gap between the pubes interferes with the normal musculature of the abdominal wall and pelvis: the exstrophied bladder itself bulges like a hernia and if a simple cystectomy is performed there is a large defect with a ventral hernia which is very difficult to control. An umbilical hernia is present in a large proportion of cases, but is simple to manage, and the same may be said of the common inguinal hernia. Rectal prolapse is commonly encountered evidence of the weakness of the pelvic floor in infants; it usually improves spontaneously or along with the surgical treatment of the exstrophy, but poor anal control often persists and is a factor to be considered in relation to urinary diversion.

The skeletal deformity

The gap between the pubes is brought about by the outward rotation of the os innominatum on each side of the sacrum: it involves some external rotation of the hip joint and produces in the early stages a waddling broad-based gait. With time and training, however, the gait becomes virtually normal and no specific orthopaedic correction is required.

The genital deformity

In the female the vaginal orifice is narrow and anteriorly placed, so that an episiotomy may be required to allow intercourse; the bifid clitoris itself does not constitute a handicap, and the rest of the genital tract is normal. A normal sexual life may be anticipated, though because of the weakness of the pelvic floor, uterine prolapse may occur after parturition.

In the male, however, the problem is more difficult: in epispadias, and even to a greater extent in exstrophy, the penis is short and upturned; occasionally it is also very small. The upward chordee is maintained chiefly by the shortness of the urethral strip, which cuts the corner between the abdominal wall and the upper surface of the penis. The corpora cavernosa are also angulated upwards by adhesions tethering them to the region of the pubic tubercles. Rarely there is an intrinsic curvature in the corpora themselves. In adult life the penis is usually more effective than its appearance in childhood would suggest, and intercourse is possible provided the chordee has been released, otherwise the erect organ is pulled tightly against the abdominal wall. The testicles, vasa and ejaculatory ducts are normal, and the ejaculation of normal semen is possible.

The urinary incontinence

In exstrophy, the urine is projected on to the surface directly by the ureteric efflux; in epispadias the bladder is formed, but the bladder neck is widely relaxed, if it is formed at all: the urethral strip is narrowest at the level of the verumontanum where there is little muscular support, while the external sphincter system is defective anteriorly. Only, therefore, in the mildest examples is there normal urinary control; a few borderline cases have no more than stress incontinence, but most children of both sexes dribble urine continuously. In considering reconstructive surgery it must be borne in mind that continence requires an active muscular bladder as well as a muscular and elastic control of the urethral outflow. In exstrophy a healthy bladder wall is unusual, a few children have an organ of potentially good capacity, but in most the bladder is small, the muscular layer defective with fibrous areas and with downgrowth of the mucosa into it. In epispadias the material is better, but by no means normal. The state of the urethral and bladder neck musculature is also variable but never wholly adequate. It thus happens that although reconstructive surgery is obviously desirable, urinary diversion is often the only means of keeping the child dry.

The ureteric abnormality and liability to pyelonephritis

This, the least obvious handicap, may be the greatest danger to life and health. In the untreated exstrophy there is some liability to urinary infection and to slight ureteric dilatation, but the dangers occur chiefly after attempts at bladder closure, or at bladder neck tightening in both exstrophy and epispadias. The ureters enter the bladder at a right angle, they have none of their normal obliquity and have therefore little capacity to prevent reflux. This may be of no great consequence in a normal bladder, or in one where there is no attempt at continence, but in the small capacity, inelastic bladder with a narrow outflow which results from surgical closure in this group, reflux is rapidly productive of ureteric dilatation, with a liability to urinary infection and pyelonephritis. It is vitally important that whether reconstructive or diversionary surgery is undertaken, the state of the upper urinary tract should be kept under review.

PLAN OF TREATMENT

It will be clear from this list of handicaps that the whole urogenital system must be taken into consideration when planning treatment in this group of deformities.

Even though surgery may be postponed for months or years a very early consultation with the parents is advisable so that the hazards and the possibilities of treatment can be sketched out. They often expect an immediate 'kill or cure' procedure: they have to accept a life-long but manageable handicap.

Epispadias. Treatment should always be postponed until the degree of incontinence is evident. Parents are often more optimistic in this respect than the facts justify, and since operative cure cannot be guaranteed it is as well to be sure of the pre-operative condition. It is, of course, desirable that the child should be dry when he goes to school, and treatment should therefore be undertaken between 3 and 5 years of age. In both sexes reconstructive treatment should be attempted, though it will have to be accepted that secondary diversion will be required in some. In the boys, penile correction should proceed along with bladder neck correction, though a two-stage operation is usually required for the penis.

Exstrophy. Reconstructive treatment is even now something of an experiment: it should be reserved for cases with a supple bladder of reasonable capacity and with healthy mucosa. Girls have a somewhat more favourable outlook than boys, and where the penis is very short attempts at bladder closure may make the genital reconstruction more difficult. The age at which closure should be attempted is uncertain, the writer's preference is for the end of the first year of life. A failed reconstruction may require urgent diversion because of damage to the upper urinary tract, or more usually a diversionary procedure for incontinence postponed by years of disappointed optimism. Where reconstruction is deemed inadvisable, diversion should be performed in the second or third year of life, and abdominal wall and genital correction undertaken subsequently.

Penile correction

In most epispadias, and all exstrophy, cases a preliminary chordee correction is required, in many ways corresponding to the first procedure in hypospadias. Additional length must be obtained for the urethral strip and the skin brought in for the purpose should be penile skin, smooth, hairless and supple. The simplest methods are probably the best: a transverse incision can be made just proximal to the coronal sulcus and carried outwards into the redundant preputial skin (Fig. **27**, 3). The proximal urethra is then dissected off the corpora cavernosa as far back as the verumontanum and allowed to retract. The upper surfaces of the corpora are freed from the adhesions which tether them upwards to the pubic tubercles. The transverse incision is then closed by a sagittal suture line with, if necessary, a relaxing incision on the undersurface of the penis. If preferred, a 'V-Y' plasty may be substituted for the simple incision and closure, or preputial flaps may be formed to bring round the skin by a staged procedure. At least three months should elapse after this operation before any further surgical correction is undertaken on the bladder or urethra.

The second stage of penile correction, the formation of a tubular urethra, is simpler than the equivalent step in hypospadias since more tissue is available and the glans, which is broad and flattened, may be safely rolled up to form a terminal urethra. The penile urethra is isolated by longitudinal incisions joined around the epispadiac meatus proximally (Fig. **27**, 4). It is mobilised laterally and rolled into a tube. The

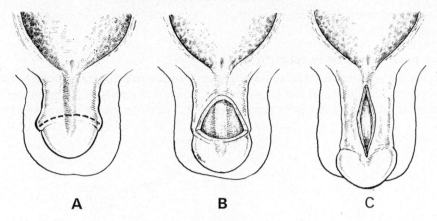

Fig. 27, 3

Operation for elongation of the urethral strip. (A) A transverse incision is made across the urethral strip just proximal to the coronal sulcus and carried laterally into the preputial tissue. (B) The urethra is stripped back proximally off the corpora cavernosa and the skin mobilised laterally. (C) The incision is closed in the vertical midline.

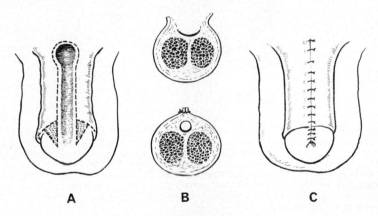

Fig. 27, 4

Closure of the urethral strip in male epispadias. (A) The outline of the incision along the muco-cutaneous junction, carried laterally into the preputial tissue and baring an area of the glans on either side of the central urethral strip. (B) Sectional view of the penis to show closure. (C) The urethra is closed in a tube and the skin approximated in the mid-line over it. The glans is rolled up to form a tube.

overlying adventitial tissue is sutured with a continuous catgut and the skin closed, with a continuous sub-cuticular nylon. On the glans, two areas are bared of their mucosa on either side of the central urethral strip and the glans is rolled up to give a terminal meatus. The only difficulty arises at the junction between the skin and the glans, but careful suturing of skin flaps to bared areas at the coronal sulcus should prevent fistula formation here. The effective construction of a tube for the passage of urine is not usually a matter of great difficulty; the sexual success of the penis depends on its size and upon the efficiency with which the first stage in correction of chordee has been carried out.

Bladder neck correction in epispadias

In both sexes, operations to achieve urinary continence are fraught with difficulties and as yet no ideal method has been devised. Success depends more upon the amount of muscular tissue present pre-operatively than upon the exact operative technique.

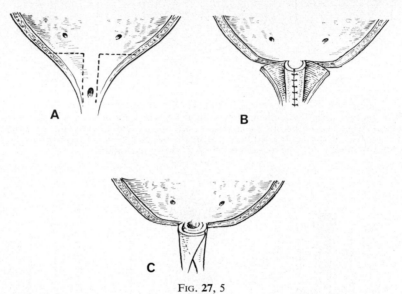

FIG. 27, 5

Bladder neck correction in epispadias cases (male and female). The bladder is approached through a Pfannenstiel incision and opened in the midline. (A) Shows the open bladder funnelled down to the level of the verumontanum. The dotted line shows the incision for removal of triangular areas of mucosa to form a central urethral strip. (B) The urethral strip has been closed as a tube and horizontal incisions are made in the muscular layer to form two flaps on either side of the mucosal tube. (C) These flaps are overlapped to form a muscular support for a new bladder neck.

Various sling techniques are possible, particularly in girls; the Millin operation (Millin, 1947) is appropriate and can follow the standard technique, although great care must be taken in defining the bladder neck area and the plane between it and the vagina. However the procedure which aims at creating a bladder neck and urethra from the lower part of the bladder as originally proposed by H. H. Young (1937) has probably the best hope of success. The bladder is approached through a Pfannenstiel incision and the area of the posterior urethra is freed from the fibrous bar uniting the pubes. The bladder and urethra are opened by a vertical mid-line incision exposing the verumontanum (Fig. 27, 5); the ureteric orifices are defined. Almost always the ureters must be re-implanted, first to move their orifices to a higher level to allow for the bladder neck reconstruction, secondly to prevent reflux, for it must be emphasised that if the bladder neck is tightened in the presence of reflux there is likely to be a serious deterioration of the upper urinary tract. The Leadbetter-Politano operation

(Politano and Leadbetter, 1958) is a suitable method to employ. Triangular areas of mucosa are excised on either side of a central strip of mucosa which should extend upwards for 2 or 3 cm from the verumontanum. This strip is then closed as a tube to form a supra-montanal urethra. Horizontal incisions are next made in the musculature at the level of the new bladder neck and flaps of muscle so formed are wrapped around the urethral tube. The urine must, of course, be diverted by supra-pubic cystostomy during the healing period. Some months of training are required before continence is achieved even in the favourable cases, and care must be taken to control any urinary infection. The writer has been able to obtain continence in only two thirds of the girls and less than half the boys treated (Burkholder and Williams, 1965).

Bladder closure in exstrophy

Attention has already been drawn to the hazards of reflux and pyelonephritis following closure of the exstrophied bladder, and it must also be recognised that the chances of continence are small. Only favourable cases with a healthy bladder of good capacity should be selected for reconstructive treatment: in them it is justifiable since abdominal wall and genital correction will be required in any event and it is of no great importance if diversion is performed after rather than before this correction.

In the male children a preliminary chordee correction is performed as already described. In infants, though not in older children, great assistance in the definitive closure may be obtained by a bilateral iliac osteotomy which allows the pubes to be brought together in the midline. The osteotomy is performed at the same time as the closure, or a few days before. The child is placed prone upon the table and a vertical incision is made parallel, and a little lateral, to the sacro-iliac joint (Fig. **27**, 6). The incision is deepened through the gluteal muscles to the bone and the periosteum is then

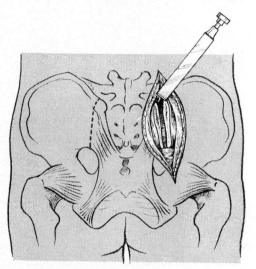

Fig. **27**, 6

Osteotomy for closure of exstrophy of the bladder. The iliac bone is exposed immediately lateral to the sacro-iliac joint. The periosteum is raised and the bone cut through with an osteotome.

stripped. A lever is placed subperiosteally in the greater sciatic notch to protect the structures emerging from the pelvis; the bone is then cut through with an osteotome. When completed, the osteotomy allows the os innominatum to hinge freely when the pelvis is compressed. The wound is sutured and the procedure repeated on the opposite side. The child's legs are suspended in a 'gallows' splint for three weeks after operation.

The closure operation on the bladder and urethra commences with an incision

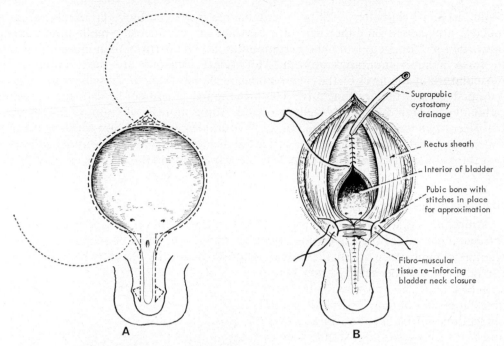

Suprapubic
cystostomy
drainage

Rectus sheath

Interior of bladder

Pubic bone with
stitches in place
for approximation

Fibro-muscular
tissue re-inforcing
bladder neck closure

A   B

FIG. 27, 7

Closure of the bladder in exstrophy. (A) Shows the incision outlining the urinary tract. An area of skin, including the umbilical scar, is also excised and triangles of mucosa at the bladder neck are removed. Triangles on the glans are also laid bare to allow rolling up as in epispadias. The faintly dotted line shows extensions of the incision which my be required for the formation of rotating skin flaps if an osteotomy has not been performed. (B) The bladder is closed by continuous midline suture with a suprapubic tube. The fibro-muscular tissue derived from the interior of the pubic bone is closed across the bladder neck, and if an osteotomy has been performed the pubes are approximated with strong catgut sutures. The urethra is closed as a tube. Subsequent skin closure can be with a vertical midline suture after osteotomy or by rotation of flaps if this is not possible.

around the muco-cutaneous junction (Fig. 27, 7). The bladder is separated from the rectus sheath and at the lower end the plane immediately behind the pubic bone is opened up, severing the fibrous bands which join the bladder to the bone. This frees the bladder and bladder neck on either side along with its nerve and blood supply and allows it to be displaced backwards to enable such muscular tissue as is available to be brought around the front of the bladder neck. The ureters are re-implanted now, or if necessary at a later operation when a saccular bladder has been formed. The construction of a bladder neck proceeds as in epispadias and the bladder neck and urethra are closed by two layers of continuous catgut. The distal urethra is again treated as in epispadias. The fibro-muscular tissue freed from the pubic bones is sutured in front of the bladder neck. The rectus sheath and pubes can then be brought together in the mid-line with strong catgut if an osteotomy has been performed and the skin is closed with a suprapubic cystostomy supplemented if necessary by ureteric catheters led out through the newly formed urethra. In the absence of an osteotomy, the abdominal wall should be reconstructed by flaps of rectus sheath, which are hinged on their medial border and turned inwards as in repair of ventral hernia. In these circumstances the skin should be closed by rotation of flaps from above and below the area of the closed bladder. Once again, the urine must be carefully checked during the months which follow operation and an intravenous pyelogram performed to ensure that there is no upper tract dilatation.

Results of functional closure of exstrophy have varied but are in general somewhat disappointing (e.g. Chisholm, 1962; Swenson, 1963; Lattimer and Smith, 1966). In a series of 51 cases reviewed in 1966 by the author only 5 achieved satisfactory continence, and of these, 3 had to be diverted because of upper tract dilatation. In a much more carefully selected group of 11 since that time, 3 have acquired reasonable continence, 3 have been diverted and four are still incontinent but otherwise well: one has been lost to follow up. It is clear that with a more selective use of reconstruction and a better control of reflux, a greater, though small, proportion of successful results has been achieved and the major dangers of the procedure have not been encountered (Williams and Savage, 1966).

Abdominal wall closure with diversion

In cases of exstrophy of the bladder where diversion is used as the primary method of treatment, the genitalia in the male are reconstructed as for epispadias. The bladder should not be excised completely, but the mucosa should be stripped off it, the muscle layer plicated by a series of catgut sutures and the skin closed by rotation of flaps over the bladder area, in this way a hernia at the site of cystectomy is avoided.

Choice of diversion

Methods of urinary diversion which employ the anal sphincter for the retention of urine involve very much less handicap for the child, but risk ascending infection and renal damage. Urinary diversions onto the skin of the abdominal wall are unquestionably safer, though not free of complications, but leave the child with the need for a permanent appliance. Many factors will influence the decision in the choice of diversion, not least amongst them the social circumstances of the child and his own and his parent's intelligence, since an appliance is only acceptable in some societies and can only be managed with success by someone who understands it well. In some exstrophy cases the anal sphincter is inadequate to retain urine in the bowel and careful tests for its competence should always be made before deciding on the operation to be performed. A decision is hard to make in very early infancy, but by the age of 2 or 3 the facts can usually be established by running some saline into the rectum as an experiment. It is clear that if the anal sphincter is incompetent then a skin diversion of urine by an isolated ileal, or an isolated colonic, segment is the method of choice. If the anal sphincter is competent and if the ureters are normal in calibre, a uretero-colic diversion is justifiable provided that the parents understand the need for careful follow-up and for re-diversion of the urine onto the skin if serious complications should supervene. Methods of diversion which attempt to use the anal sphincter for the separate control of two channels, one faecal and one urinary, although superficially attractive are difficult to accomplish with success and probably have little advantage over a straight uretero-sigmoidostomy.

D. INNES WILLIAMS

REFERENCES

BURKHOLDER, G. V. & WILLIAMS, D. I. (1965). *J. Urol.* **94**, 764.

CHISHOLM, T. D. (1962). In *Paediatric Surgery*. Ed. Mustard, W. T. *et al.* Chicago: Year Book Medical Publishers.

LATTIMER, J. K. & SMITH, M. J. V. (1966). *J. Urol.* **95**, 356.

MILLIN, T. (1947). *Retropubic Urinary Surgery*. Edinburgh: Livingstone.

POLITANO, V. A. & LEADBETTER, W. F. (1958). *J. Urol.* **79**, 932.

SWENSON, O., MOUSSATOS, G. H. & FISHER, J. N. (1963). *Surg. Clins N. Am.* **43**, 151.

WILLIAMS, D. I. & SAVAGE, J. (1966). *Br. J. Surg.* **53**, 168.

YOUNG, H. H. (1937). *Genital Abnormalities, Hermaphroditism and Related Disorders*. Baltimore: Williams and Wilkins.

CHAPTER XXVIII

VAGINAL AGENESIS

Congenital absence of the vagina and obliterative conditions of the external genital tract in females are due to various degrees of maldevelopment of the Mullerian ducts and the urogenital sinus.

Most of the malformations belonging to this category do not necessarily need correction in infancy or childhood and therefore do not, strictly, fall under paediatric plastic surgery. However, the paediatric as well as the plastic surgeon very often gets these patients referred for examination, and sometimes also for treatment.

A short description of these anomalies and the principles of their correction is, therefore, not out of place in this book on paediatric plastic surgery.

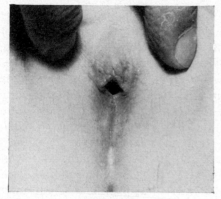

Fig. 28, 1
Adhesion of posterior three-quarters of labia minora.

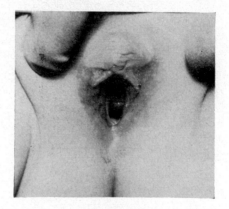

Fig. 28, 2
After blunt separation.

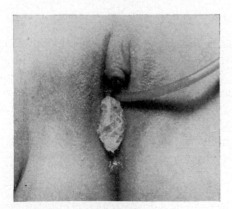

Fig. 28, 3
Vaseline gauze pad (4 to 5 days) prevents new adhesion.

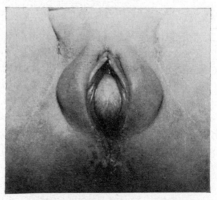

Fig. 28, 4
Mucocolpos in newborn, due to imperforate hymen.

ADHESION OF THE LABIA

This condition may exist as a congenital abnormality, and is found in all degrees from a posterior, partial adhesion of the labia minora (Fig. **28**, 1) to a complete fusion of both labia minora and majora. In most cases, however, the adhesion is apparently due to a mild inflammatory process. The treatment is simple and consists in blunt separation of the labia (Fig. **28**, 2); very rarely, a knife or scissors are necessary. To prevent recurrence of the adhesion, a pad of vaseline gauze is introduced between the separated labia for a period of four to five days (Fig. **28**, 3) and at the same time it is advisable to leave a catheter in the urethra.

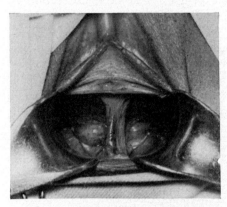

FIG. **28**, 5
Congenital sagittal septum of the vagina.

IMPERFORATE HYMEN AND VAGINAL SEPTA

An imperforate hymen or a transverse vaginal septum are rarely discovered until after the onset of the menarche. In some cases of imperforate hymen a mucocolpos may develop at an early stage, even in the newborn (probably due to maternal hormones), appearing as a cystic mass protruding in the vulva (Fig. **28**, 4), requiring immediate incision and evacuation. When otherwise discovered in infancy or childhood the imperforate hymen or transverse vaginal septum should be excised to prevent haematometra and haematocolpos formation at the onset of puberty. A sagittal vaginal septum (Fig. **28**, 5) is a rare condition and easily corrected by splitting or excision.

VAGINAL APLASIA IN OTHERWISE NORMAL GIRLS

Congenital absence of the vagina in otherwise normal women is, like the imperforate hymen, usually not discovered prior to the onset of puberty, and in most patients does not require any treatment until that time. In most cases the patients' appearance at the age of puberty is otherwise completely feminine with female breast development and pubic hair growth. A uterus is usually not found, or is rudimentary; only a few cases of functioning uteri have been described. The ovaries are normal and sex chromatin present. Congenital anomalies of the urinary tract are demonstrated in a significant number of the patients, for instance absence or ectopia of one kidney.

Treatment

It is not of value to describe here the old, more or less historical methods of constructing an artificial vagina, i.e. intestinal transplantation, pedicled flaps from neighbouring skin, progressive intermittent pressure of an external mould, and, in theory, the simplest of all techniques—keeping a dissected cavity open by an inserted mould for spontaneous epithelialisation.

All plastic surgeons and most gynaecologists, however, agree that nowadays the method of choice is the inlay skin grafting technique. The principle of the operation has been known since the days of Abbe (1898), and many surgeons have contributed to the development of the procedure. Credit should be given primarily to McIndoe (1950) who popularised the technique and in a series of papers published his experiences from the treatment of a large number of patients, partly in collaboration with a gynaecologist.

Operative technique

With the patient in the lithotomy position, and with a Foley catheter in the urethra, a sagittal incision is made from 1·5 cm posterior to the urethral meatus through the vaginal depression between the labia to 2 cm in front of the anus, so dividing the fourchette. A vaginal cavity is created by blunt dissection between the urethra and bladder anteriorly and the rectum behind; it should be carried up to the pouch of Douglas, which should, however, not be opened. Haemostasis is important, but if the correct plane of cleavage is entered bleeding is usually slight.

The next step of the operation is insertion of a skin graft fixed on a mould. The skin graft is removed as a thin split-skin graft in one large piece, either with a Humby or similar knife or as a full drum dermatome graft from the lower part of the

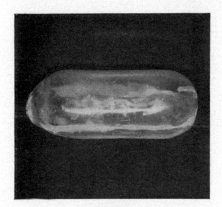

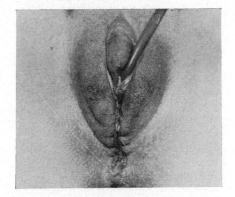

FIG. **28**, 6
Vaginal mould of original McIndoe type.

FIG. **28**, 7
Labia split and sutured across lower end of mould.

abdomen or from the inner side of the thigh. The original McIndoe mould (McIndoe, 1950) is oval in shape (Fig. **28**, 6), 10 cm long and 7 cm in circumference, made of two thin, polished acrylic shells sealed together. After painting with mastisol the mould is draped with the graft, raw surface outwards, and slid into position in the prepared cavity. The labia minora are split longitudinally and sutured across the lower end of the mould to keep it into position, leaving a small hole anteriorly for drainage (Fig. **28**, 7). According to McIndoe, the mould should remain *in situ* for about 4 to 6 months and then be removed. In most cases the major part of the graft will have taken, and any remaining granulations are curetted away. After removal of the mould a period of constant dilatation (i.e. day and night) with plastic or glass dilators is necessary to prevent shrinkage until marriage or regular intercourse has taken place.

Sometimes, however, complications occur, mostly due to haematoma formation and subsequent infection resulting in partial or even total loss of the graft. To avoid

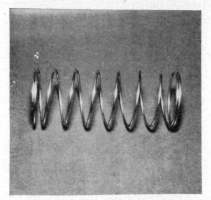

FIG. 28, 8
Metal spiral from ladies' hair-curler.

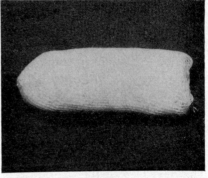

FIG. 28, 9
Spiral covered with tube gauze and filled up with gauze pads.

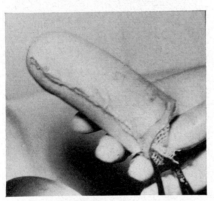

FIG. 28, 10
'Curler-mould' covered with jelonet and split-skin graft.

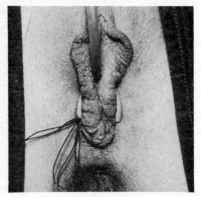

FIG. 28, 11
Labia minora temporarily united with mattress suture after insertion of mould.

this, several modifications of the inlay grafting technique have been designed. Stabler (1966), for instance, suggested delayed grafting, i.e. dissection of the cavity and insertion of a naked mould as a first stage, and three days later a graft is cut and inserted on the lenticular-shaped mould.

Another modification has proved useful at the Deaconess Hospital in Copenhagen (Jemec and Fogh-Andersen, 1967): a mould is made of a metal spiral (for instance from an old-fashioned ladies' hair-curler (Fig. 28, 8) covered with tube gauze and filled up with gauze pads (Fig. 28, 9). After creation of the raw vaginal cavity the dry-sterilised 'curler-mould' is first dressed with vaseline gauze (Jelonet) and then covered with a split skin graft (Fig. **28**, 10) and placed in the cavity. The labia minora are temporarily united with a mattress suture tied through a rubber tube (Fig. **28**, 11), and a Foley catheter is inserted into the bladder. The gauze packing is changed for the first time five days postoperatively. The curler-mould is removed on the tenth day together with the catheter, and the curler-mould is then exchanged for an acrylic mould, which the patient keeps inserted for about two to four months. Advantages of the curler-mould are: It is flexible and elastic and therefore does not cause pressure sores. It will enable satisfactory drainage to take place in combination with changes of the gauze pad packing.

VAGINAL APLASIA IN MALE PSEUDOHERMAPHRODITISM

In male pseudohermaphroditism, as for instance in the so-called testicular feminisation or Morris' syndrome (Morris, 1953), a normal or a hypoplastic vagina may be present, or the vagina may be completely absent. The gonads in these inter-sexual patients are testicles, situated in the abdomen or in the inguinal canal, and the sex chromatin is lacking. Phenotypically they are female at birth, except that the clitoris is sometimes slightly enlarged. At puberty they will develop either in the

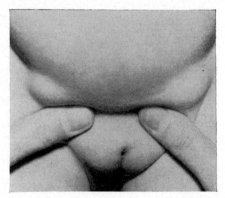

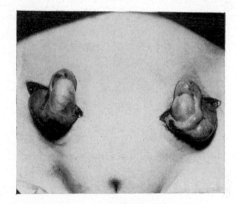

FIG. **28**, 12	FIG. **28**, 13
Palpable and visible gonads in both inguinal canals in 3-year-old girl.	Gonads which at operation appear to be testicles, before transposition into the abdomen.

feminine direction, 'total testicular feminisation', or more or less in the masculine direction, 'partial testicular feminisation' (Morris and Mahesh, 1963) (Chap. XXIX).

Occasionally the condition is discovered in infancy or childhood, usually in a girl who presents with an inguinal hernia, most often bilateral, containing a gonad (Fig. **28**, 12) which surprisingly proves to be a testicle (Fig. **28**, 13). This could either be transposed upwards through the inguinal canal into the abdomen for protection, awaiting the future development of the patient at puberty, or it could be removed on both sides, and later replacement hormone therapy instituted.

The treatment of vaginal aplasia in Morris' syndrome should follow the same principles as in otherwise normal girls, i.e. no attempt at reconstructive procedures until after puberty. A uterus is never found in these cases. For psychological reasons it is advisable not to tell these intersexual patients about the true character of their gonads or genetic sex. Correctly treated most of the patients will be able to have a normal life and be happily married—but will of course never be able to have children.

P. FOGH-ANDERSEN

REFERENCES

ABBE, R. (1898). *Med. Rec.* **64**, 836.
JEMEC, B. & FOGH-ANDERSEN, P. (1967). *Nord. Med.* **77**, 830.
McINDOE, A. H. (1950). *Br. J. plast. Surg.* **2**, 254.
MORRIS, J. M. (1953). *Am. J. Obstet. Gynec.* **65**, 1192.
MORRIS, J. M. & MAHESH, V. B. (1963). *Am. J. Obstet. Gynec.* **87**, 731.
STABLER, F. (1966). *J. Obstet. Gynaec. Br. Commonw.* **73**, 463.

CHAPTER XXIX

HERMAPHRODITISM AND PROBLEMS OF SEXUAL DEFINITION

Hermaphroditism and problems of sexual definition are more frequently recognised and better understood. The incidence of these anomalies has been reported as high as 1 per 1,000 births, approximately equal to the incidence of cleft lip and palate (Snyder, 1964). The multidiscipline approach which includes the plastic surgeon, endocrinologist, gynaecologist, urologist and psychiatrist has improved the care of these patients and appears to be the most promising way of establishing optimal functional and psychological satisfaction.

SEX ASSIGNMENT

Generally the sex of any individual is determined by the external expression (phenotype) of that individual's genetic constitution (genotype). The normal human cell has 46 chromosomes, 44 autosomes and 2 sex chromosomes, X and Y. XX is the normal female genotype, XY the normal male. Certain variations are known to exist in specific abnormalities. For example, XO is found in ovarian dysgenesis (Turner's syndrome) and XXY in testicular dysgenesis. Normal chromosomal arrangement is necessary for normal gonadal development. Development of the external genitalia is in turn determined by the type of gonadal development. Growth of the (sex primordia) genital tubercle and paired scrotolabial folds is influenced by androgenic steroids from the fetal gonads. In the absence of significant androgens, the female vulva develops. When androgens are produced, phallic enlargement and scrotal formation ensue (Barclay and Sternberg, 1966). Between these normal variations lies the spectrum of ambiguous sexual developments which result in problems of sex assignment that may vary from simple to the extremely complex.

Jones (1968) lists seven characteristics which are useful in establishing proper sex identification:

1. Sex chromatin and sex chromosomes
2. Gonadal structure (microscopic)
3. Morphology of external genitalia
4. Morphology of internal genitalia
5. Hormonal status
6. Sex of rearing
7. Gender (role) (patient's role as he acts it—not applicable in infants under two years of age).

Consideration should be given to all of these characteristics; depending on the individual problem, as many as necessary are thoroughly studied. The history and physical examination can supply information of the sex of rearing, gender role, and the morphology of the external genitalia. Chromosomal and chromatin studies may be done on peripheral blood smears, skin biopsy or by scraping the buccal mucosa,

Exploratory laparotomy is necessary to obtain the morphology of the internal genitalia. The hormonal status may be determined by studies of urinary 17-keto-steroids, oestrogens and pregnanetriol and blood determinations of 17-hydroxy-corticoids, ACTH and ICSH (Jones, 1968). In difficult cases, X-ray studies should include sinograms of all genital orifices, urethrography and intravenous pyelograms.

The decision of sex assignment is often most perplexing. With patients over two years of age and older, greater importance is given to the gender role and sex of rearing. In borderline cases where treatment could theoretically establish either sex, it must be remembered that it is easier to surgically construct a functioning female than a functioning male (Snyder, 1964).

While each case must be evaluated separately, some principles and guide lines are helpful. It is most important that the sex assignment be made as early as possible. Temporising does not help clarify the problem. A change made later in life may be very psychologically traumatic for the patient and family. Unfortunately, not all cases are diagnosed in infancy, for with minor ambiguities of the external genitalia, the actual intersex problem frequently does not become apparent until adolescent years. In these older cases, any change contrary to the sex already established should await an evaluation by a psychiatrist familiar with intersex problems. It is empha-sised that the sex of rearing is the most important consideration in the formation of the gender role. This has been shown to be more important than even the morpho-logy of the external genitalia, the hormonal dominance or the gonadal sex (Jones, 1968).

CLASSIFICATION OF INTERSEXES

The classification outlined by Barclay and Sternberg (Barclay and Sternberg, 1966) is uncomplicated and practical with only four major categories: (1) true herma-phroditism; (2) female hermaphroditism; (3) male hermaphroditism, and (4) chromo-somal abnormalities. True hermaphrodites have gonadal tissue of both sexes (ovarian and testicular). Female hermaphrodites are genetic females with two similar sex chromosomes (XX) and ovaries, but ambiguous external genitalia. Male herma-phrodites are genetic males (XY) with testicular tissue and poorly developed or feminised genitalia. The chromosomal aberrations include those syndromes with abnormal sexual development related to specific chromosomal abnormalities such as in Turner's and Kleinfelter's syndromes. Barclay and Sternberg are careful to point out that the chromosomal aberrations are not always true intersex problems.

True hermaphroditism

This is the rarest of types with fewer than 100 cases documented (Wakefield, 1967). There are no exclusive characteristics and it must be considered as a possibility in almost all problem cases (Jones, 1968). The diagnosis of a true hermaphrodite is established by the histologic demonstration of both ovarian and testicular gonadal tissue. Most are reared as males because of the masculine appearance of the genitalia, but almost all will develop female breasts and many will menstruate (Jones, 1968). Examination of a true hermaphrodite will usually reveal an enlarged phallus with what appears to be a marked perineal hypospadias. The principles of treatment involve medical and surgical efforts to remove contradictory organs and to reconstruct the external genitalia in keeping with the assigned sex. In the patient that has been reared as a male, this frequently includes removal of uterine and ovarian tissue, bilateral gynaecomastia procedures, obliteration of the vagina, and hypospadias repair. In the patient to be made a female, this surgery would consist of an orchiectomy, contouring of the phallus into an appropriate-sized clitoris, and later construction of an adequate vagina. The ideal time for final vaginal reconstruction in these patients may vary. We recommend that this surgery usually be deferred until six months prior to marriage.

True hermaphroditism diagnosed before the age of two could theoretically be assigned to either sex, but for practical purposes it should be the sex which medical and surgical therapy can more nearly establish.

Female hermaphroditism

This is the most common of all intersex anomalies and should be suspected in any newborn with abnormal genitalia (Wakefield, 1967). With rare exceptions, these patients should be reared as females. The deformity is most often related to adrenocortical hypoplasia with abnormal production of androgens and hydrocortisone. Chromosomal studies showing a positive chromosomal sex mass (only in females), elevated urinary 17-ketosteroids and pregnanetriol, subnormal urinary 17-hydroxysteroids and their correction to normal levels by the administration of cortisone are diagnostic. Other causes are the administration of androgenic steroids to the mother during the first trimester of pregnancy or an androgen producing ovarian tumour in the mother. Clitoral hypertrophy and fusion of the labia to simulate a male scrotum may be misleading to casual inspection. There are no gonads in the false scrotum. A urethra may be found in a urogenital sinus with a small vaginal meatus, or there may be a normal vagina with a vesicovaginal or urethrovaginal fistula. Diagnosis and treatment early in infancy can prevent the serious electrolyte and bone growth abnormalities seen in the late untreated cases. Surgical therapy, when indicated, is usually directed towards reducing the size of the enlarged clitoris and reconstruction of the vaginal vault. Wakefield (1967) feels this vaginal vault reconstruction is best left until shortly after the onset of puberty.

Male hermaphroditism

Although these individuals have unilateral or bilateral testicular tissue, only approximately one-third of all male hermaphrodites are suitable for male rearing (Jones, 1968). Those born with entirely female appearing genitalia generally feminise at puberty, while those born with ambiguous external genitalia will probably viralise (Jones, 1968). Inguinal hernias and ectopic testes are common. The phallus is frequently short and hypospadiac. There is sometimes a separate vaginal opening.

When the male sex is assigned, an orchipexy is indicated, the hypospadias is repaired, and the vagina (if present) obliterated. When the patient is to be made a female, an orchiectomy, vaginal reconstruction and reduction of the phallus will be required.

Chromosomal abnormalities

Most of these cases have gonadal dysgenesis or agenesis represented by small or rudimentary genitalia and undeveloped sex characteristics (Snyder, 1964). There are fewer opportunities for reconstruction in these cases, as many have decreased mentality, sterility, etc. Some may benefit by surgery designed to improve the appearance of the external genitalia to conform with the sex of rearing.

R. A. MLADICK, C. E. HORTON AND J. E. ADAMSON

REFERENCES

BARCLAY, D. L. & STERNBERG, W. H. (1966). A classification of intersexes. *Sth. med. J.* **59**, 1383–1392.
JONES, H. W. (1968). The intersex states. In *The Encyclopedia of Urology*, Vol. VII, Malformations, pp. 357–456. Ed. Amar, A. D. *et al.* Berlin: Springer.
SNYDER, C. C. (1964). Intersex problems and hermaphroditism. *Plastic and Reconstructive Surgery*, Chap. 72. Ed. Converse, J. M. Philadelphia: Saunders.
WAKEFIELD, A. R. (1967). Intersex and related problems. *Surg. Clins N. Am.* **47**, 505.

CHAPTER XXX

SACROCOCCYGEAL TERATOMA, DERMAL SINUS AND POSTANAL PITS

SACROCOCCYGEAL TERATOMA

Sacrococcygeal teratoma only occurs in about 1 in 40,000 births but is of some importance because prompt, adequate treatment gives expectation of normal life whereas delay or incomplete operation increases the risk from malignancy.

The tumour arises from totipotent cells and is presumably always present at birth. It is four times as common in the female, and some series have shown an increased incidence of twinning in the families. Elements from all layers are present—neural, glial, alimentary and respiratory epithelial; pancreatic, bony, cartilaginous and muscular tissues are common. It is often multicystic. In about 15 per cent. of those presenting at birth a solid element may be malignant. In those presenting later, up to 50 per cent malignancy has been reported. It seems that malignancy may be present at birth or may develop later in a previously benign tumour. Of 74 teratomas at Great Ormond Street, 41 were sacrococcygeal and, of these, 12 were malignant. Chromosome studies of 10 showed the same sex as the host in 9, different in 1 (Taylor, 1966).

The tumour arises from the region of Henson's node and is hence attached to the coccyx. Its early onset causes enlargement of the pelvic outlet and, following the line of least resistance, it extends backwards and downwards. There is always a nodule between the coccyx and rectum. The gluteal muscle is stretched over the tumour which may extend between muscle bundles. The levator is stretched so that the rectum is lengthened and the anus rotated so that it points forward. The tumour develops a fibrous, false capsule.

Clinical presentation

The tumour usually presents as a large swelling at birth. It may be large enough to cause difficulty in delivery. The swelling back and down from the sacral region displaces the sacrum and coccyx to produce the typical 'duck bottom' appearance (Fig. **30**, 1). The tense skin over the tumour may ulcerate. There are commonly large, subcutaneous veins from which bleeding may be troublesome. The anus is displaced to point forward, but nevertheless function is normal. Rectal examination reveals the extent of the presacral element of the tumour. Occasionally it extends far up towards the abdominal cavity.

Cases presenting later are more often malignant (Fig. **30**, 2). Metastasis may take place by local lymphatics or by blood spread to lungs or liver, and spinal metastases occur.

Occasionally the tumour may be unilateral (Fig. **30**, 3), or may arise from the coccygeal region by a narrow pedicle.

X-ray examination frequently reveals calcification and may even show formed bony elements.

Differential diagnosis

A sacral meningomyelocele covered by normal skin may look similar. It is usually recognisably cystic. Because it is so low down neurological deficit may not be recognisable and in the neonatal period the X-rays may not reveal the spina bifida. Occasionally a sacral meningomyelocele may be associated with a teratoma (Fig. 30, 4).

Other tumours which may arise in the area include neurofibroma (which may be associated with grossly enlarged exit foramina), ganglioneuroma, neuroblastoma and chordoma.

The author has seen a truly 'dermoid' cyst in this area associated with an abnormal anus of the 'covered' variety and a bifid distal sacrum. Rarely an excrescence in this region may represent a rudimentary tail (Fig. 30, 5). This may even have muscle and be capable of movement (Blaxland, 1950). Such is a malformation rather than a true tumour. A hamartomatous haemangioma may also occur here but should always be suspected of being part of a true teratoma.

Management

Prompt, complete operation is required in the first few days of life because

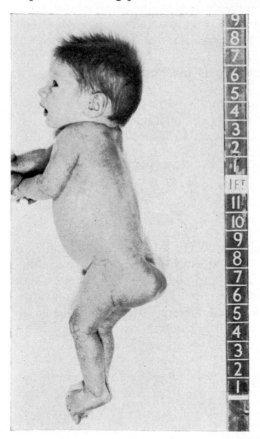

FIG. 30, 1

Typical 'duckbottom' appearance of sacro-coccygeal teratoma.

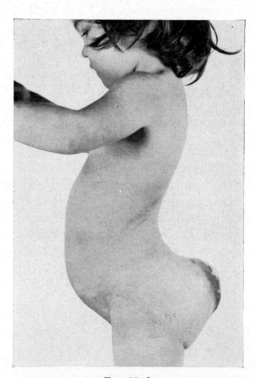

FIG. 30, 2

Sacrococcygeal teratoma presenting later. Malignant with overlying ulceration (spinal metastases developed).

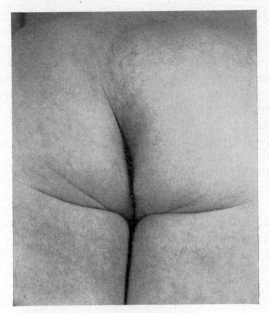

Fig. 30, 3

A sacrococcygeal teratoma presenting atypically as a mainly unilateral buttock swelling.

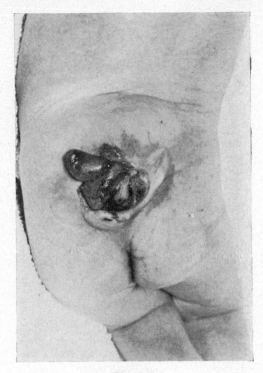

Fig. 30, 4

Unusual sacrococcygeal teratoma associated with meningocele.

of the increased hazards, including malignancy, with delay. With present-day neonatal surgical and nursing techniques the mortality should be negligible and there is no justification for delay.

The operation

Is carried out under endotracheal anaesthesia, having an intravenous infusion running and blood available, with the baby over a heating blanket.

A perineal approach is used with the baby prone. (In the unusual case having extension high in the pelvis the author prefers to begin with a laparotomy to mobilise the upper part of the tumour. Special care is taken to avoid damage in the region of the bladder neck.)

The baby is placed face down with a folded towel under the shoulders and a larger one under the lower abdomen to elevate the pelvis. The rectum is packed with vaseline gauze to assist recognition during dissection.

Gross' 'chevron' incision is used with the apex near the coccyx. The V-shaped flap is dissected back (Fig. 30, 6). The false capsule of the tumour allows a plane to be found and care may be needed to free gluteal fibres intermingled with extensions of the tumour. Some of these bundles can be safely removed with the tumour if necessary. If the overlying skin is damaged or ulcerated at the apex an ellipse may be excised as there is always an excess. The coccyx is then excised giving entrance to the

PS Q

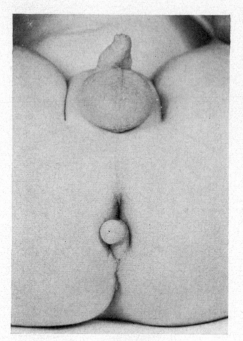

FIG. 30, 5
A rudimentary 'tail'.

plane in front of the sacrum and the tumour cleared above. It separates well from the elongated rectum. If there is any doubt about the plane the surgeon can put on a second left glove and continue dissection with the right hand whilst the left index is placed in the rectum. The extra glove can then be discarded to continue. When the tumour is freed above, laterally and anteriorly great care should be taken at the lower part to avoid damage to the stretched levatores ani whilst excision is completed.

The levators and raphe should be re-attached to the coccygeal region and it may be helpful to take in a tuck. The flap is trimmed and sutured in the usual way with a suction drain on either side of the rectum brought out through the stab wounds above the suture line away from the perineum. The author prefers the known low negative pressure suction of the Denis Browne method to the convenient but less controlled pressure of the more recently developed apparatus.

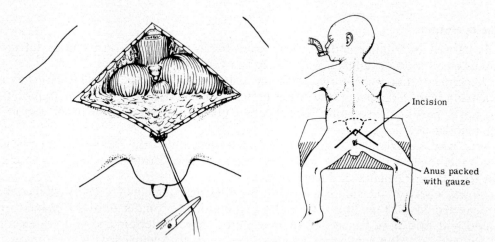

FIG. 30, 6
Showing exposure of tumour by freeing tip of coccyx and peeling down from the rectum. Inset shows incision.

Blood loss is not great in a straightforward excision. With prompt quantitative replacement there should be no need for postoperative intravenous fluids and oral feeding can begin next morning unless an abdominal phase has been necessary.

Results

Results are excellent with neonatal excision even if malignant areas are found. Nerve damage is rare but a careful watch should be kept on bladder function.

Operations later in childhood are less satisfactory with a great incidence of malignancy (Hatteland and Knutrud, 1960: 15 per cent malignancy under 3 months, 50 per cent over 3 months). The tumours are not very sensitive to radiotherapy and chemotherapy has not yet given significant benefit.

DERMAL SINUS

A dermal sinus can arise in the midline dorsally anywhere from occiput to sacrum. The orifice is insignificant but a related angioma may give a clue to its presence. It is an important lesion because the track leads into the vertebral canal, where there may be a cystic termination. Infection of the track causes recurrent spinal meningitis and, therefore, prophylactic excision is required.

POSTANAL PIT

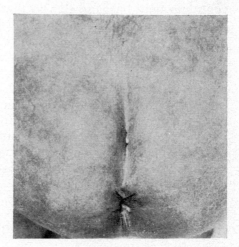

FIG. 30, 7
Postanal pit.

These pits occur over the coccyx which may be back tilted. They are commoner and less important. The sinus is short and one can often push back the surrounding skin to see the apex without any further track. They are often called 'pilonidal' but hair nests are not seen and their connection with the adult lesion seems arguable. If symptomless, as is usual, they can be left. They may become inflamed as a result of difficulty in hygiene (Fig. **30**, 7).

It is then simple to excise them (along with the tip of the coccyx if this is back tilted). Deep, slack mattress sutures are used which also pick up the base of the wound to close the dead space. Their ends are used to tie a collodion dipped gauze roll dressing over the wound. A 'Sleek' watershed is fixed between the anus and the wound as further protection against soiling.

H. H. NIXON

REFERENCES

BLAXLAND, P. J. (1950). *Brit. med. J.* **2**, 870.
HATTELAND, K. & KNUTRUD, O. (1960). *Acta chir. scand.* **119**, 444.
TAYLOR, A. (1966). *Ph.D. Thesis*. University of London.

CHAPTER XXXI

PLASTIC SURGERY OF THE INFANTILE AND ADOLESCENT BREAST

EMBRYOLOGY AND DEVELOPMENT

The mammary gland develops from both ectoderm and mesoderm. Although some authors feel that mammary gland tissue is similar to the sweat glands, breast formation actually precedes the latter in development by several months. During the sixth week of intrauterine life, two parallel ridges of thickened epithelium along the ventral surface of the embryo become recognisable. These bilateral ectodermal bands, oriented longitudinally, extend from the axillary to the inguinal regions and are called 'milk lines'. As the embryo develops, these ectodermal milk lines enlarge and begin to push into the subcutaneous mesoderm. Normally, the milk lines disappear except in those two areas of the mammary anlage which are destined to become normal breast tissue. Beginning at about the eighth week, epithelial cells begin to form a localised cluster around the level of the fourth rib. These cells proliferate to form buds and cords of breast tissue which ramify through the subjacent tissue. This process continues until birth, so that at that time all the main glandular ducts have been formed. At birth, and continuing for a few weeks following delivery, the normal infantile breast of both sexes may be engorged as a result of hormonal stimulation from the mother. This enlargement disappears spontaneously as excess circulatory placental oestrogen is destroyed. The normal male breast remains relatively quiescent, unless, for various reasons, gynaecomastia occurs. In sharp contrast, the female breast shows amazing proliferative activity. Beginning with the prepuberal elevation of the areola, the female mamma progressively enlarges through the puberal period by a process of periductal fat deposition. Acini are established and the ductal system gradually appears; however, this system achieves a completed status only after the development of pregnancy. All phases of mammary development are directed by hormonal stimuli (Arey, 1947).

THE DEVELOPING FEMALE BREAST

Polythelia (the presence of multiple nipples) occurs when the ectodermal tissue of the milk line does not degenerate or disappear and as a result multiple pigmented areas simulating nipple and areola formation may occur along the chest and abdomen. These are of concern to the paediatric patient for cosmetic reasons only and it is not mandatory that they be removed. Usually, however, excision of this tissue prior to puberty is necessary because of the desire of the parents and patient to be rid of the cosmetic deformity.

Polymastia (the presence of multiple breasts) occurs when both mesodermal tissue and ectodermal tissue of the milk line persists in abnormal positions. Some authors recommend that this tissue be removed to 'prevent the formation of a malignancy', however, this appears to be a theoretical rather than a practical concern. Accessory breast tissue can be removed for cosmetic and psychological reasons at any age and probably should be done prior to puberty (De Cholnoky, 1939).

When all of the ectodermal and mesodermal tissue of the milk lines disappear, *athelia* (absence of the nipple) or *amastia* (absence of the breast) may occur either bilaterally or unilaterally (Trier, 1965). More common is the condition of unilateral *hypomastia*. The true incidence of unilateral breast hypoplasia is relatively rare, although it is difficult to assess accurately. It is common knowledge that in the normal adult female one breast may be larger than the other, and that nipple height, level and position may be asymmetrical. These observations would indicate a variable end-organ potential acquired at some point in development, since embryologically the mammary anlagen begin as symmetrically paired structures. Unilateral breast hypoplasia usually is not difficult to diagnose. Because nipples are normally present in the infant, no abnormality is noted until puberty. At that time the patient tends to develop one normal breast but the abnormal side does not develop or does not develop adequately. No treatment is recommended for athelia, amastia and unilateral hypomastia until the patient is past adolescence. At that time, reconstructive procedures employing tubed pedicles, synthetic implants, vaginal mucosal grafts (and other procedures) may be utilized to reconstruct the missing breast substance and to simulate areola and nipple appearance.

Gigantomastia or virginal hypertrophy occurs infrequently in the adolescent female (Auber, 1923). This condition is manifested by excessively large breasts bilaterally. On palpation, the breast tissue appears normal and no tumour formation is noted. These breasts may become so large that reduction mammaplasty is desirable for cosmetic reasons. Only rarely will symptoms of backache, ulceration and difficulty in breathing be encountered in the young patient. In the young female, soon to potentially lactate, an amputation type of reduction mammaplasty is not indicated. Here the Biesenberger-McIndoe technique (Biesenberger, 1931) of breast reduction or the Strombeck procedure (Strombeck, 1960) for breast reduction is theoretically desirable. These techniques allow the ductal system of the nipple and areola to remain attached to underlying tissue and lactation is possible following such surgery (Figs. **31**, 1 and **31**, 2). Occasionally breast hypertrophy may recur after surgery, and in some circumstances simple mastectomy is indicated to prevent virginal hypertrophy regrowth.

Tumours of the breast in female children

Benign tumours of the breast area are not infrequent. These may pathologically involve any of the tissues around the breast area and the differential diagnoses may include haemangiomata, naevi, papillomata, and more infrequently, large benign fibroadenoma of the breast tissue itself. Potential damage to the underdeveloped breast tissue should be considered at all times in treating benign lesions of the breast. When small naevi and papillomata occur and must be excised in infancy, resection of these lesions should be performed with a dissecting microscope in order to preserve as much areola, nipple and breast tissue as possible. If these lesions appear benign and it is felt that no difficulty would ensue until the breast is developed, it is best to

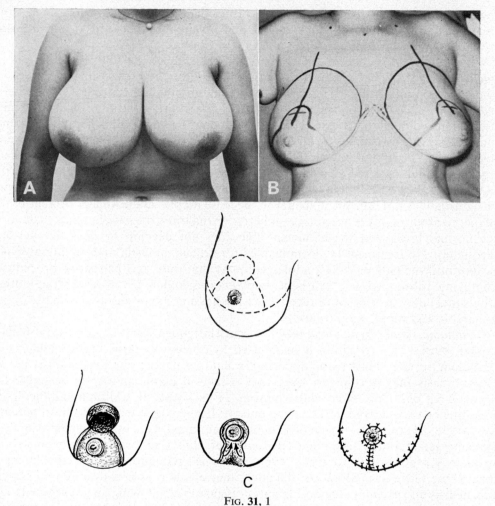

Fig. **31**, 1

(A) A 13-year-old female with virginal hypertrophy of both breasts. (B) Pre-operative markings for Strombeck reduction mammaplasty. (C) Strombeck reduction mammaplasty: schematic representation.

leave these untreated. After the breast is developed and when the structures are larger, adequate excision can be performed. In the past, many haemangiomata on or around the infantile breast have been treated with radiation. Iatrogenic unilateral mammary hypoplasia has been produced in many such cases and we feel X-ray of any kind to the infantile breast area for benign lesions is contraindicated. Our treatment for haemangiomata of the breast area consists of watchful waiting for spontaneous resolution of the haemangioma. If the haemangioma is large and ulceration with infection occurs, the plastic surgeon should determine whether excision and control of the disease with surgery would produce less damage to the breast then allowing the ulceration and infection to continue (Figs. **31**, 3 and 4).

In prepuberal and puberal females, *giant fibroadenoma* and *cystosarcoma phyllodes*

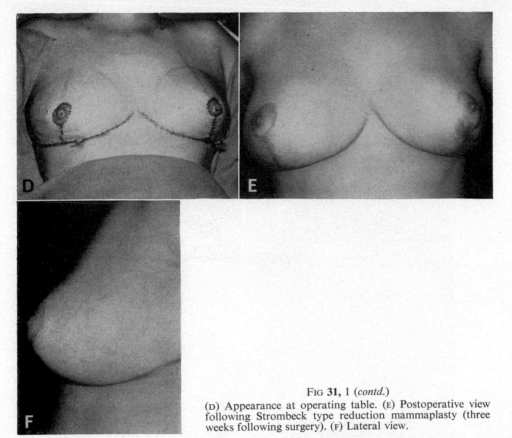

FIG **31**, 1 (*contd.*)

(D) Appearance at operating table. (E) Postoperative view following Strombeck type reduction mammaplasty (three weeks following surgery). (F) Lateral view.

may occur. This is differentiated from virginal hypertrophy or gigantomastia by the fact that a definite tumour mass can be palpated. The tumour mass may grow, become tender, and impending ulceration near the tumour mass may occur. Excision of this tumour should be performed as soon as the diagnosis is suspected. Occasionally the tumour may distort the remaining normal tissue of the breast so that a mastopexy must be performed in combination with the excision of the tumour. These specimens should be examined carefully by the pathologist as malignant varieties of cystosarcoma have been reported (Geschickter, 1943).

Malignant tumours of the breast in children are infrequent. McDivitt and Stewart from the Memorial Hospital for Cancer and Allied Diseases in New York reported (1966) that no case of breast malignancy in children was found in a sample of over 10,000 breast cancer cases treated at Memorial Hospital in a period of 15 years. During that time, they examined seven cases of breast tissue carcinoma in children sent from elsewhere to the Pathology Department; the patients ranged in age from 2 to 15 years. They point out that cancer of the breast in children is different from cancer in the adult breast. They saw no cases of regional or distant metastasis in children and the five year survival rate was 100 per cent. even in those treated only by excisional biopsy. From these and other statistics, it can be concluded that malignancy

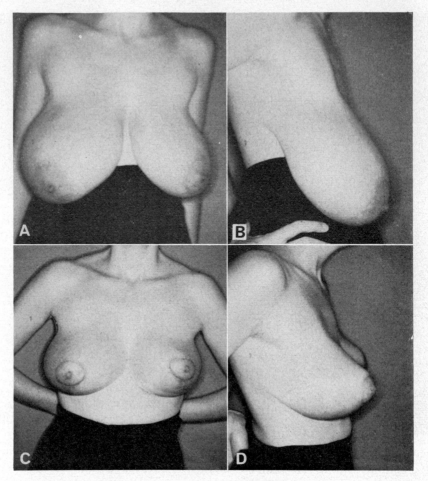

FIG. 31, 2

Gigantic breasts in teenager. (A) Pre-operative—front. (B) Pre-operative—side.
(C) Immediately postoperative—front (Biesenberger-McIndoe technique). (D) Immediately postoperative—side (nipple sensation and lactation function preserved).

of the breast in children is extremely rare; however, it must be included in the differential diagnosis of any breast mass in a child. Local excision seems to be the treatment of choice in this particular disease.

Trauma to the breast may produce skin-scarring which can restrict the growth of the breast by compression. Burns or avulsions of the skin of the chest wall and surgical scars over the breast may produce severe growth disturbances. Burn scar contractures of the breast area should be corrected early in puberty during the time the breast begins to develop in order to allow unrestricted growth. Several split-thickness skin grafts or various types of flaps at different time-periods may be necessary in order to totally free the breast for growth. If heavy scar contractures are not removed, the breast tissue will be compressed beneath the dense layer of scarred chest wall, and

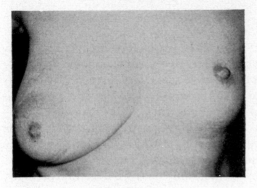 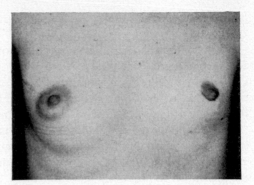

FIG. 31, 3	FIG. 31, 4
Iatrogenic unilateral mammary hypoplasia caused by surgical excision of a tumour of the breast in infancy.	Iatrogenic unilateral mammary hypoplasia caused by treatment of haemangioma of infantile breast with radiation.

normal development will not occur. Reconstruction of the breast wall with split-thickness skin grafts should begin at 10 to 12 years of age and continue until the breast has developed normally to its full potential. If the nipple was destroyed by the trauma, it is not necessary to reconstruct the nipple until the breast size and position has been ascertained, at which time a vaginal mucous membrane graft can be performed (Adams, 1949) to simulate the missing areola and nipple (Fig. 31, 5).

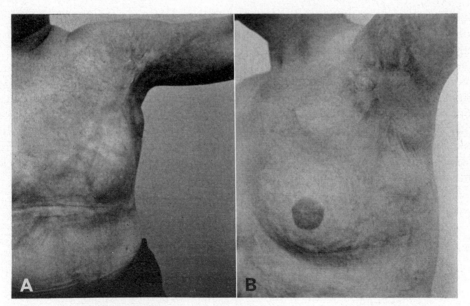

FIG. 31, 5

(A) Pre-operative burn scar of axilla and chest. Breast cannot develop because of dense scar. The nipple has been destroyed by the burn. (B) Postoperative appearance after split-skin grafts and flaps to the axilla and breast area. The nipple has been reconstructed from labial mucosa. This surgery should be strarted in the growing child to allow normal breast growth.

PS Q 2

THE MALE BREAST

Developmental anomalies consisting of *polythelia, polymastia* and *athelia* may occur in the male. Since the male breast does not normally enlarge as does the female in puberty, unilateral hypomastia does not occur. If accessory nipples or breasts occur in the male, these should be excised at a time convenient to the patient and his family, usually prior to school age to avoid embarrassment for the patient.

Benign tumours of the male breast occur infrequently. The most common benign tumour is *gynaecomastia*, meaning 'womanly breasts', a term frequently used to describe excessive breast formation in the male. This condition often occurs at puberty, due probably to an oestrogen-androgen imbalance and is self-correcting in many cases as testicular function becomes dominant.

Gynaecomastia is usually a unilateral problem and about 20 per cent. of the patients complain of pain. It should be emphasised that gynaecomastia in the puberal male will usually disappear without treatment; however, if it persists for more than two years, a thorough investigation of the body should be performed. Pathological gynaecomastia is a manifestation of an abnormality which has created a hormonal imbalance. Tumours of the testes as well as hypogonadism, as in Klinefelter's syndrome, may cause breast enlargement as both androgens and oestrogens may be mammotropic. Liver disease, when normal destruction of oestrogens is impaired, may be found frequently with gynaecomastia. Malnutrition and vitamin deficiency may cause liver impairment and may also be associated with gynaecomastia (Nydick *et al.*, 1961).

Once gynaecomastia has been diagnosed and systemic illness eliminated, the condition may be treated if abnormal lengthy persistence occurs. Surgical excision should be performed using either local or general anaesthesia. Preservation of the nipple and areola is important. A peri-areolar incision (Webster, 1946) or a trans-areolar incision (Pitanguy, 1966) will allow resection of the breast tissue with minimal residual scarring after healing. In most cases it is not necessary to extend the incision beyond the pigmented areola and skin border; however, if necessary, a small lateral extension (Lynch, 1954) may be utilised (Fig. **31**, 6). Only in extreme cases will a simple mastectomy and free nipple transplant be necessary. Postoperative suction or compression to the wound is recommended as one of the frequent complications in this surgery is postoperative haematomata (Von Kessel *et al.*, 1963).

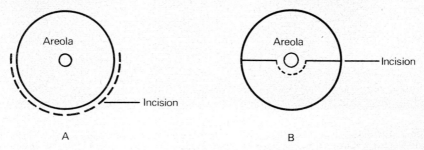

FIG. **31**, 6

(A) Circumareolar incision for gynaecomastia. (B) Transareolar incision for gynaecomastia.

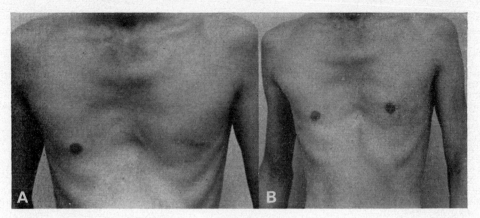

FIG. 31, 7

(A) This adolescent male had an enlarged breast removed with the nipple, leaving a cosmetic deformity causing psychological changes. (B) Postoperative appearance. A scrotal graft has been used to reconstruct the nipple. As the patient grows older, hairs may occur in this graft but are usually not objectionable.

Malignancies of the prepuberal or adolescent male breast are rare. This condition, however, must be kept in mind in the differential diagnoses of breast enlargements in the prepuberal male.

Trauma to the male breast will usually not result in asymmetry unless the areola and nipple are destroyed. Such destruction may result from burns, avulsions in accidents, and from surgical excision of the breast and nipple. Loss of the areola and nipple in the male is psychologically disturbing to the normal person and should (if at all possible) never be produced surgically. When nipple and areola loss has occurred, three procedures are available to simulate a nipple on the involved side. Tattoo pigment may be utilised to colour the skin of the nipple-areola area. This is usually not satisfactory since the skin of this area remains flat and the disguise is not adequate. A second method using a split thickness skin graft from the opposite normal areolar area may be considered. These grafts take well and provide a flat pigmented skin areola for the damaged chest wall. Occasionally, tattooing may be necessary to supplement the skin graft since it is difficult to take a graft from an irregular area, particularly if the nipple is protruding. Tattoo pigment can be used to supplement this graft with great success.

A third way to simulate a missing nipple in the male is to graft a circular portion of the scrotum on to the desired position of the chest. Scrotal skin is pigmented and will simulate quite nicely the missing areola and nipple. Full-thickness grafts are the easiest to procure, and since the scrotum will ultimately bear hairs the follicles are transplanted in the graft material. Ordinarily the adult male has some hair around the areola, therefore the transplantation of a few scrotal hairs does not detract from the graft. Again, it may be necessary to supplement the scrotal graft with tattoo pigment. Since psychological disturbances can be induced by nipple and areolar absence in the young male, we feel that the reconstruction of these defects should be done prior to adolescence if possible (Fig. 31, 7).

C. E. HORTON, J. E. ADAMSON AND R. A. MLADICK

REFERENCES

ADAMS, W. M. (1949). Labial transplant for correction of loss of the nipple. *Plastic reconstr. Sur.* **4**, 295.

AREY, L. B. (1947). *Developmental Anatomy*, 5th ed. pp. 409–412. Philadelphia: Saunders.

AUBER, V. (1923). Hypertrophie mammaire de la puberté, resection partielle restauratrice. *Archs fr.-belg. Chir.* **3**, 287.

BIESENBERGER, H. (1931). *Deformitaten und Kosmetische Operationen der Weiblichen; Brust.* Wein: Maudrich.

DE CHOLNOKY, T. (1939). Supernumerary breast. *Archs Surg.* **39**, 926.

GESCHICKTER, C. F. (1943). *Diseases of the Breast.* Philadelphia: Lippincot

LYNCH, R. C. (1954). An operation for correction of gynecomastia through an areolar incision; *Plastic reconstr. Surg.* **13**, 412–416.

McDIVITT, R. W. & STEWART, F. W. (1966). Breast carcinoma in children. *J. Am. med. Ass.* **195**, 388.

NYDICK, M., BUSTOS, J., DALE, J. H., Jr. & RAWSON, R. W. (1961). Gynecomastia in adolescent boys. *J. Am. med. Ass.* **178**, 109.

PITANGUY, I. (1966). Transareolar incision for gynecomastia. *Plastic reconstr. Surg.* **38**, 414–419.

STROMBECK, J. G. (1960). Mammaplasty: report of a new technique based on the two-pedicle procedure. *Br. J. plast. Surg.* **13**, 79.

TRIER, W. C. (1965). Complete breast absence. *Plastic reconstr. Surg.* **36**, 430.

VON KESSEL, F., PICKRELL, K. L., HUGER, W. E. & MATTON, G. (1963). Surgical treatment of gynecomastia. *Ann. Surg.* **157**, 142.

WEBSTER, J. P. (1946). Mastectomy for gynecomastia through semicircular intra-areolar incision. *Ann. Surg.* **124**, 557.

SECTION 3

LIMBS

CHAPTER XXXII

THE UPPER EXTREMITY

CONGENITAL MALFORMATIONS OF THE HAND

General considerations

Congenital malformations in the human being are a heterogeneous group. A certain percentage of congenital malformations appears to be genetic (intrinsic) in origin, and the remainder almost entirely environmental (extrinsic). The pathologic mechanism of both types need not necessarily be the same, and there are probably important differences that remain undiscovered.

In discussing the development of congenital malformations, Waddington (1963) distinguishes between what might be called the *primary* lesion, the state at which the developmental processes begin to deviate from their usual course, and the *secondary* lesions which are the consequences of this disturbance of the normal course. The morphogenetic basis of developmental mechanisms is an enormously complicated physico-chemical process.

The primary lesion may be caused either by an abnormal genetic factor in the developing embryo or by unusual environmental circumstances, including the presence of specific deleterious drugs. Further, there may be a complex interaction of the intrinsic and extrinsic factors. The majority of congenital malformations of the limb do not in general conform to any simple genetic hypothesis, nor are they attributable to known factors in the environment except in certain specific instances.

The primary lesion is always at the cell level of organisation. Here all developmental processes can be altered by the genes, which are intracellular structures, and their activities occur within the cell itself.

The secondary lesion, the manifestation of the congenital malformation, is the result of disturbances of the morphogenetic processes, in which huge numbers of cells are involved. To put it simply, the malformation is the result of malfunction somewhere in the delicate process whereby a mass of early embryonic cells are moulded into a characteristic form.

The developing structure progresses through a series of changes which are activated by the synthesis of particular proteins within the cells. Thus the properties of the cytoplasm within the developing cell may be changed; or the properties of the cell surface may be altered and thus its morphogenic properties change. The newly appearing substances will be formed under the influence of the nuclear genes of the cell (Waddington, 1963). This is an enormously complex mechanism involving DNA, RNA, various ribosomes, etc. The primary lesion which becomes the ultimate congenital malformation is the result of the abnormal functioning of 'gene-ribosome' systems, the presence of an unusual gene.

Malformations can be shown in many instances to be due to the influence of hereditary factors following Mendelian laws, as for example arachnodactyly and polydactyly. The trait may skip one generation, may alter its form of expression or otherwise behave in an atypical manner. To explain these failures of expected ratios, geneticists use many explanatory and qualifying terms, such as 'variable expression,' 'reduced penetrance', 'inhibiting or modifying genes', 'environmental factors' or 'incomplete dominance'. The penetrance concept measures the percentage of affected among subjects carrying a deleterious dominant gene. This reduced penetrance may perhaps be caused by environmental conditions. Even if we cannot, in a population study, find sufficient genetic cause for a malformation, we may sometimes be able to detect the presence in the mother of a deleterious drug or virus. The tragic thalidomide incident in causing phocomelia is a classic example of the effect of a deleterious drug, and the following virus infections have been strongly associated with congenital abnormalities: rubella, herpes zoster, mumps, Coxsackie, and vaccinia. Nevertheless, one must remember that the primary lesion is on the gene, which affects the synthetic process activated in the cell cytoplasm environment.

Genetic factors are by far the most important in this field and several long pedigrees are recorded showing the same anomaly appearing generation after generation. It must be remembered that all genes participate in the environment of cell protoplasm and this environment is to a certain extent dependent upon external conditions such as temperature, oxygen supply, and other metabolites, and the presence or absence of deleterious chemicals.

There is evidence that genetic factors are modified by environmental factors, as is seen in cases of single-ovum twins in which one is born with a cleft lip and/or cleft palate and one is normal, despite their identical genetic constitution. Genetic factors may act after birth, producing dynamic or progressive lesions as reported by Hiller (1927) in the case of a constricting band that later appeared proximal to the amputation stump, which was the result of a previous constriction.

Precisely how deleterious agents, drugs or viruses, act upon the genes has not been discovered. It is unlikely that the teratogenic drugs reach the gene, although some of the abnormal analogues of amino acids or of the nucleic acid bases may affect the synthetic process more or less directly.

The effect of radiation has been studied widely in the laboratory. In the mouse embryo, its effect is highest immediately after fertilisation, during the morula and blastula stages. In the human, we have not yet discovered the smallest dose that can harm the foetus, nor do we know what is the largest dose the human foetus receives from diagnostic medical radiology. In the laboratory, it has been shown that a dose as small as 50 r will reliably produce malformations of the skull and brain in a large percentage of rats. It has been assumed that a much smaller dose suffices to produce leukemia. This appears to be confirmed by the experience of the Hiroshima explosion (Neel, 1958).

In our own personal experience with the Hiroshima patients, in a group of 25 young women exposed, who sustained confirmed radiation illness, there have thus far been no known cases of leukemia nor have any of the offspring, which I believe to be 16 in number at present, shown any congenital malformations.

The gonadal effect of radiation is well realised and hence precautions should be taken in medical radiography, television viewing, and occupation.

The timing of the effect of the noxious agent is of paramount importance. This point is the application at the *critical period*, the period when the region is developing most actively. In the human, the critical time might be expected to occur between the fourth and seventh weeks, which includes the period between the appearance and the differentiation of the arm bud.

The overall incidence of malformations is approximately the same in different parts of the world and in different racial groups. However, specific types of abnormality do differ in different racial groups.

Incidence is also related to sex, parental age, associated defects, and a variety of unknown environmental factors. For example, the increased occurrence in consanguineous parents has been demonstrated in Schull's study of the Japanese population. Incidence in unrelated parents is about 1 per cent., as compared to 1·75 per cent. in children of first cousins.

No comprehensive world-wide or completely reliable statistics are extant. The attempt to explore this question which comes closest to being useful is Birch-Jensen's monograph published in 1949, a careful study of all living patients in Denmark with hand anomalies. There are 625 cases, representing an incidence of one anomaly in each 6438 persons. Unfortunately, the study did not include polydactyly or simple uninvolved syndactyly, which are the most common types of deformity. Furthermore, the population of Denmark is homogeneous and stable with practically no immigration or emigration. For these reasons the figures given cannot be applied to other countries with less homogeneous populations.

SYNDACTYLY

In our own experience syndactyly has been the commonest congenital hand malformation. However, polydactyly has been reported as the most frequent. Probably this is so, but in many cases, the defect is so minimal that the patient is not referred to the surgeon for treatment, and the obstetrician or the paediatrician removes or ties off the rudimentary accessory digit. In humans, syndactyly is associated with polydactyly and with other complicated hand malformations as well as with malformations of the extremity.

Pathogenesis and Aetiology

In the 4-week-old embryo, there are indications of the developing digits on the upper extremity. (The lower extremity is delayed for about an additional week.) The finger buds grow rapidly between the sixth and seventh weeks, when webbing between the fingers disappears and the fingers become digitated, being completely formed at about the eighth week. When, during this period, there is disturbance of some phase of digital development, the webbing may persist, while the webbed fingers continue to grow at a uniform rate.

Experiments on rats carried out by Warkany and Nelson in 1941 have shown that dietary deficiency may cause foetal anomalies including syndactyly. Riboflavin deficiency has been cited as the cause of this maldevelopment. The relative importance of genetic and environmental influences in humans has not been clearly determined, but it is generally felt that genetic factors are the more important.

It has been suggested (Alvord, 1947) that syndactyly may be attributed to one or more mutant genes, but because of the great plasticity in the development of the digits, many different genes may affect them in different ways. Studies of pedigrees by Penrose (1946) have demonstrated that paternal genes are more influential than maternal, and he concluded that syndactyly may be due primarily to incompatibility between the mother and a foetal antigen derived from the father. Hicks (1953) concluded that most malformations of the fingers in the skeleton, especially syndactyly, originate in abnormal genes. Gates (1946) found that webbing between the second and third toes is about twice as common in men as in women and attributed the condition to a simple dominant gene probably in sex chromosomes. Montague (1953) described a history of middle and ring finger syndactyly transmitted through four generations in both male and female lines. He concluded that the anomaly is due to a dominant gene carried in the X chromosome. On the other hand, studies have shown high familial incidence of syndactyly which varies greatly in form and degree over a number of generations. Thus it can be seen that the genetic transmission is not rigid, but may be a Mendelian dominant, a sex-linked dominant, or sometimes a recessive or even occasionally a mutant gene.

Incidence

MacCollum (1940) reported that syndactyly occurs once in about every thousand to three thousand births. Bunnell (1956) made a similar observation. It is generally agreed that the condition is commoner in male than in female children, and in our own series 56 per cent. were males. In MacCollum's series, 48 per cent. of the patients had the condition bilaterally and the toes were affected in 35 per cent.

Schurmeier (1922) reported that syndactyly was the commonest hand deformity found in white men, while polydactyly was more frequent among Negroes. In our own series reported in 1958, 38 per cent. of the patients with syndactyly were affected bilaterally, the malformation most commonly affecting the ring and middle fingers. It was most likely to be symmetrical on both sides.

Syndactyly frequently is found together with other hand malformations, especially ectrodactyly, brachydactyly, or annular bands; 42 per cent. of our syndactyly patients had other hand malformations. Syndactyly is often found with various deformities of the skull, such as oxycephaly or Apert's disease (see Chap. XII).

FIG. 32, 1

Partial (or incomplete) syndactyly involving the ring and middle fingers. These are the digits most commonly affected. The surgeon should not be misled into thinking there is enough tissue present in this type of case to resurface the denuded areas on the separated fingers. A supplementary skin graft will be necessary. The same type of operation as shown in Figure 32, 6 can be used.

Varieties

There are various forms of syndactyly. When only two digits are webbed, this would be called a 'single syndactyly'; when more than one web is affected, it would be referred to as a 'multiple syndactyly'—double, triple, etc. A web that extends only part way up the finger from the base would be called 'partial syndactyly' (Fig. **32**, 1) and when it extends from base to finger tip—'complete syndactyly' (Fig. **32**, 2). A webbing that consists only of the skin is called a 'simple syndactyly'; when bones or finger nails of the adjacent fingers are fused, the condition may be referred to as 'complicated syndactyly' (Fig. **32**, 3). In some cases the nerves and even the tendons may be joined.

Simple, complete, single syndactyly involving only one web, usually between the ring and middle fingers, is the commonest type. The multiple types (Fig. **32**, 4) are much less frequent and thumb involvement is the least frequent.

Treatment

Didot's (1850) flap operation is mentioned only to be condemned. In this operation, flaps were designed to cover both the separated fingers. The flaps were rarely if ever wide enough to resurface the fingers, the incisions had to be closed under great tension, and the resultant scar and frequent breakdown prevented functioning of the fingers and made secondary repair more difficult.

The surgical treatment for syndactyly will achieve best results if the operation can be delayed until the child is at least 2 years or older. It is difficult to mobilise the tiny infant fingers in extension. However, one should not be too rigid about the age of operation, for if the webbing is retarding the growth of fingers, earlier operation may

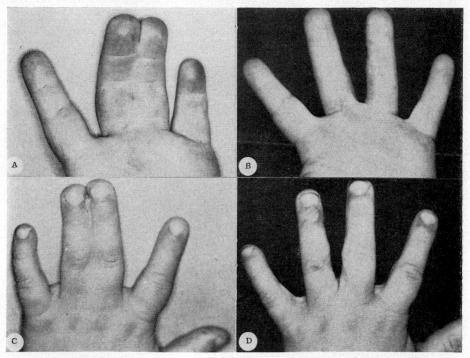

FIG. **32**, 2

Complete uncomplicated syndactyly. (A and C) Palmar and dorsal view pre-operatively. (B and D) Palmar and dorsal views postoperatively. A normal-appearing web is most desirable, and it should be deep enough. Operative procedure shown in Figure **32**, 6 used for correction.

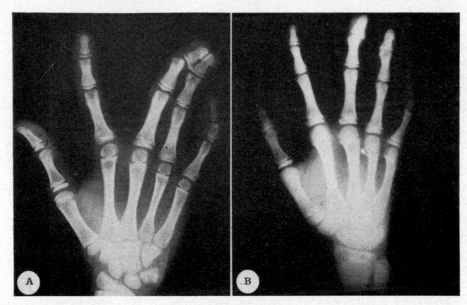

FIG. **32**, 3

Single complete complicated syndactyly. The condition was bilateral and symmetrical. The patient is a 15-year-old male. (A) Pre-operative; bony union is present between the epiphyseal plates and the distal ends of the phalanges. One is justified in this type of case in operating at an early age to prevent deviation of the fingers. (B) Postoperative. The deviation of the fingers was corrected spontaneously. Deviation is invariably toward the shorter finger.

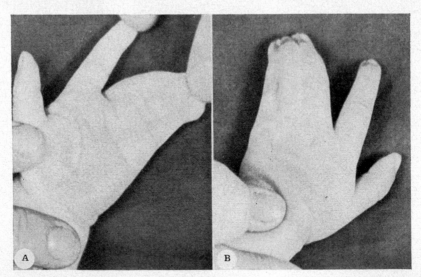

FIG. **32**, 4

Double syndactyly. The middle, ring and little fingers are involved. (A) Palmar view. (B) Dorsal view. Note the tendency of the ring finger toward contracture. This type of syndactyly is far less common than the single variety. All three digits should not be separated at the same operation lest the circulation to the ring finger be seriously compromised. The same precaution holds in syndactyly of a more advanced nature, such as when all four fingers are involved.

be indicated (Fig. **32**, 5). We have found that in cases such as illustrated in Figure **32**, 3, even when the procedure is carried out at the age of about 15 years, the curvature of the long finger caused by the attachment to the shorter finger may spontaneously correct itself after operation and the fingers achieve normal length and straightness.

Surgical treatment consists of separating the fingers and skin grafting denuded surfaces. In multiple syndactyly, one should perform the operation in stages rather than take a chance and denude both sides of a digit at the same operation. The basic principles of operation are the use of flaps in the depth of the commissure to permit full abduction of the fingers, the use of zigzag incisions in order to minimise secondary contraction, and wherever possible utilisation of flaps to cover one finger so that only the other finger will require a free skin graft. It is felt that the radial side of a digit is functionally more important than the ulnar side and hence the flap should be utilised to cover the radial side of the digit and free graft applied to the ulnar side of the other digit.

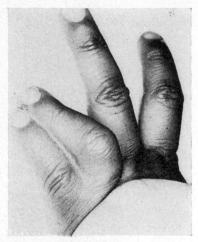

Fig. **32**, 5

Single complete syndactyly of the ring and little fingers. The patient is a 3-year-old male. There is a flexion deformity of the ring finger. One is justified in operating on this type of case at an early age with the hope of avoiding adverse effect on growth and development of the ring finger. The prognosis should be cautious in view of the fact that very often it is almost impossible to correct the contracture of the ring finger. Note that syndactyly between the ring and little finger alone is rare.

AUTHOR'S TECHNIQUE

Pre-operative X-ray studies should always be carried out so as to determine the condition of the bony structures. Operations should always be performed under tourniquet.

The procedure that follows is one utilised for simple syndactyly. When the condition is multiple, it is not advisable to denude both sides of a finger at the same operation. This may interfere with the blood supply of the digit. For example, if the four fingers are webbed, it will be advisable only to separate the radial digit and the ulnar digit, leaving the web between the ring and middle fingers to be treated at another stage. Figure **32**, 6 shows the design of a flap that has produced the best results in the author's hands. Two points are to be emphasized: (1) the flap design should provide adequate coverage for the commissure and (2) incisions are never straight, but always zigzag or curved. The use of a zigzag incision will prevent secondary linear contraction. It should be borne in mind when making incisions and carrying out dissection that the nerve supply may be anomalous, as indicated in Figure **32**, 7. Thus one should always identify the common digital nerve proximally and dissect it digitally to make sure that an adequate nerve supply is retained.

In the event that bones are fused, they must be separated. Should a joint be opened, it should be closed with very fine absorbable sutures. When a double nail is present, it should be split and part of the adjacent nail matrix should be ablated.

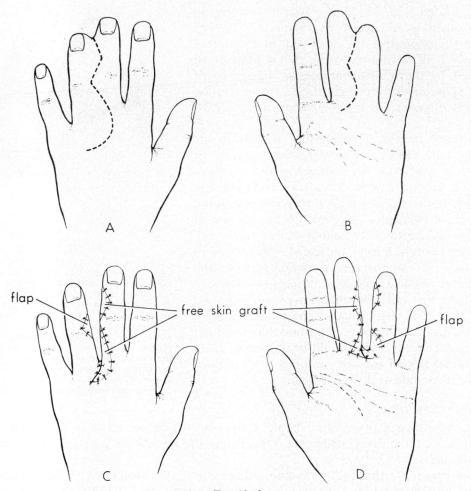

Fig. 32, 6

Operation for syndactyly. (A) Incision on the dorsum of the hand. The proximal part of the flap should be sufficiently large to cover the radial surface of the ring finger and also to provide adequate covering for the depth of the commissure. (B) Volar incision. Every effort must be made to avoid damaging the nerve supply to the digit (see Fig. 32, 7). (C) After reflection of the flap, the ring finger is covered and the remainder of the defect on the ulnar side of the long finger is resurfaced with a free skin graft. (D) Note the use of zigzag incisions and flap coverage in the commissure.

In the procedure shown in Figure 32, 6, one finger will be covered with flaps, leaving only the denuded side of the remaining finger to be covered. For this purpose a thick split graft, or better a full-thickness skin graft should be utilised. Grafts should be cut to pattern and carefully sewn in place. The fingers and hand are immobilised by a light pressure dressing. It is advisable to use a plaster splint.

Every effort should be directed toward a successful primary operation, otherwise secondary contraction will occur and this will be extremely difficult to correct (Figs. 32, 8 and 32, 9).

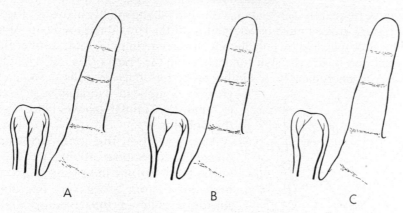

FIG. **32**, 7

When two digits are joined, as in syndactyly or polydactyly, anomalies of the nerves are found. These anomalies are similar in both conditions and the precautions advised apply equally, although the drawings illustrate only polydactyly. (A) The preservation of a nerve supply to each side of the retained finger is easily accomplished in polydactyly, but in syndactyly it will be necessary to split the central nerve trunk in order to supply innervation to both sides of the separated digits. (B) In polydactyly, if one did not identify the nerve proximally, one could easily ablate the nerve leaving one side of the finger desensitised. Again, in syndactyly, the nerve should be split so as to retain nerve supply on both sides of the digits. (C) In polydactyly one should transplant the entire nerve trunk to the retained digit and in cases of syndactyly, the digits would have only one nerve trunk on one side of the digit with spreading at the distal ends.

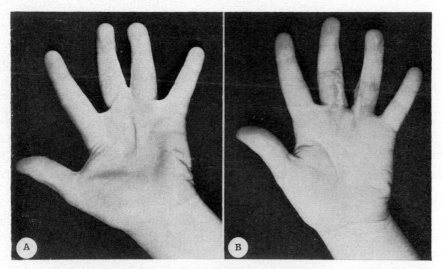

FIG. **32**, 8

(A) Residual deformity following improperly performed primary operation. The commissure is located too far distally and there are contracted scars on the palmar surfaces of the fingers, causing a flexion deformity. (B) Postoperative result showing reconstruction of the commissure. Note that the scar is zigzag. This avoids the possibility of a secondary contracture. An extensive free graft is necessary to correct this condition, as shown in Figure **32**, 9.

Syndactyly is frequently associated with other hand malformations (Fig. **32**, 10) and the procedure utilised must be adapted to fit the special requirements of the case. If syndactyly is complicated by polydactyly, it is sometimes possible to fillet the supernumerary digit and to use the skin for separating the fingers (Fig. **32**, 11). Occasionally, in a case of macrodactyly, a similar procedure may be utilised. When annular grooves complicate syndactyly, it is advisable to repair the annular grooves before correcting the webbing.

After operation free grafts are usually not dressed for a period of about a week to 10 days unless there is some indication to do so. It has been our custom to use very fine absorbable sutures in children, thus avoiding the troublesome problem of removing sutures in an apprehensive child. Grafts and flaps are generally taken and applied in the usual manner. Later, when healing is complete, exercise and massage keep the grafts supple. We have rarely found it necessary to utilise prolonged postoperative splinting. Occasionally children develop hypertrophic scarring. In these cases, prolonged splintings may be of use although secondary contracture usually regresses; postoperative massage is helpful.

FIG. **32**, 9

Secondary correction after unsuccessful syndactyly operation. (A) Zigzag incisions are necessary; the commissure should be deepened to the proper depth and a pleat fashioned on the dorsum. (B) The free skin graft should be generous in size.

POLYDACTYLY

Polydactyly is a phenomenon of duplication of parts, and it varies from duplication of a single phalanx to the duplication of an entire extremity. It is also found in monkeys and other animals. The malformation is indigenous in certain localities. In 1898, Boinet reported the presence of hetrodactyly in an Arabian tribe, the Hyabrites. A five-fingered child was considered abnormal and was sacrificed.

Aetiology

Polydactyly is considered an inherited malformation frequently associated with other anomalies. It may originate in mutation. It may be a dominant, recessive or intermediate trait tending to be recessive at first and becoming increasingly dominant through succeeding generations. The failure to appear regularly in family histories is apparently due to 'lack of penetrance'. Thus, the gene causing polydactyly is present but is not expressed, either because the genes vary in strength or because there is some inhibiting factor which is active in the particular case. Gates postulated that different genes probably control radial and ulnar polydactyly.

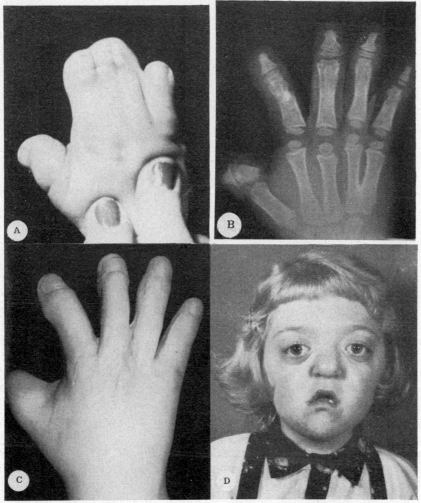

FIG. **32**, 10

Acrocephalosyndactyly. (A) Pre-operative dorsal view. The fingers are shortened and all four fingers are webbed. The thumb deviates radially. (B) Roentgenogram. Note the characteristic deviation of both phalanges of the thumb. No attempt should be made to correct this until the epiphysis has closed and the possibility of interference with growth and development is avoided. Note that there are only two joints in each digit, the metacarpophalangeal joint and an interphalangeal joint, probably the distal phalanx. I have not seen good function in these interphalangeal joints. Only satisfactory meta-carpophalangeal joint function is usually present. The appearance of the index finger suggests that symphalangism of the middle and proximal phalanges exists. (C) Post-operative appearance after a syndactyly operation in two stages. The patient is able to carry out ordinary functions such as dressing, writing etc. (D) Facial appearance in acrocephalosyndactyly.

Varieties

Polydactyly appears in a wide variety of forms. The most minor manifestations are small nubbins of skin with or without bone, usually attached to the ulnar side of the hand. The supernumerary digit of this kind is rudimentary and contains no tendon.

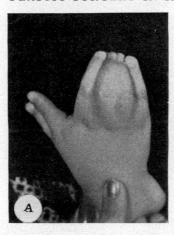

FIG. 32, 11
Multiple syndactyly (four fingers are webbed) and polydactyly of the thumb, bilateral. (A) Dorsal view, pre-operatively. Note that all fingers are approximately the same length, and that contracture of the middle and ring fingers is present.

Occasionally one finds a complete extra digit with metacarpal, tendons and nerves (Fig. 32, 12). When a supernumerary digit originates at the metacarpophalangeal joint, an extra articular facet is usually found on the metacarpal.

Polydactyly is sometimes complicated by syndactyly. Polydactyly is usually radial or ulnar. However, the supernumerary digit may be interposed between the normal digits. Sometimes it is difficult to determine which is the normal digit and which the supernumerary digit. Müller (1937) reported that radial duplication is the most frequent. In our own experience, radial duplication is nearly twice as common as ulnar. Duplication of the little finger is next in frequency, followed by that of the ring and middle fingers. We have never seen duplication of the index finger. This observation coincides with those of Kanavel (1931, 1932) and Handforth (1950). Supernumerary fingers tend to be bilateral and on the ulnar side. One-third of our cases are bilateral. Involvement of the feet is very frequent.

Polydactyly of the little finger is often the simplest (Fig. 32, 13). As stated previously, usually the finger contains no tendons and is aplastic, but complete duplication of the digit with function is occasionally found. When the middle or ring finger is duplicated, the form is likely to be atypical and the condition obscured by the associated syndactyly. Repair in these cases is complicated by distorted joints and by a metacarpal often enlarged and bifurcated distally, or fused at its base (Fig. 32, 14). Prognosis as to joint motion in digits of this type should be guarded.

Polydactyly of the thumb (Fig. 32, 15) takes a variety of forms. The simplest form is that in which the distal phalanx is much broader than normal, and there is a suggestion of bifurcation at the tip. At the other extreme from this condition, one finds occasionally a fully developed second thumb. Although duplication of the distal phalanx is most common in the thumb, we have found it in the ring and middle fingers. When the supernumerary thumb articulates at the metacarpophalangeal joint, rarely if ever is either the normal or supernumerary part in the proper axis or of normal size.

Triphalangism of the thumb may be regarded as a form of polydactyly. Although the general shape of the thumb may be normal, there is usually a tendency toward

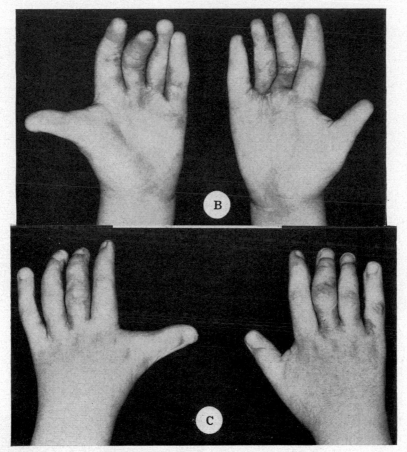

FIG. **32**, 11 (*contd.*)

(B and C) Postoperative palmar and dorsal views. Note that the contracture of the middle and ring fingers has not been completely corrected. All the fingers are still approximately the same length. At the first operation, the supernumerary thumbs were removed and their tendinous attachments transferred to the retained thumb. At the same operation, the little finger and the index finger were separated and skin-grafted. At the next operation, the middle and ring fingers were separated and skin-grafted. When a supernumerary digit is removed, or when the fingers are separated in syndactyly, close attention must be paid to preserving the nerve supply. Figure **32**, 7 shows some varieties of nerve anomaly found. The necessity for splitting the nerve or actually transferring it is evident.

curvature. There is some question as to whether the extra phalanx is a proximal phalanx or a metacarpal. Cohn (1932) expressed the belief that the first metacarpal disappeared in the process of evolution and what is usually considered the first metacarpal is actually a proximal phalanx. To support this theory, it should be noted that the epiphysis of the first metacarpal is at the proximal end of the bone as in the phalanges, instead of at the distal end as in the other four metacarpals.

The entire thumb ray was duplicated in one of our cases and each ray had three phalanges. All the digits in this patient's hand were webbed in the form of a mitten hand, and on the other margin there was an extra little finger with two phalanges and

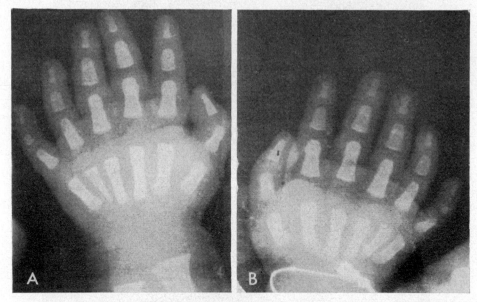

Fig. **32**, 12

Bilateral ulnar symmetrical polydactyly. There are six digits on each hand and the supernumerary little finger is completely functional and has a full range of motion and normal sensation. It is rare in polydactyly to find a completely functional supernumerary digit. When removing the ulnar digit, its hypothenar muscular attachments should be shifted to the retained little finger.

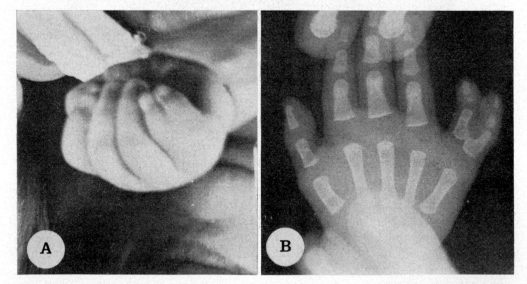

Fig. **32**, 13

(A) Ulnar polydactyly associated with syndactyly. (B) Roentgenogram showing the accessory digit interposed between the little finger and the ring finger.

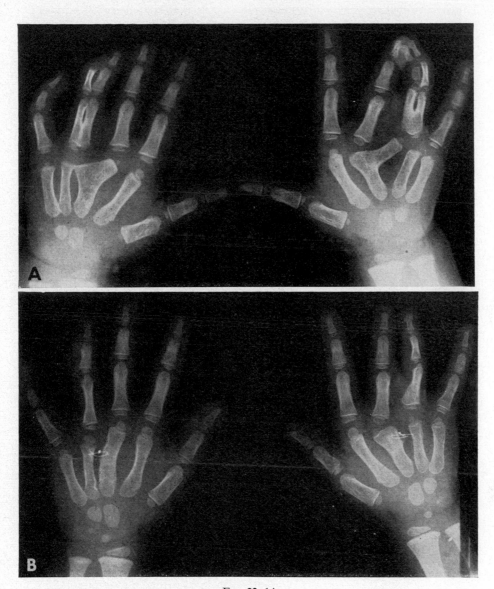

FIG. **32,** 14

Complicated polysyndactyly, bilateral, symmetrical. This is an uncommon malformation, observed in totally unrelated individuals. It is probably caused by a chromosomal aberration. Duplication of the ring finger is uncommon. (A) Pre-operative roentgenogram. The third metacarpal is malformed and has two articular facets, one for the middle finger and the other for the ring finger. (B) Postoperative correction. The metacarpal has been revised, retaining one head in the proper axis. Its alignment has been corrected by the use of a stainless steel wire and the supernumerary digit removed. Prognosis as to movement in the joints should be guarded, as full motion is practically never obtained in these cases. (Surgery performed by Dr Bernard E. Simon.)

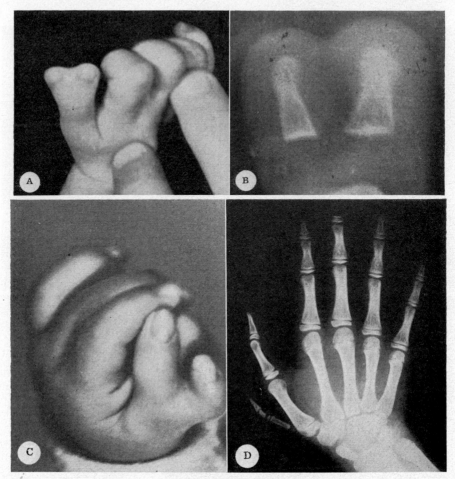

FIG. 32, 15

Varieties of radial polydactyly. (A) Duplication of the distal phalanx of the thumb. (B) The roentgenogram. Note that rarely, if ever, is either one of the phalanges in the proper axis. (C) Another variety of radial polydactyly in which the supernumerary digit arises at an acute angle and articulates with the metacarpophalangeal joint. (D) Small triphalangeal accessory thumb arising at the base of the metacarpal.

an extra phalanx situated distally between the genuine little finger and the ring finger.

Treatment

Often after delivery the obstetrician or even the paediatrician may ligate the rudimentary accessory digit. Such treatment is satisfactory only for very small nubbins or appendages with thin pedicles and without cartilage or bone. Sometimes, small remnants of cartilage are left at the site of ligation and may be regarded by the parents as a stigma of sufficient importance as to warrant surgical correction. Operation is the procedure of choice for all but the simplest and most rudimentary types.

In uncomplicated polydactyly, the decision as to which digit to retain is usually an easy one. However, in some cases, most careful study is necessary before deciding which digit to retain. Innervation, blood vessels and tendons are likely to be atypical. Most careful pre-operative examination is essential. At operation exploration is essential to assure properly retained nerve supply and tendon attachment. The attachments of the tendons and intrinsic muscles in the retained thumb must be preserved. It may be necessary to transfer a tendon or a muscle from one accessory digit to a retained part.

When a bifid thumb is present, wedge incision of the central portion and joining of the segments usually produces an acceptable result. If the entire phalanx is duplicated and one is removed, it is often necessary to correct the axis of the remaining phalanx by reefing in the capsule on one side.

On the whole, removal of a supernumerary digit is usually a simple procedure, but sometimes it is extremely complicated and difficult. The skin of the filleted digit should be left for trimming. Loose cooptation should be carried out to avoid scar contraction. A midlateral suture line is advisable.

BRACHYDACTYLY

The term 'brachydactyly' simply means 'short finger'. However, we restrict the use of the term brachydactyly to fingers in which the shortness is due to a shortness of the phalanx or metacarpal (Fig. 32, 16). In other words, the normal number of bones are present but they are reduced in size. This term differentiates brachydactyly from ectrodactyly, in which the shortness is caused by the absence of one or more phalanges or metacarpals. A single digit in a hand may be affected or all the digits.

Finger flexion will depend on the presence of the profundus tendon insertion at the distal phalanx. When normal insertion is present and finger flexion is active and strong, function will be good. On the other hand, if distal insertion is absent, the distal phalangeal joint is flail and the patient will have to back up or reinforce the flail finger tips with other fingers if these are normal.

Incidence

Brachydactyly is not nearly so frequent as are syndactyly and polydactyly. The condition is often associated with simple, partial syndactyly.

Pathogenesis

It is of interest to note that brachydactyly is reported to be the first example of Mendelian inheritance to be demonstrated in man. Although it is commonly considered a simple Mendelian dominant, Gates (1946) and others do not feel that the malformation is necessarily dominant. In 1943 Villaverde reported that he believed the endocrine system was involved in brachydactyly of the thumb and at the same time he found other skeletal deformities in at least 75 per cent. of his cases. Burrows (1938), in 108 collected cases of shortened terminal phalanx of the thumb found no associated skeletal abnormalities. He reported that the condition was transmitted irregularly by both sexes as a Mendelian dominant with some skipping. In 1951, Bell reported 124 cases of brachydactyly and symphalangism among 1336 individuals. Premature union between the metaphysis and epiphysis and obliteration of the

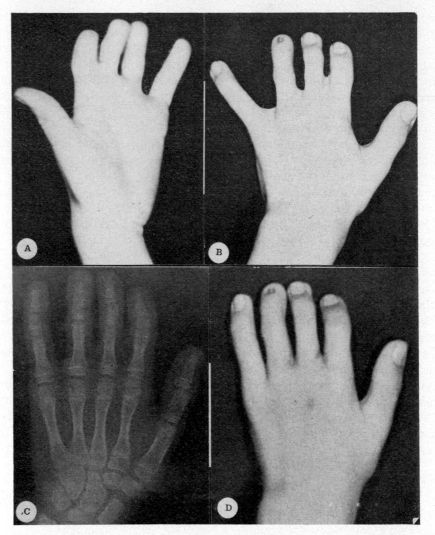

FIG. **32**, 16

Brachydactyly. (A and B) Pre-operative views. The web is higher on the palmar aspect and limits abduction of the index finger. Note also the shortness of the index, middle, and ring fingers. All of them are shorter than the normal little finger. (C) Roentgenogram. Note the shortness of the middle and distal phalanges, the proximal phalanx apparently being of normal length. This is a case of true brachydactyly. One will usually find in this type of case that the profundus tendon is attached to the distal phalanx and these patients have good flexion. (D) A postoperative view with the finger clefts deepened This improves the appearance of the hand and will permit better abduction of the index finger.

epiphyseal line was found in many of these patients. Bell also believed the inheritance was dominant.

Surgical treatment

When partial syndactyly is present in brachydactyly, deepening of the webs will improve the appearance of the hand but not the function. In cases where flail joints are present, they must be arthrodesed at the proper age.

Symphalangism

This is defined as an end to end fusion of phalanges with fixed interphalangeal joints (Fig. **32**, 10B). Though the finger may be of normal length, usually the only joint that will function is the metacarpophalangeal joint. In our own series symphalangism has always been associated with one of the more complex types of syndactyly, with additional phalanges and/or with brachydactyly.

Pathogenesis

In 1943, Freud and Slobody reported their conclusion that symphalangism is due to the failure of differentiation of the interphalangeal joints in embryonic life. In serial roentgenographic studies of foetal development, these authors demonstrated that the articulations became differentiated through constriction of the phalangeal beam. The progressive constriction continues until only a central bridge of bone remains and this finally becomes less and less distinct until it disappears, with a resultant normal interphalangeal space. If the process is interrupted before differentiation is complete, the result is symphalangism.

This condition is considered to be a Mendelian dominant. In 1907 Drinkwater traced fused proximal and middle finger phalanges through 14 generations of the family of John Talbot, the First Earl of Shrewsbury, who was killed in 1453. When his tomb was opened in 1874, his finger bones were found to have the same malformation as those of his living descendants.

Treatment

The only treatment for the condition is arthrodesis of the proximal and distal interphalangeal joints to give them a more functional position. Although arthroplasty has been suggested, the results of treating interphalangeal joints by arthroplasty are notoriously poor. However, arthroplasty can be used for reconstructing the metacarpophalangeal joint.

Annular Grooves (Ring Constrictions) and Bands

Annular grooves vary from simple, small, shallow grooves partly encircling a single finger to multiple, deep, constricting, encircling grooves which may extend almost down to the bone and severely affect the circulation (Fig. **32**, 17). Oedema is sometimes caused by impairment of lymphatics and venous drainage. Annular grooves are also found in the forearm, the toes, and the legs.

In our own series, there was only one case of annular grooves of the fingers without any other defects. Most of our cases of annular grooves showed some additional type of malformation, such as syndactyly or ectrodactyly. The condition is often associated with annular bands of the lower extremities (Fig. **32**, 18).

Aetiology

The pathogenesis of congenital grooves have never been definitely established. At

PS R

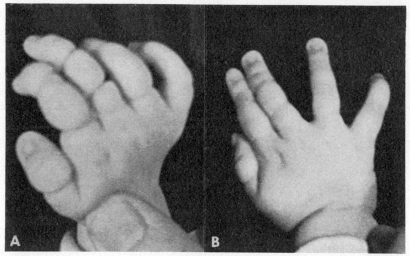

FIG. 32, 17

Multiple annular grooves or bands in a 1-year-old child. (A) Pre-operative view. The condition is unilateral. (B) Postoperative. It is best not to encircle a finger completely at operation. One might, however, go half-way around the ulnar side of the proximal groove and half-way around the radial side of the distal groove. At a second operation, the remaining bands may be excised. One should go as deep as necessary, removing all constricting and fibrous tissue. Z-plasties will be useful in preventing secondary contraction.

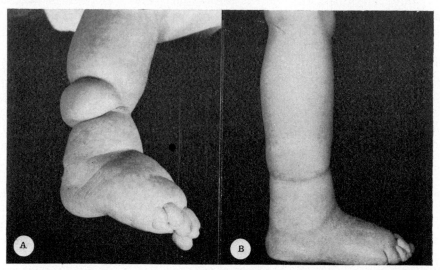

FIG. 32, 18

Annular grooves or bands on the leg of a patient whose hand had a condition similar to that shown in Figure 32, 21 A and B. (A) Pre-operative. (B) Postoperative.

one time it was believed that a constricting band of amnion might possibly cause both the annular grooves and the more advanced defect, intrauterine amputation. Some writers believe that the amniotic adhesions are the result rather than the cause of the constricting bands. In 1952, Brindeau *et al.* reported that inflammation, intoxication, or arrested development can cause distinct malformations. In 1961, Patterson expressed the belief that the grooves are caused by intrinsic factors and that their development was analogous to that of cleft lip; that is, both are caused by failure of the development of mesodermal masses underneath the skin, secondary ulceration of the skin, and finally by adhesion of adjacent ulcerated parts which form the amniotic 'band'. Patterson observed that the ulcers may persist at birth but usually heal during foetal life, leaving only the mesodermal defect and the extrinsic bands adherent to the deep groove. Inglis, in 1952, expressed the belief that the grooves are not caused by extrinsic factors or hormonal defects or disturbed innervation, but are simply due to 'inferiority of tissue in various parts of the body resulting from influences transmitted in the germ plasm and determined by fundamental biological laws of growth and development'.

Treatment

If the grooves are shallow, do not interfere with circulation, and are not unsightly, they may be left alone. Deeper rings should be excised down to the normal structure. In the presence of a well-defined digital vessel capable of maintaining circulation in the finger tip, the entire encircling groove can be excised in one operation. Nevertheless, unless one is absolutely certain of the circulation of the distal part, this should not be done and the groove on one side only of a digit should be excised at one operation. If, for instance, there are two grooves on a digit, one may excise opposite halves of each; e.g. the ulnar half of the proximal groove, and the radial side of the distal groove. At the following operation, the remaining bands could be removed. Z-plasties are often utilised to prevent secondary contraction. A small unstable nubbin of tissue at the finger tip should not be retained especially if it has no sensation and cannot be stabilised surgically. In the event that the distal interphalangeal joint is flail, the terminal phalanx should be removed unless it can be made functional by arthrodesis at the proper age.

ECTRODACTYLY

The term ectrodactyly was introduced in 1832 by Isidore Geoffrey Saint-Hilaire, who published a three-volume work on congenital malformations in men and animals. He also cited cases of cleft hand.

This ectrodactyly is characterised by the absence of a part or all of a digit (Fig. **32**, 19). All the phalanges may be absent as well as the metacarpal of a single digit, or else several fingers may be affected in part or entirely. Partial ectrodactyly involving only the absence of one or more phalanges is illustrated in Figure **32**, 19A. This represents the mildest form. When all the fingers are absent, the hand has the appearance of a small paw, which contains hypoplastic metacarpals. In such cases, the fingers may be represented by small nubbins which sometimes have fingernails. In very young infants the metacarpals may not appear on the roentgenogram, but can be palpated. Such cartilagenous metacarpals may be seen on the roentgenogram when the child is older and the bones are ossified.

In planning a restoration in these cases parts should not be ablated unless one is certain that they cannot be utilised.

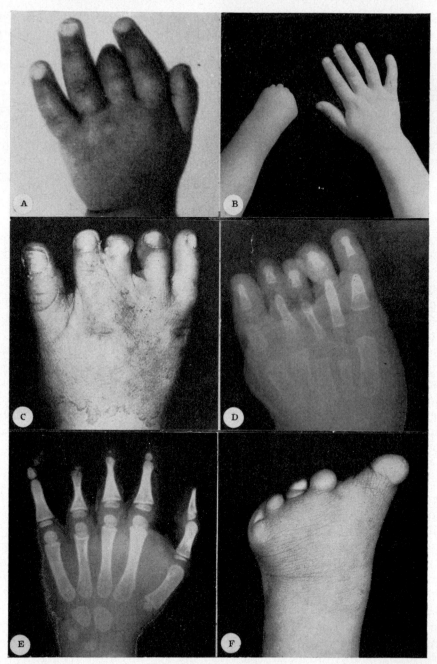

Fig. **32,** 19

Forms of ectrodactyly. (A) The mildest form; absence of the distal phalanx of the middle finger. (B) Severe form; all the digits are missing, with small nubbins present on the ulnar side of the hand; even the carpus is greatly reduced in size. (C and D) In this case only the thumb is normal in size and function; the remaining digits have only two phalanges, with the middle one lacking. There is marked disproportion in size of the metacarpals of the middle and ring fingers. In this type of case these are often functionless. (E) Here only the proximal phalanges of the index, middle, and ring fingers are present. (F) All four fingers are missing, represented only by residual nubbins. The thumb is short but functional. Function of the hand will be greatly improved in these cases if it is possible to build up a post for the thumb to pinch against.

Birch-Jensen (1949) reported defects of the distal phalanx present in one out of 90,000 persons in the general population in Denmark. Sex distribution was even, and half the patients had other malformations. The appearance of the defect in siblings and offspring was not unusual. Ectrodactyly is considered a sporadic anomaly, but when there is a dominant trait, it can of course be inherited. In 1932, Klein reported that ectrodactyly is a recessive trait, which would account for its sporadic appearance.

Treatment

This is dictated by the precise condition (Fig. **32**, 20). In ectrosyndactyly, when all the digits are webbed and the finger tips clumped, with overlapping, orientation is difficult for the surgeon (Fig. **32**, 21). In these cases, after careful X-ray study, either

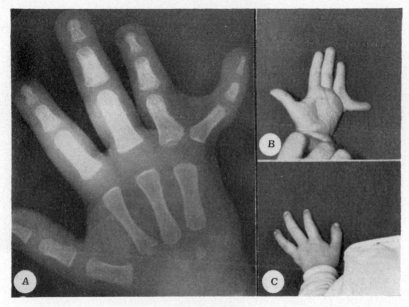

FIG. **32**, 20

Ectrodactyly. (A) This should more properly be called ectrometacarpia. Both the ring and little fingers articulate with the fourth metacarpal. (B) Pre-operative palmar view. The wide ulnar angulation of the little finger and its lack of muscular attachment dictated its ablation. (C) Postoperative dorsal view, with marked cosmetic improvement.

the radial or the ulnar component should be separated at the first operation. When annular grooves complicate ectrodactyly they should be treated as previously described.

In ectrosyndactyly the entire upper extremity is sometimes smaller than the opposite side (Fig. **32**, 22) and this is sometimes called Poland's syndactyly. One often finds in these cases that the pectoral muscles are missing on the affected side and occasionally there may be a skin web present (Fig. **32**, 23). This may be corrected by a Z-plasty.

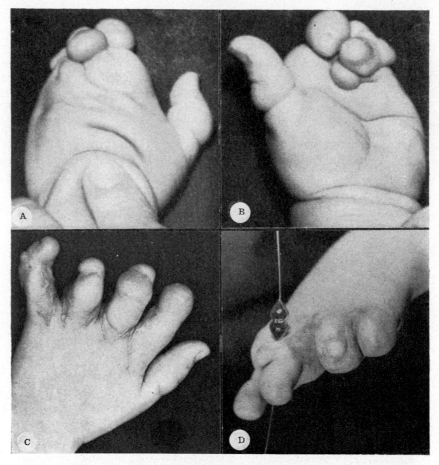

FIG. **32**, 21

Ectrodactyly complicated by annular grooves and syndactyly. (A and B) Palmar and dorsal views pre-operatively. The fingers are crossed, overlapped, and clumped. Deep annular grooves are present. These grooves should be eliminated at an early age, during infancy if possible. Parts of the digits distal to the groove should be retained only if they are of sufficient size to be of practical use, if they have good sensation, and if they are stable, or if there is a possibility of stabilising them later. (C) Postoperative dorsal view. (D) At the base of the crease between the digits, an epithelial tract is frequently found that leads from the palmar to the dorsal surface. These tracts should be very carefully dissected out at operation. If, at operation, they are covered with a skin graft, secondary infection usually follows.

CLEFT HAND

Cleft hand is a form of ectrodactyly characterised by absence of one or more of the central rays of the hand. It is sometimes called 'split hand' or 'lobster claw hand'. The condition appears in two main types, typical and atypical.

The typical form of cleft hand (Fig. **32**, 24) is sometimes familial and accompanied by a similar deformity of the foot. It is characterised by a deep V-shaped or funnel-shaped defect in the central part of the hand with the terminal parts affected. In this

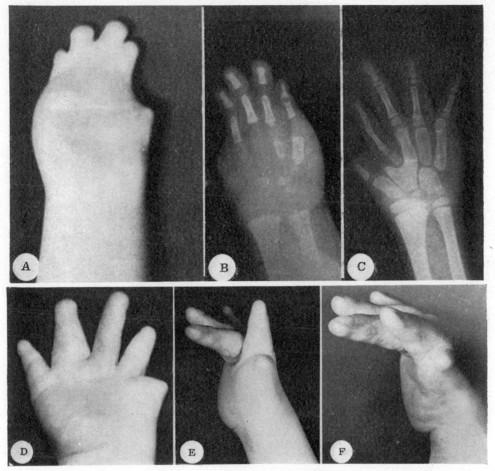

FIG. **32**, 22

Ectrosyndactyly (so-called Poland's syndactyly). (A) Pre-operative palmar view. The entire hand is much smaller than the opposite side. The four fingers are webbed and a rudimentary thumb stump can be palpated. (B) Early roentgenogram does not indicate osseous metacarpal support for the thumb, index, and middle fingers, although some supporting structures could be detected by palpation. (C) Later development of bony support structures with fusion of the first and third metacarpal and carpal bones. (D) Result obtained after separating the fingers, providing four fingers which extend only at the metacarpophalangeal joint. A thumb stump is also present. (E) The little, ring, and middle fingers flex at the metacarpophalangeal joint, the index finger extends at this joint but does not flex. (F) Improved flexion was obtained, using the palmaris longus as a motor, prolonged into the finger by a tendon graft. Subsequently the thumb-index cleft was deepened by a skin flap.

deformity, one never finds a distal phalanx present with the intermediate parts missing. More severe forms show the entire third ray missing, sometimes the adjacent index ray as well, with a deep cleft dividing the hand into radial and ulnar components. Each component may have two digits, and these are sometimes webbed.

The atypical form of cleft hand is a more severe anomaly, described by Lange in 1936. Three central rays of the hand including the metacarpals are missing and only the marginal rays, the thumb and little finger, are present, sometimes in attenuated form (Fig. **32**, 25). This form of cleft hand is usually unilateral and without associated foot involvement or family history. Lange believed it to be an independent deformity.

Jan Jacob Hartsinck (1716–1779) of the East India Company and an important person in the Netherlands Admiralty, in 1770 published a two-volume report on Dutch Guiana in which he gave a detailed report of the Touvingas or 'two-fingered Negroes'. The illustration from his book shows clearly that this condition was cleft hand. Hartsinck appears to be the first to have used the term 'claw hand'.

Incidence

In 1964, the author reported his cases of cleft hand and compared them with those of Birch-Jensen.

Table **32**, 1

STATISTICAL ANALYSIS

	Birch-Jensen	Barsky
Total no. of hand anomalies	625	400
Cleft hands	36	19
Percentage of cleft hands	5·76	4·75
Typical	16	10
Atypical	20	9
Incidence at birth	Typical 1:90,000 Atypical 1:150,000	
Heredity	15	3

Table **32**, 2

STATISTICAL ANALYSIS

	Birch-Jensen	Barsky
Bilateral	21	10
Unilateral	R.11	R.4
	L. 4	L.5
	—	—
	15	9
Sex	♂20	♂ 9
	♀16	♀10
Cleft foot	18	5
Cleft lip and palate	1	3

Treatment

Treatment of the cleft hand varies according to the severity of the case. The appearance of the hand is so bizarre that the patient becomes a curiosity and treatment may be indicated for cosmetic reasons rather than for functional improvement. Syndactyly, when present, should be treated in the usual manner, observing preservation of the nerves, tendons, etc. The denuded surfaces will, of course, require a skin graft. In some instances the skin excised from the cleft may be used as a free graft. Figure **32**, 26 shows the author's operation to close the cleft. At about the level of the proposed new commissure the diamond-shaped flap is elevated from one side to be implanted on the opposite side. This flap will restore the commissure between the

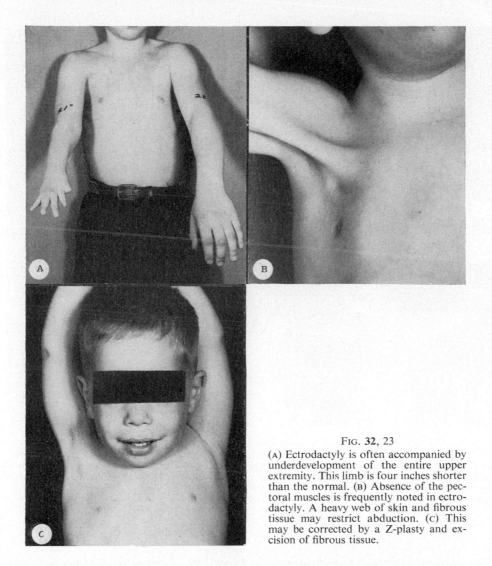

Fig. **32**, 23
(A) Ectrodactyly is often accompanied by underdevelopment of the entire upper extremity. This limb is four inches shorter than the normal. (B) Absence of the pectoral muscles is frequently noted in ectrodactyly. A heavy web of skin and fibrous tissue may restrict abduction. (C) This may be corrected by a Z-plasty and excision of fibrous tissue.

fingers nicely. Subperiosteal exposure of the metacarpals is carried out and holes drilled through both just proximal to the metacarpal head. Heavy chromic sutures may be inserted through these holes or stainless steel wire may be used to correct the divergence of the metacarpals. It is not necessary to perform osteotomies to align the metacarpals. A non-functional metacarpal, one without phalanges, may be used as a bone graft to correct the divergence. Then the second or third metacarpals or both are removed, the attachments of the adductor pollicis are transferred to the fourth metacarpal. The cleft should never be decreased to the point where function is impaired. A zigzag closure, excising superfluous skin, should be used both on dorsal and volar surfaces.

PS R 2

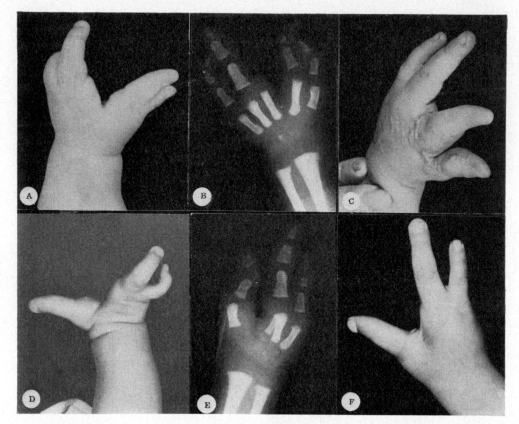

FIG. **32**, 24

Typical cleft hand, bilateral, asymmetrical. (A) Left hand, pre-operative. Note the syndactyly of the index finger and thumb, which is rarely found except in cleft hand. (B) Roentgenogram showing a third metacarpal. (C) Postoperative view after correction of syndactyly and carrying out of operative procedure described in Figure **32**, 26. (D) Right hand pre-operatively. Note the deep cleft. The middle and index fingers are absent but a small third metacarpal is present. (E) Roentgenogram. The small third metacarpal and wide fourth metacarpal are clearly shown. (F) Postoperative view.

The atypical cleft hand as illustrated in Figure **32**, 25 may require no treatment. Function may be improved simply by use and exercise. If the web between the thumb and little finger restricts function, a Z-plasty will increase the range of motion. These little patients usually develop a surprising degree of dexterity. In the atypical cleft hand, rotatory osteotomy on the ulnar digit will sometimes be required when the child is older to make it possible to oppose the little finger and thumb. When a complete digit is present on one side of the hand, but only a metacarpal on the other, it is possible to build up a post on this metacarpal upon which the functional digit can pinch. This will require a tube pedicle and a bone graft. No procedure should be carried out on the hand which will interfere with the growth and development of the existing parts.

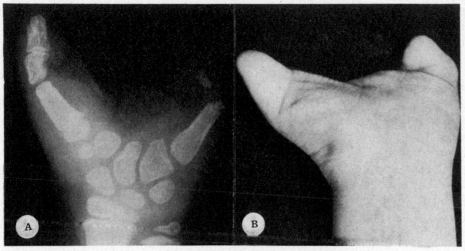

FIG. **32**, 25

Cleft hand, atypical. (A) Only the thumb is normal. In the little finger the metacarpal is present and a small radially deviated phalanx. (B) Palmar view. There is often a web extending from the thumb to the little finger in these cases. This can be relieved by a Z-plasty, which will permit the patient to grasp large objects.

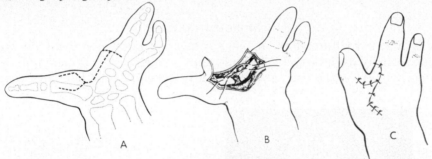

FIG. **32**, 26

Operation for cleft hand. This is intended primarily to improve the appearance of the hand. If syndactyly is present between the thumb and index finger, this will require correction. (A) A diamond-shaped flap is elevated on the radial side of the cleft and a T-shaped incision made on the other side of the cleft. (B) The metacarpals are exposed subperiosteally and holes drilled proximal to the head. (A metacarpal without phalanges should be removed and the muscular attachments transferred.) Stainless steel wire sutures are used to align the metacarpals. (C) The diamond-shaped flap restores the commissure and zigzag closure is carried out on the dorsal and volar surfaces.

ECTRODACTYLY OF THE THUMB

This may vary from partial absence of the distal phalanx to complete absence of the entire ray. The mildest form, of course, requires no surgical correction. If both phalanges are missing, deepening the web between the thumb metacarpal and adjacent finger will improve the grasp. Occasionally one finds a small thumb in the normal position with normal long flexor and extensor tendons, but the thenar muscles are absent. If the soft tissues will permit opposition, an opponens transfer may be carried out to improve the function. If the soft tissues do not permit opposition, it may be necessary to insert either a flap or a free graft in the web space.

In some instances the thumb is abnormally small, but the bones and muscles are normal. This type of thumb is likely to be located far more distal than its normal position. There is reduced range of motion and ability to oppose the other fingers. The practicability of improving the function of this type by operation is questionable.

Floating thumb (pouce flottant)

In this condition, the phalanges are present, but the metacarpal (or most of it) is absent and the thenar muscles, long extensors and flexors of the thumb are also missing. This type of thumb is located far more distally and radially than is normal and has no opposition.

In the past, I have migrated this *pouce flottant* to a more functional position on the hand. When completely healed, a free transplant of a metatarsophalangeal joint was performed. Subsequently tendon transfers were carried out for flexion, opposition and extension. The patients developed a surprising range of motion. However, although the joint transplant survived, it did not maintain proper growth and development, resulting years later in a miniature bizarre thumb much smaller than its mate on the opposite side (Fig. **32**, 27). I feel, therefore, that it is not advisable to attempt to treat floating thumbs by surgery, but to ablate them and possibly migrate the radial digit into the position of the thumb.

MONODACTYLY

This is a rare malformation in which only one digit is present, in our own experience usually the little finger. In these cases the entire radial portion of the hand, including the metacarpals, was absent. No involvement of the feet has been noted.

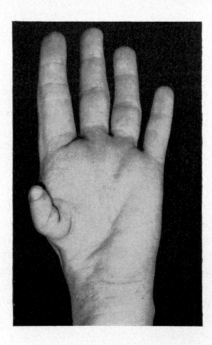

Fig. **32**, 27
Pouce flottant. Photograph taken 10 years after migration of the thumb to a more functional position, free metatarsophalangeal joint transplant, and tendon transfers. The patient has good range of motion but proper growth and development have not taken place.

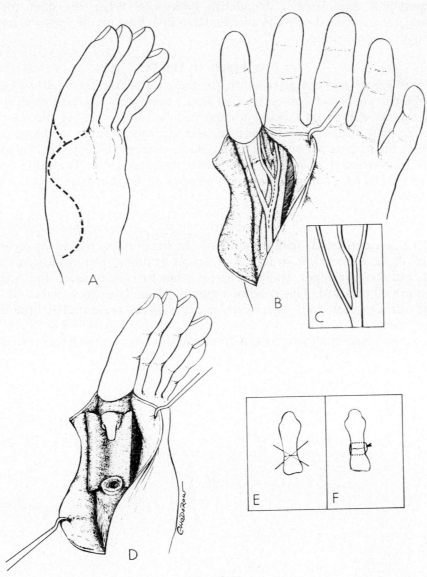

FIG. **32,** 28

Pollicisation. The operation is suitable for the five-fingered hand or the four-fingered hand of congenital or traumatic origin. (A) The incision. (B) Exposure. It should be noted that in the four-fingered hand there is often one common digital vessel that supplies the entire radial digit and the radial side of the adjacent digit. Occasionally this vessel may perforate the digital nerve. Maintenance of vascular supply to the radial digit requires tying off the branch to the radial side of the adjacent digit. (C) The common digital nerve must be split proximalward to permit mobilisation. (D) The metacarpal ligament on the ulnar side must be split and the metacarpal exposed subperiosteally. As much of the metacarpal as possible should be ablated to provide a properly shortened thumb. A peg or strut (Littler) may be formed on the distal part of the metacarpal and a hole drilled proximally into the base of the metacarpal or carpal bone to receive the strut, which is secured by Kirschner wires. (E and F) Alternate methods of fastening the shortened metacarpal.

Monodactyly is considered a Mendelian dominant. When the digit present is functional, the surgeon should consider building up a post on the opposite margin of the hand to pinch against.

Five Fingered Hand

This malformation is characterised by the presence of five digits, all triphalangeal and in the palmar plane. The radial digit is not opposable. In these cases one may migrate the radial digit on a neurovascular pedicle, shortening the metacarpal and placing the digit on the thenar eminence, and securing it either to the base of the remnant of the metacarpal or to the carpal bones present. Figures **32**, 28 and **32**, 29 illustrate the one-stage operation suitable for this procedure. The same operative procedure can be used for pollicisation in absence of the thumb or in pouce flottant (Fig. **32**, 30).

Macrodactyly

This is a rare congenital malformation of the hand characterised by an increase in size of all the elements or structures of a digit or digits. The metacarpals are not affected, but the phalanges, tendons, nerves, vessels, subcutaneous fat, fingernails and skin are all enlarged. This condition may occur unilaterally or bilaterally, symmetrically or asymmetrically. Syndactyly is occasionally present. The little finger is rarely involved.

It should be noted that there are similar conditions wherein the fingers are enlarged

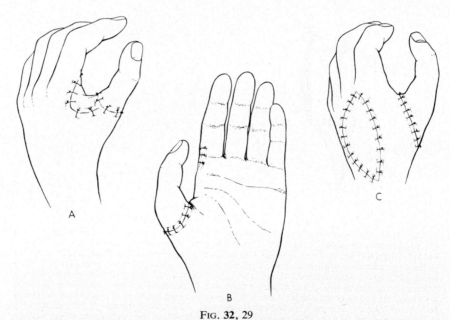

Fig. **32**, 29

Pollicisation, concluded. It is essential that the closure be loose. (A) Dorsal view of the closure. (B) Volar view. (C) An alternate method of closure utilising a double pedicle flap dorsally and a free skin graft to the donor area of the flap.

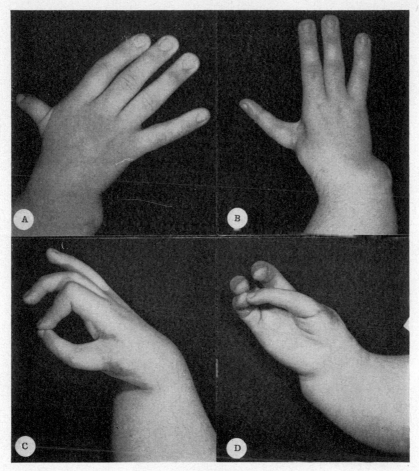

FIG. **32**, 30

Radial club hand with pouce flottant. (A) Pre-operative view showing the floating thumb, which was removed. The alignment of the hand on the forearm is satisfactory. (B) Dorsal view after pollicization of the index finger. Abduction is satisfactory. (C) Good pinch between the 'thumb' and middle finger. (D) Tip to tip opposition between the thumb and little finger.

but do not represent true macrodactyly; usually the enlargement is due to haemangioma, only the skin and soft tissues are enlarged and roentgenograms do not show any increase in size of the bony structures.

There are two forms of genuine macrodactyly. In one, the enlargement is noted at birth, and the increase in size as the child grows is not disproportionate (Fig. **32**, 31). De Laurenzi called this the static type. In the second type, the progressive type, there is a disproportionate growth of the involved digit or digits, and these increase at a faster rate than a normal growth pattern. This progressive type is further complicated by a fatty overgrowth of tissue in the palm and dorsum of the hand and the forearm

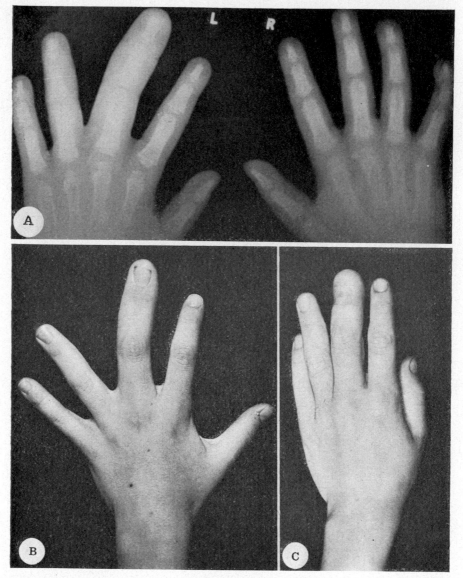

FIG. **32, 31**

Macrodactyly, static type. (A) Pre-operative roentgenogram. Only the middle finger of the left hand is affected, in both its length and bulk. (B) Pre-operative appearance. (C) Postoperative appearance.

(Fig. **32, 32**). A survey of the literature shows that true macrodactyly is one of the rarest congenital malformations of the hand.

Aetiology, pathology and findings

The aetiology of this curious malformation is not known. Hereditary factors are not involved either in our own cases or in those reported in the literature. The

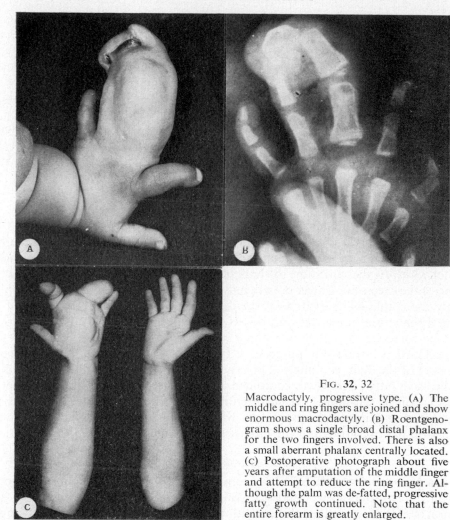

Fig. **32, 32**
Macrodactyly, progressive type. (A) The
middle and ring fingers are joined and show
enormous macrodactyly. (B) Roentgenogram shows a single broad distal phalanx
for the two fingers involved. There is also
a small aberrant phalanx centrally located.
(C) Postoperative photograph about five
years after amputation of the middle finger
and attempt to reduce the ring finger. Although the palm was de-fatted, progressive
fatty growth continued. Note that the
entire forearm is greatly enlarged.

condition does not appear to be associated with other congenital abnormalities.
Chromosomal studies in our own cases have not demonstrated any abnormalities.

Biopsies have revealed normal skin with fatty fibrocellular tissue which is dense
and abundant, vessels apparently normal but the nerves enlarged. The enlargement
of the nerves is quite noticeable and startling. The nerves are infiltrated with a fibro-
fatty tissue. The fatty tissue present in the subcutaneous areas of the hand resembles
adult subcutaneous tissue rather than that of the child. Globules of the fat are large
and dark and difficult to remove. They are unlike the globules of normal fat which
can be extruded under pressure. The fat appears to be traversed by many fine vessels.

Macrodactyly may be the result of the interaction of two or more extrinsic agents,
each by itself unable to produce a teratologic effect. My personal opinion is that
macrodactyly is caused during foetal development by a disturbance of the growth-

limiting factor in the local area affected. This lack of inhibition locally continues the increase in size and this will account for the progressive overgrowth in later years. Moore (1942) expressed his opinion that the local hypertrophy was so consistently associated with peripheral nerve pathology that there must be some relationship between them. He felt that the nervous system exerts some controlling action on the process of growth and that the impaired nerves fail in this function, resulting in an uncontrolled or uninhibited growth.

In support of Moore's view, it should be noted that when more than one digit is involved, the digits are invariably adjacent to each other. In one of our cases only the left index finger was affected, and this on the radial side alone. The digital nerve on the radial side of the index finger was about twice the normal size.

Treatment

The surgical treatment depends upon the severity of the malformation. In the static type, finger length may be reduced by ablation of the distal interphalangeal joint and arthrodesis of the remnants of the distal and middle phalanges using Kirschner wires. At the same time the bulk of the finger may be reduced by dissecting out some of the excess fat. Finger growth may be retarded by destroying or by stapling or wiring the epiphysis. Curvature of the digit may be corrected by ablation of the distal interphalangeal joint and arthrodesis with correction of deviation. Deviation can also be corrected by wedge osteotomy.

Figure **32**, 32 illustrates the progressive type of macrodactyly with an enormous enlargement of the digit, complicated by syndactyly. Despite amputation of the digit, the progressive fatty overgrowth continued and it is not possible to predict whether the process will be self-limited. It has been impossible in this case to defat the hand completely. In extreme cases amputation will have to be resorted to, but even this may not stop the overgrowth of the fatty tissue proximal to the site of amputation.

ARTHROGRYPOSIS

This is a congenital muscle deficiency complicated by joint contracture. It is sometimes called 'arthrogryposis multiplex congenita' or 'multiple articular rigidity'. Middleton (1934) has described this condition in lambs and has compiled a good deal of information. He considered the defect a fatty degeneration of muscle during intrauterine life and regarded it as analogous to muscular dystrophy in later life. He found muscle fibre remnants containing adipose tissue and fibrous strands replacing extensor pollicis longus. We have performed an autopsy on a stillborn foetus with bilateral subcontractures, and the following has been noted: (1) the extensor pollicis longus ended as a fibrous band at the base of the proximal phalanx of the thumb; (2) the metacarpophalangeal joint of the thumb was fixed in flexion subluxation with the base of the proximal phalanx displaced towards the palm; (3) the interphalangeal joint of the thumb was fixed in flexion. All joints appeared normal in microscopic examination. Musculature, including dorsal and volar muscles of the forearm, was abnormal: the muscle fibres were small with a relative increase in the sarcolemma, an increase in the number of nucleii, and a relative increase in the amount of interstitial mesenchymal tissue. The spinal cord was normal.

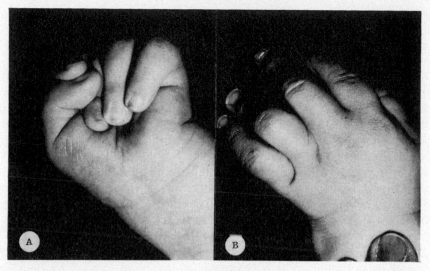

FIG. 32, 33

Arthrogryposis. Both hands were involved. (A) Before treatment. When the patient was first seen at 2 months of age, the hands were held tightly closed. (B) The result achieved after stretching with progressive splinting for six months.

Arthrogryposis may affect only a single digit or many joints, even all the joints of all the extremities. It is usually bilateral rather than unilateral. If the cases are treated early in infancy, early splinting will counteract the muscular contracture (Fig. 32, 33). If there are enough normal muscle fibres left to function, this method will result in improvement. Weckesser and his co-workers also have reported successful results. If the condition is allowed to persist for many years into adolescence or beyond, complicated operative procedures are required and the results are not nearly as satisfactory.

CLINODACTYLY

Clinodactyly means 'bent fingers'. We are, however, reserving the use of this term to indicate a lateral deviation of the fingers, not a congenital flexion contracture. Clinodactyly may often be caused by a rudimentary wedge-shaped bone which takes the place of a normal phalanx or supernumerary. Clinodactyly may be present as a single malformation or may be found as part of a more complicated one. Early treatment in infancy should be conservative and should consist of straightening the finger by manipulation and by progressive splinting. Unsuccessful results or residual deformity may be corrected by surgery but this should be delayed until the child is older. If the deviation is due to curvature of the bone, wedge osteotomy will correct it. If an extra bone is interpolated, it should be excised if such excision would not interfere with function.

CAMPTODACTYLY

This is a non-traumatic, idiopathic flexion contracture of a finger. Conditions such as radial club hand, absence of extensive tendons, arthrogryposis and Dupuytren's contracture are not considered as camptodactyly.

This condition occurs more frequently in girls than in boys and most commonly in the little finger. Two forms are recognised: (1) A congenital form discovered at or shortly after birth. This form appears to be hereditary. (2) A second form which is noted in childhood and appears to progress during growth. Among the causes postulated for camptodactyly are shortness of the sublimis tendon, and attachment of the lumbrical muscle to the sublimis tendon restricting extension. If the contraction is due to shortness of the sublimis tendon, this may be determined by flexing the wrist which should in this position permit the finger to extend. If a short sublimis is the cause, severing it will improve the condition. If it is due to an abnormal lumbrical attachment, this may be dissected out.

One should be cautious about severing the sublimis tendon in the index finger as it contributes greatly to the strength and function of this digit. If it is felt that the sublimis to the index finger is the cause of the condition, its tendon may be lengthened in the forearm.

CLUB HAND

Club hand or talipomanus is a deviation of the hand caused by hemimelia or absence of a part of a forearm. It may be unilateral or bilateral. Radial hemimelia is more common than ulnar, hence radial club hand is seen much more frequently. In these cases the radius may be missing entirely or in part. It should be noted in passing that the radius may appear to be completely absent at birth, but as the child grows, the proximal part of the radius appears to ossify.

The soft parts on the radial side of the hand and arm are often missing as well and the thumb is often absent. Carpal bones may be absent or fused, and the ulnar bowed markedly. In a well-defined radial club hand the hand itself appears to deviate radially at an acute angle.

As stated previously, the ulnar is less frequently missing than the radius, and in these cases elbow function is affected.

Pathogenesis

Various experimental means have been utilised to produce hemimelia. Warkany and Nelson, in 1941, used deficient maternal diet in rats to produce the condition. Warkany and Schraffenberger in 1947 utilised intrauterine radiation. It should be noted that when the growth of one of the forearm bones has been arrested, the development of the other bone is disturbed in accordance with Ollier's Law. The curvature of this remaining bone may be marked or slight.

In radial club hand, curvature of the ulna is usually present, sometimes to a marked degree. This may be due to the presence of the fibrous tissue band which develops in place of the absent radius. It is felt that this band does not grow proportionately with the ulna and consequently restricts development of the ulna, acting like a bowstring. The strong muscular pull of the hand flexors also tends to accentuate the displacement.

It should be noted that stiffness of the index and sometimes the middle finger is often found in radial club hand.

In the absence of one of the forearm bones, the forearm itself is abnormally short.

Treatment

No surgical procedure should be attempted which will interfere with the growth and development of the normal remaining bone. One of the mechanical difficulties to be overcome is to correct and maintain the hand in the proper axis on the forearm. When a bone graft is used to provide stability and to support the hand in its proper position, the graft will not continue to grow as the limb develops. However desirable early operation may be to correct position of the hand, no procedure should be undertaken that could possibly damage the growth centre.

As soon as possible, splinting should be undertaken to maintain proper alignment of the hand. Splinting of a small infant's hand is a difficult procedure and will require frequent change of the splint. Early operation on the soft tissue is advisable (Fig. 32, 34). A Z-plasty may be carried out on the concave side of the wrist and forearm as suggested by Bunnell and Dehne (1955). In radial club hand, tendon lengthening on the radial side of the hand may be required. If sufficient relaxation is not accomplished

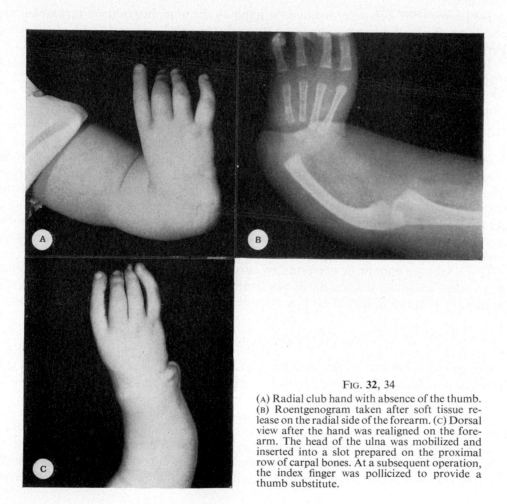

FIG. 32, 34

(A) Radial club hand with absence of the thumb. (B) Roentgenogram taken after soft tissue release on the radial side of the forearm. (C) Dorsal view after the hand was realigned on the forearm. The head of the ulna was mobilized and inserted into a slot prepared on the proximal row of carpal bones. At a subsequent operation, the index finger was pollicized to provide a thumb substitute.

with the Z-plasty, a free skin graft may be required as a supplement. Kirschner wire immobilisation through the palm into the forearm can be utilised to maintain alignment until further surgery is carried out.

At a second stage, the hand may be realigned on the forearm by mobilising the distal end of the ulna, without disturbing its epiphysis, cutting a slot into the proximal carpal bones and placing the ulna in this position, and immobilising it with Kirschner wires. It is advisable to carry out this procedure before bowing of the remaining ulna becomes too marked.

In 1955 Riordan advised osteotomy to correct curvature of the ulna and free transplantation of the upper end of the fibula with its epiphysis into the forearm, inserting it between the extensor muscles through an incision on the radial side of the wrist. He abutted the distal end of the graft against the carpus and inserted the proximal part obliquely into the shaft of the ulna. This procedure has not resulted in the permanent correction expected for continued growth of the epiphysis did not take place.

De Lorme (1969), in order to align the hand on the ulna, inserted an intramedullary rod through the third metacarpal and through the epiphyses and shaft of the ulna, performing an osteotomy of the ulna if it is badly bowed.

If the thumb is absent the radial digit may be pollicised.

PHOCOMELIA

This is a congenital malformation in which the hand is present, but the remainder of the extremity is missing. There were very few cases of this deformity until the recent thalidomide incident when a large number of cases of phocomelia were reported in Europe in which the mother used the drug thalidomide in the early months in pregnancy. There were relatively few cases in the United States. We had the opportunity of studying an adult case, a male 51 years of age, whose twin sister had the same anomaly but died shortly after birth. No other member of the family had a similar condition. Sensation of the hand was good, the skin was unusually smooth, but this is to be expected, since it was not used to any great extent. The fingers were small and had a good range of motion except for the thumb which was flexed.

This condition cannot be corrected by surgery. Before advising the use of a prosthesis, the functional evaluation of the hand should be carefully estimated and the possibility of training should also be considered.

AXILLARY CONTRACTURE

Congenital webbing of the anterior axillary fold together with absence of the pectoral muscle is sometimes associated with ectrodactyly. This type of webbing is easily corrected by a Z-plasty.

Almost invariably, axillary contractures are the result of burns when the area has been permitted to heal by scar. This should be avoided. It is extremely important in burn cases to graft the axillary areas as soon as local and general conditions permit.

Axillary contractures vary greatly in extent and character, from contractures so slight that they interfere little or not at all with the abduction of the arm, to massive

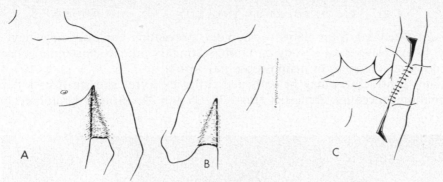

Fig. 32, 35

Z-plasty for axillary contracture. Local tissue should be used only when it is soft, pliable and elastic. (A) Anterior incision. (B) Posterior incision. (C) Closure.

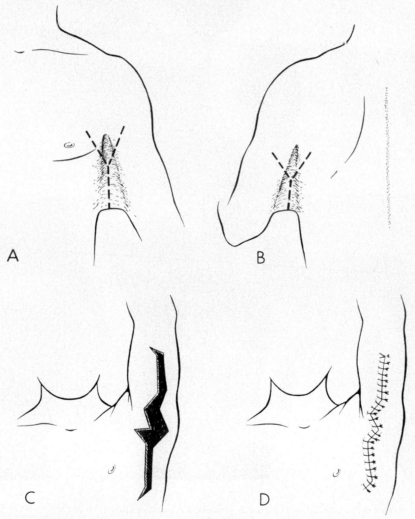

Fig. 32, 36

Utilisation of triangular flaps. (A and B) Incision. (C and D) Closure.

adhesions extending from elbow to shoulder, preventing any arm movement whatsoever. In extensive cases of long duration, secondary muscle shortening consequent to the long maintenance of malposition may result.

Axillary contractures may be corrected either by a free skin graft or a flap or a combination procedure. Z-plasties (Figs. **32**, 35 and **32**, 36) may be utilised in mild

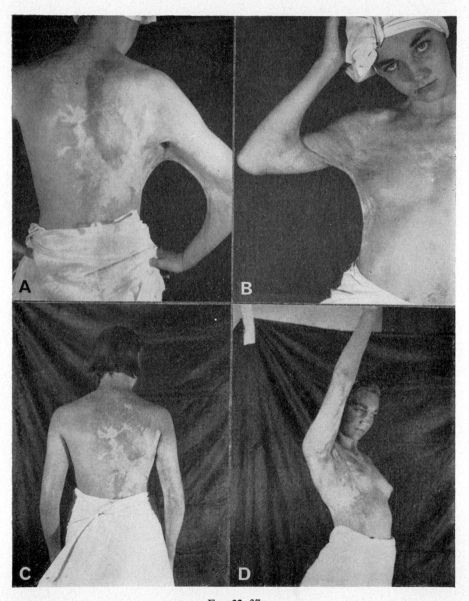

FIG. **32**, 37

Contracture of the axilla due to burn scar repaired by split-thickness skin grafts. (A and B) Preoperative. (C and D) Postoperative.

cases of axillary contracture in which abductor action has stretched the scar into a soft, pliable web. Dense, heavy, inelastic scar tissue should not be used. If scar flaps are of doubtful viability, they should not be used and free graft should be resorted to (Fig. **32**, 37).

When an extensive adhesion exists one should not even consider the use of local tissue. If the adjacent tissue is satisfactory, one may use a combined flap and free graft procedure (Fig. **32**, 38). The flap should be applied over the deep axillary contents and the supplementary skin graft used to recover the remaining denuded areas and the donor areas of the flap. Vessels and nerves that bowstring are best covered with flaps.

Whatever method of resurfacing is utilised, basic principles must be followed. At operation the web should be carefully incised by the surgeon as the assistant abducts the arm. All superficial and deep scars should be excised to permit abduction. The

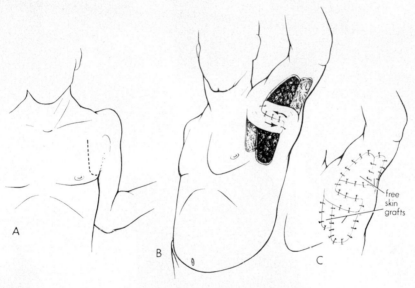

FIG. **32**, 38

Combined use of local flaps and free skin grafts to correct axillary contracture. (A) Pre-operative. The broken line indicates the pectoral flap. (B) Both local flaps are reflected to cover the axillary contents. (C) Closure utilising free skin grafts to cover the remaining denuded surfaces.

loss of skin in some of these cases will be surprisingly great. Important vessels and nerves must not be damaged. Viable tissue only should be used for flaps (especially to cover exposed vessels and nerves), flaps should not be too long nor too pointed, they should be fitted accurately and anchored upon the deep surfaces with absorbable sutures.

When split skin grafts are used, they should be taken in as large pieces as possible (Fig. **32**, 39). Junction lines should extend in an anterioposterior direction rather than along lines that parallel the axillary borders. Here zigzag junction lines should be used in order to avoid subsequent linear contracture. Postoperatively the area should

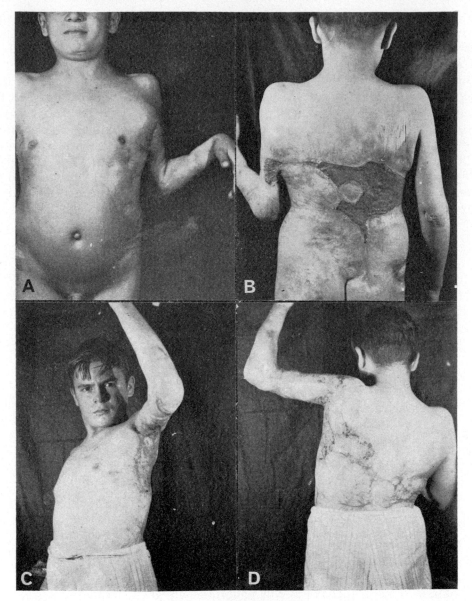

FIG. **32**, 39
Extensive axillary contracture repaired by split-thickness skin grafts. (A and B) Pre-operative.
(C and D) Postoperative.

be held in abduction with a light pressure dressing to maintain the free graft or flap
in contact with the base.

In children, after proper resurfacing has been carried out it is possible to stretch
out contracted muscles. Physio-therapy should not be utilised until the area is
completely healed and there is no possibility that the graft will separate from its base.

THE ELBOW

The general principles applying to axillary contractures are valid for the elbow joint. The avoidance of longitudinal scars on the surface of the antecubital area is extremely important (Fig. **32**, 40). Flaps may be used, provided that the tissue so

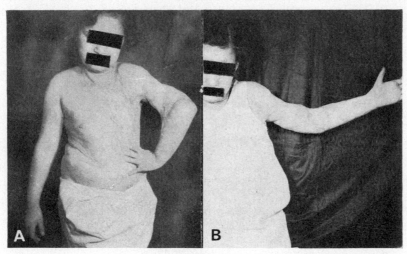

FIG. **32**, 40
Contracture of the elbow corrected by split-thickness skin grafts. (A) Pre-operative. (B) Postoperative.

utilised is pliable and viable, or free graft may be used. Tendon lengthening and joint surgery are contraindicated at the time of applying a free graft. In children (except in the case of spastic paralysis), when a normal muscle belly is present, tendon lengthening will rarely be required.

A. J. Barsky

REFERENCES

Alvord, R. M. (1947). Zygodactyly and associated variations. *J. Hered.* **38**, 49–53.
Barsky, A. J. (1938). *Plastic Surgery*. Philadelphia: Saunders.
Barsky, A. J. (1948). Restoration of the thumb. *Surgery, St. Louis* **23**, 227–247.
Barsky, A. J. (1950). *Principles and Practice of Plastic Surgery*. Baltimore: Williams & Wilkins.
Barsky, A. J. (1951). Congenital anomalies of the hand. *J. Bone Jt Surg.* **33A**, 35–64.
Barsky, A. J. (1958). *Congenital Anomalies of the Hand and Their Surgical Treatment*. Springfield, Illinois: Thomas.
Barsky, A. J. (1959a). Congenital anomalies of the thumb. *Clin. Orthop.* **15**, 96–110.
Barsky, A. J. (1959b). Reconstructive surgery in congenital anomalies of the hand. *Surg. Clins N. Am.* **39**, 449–467.
Barsky, A. J. (1964). Cleft Hand. *J. Bone Jt Surg.* **46A**, 1707–1720.
Barsky, A. J. (1967). Macrodactyly. *J. Bone Jt Surg.* **49A**, 1255–1266.
Barsky, A. J., Kahn, S. & Simon, B. E. (1964). *Principles and Practice of Plastic Surgery*. New York: McGraw-Hill.
Bell, J. (1951). On hereditary digital anomalies, Part I: On brachydactyly and symphalangism. In *The Treasury of Human Inheritance*, Vol. 5. London: Cambridge University Press.
Birch-Jensen, A. (1949). *Congenital Deformities of the Upper Extremities*. Copenhagen: Munksgaard.
Boinet, E. (1898). Polydactylie et atavisme. *Revue Méd.* **18**, 316–328.

BRINDEAU, A., LANTUÉJOUL, P. & CHAPPAZ, G. (1952). Des malformations d'origine amniotique. *Sem. Hôp. Paris*, **28**, 2769–2775.

BUNNELL, S. (1956). *Surgery of the Hand.* 3rd ed. Philadelphia: Lippincott.

BUNNELL, S. & DEHNE, E. (1955). Z-plasty for clinarthrosis of the wrist. *Plast. reconstr. Surg.* **16**, 169.

BURROWS, H. J. (1938). Developmental abbreviation of terminal phalanges. *Br. J. Radiol.* **11**, 165–176.

COHN, I. (1932). Skeletal disturbances and anomalies. *Radiology*, **18**, 592–626.

DE LORME, T. L. (1969). Treatment of congenital absence of the radius by transepiphyseal fixation. *J. Bone Jt Surg.* **51A**, 117–129.

DIDOT, A. (1850). Note sur la séparation des doigts palmés. *Bull. Acad. r. Méd. Belg.* **9**, 351–356.

DRINKWATER, H. (1907). An account of a brachydactylous family. *Proc. R. Soc. Edinb.* **28**, 35–57.

FREUD, P. & SLOBODY, L. B. (1943). Symphalangism. *Am. J. Dis. Child.* **65**, 550–557.

GATES, R. R. (1946). *Human Genetics.* New York: Macmillan.

GEOFFROY SAINT-HILAIRE, I. (1832). *Histoire générale et particulière des anomalies.* Vol. 1, 676–681. Paris: Baillière.

HANDFORTH, J. R. (1950). Polydactylism of the hand in southern Chinese. *Anat. Rec.* **106**, 119–125.

HARTSINCK, J. J. (1770). *Beschryving van Guiana.* Vol. II: 811–812. Amsterdam: Gerrit Tielenburg.

HICKS, S. P. (1953). Developmental malformations produced by radiation. *Am. J. Roentg.* **69**, 272–293.

HILLER, B. (1927). Congenital constriction of limbs. *Med. J. Aust.* **1**, 283.

INGLIS, K. (1952). The nature of agenesis and deficiency of parts. *Am. J. Path.* **28**, 449–475.

KANAVEL, A. B. (1931). Congenital malformations of the hands. *Trans. Sect. Surg. Am. med. Ass.* 17–121.

KANAVEL, A. B. (1932). Congenital malformations of the hands. *Archs Surg.* **25**, 1–53 and 282–320.

KLEIN, I. J. (1932). Hereditary ectrodactylism in siblings. *Am. J. Dis. Child.* **43**, 136–142.

LANGE, M. (1936). Grundsätzliches über die Beurteilung des Entstehung und Bewertung atypischer Hand- und Fussmissbildungen. *Verh. dt. orthop. Ges.* **31**, 80–87.

MACCOLLUM, D. W. (1940). Webbed fingers. *Surgery, Gynec. Obstet.* **71**, 782–789.

MIDDLETON, D. S. (1934). Studies on prenatal lesions of striated muscle. *Edinb. med. J.* **41**, 401–442.

MONTAGU, M. F. A. (1953). A pedigree of syndactylism. *Am. J. hum. Genet.* **5**, 70–72.

MOORE, B. H. (1942). Macrodactyly and associated peripheral nerve changes. *J. Bone Jt Surg.* **24**, 617–631.

MÜLLER, W. (1937). *Die angeborenen Fehlbildungen der menschlichen Hand.* Leipzig: Thieme.

NEEL, J. V. (1958). A study of major congenital defects in Japanese infants. *Am. J. Hum. Genet.* **10**, 398–445.

PATTERSON, T. J. S. (1961). Congenital ring constrictions. *Br. J. plast. Surg.* **14**, 1–31.

PENROSE, L. S. (1946). Inheritance of zygodactyly. *J. Hered.* **37**, 285–287.

RIORDAN, D. C. (1955). Congenital absence of the radius. *J. Bone Jt Surg.* **37A**, 1129–1140.

SCHULL, W. J. (1959). Consanguinity and the etiology of congenital malformations. *Pediatrics, Springfield* **23**, 195–201.

SCHURMEIER, H. L. (1922). Congenital deformities in drafted men. *Am. J. phys. Anthrop.* **5**, 51–60.

VILLAVERDE, M. (1943). Sistema endocrino y anomalías congénitas. *Vida nueva* **51**, 228–254.

WADDINGTON, C. H. (1963). Developmental mechanisms. In *Second International Conference on Congenital Malformations*, pp. 213–218. Ed. International Medical Congress Ltd. New York.

WARKANY, J. & NELSON, R. C. (1941). Skeletal abnormalities in the offspring of rats reared on deficient diets. *Anat. Rec.* **79**, 83–100.

WARKANY, J. & SCHRAFFENBERGER, E. (1947). Congenital malformations induced in rats by roentgen rays. *Am. J. Roentg.* **57**, 455–463.

CHAPTER XXXIII

THE LOWER EXTREMITY

CONGENITAL MALFORMATIONS

Polydactyly and Syndactyly

Polydactyly and syndactyly of the foot are treated in a manner similar to those in the hand (polydactyly, page 472; syndactyly, page 465). Polydactyly may be corrected quite early. So far as syndactyly is concerned, this does not require any treatment except for aesthetic reasons since there is no functional disability.

Annular Constricting Bands

Annular constricting bands of the lower extremities are usually found at the junction of the lower and middle thirds of the leg. They are generally unilateral and may completely circle the limb. Circumferential congenital annular band at the upper part of the lower limb is much less common than that of the lower part (Fig. 33, 1).

These constricting annular bands sometimes extend almost down to the bone, leaving only a very small space for the passage of nerves, muscles, tendons and vessels. The limb distal to the constriction band, especially the dorsum of the foot, will show oedema, sometimes to a marked degree. Since the soft tissues above and below the

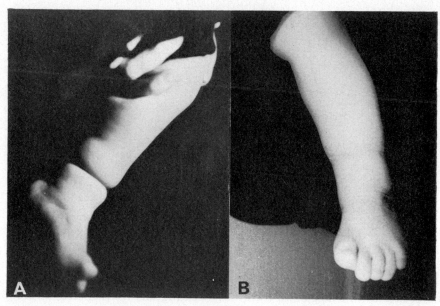

FIG. 33, 1

Annular constricting band of the lower extremity. (A) The most common site of the constriction is at the junction of the middle and lower thirds of the leg. (B) Postoperative result obtained in two stages, excising the band and using several Z-plasties.

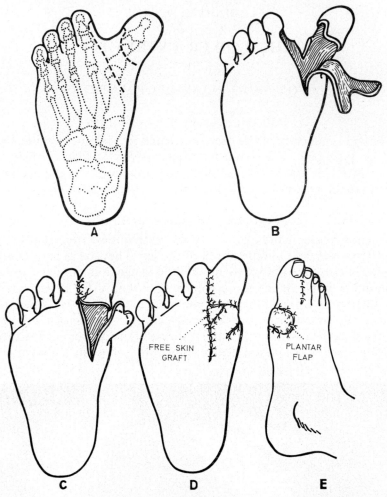

FIG. 33, 2

Congenital hallux varus repaired by the method described by Farmer. (A) Plantar
flap outlined extending along adjacent surfaces of the great and second toes.
(B) Elevation of the flap. (C) The great toe is brought into proper alignment; a
capsulotomy of the metatarsophalangeal joint is necessary. (D) Surgical syndactyly has been created and the denuded surfaces covered with a free skin graft.
(E) Extension of the plantar flap to cover the defect on the medial side of the foot.

band are usually adequate, the condition can be corrected by excising the band and
uniting the subcutaneous tissue in layers, utilising a Z-plasty for the skin to prevent
possible recurrence of secondary linear contracture of the scar. It is not advisable to
encircle the limb completely at one operative procedure but it is better to do half the
circumference at one stage and then, after healing has taken place, to complete the
remainder of the constriction. Usually the peripheral oedema will improve, although
in some cases it may be necessary to maintain gentle compression on the distal part
to control the oedema.

Macrodactyly of the Toe

Macrodactyly of the toe is much less common than that of the hand. If not of extremely large size, it may be left alone unless cosmetic improvement is desired. The treatment outlined for macrodactyly in the hand (p. 494) can be utilised. However, in the foot (especially in the great toe) it is advisable in all cases to leave the proximal phalanx after resecting the distal two phalanges in order to preserve appearance and function.

Congenital Hallux Varus

This condition may be corrected by utilising a dorsal or a plantar flap after realigning the great toe in its proper position. The flap, dorsal or plantar, will have to be rotated immediately to cover the defect left on this surface. The noted areas may require resurfacing with free split-thickness skin grafts. Figure **33**, 2 depicts the operation described by Farmer (1958) utilising a plantar flap.

Cleft Foot

Cleft foot is rarely found by itself but usually in conjunction with cleft of the hand. The only reason for correcting the condition is cosmetic and the type of operation described for the hand (p. 485) may be utilised.

A. J. Barsky

REFERENCE

Farmer, A. W. (1958). Congenital hallux varus. *Am. J. Surg.* **95**, 274–278.

SECTION 4

GENERAL

CHAPTER XXXIV

PIGMENTED NAEVI

It is extremely rare for any pigmented skin lesion to show malignant melanomatous change before puberty and therefore the only aim of surgical treatment in children is cosmetic improvement. The sole exception to this rule is the *giant hairy naevus* which will be discussed later. In a sense it is true that excision of a simple pigmented tumour avoids future malignancy but the risk is only one in many millions and is no justification for the wholesale removal of moles in children. At one time it was customary to excise pigmented naevi from the beard area in boys on the assumption that the recurring irritation of shaving would induce malignant change; but there is little evidence to support the idea that chronic irritation is an important factor in inducing malignant change in pigmented lesions and furthermore, the beard area is not a common site for malignant melanoma. In children therefore operation should be reserved for those lesions large enough to constitute a cosmetic handicap.

There are many different varieties of pigmented skin lesions, flap or raised, hairy or non-hairy, dark or light, tiny or involving most of the skin surface and many descriptive names have been applied to them. There is no point in cataloguing these since the techniques of surgical removal are unaffected by the type of lesion with one minor exception. Warty naevi of the hystrix variety (Fig. **34,** 1) may be treated by shaving the lesion flush with the surrounding skin. There may be some recurrence and

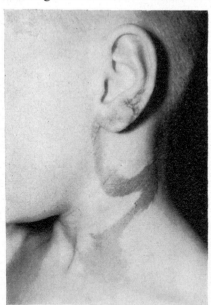

FIG. **34,** 1
This type of naevus responds well to shaving. There was some recurrence which was shaved off a second time. Only a faint trace of pigment remains.

treatment may have to be repeated; the case illustrated was shaved twice and only a faint trace of pigment now remains. Most other varieties are unsuitable for shaving because of the virtual certainty of recurrence. The methods available for removing those too large for excision and suture are excision and grafting, or serial excision with advancement.

Excision and grafting

Hynes (1956) recommended that the lesion should be excised through the deep layer of the dermis. This he accomplished with a skin grafting knife so that the excised lesion thinned out at the margin into normal skin. A split skin graft similarly cut, i.e., thicker at the centre and tapering to the edges, and of the same size as the defect, was used for cover. The immediate result of this procedure is good and a smooth surface results. It is not, however, suitable for hairy naevi as many hair bulbs remain behind and hairs grow through the graft. Furthermore, spots of pigmentation appearing

514

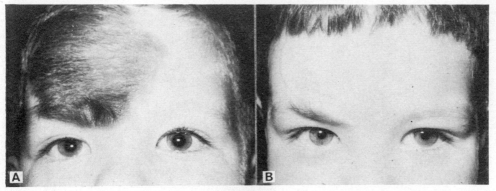

Fig. **34**, 2

(A) Extensive hair-bearing naevus of the forehead. (B) After excision and split skin grafting. A better cosmetic result could be obtained by segmental excision and grafting of all the forehead skin.

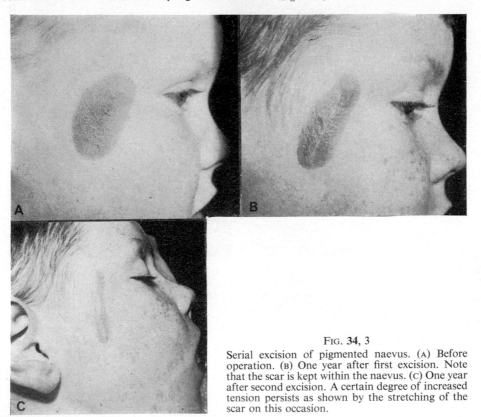

Fig. **34**, 3

Serial excision of pigmented naevus. (A) Before operation. (B) One year after first excision. Note that the scar is kept within the naevus. (C) One year after second excision. A certain degree of increased tension persists as shown by the stretching of the scar on this occasion.

on the graft are common later. Indeed as Whimster (1967) has shown, pigmented areas may continue to appear for some years in skin grafts used to resurface defects left by excising naevi even when full thickness skin and subcutaneous fat have been removed with the lesion. Whether a deep layer of dermis is retained or not, the

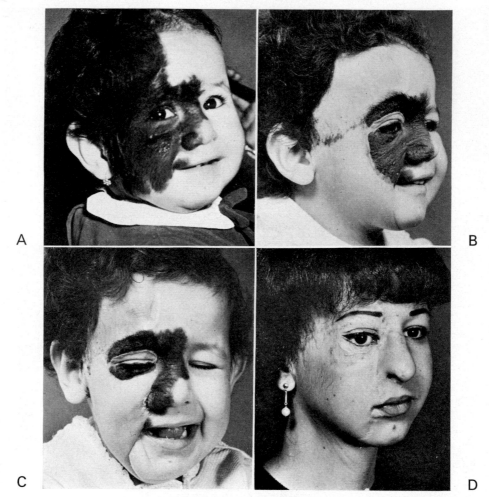

FIG. 34, 4

(A) Giant hairy naevus of the face covering approximately one half of the facial area in an 8-month-old baby girl. (B) Appearance after split-thickness grafting of the forehead and of the upper eyelid and rotation-advancement of the cervical skin in two stages. (C) Appearance after further advancement-rotation of the cervical skin. (D) Final result. The patient is now 16 years of age. The nose has been resurfaced by a median forehead flap, the lower eyelid by split-thickness graft and the eyebrow has been excised. The patient uses an eyebrow pencil to simulate the eyebrow. (From Converse *et al.* (1969). *Br. J. plast. Surg.* **22,** 303, by kind permission of the authors.)

excision should be kept superficial to avoid a depressed grafted area. The donor site needs careful selection. On the face, post-auricular skin is obviously first choice but the supply is limited. When leg or arm skin must be used, a good colour and texture match is unlikely but the result may be improved by segmental replacement later (Fig. **34**, 2).

Serial excision and advancement

The extensibility of skin, the amount by which it will stretch when any given force is applied to it, is greatest in infancy and gradually declines with increasing age (Gibson and Kenedi, 1967). It is also observable that if a wound is stitched under tension in a child that a certain amount of relaxation of the increased tension in the surrounding skin occurs with time. It is therefore possible to excise as much of a naevus as will just allow the defect to be pulled together with sutures, leave it for a year, excise a further area and repeat this process until the lesion is completely removed. Preferably the elliptical excision is kept within the confines of the naevus until the final excision (Fig. **34**, 3). The author makes a practice of sending subsequent excisions for histological examination; on no occasion has any increased activity of the melanocytes next to the scar been observed.

In many cases this technique gives admirable results but it must be remembered that total relaxation of the surrounding skin probably does not occur and a certain increased tension persists. Thus, it is not uncommon to find the final scar stretching and requiring further excision. In the case illustrated, the tension required to close the wound was measured at the first excision and then one year later after excision of the scar and undermining; only 60 per cent. relaxation had occurred, i.e., the tension across the wound was still 40 per cent. higher than normal. In many areas this is of little moment but it may cause some deformity if the lesion is near the mouth or eyelids.

In larger naevi around the face a combination of grafting and serial excision and much ingenuity may be required for the best result. Neck skin can be advanced to quite an astonishing degree and Converse *et al.* (1969) have made full use of this in the treatment of the patient shown in Figure **34**, 4.

GIANT HAIRY NAEVUS

This term is usually applied to a lesion which covers most of the trunk or an extremity (Fig. **34**, 5). It differs from other pigmented lesions not only in extent but

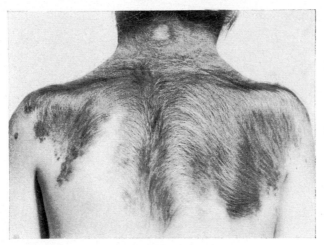

Fig. **34**, 5
Giant hairy naevus of neck and shoulders.

in the considerably increased risk of malignant change before puberty. There have now been 26 instances reported (Greeley *et al.*, 1965) and thus prophylactic excision of the whole lesion is desirable. However, the naevus may cover more than half the body surface with insufficient normal skin available for grafts. In such cases the surgeon must excise as much as the available skin grafts will permit, selecting those areas where the best cosmetic improvement can be gained. Thereafter the remainder must be kept under careful observation. Shaving off the surface layer is beneficial in some particularly when the surface is warty and difficult to keep clean; it may also reduce the intensity of the pigmentation.

T. GIBSON

REFERENCES

CONVERSE, J. M., GUY, C. L. & MOLENAAR, A. (1969). *Br. J. plast. Surg.* **22**, 302.
GIBSON, T. & KENEDI, R. M. (1967). *Surg. Clins N. Am.* **47**, 279.
GREELEY, P. W., MIDDLETON, A. G. & CURTIN, J. W. (1965). *Plastic reconstr. Surg.* **36**, 26.
HYNES, W. (1956). *Br. J. plast. Surg.* **9**, 47.
WHIMSTER, I. W. (1967). *Annali ital. Derm. Clin. e. Sper.* **19**, 168.

CHAPTER XXXV

HAEMANGIOMA

There are basically three varieties of haemangiomas which affect children, the capillary and cavernous types which are usually present at birth and are easily distinguished clinically and histologically, and the strawberry naevus which commonly appears in the first week or two of life. Whether true benign tumours or haemartomata is a matter for debate but all are simple although both the cavernous type and the strawberry naevus in its early growth phase may be locally invasive.

Capillary haemangiomas

These lie in, or rarely immediately under the dermis, and discolour the skin without distorting it. The colour varies from the light *salmon patch* to the deep red or purple of the *port wine stain* (naevus flammeus). They may affect only small areas or cover almost the entire body; when widespread, it is not uncommon to find deep structures infiltrated with haemangiomatous tissue and arterio-venous fistulae may be present. Gigantism of an affected limb often follows and if many arterio-venous shunts exist, there is a real danger of cardiac failure arising as the child grows. Capillary haemangiomas of the face are associated with angiomas of the lepto-meninges in Sturge-Weber's syndrome and hemiplegia or epilepsy may result, while Maffuci's syndrome is a combination of haemangiomas with dyschondroplasia. The *spider naevus*, a tiny red spot with radiating capillaries may occur in older children though it is commoner in adults. It is easily corrected by cauterising or excising the central core.

The type commonly referred for plastic surgery is the port wine stain affecting the face. If small enough for the defect to be covered with a post-auricular skin graft, it may be excised; some small lesions are also suitable for the technique of serial excision and advancement discussed for pigmented naevi. For larger lesions there is as yet no ideal treatment. Various forms of cauterisation and irradiation will sclerose the angioma but replace it by an obvious scar. Excision and grafting with skin grafts taken from sites other than the post-auricular region, produce a patch of white, yellow or brown skin which can be as obtrusive as the original naevus; there may be occasions when it is appropriate in adults who can appreciate the problems involved but it is unsuitable for children.

The technique of tattooing pigments into the skin to camouflage the lesion was introduced by Brown *et al.* (1946) and has been on trial since. Conway *et al.* (1968) have now published their experience of the method in over a thousand patients and their published results are such that tatooing must now be accepted as the best treatment at present available for port wine stains. The lesions may be subdivided into three varieties, subepidermal, dermal and subdermal depending on the depth at which they lie. The deep dermal and subdermal varieties (which make up 85 per cent. of cases) are suitable for tattooing since the pigment can be injected into the normal part of the dermis and mask the underlying angioma. Although a range of pigments was originally used, only white (titanium dioxide) is now usually injected. Since the

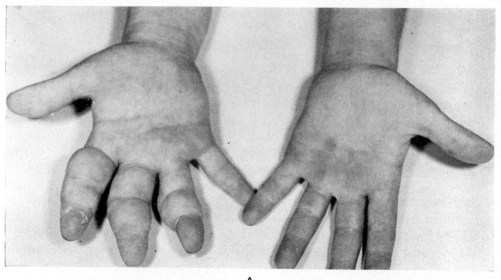

A

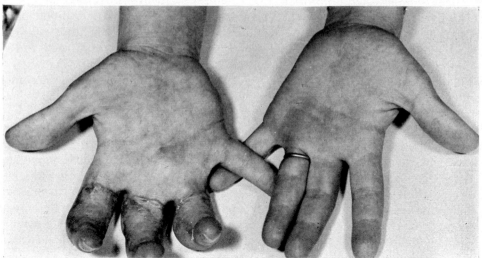

B

FIG. 35, 1

(A) Pre-operative view of cavernous haemangiomas on volar aspect of fingers. (B) Postoperative condition. Split skin grafts were used to resurface the defect after excision of the haemangiomas.

pigment lies deep to the melanin-carrying cells of the basal layer, this part of the patient's complexion is intact and there is no need to mix shades to try to simulate it.

Several motor driven tattooing devices with single or multiple needles adjustable for depth of penetration, are available commercially. The needles are coated with pigment and held so that they penetrate at an angle of about 60°. Care must be taken to inject the pigment right to the margin of the lesion but not beyond; otherwise there will be

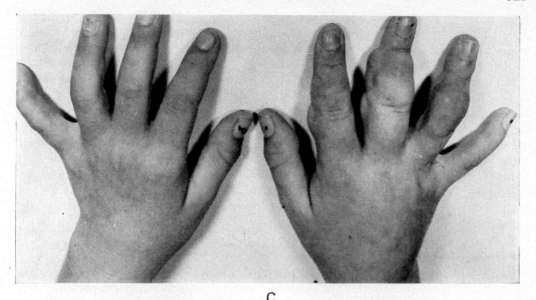

C

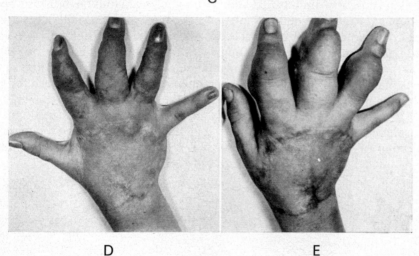

D   E

FIG. 35, 1 *(contd.)*

(C) Dorsum of same hand showing expanding haemangiomas of dorsum and fingers. (D) Postoperative split skin graft over dorsum, fingers untreated. (E) Final result following excision and split skin grafting of fingers. Note scar at wrist, the site of secondary resection.

Reproduced by permission of the author, editor and publishers from the paper by Glanz, S. (1969), *British Journal of Plastic Surgery*, **22**, 297–298.

a rimmed effect from the unmasked margin or a third colour introduced from the pigment in normal skin. Since it is not always easy to distinguish the margin while treatment is in process, it should first be delineated with carefully cut and applied adhesive tape or with tattooed dots of methylene blue.

Satisfactory results are claimed by Conway *et al.* in 84 per cent of cases.

Unsatisfactory results obtained particularly in the subepidermal variety in which the affected dermis would not retain enough pigment for camouflage. Occasionally small excisions may be required later if too much pigment is inserted or accurate tattooing of the margin is not achieved.

How far this technique is applicable in children will depend on many individual factors. An average of five treatments is required and while the method is suitable for local anaesthesia and out-patient care in older children and in adults, general anaesthesia and hospital admission are required in the young. If the patient and the parents are not too emotionally disturbed about the blemish, treatment is better delayed until the early teens.

Much can be achieved by skilfully applied cosmetics to mask port wine stains since these are usually free from surface irregularities and in some cases this may be the treatment of choice. Even after successful tattooing some make-up will greatly enhance the result.

Cavernous haemangiomas

These are much less common than the capillary type. They may occur on any part of the body as irregular lobulated swellings which compress easily on pressure; the overlying skin is usually discoloured and the diagnosis obvious. A bruit is only heard when there is an arterial feeder and most are fed by veins. Internally they consist of large inter-communicating blood spaces which make surgery hazardous because of difficult-to-control haemorrhage. Although they may remain quiescent for years, they may at any time begin to enlarge and invade neighbouring structures and in certain areas, particularly the hand, any evidence of enlargement is an indication for surgical excision before essential structures become involved.

Surgery is dangerous and difficult unless the lesion is small or situated on a limb where tourniquet haemostasis is available (Fig. 35, 1). Non-operative techniques such as the injection of sclerosing agents (Owens and Stephenson, 1948) or the insertion

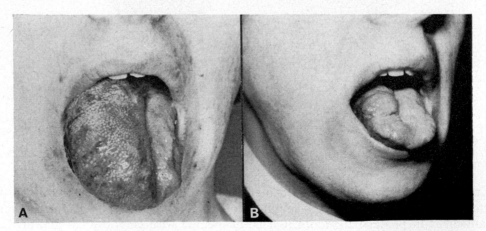

FIG. 35, 2

(A) Cavernous haemangioma of tongue. (B) Result of the insertion of multiple transfixing mattress sutures tied over rubber tubing on four occasions.

of radon seeds (Figi, 1948; Brown and Fryer, 1953) designed to induce thrombosis have been used with varying degrees of success. The lesion illustrated in Figure **35**, 2 was reduced to a more normal size by inserting a series of mattress sutures tied over rubber tubing on four occasions. In cases where infiltration of essential structures make radical excision impossible, ligation of all accessible peripheral feeders may result in diminution in size.

Strawberry naevi

The strawberry naevus has been variously labelled a 'capillary' haemangioma (Martin and MacCollum, 1961; Phelan and Grace, 1963; O'Brien, 1964) and a 'cavernous' haemangioma (Lister, 1938; Simpson, 1959); indeed, both types of vessel are often present and the histological picture depends entirely on whether the lesion is in the proliferative, static or regressive phase. The unique nature of the lesion was for long obscured by this confusion in pathological nomenclature and the attempt by many authors to fit the strawberry naevus into a general classification of angiomas.

The strawberry naevus behaves like no other simple tumour and its behaviour is fascinating and at present inexplicable. It appears as a tiny red spot within a few days of birth and grows rapidly in subsequent weeks invading and replacing the skin and destroying its normal architecture. Growth usually ceases before the child is 6 months old and the raised lobulated swelling whose colour varies from vivid scarlet to deep

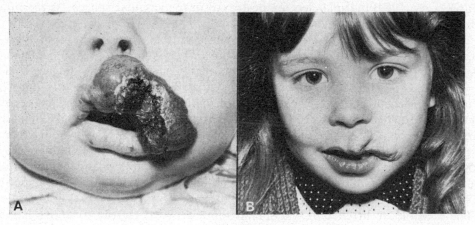

Fig. 35, 3

(A) Large strawberry naevus of upper lip with central area of ulceration. (B) At age 6 regression continues but treatment will be required for the scar of the ulcerated lesion.

purple persists unchanged for two to three years. Then it slowly regresses; the colour pales and disappears, the swelling subsides. Finally the miracle is complete; all trace of the tumour vanishes and even skin which was extensively involved, regains its normal appearance.

Some mothers claim that the tumour was present at birth but it is doubtful if it is often congenital. Walsh and Tompkins (1956) offered rewards to the medical and nursing staff of two large maternity hospitals for a record of any child born with a strawberry naevus. In almost 5,000 deliveries no case was reported although at least 77 strawberry naevi later appeared in the same group. Even when the mother is convinced that it was there when the child was born, it is always reported as being tiny and the typical growth follows; angiomas fully formed at birth are not strawberry naevi.

They may develop on any part of the body and are usually confined to the skin. Some, however, have a large subdermal element and Lister (1938) described this as the 'poached egg' type. They rarely cause symptoms although ulceration may occur particularly in lesions near the mouth, perineum or thighs, Even when ulcerated, serious haemorrhage is rare and the ulcer will usually heal with appropriate local hygiene and antibiotics. Ulceration often appears to initiate regression but it is in no way beneficial; permanent scarring remains when the ulcer heals (Fig. **35**, 3).

Strawberry naevi rarely exceed a few centimetres in diameter, but an occasional 'wildfire' growth has been reported in which, for example, the skin of a whole arm and the neighbouring trunk was involved (Matthews, 1953) or the face extensively infiltrated (Brown *et al.*, 1953). Thrombocytopenic purpura has been described in a number of cases of giant blood vessel tumours (Good *et al.*, 1955; James and Tuttle, 1961; Inglefield *et al.*, 1961) probably of the strawberry naevus type since they grow rapidly after birth and regress either spontaneously (Weissman and Tagnon, 1953) or after ulceration (Wallerstein, 1961) or irradiation (Southard *et al.*, 1951). It appears (Gilon *et al.*, 1959) that platelets are destroyed in the vascular spaces; as the tumour subsides the thrombocytopenia disappears.

Lister (1938) was the first to show conclusively that strawberry naevi regressed spontaneously; 92 out of 93 lesions in children whose mothers he had persuaded to leave them alone, had either disappeared completely or were well on the way to doing so. In spite of this and many subsequent similar reports many doctors have been reluctant to accept this overwhelming proof of natural regression and its corollary that no treatment was required. Not only is treatment unnecessary; it is positively harmful since in almost all cases it leaves a permanent scar in what would otherwise be normal skin. There is no need to detail all the sclerosing agents recommended. The most widely used was X-irradiation and the reported complications include cataract (Bek and Zahn, 1960), carcinoma (Brunner, 1961; Kolar *et al.*, 1962) and hypoplasia of the breast (Gregl and Weiss, 1961).

The possible occurrence of widespread rapid growth referred to above has been the main reason for advocating early treatment but such cases are excessively rare and no justification for active treatment of the very common strawberry naevus.

There are, however, a few indications for treatment. As Browne (1960) pointed out, if the growing red spot can be diagnosed when still tiny, it might be excised with virtually no scar and the parents spared a disfiguring blemish.

Occasionally involution seems incomplete; the skin is wrinkled and small telangiectases persist. These often continue to improve and it is wrong to consider a time limit of five, seven or more years in which all regression occurs. But pressure may be brought to bear by the parents or even the child to an extent when it is wiser to excise the excess skin and coagulate the telangiectases. Some parents from the outset are reluctant to accept the waiting period and situations can arise when it seems better to treat the tumour, particularly if small and in an area where a scar is unimportant.

Finally, thrombocytopenic purpura from a giant naevus demands treatment. Irradiation is probably preferable to excision and grafting because of the extensive area involved but the final decision might well depend on the site.

T. GIBSON

REFERENCES

BEK, V. & ZAHN, K. L. (1960). *Acta radiol.* **54**, 443.
BROWN, J. B., CANNON, B. & MCDOWELL, F. (1946). *Plastic reconstr. Surg.* **1**, 106.
BROWN, J. B. & FRYER, M. P. (1953). *Plastic reconstr. Surg.* **11**, 197.
BROWN, J. B., FRYER, M. P. & MCDOWELL, F. (1953). *Ann. Surg.* **137**, 652.
BROWNE, D. (1960). *Lancet* **1**, 55.
BRUNNER, K. (1961). *Schweiz med. Wschr.* **91**, 389.
CONWAY, M., MCKINNEY, P, & CLIMO, M. (1968). *Plastic reconstr. Surg.* **40**, 457.
FIGI, F. A. (1948). *Plastic reconstr. Surg.* **3**, 1.
GILON, E., RAMOT, B. & SHEBA, C. (1959). *Blood*, **14**, 74.
GOOD, T. A., CARNAZZO, S. F. & GOOD, R. A. (1955). *Am. J. Dis. Child.* **90**, 260
GREGL, A. & WEISS, J. W. (1961). *Fortschr. Geb. RöntgStrahl. NukleMed.* **94**, 244.
INGLEFIELD, J. T., TISDALE, P. D. & FAIRCHILD, J. P. (1961). *J. Pediat.* **59**, 238.
JAMES, D. H. & TUTTLE, A. H. (1961). *J. Pediat.* **59**, 234.
KOLAR, J., VRABEC, R. & KRAL, Z. (1962). *Strahlentherapie*, **117**, 147.
LISTER, W. A. (1938). *Lancet*, **2**, 1429.
MARTIN, L. W. & MACCOLLUM, D. W. (1961). *Am. J. Surg.* **101**, 571.
MATTHEWS, D. N. (1953). *Br. J. Plast. Surg.* **6**, 83.
O'BRIEN, B. M. (1964). *Med. J. Aust.* **1**, 381.
OWENS, N. & STEPHENSON, K. L. (1948). *Plastic reconstr. Surg.* **3**, 109.
PHELAN, J. T. & GRACE, J. T. (1963). *J. Am. Ass.* **185**, 246.
SIMPSON, J. R. (1959). *Lancet*, **2**, 1057.
SOUTHARD, S. C., DE SANCTIS, A. G. & WALDRON, R. J. (1951). *J. Pediat.* **38**, 732.
WALLERSTEIN, R. D. (1961). *Am. J. Dis. Child.* **102**, 111.
WALSH, T. S. & TOMPKINS, V. N. (1956). *Cancer, N.Y.* **9**, 869.
WEISSMAN, J. & TAGNON, H. J. (1953). *Archs intern. Med.* **92**, 523.

CHAPTER XXXVI

LYMPHANGIOMA

Lymphangiomata are not commonly seen outside a large children's hospital. Attempts at classification (Paletta, 1966) are confusing. They are probably all hamartomatous in origin and in paediatric practice they commonly present as a cystic hygroma. In the lip and tongue they may be capillary in structure and cause one type of machrocheilia (Fig. **36**, 1) or macroglossia (Fig. **36**, 2) respectively. In the skin, mucous membranes, neck, axilla and groins, they are usually cavernous and are called cystic lymphangiomas or cystic hygromas. They vary greatly in size and the diameter varies from 1 or 2 mm to large cystic swellings filling one or both posterior triangles of the neck, often extending into the mediastinum.

Most cystic hygromas appear in the posterior triangle of the neck and they often occupy the supra-clavicular fossa. They also occur in the axilla and the lesion may extend from one region to the other (Fig. **36**, 3A). The swelling is often present at birth and most become obvious during the first year of life. The overlying skin is normal in texture with a bluish tint due to the underlying fluid. The mass can be transilluminated but either haemorrhage or infection can alter the size and consistency of the swelling—often in a dramatic fashion. Very rarely, hygromas regress spontaneously but

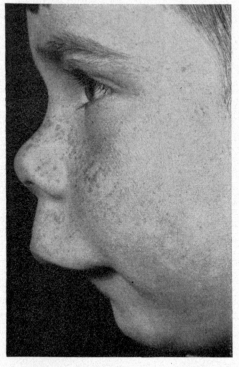

Fig. **36**, 1
Macrocheilia due to lymphangioma.

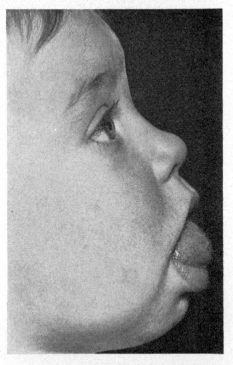

Fig. **36**, 2
Macroglossia due to lymphangioma.

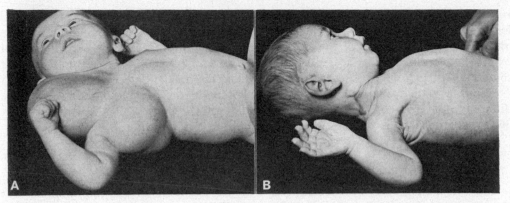

FIG. 36, 3

(A) Cystic hygroma of neck and axilla causing respiratory distress. (B) Ten days after operation.

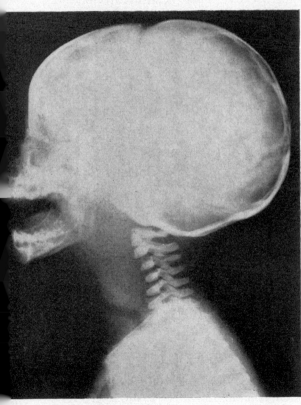

FIG. 36, 4

re-vertebral lymphangioma displacing trachea forward and using severe respiratory distress in first day of life.

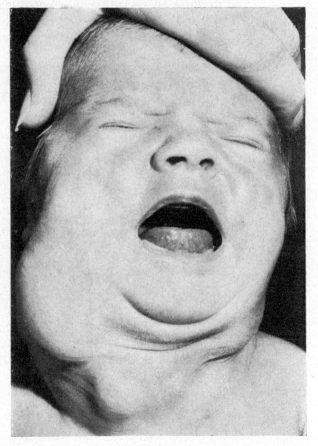

FIG. 36, 5

Cystic dysplasia of thyroid gland in newborn infant causing severe respiratory distress and simulating multi-loculated cystic hygroma.

regression occurs with sufficient frequency to warrant delay in surgical intervention in lesions of the cheek and lesions of the breast in the young female. Less common sites are the anterior triangle of the neck in the submandibular region with intra-oral extensions. As in the cervical pre-vertebral region (Fig. **36**, 4), hygromas in such regions often present with severe respiratory distress in the newborn.

The differential diagnosis is rarely difficult but in the neck, the lesions must be differentiated from branchial cyst, dermoid, cystic dysplasia of the thyroid (Fig. **36**, 5), deep haemangioma and the very rare lipoma of childhood.

TREATMENT

There is no place for radiation therapy in the treatment of lymphangiomas. Not only has it little effect on the size of the swelling but such treatment makes subsequent attempts at surgical excision difficult or impossible. Incision and drainage and injection of sclerosing agents also lead to fibrosis and make excision difficult.

Despite the reiterated pessimism in the literature about the difficulties of complete excision of lymphangiomas in the neck and axilla because of ramifications around the

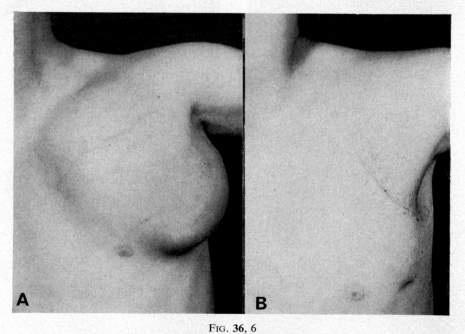

FIG. **36**, 6

(A) Cystic hygroma of axilla extending on to chest wall. (B) Seven days after operation. Note scar of drainage tube lateral to nipple.

vessels, nerves and other vital structures, it is remarkable how often cystic hygromas shell out with ease (Figs. **36**, 3 and **36**, 6). Nevertheless the surgeon must be prepared for a painstaking dissection—sometimes to remove as many cysts as possible and to open the remainder. Matched blood for transfusion is always available.

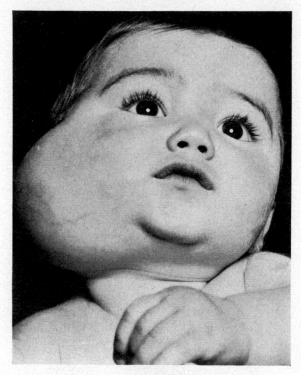

FIG. **36**, 7
Lymphangioma of parotid region.

Face and lip

The lesions are usually slow-growing and fractional or complete excision is carried out at any time after the age of 3 months. In the parotid region (Fig. **36**, 7) the facial nerve is displayed and meticulous dissection is carried out.

Tongue

While one is always prepared to perform a tracheostomy, I have never found this necessary after wedge resections from the tongue in macroglossia due to lymphangioma. With traction sutures in position blood loss is minimal. Repeat excision may be necessary when a large tumour is deforming the palate and dental arches.

Neck

The patient is X-rayed to exclude mediastinal extensions. After intubation, the swelling is excised through a simple transverse cervical incision. The great vessels and nerves may be closely involved. It is wise to drain the wound for 24 hours postoperatively.

Axilla

Here too (Fig. **36**, 6), the lymphangioma may involve the great vessels and nerves and complete excision may be impossible.

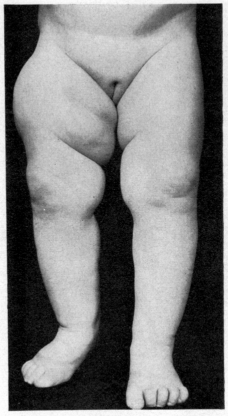

Fig. **36**, 8
Fibrous haemo-lymphangioma of right thigh.

Other sites

I do not attempt to excise breast lesions in the female during infancy and childhood. Only after puberty is the breast tissue easily recognised when the lymphangioma can be excised without risk of damage to the tiny nodule which represents the entire breast tissue of the child. Lesions of the limbs (Fig. **36**, 8) and buttocks are often haemolymphangiomas and radical excision may be impossible or mutilating.

Lymphangiomas of the neck and upper mediastinum which present as respiratory neonatal surgical emergencies are best dealt with in a neonatal surgical unit where skilled paediatric nursing is available.

W. M. Dennison

REFERENCES

Benson, C. D., Mustard, W. T. *et al.* (1962). *Pediatric Surgery*. Chicago: Year Book Medical Publishers.
Dennison, W. M. (1967). *Surgery in Infancy and Childhood*. Edinburgh & London: Livingstone.
Paletta, F. X. (1966). Lymphangioma. *Plastic reconstr. Surg.* **37**, 269.

CHAPTER XXXVII

THE TREATMENT OF BURNS IN
INFANCY AND CHILDHOOD

INTRODUCTION

The great majority of thermal injuries admitted to hospital in this country are due to accidents in the home, and at the Roehampton Burns Centre, which treats adults and children, approximately 80 per cent. of all admissions are domestic in origin. Children and the elderly are the two main groups at risk, and out of a total of 1,640 patients admitted to Roehampton between April 1959 and March 1968, 714 were under 15 years of age. Of these last, 501 (70 per cent.) were less than 5 years old and it may be noted that the susceptibility to these injuries begins at birth (Fig. 37, 1).

Helpless babies may suffer from such careless actions as being placed in too hot a bath or the placing of a cot near an unguarded coal fire where a spark may ignite

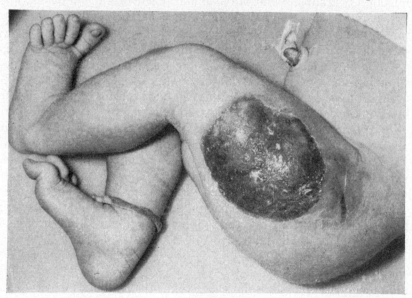

FIG. 37, 1

New-born baby with contact burn from unprotected hot-water bottle. The burn was excised and grafted when the baby was 14 days old.

the bedclothes. The crawling or toddling infant is in danger from unguarded open fires, gas and electric heating appliances, kettles, saucepans or teapots left within their reach, or the presence of faulty electric wires and plugs. The older and more venture-some child may fall to the temptation of playing with matches, pushing paper into the fire, playing near bonfires and other forbidden activities.

In recent years there has been considerable propaganda aimed at reducing the incidence of domestic burning accidents, and regulations have been introduced con-cerning the safeguarding and improved design of heating appliances and limiting the sale of inflammable children's nightwear. While there has been a slight fall in the number of children's clothing burns, especially those due to electric fires, there has been little change in the overall incidence and mortality, and continuing efforts are necessary in this important field of prevention. The mortality, lengthy periods of surgical salvage, residual disablement and disfigurement arising from these accidents provide a world-wide problem and it is noteworthy that the International Society for Burn Injuries has as its first aim—'To disseminate knowledge and to stimulate prevention in the field of burns.'

THE THERMAL INJURY

The severity of the tissue damage depends on the temperature to which the tissues are raised and the length of time for which this rise is maintained. Where the thermal effect is greatest cells will be destroyed but adjoining or deep to this area there will be a zone where cellular damage is reversible, and in the absence of adverse factors such as infection or trauma, tissue survival and regeneration will occur. The effect of heat is greatest on the surface and diminishes as the temperature falls through successive layers, as distinct from the electrical injury where the passage of current releases heat in the depth of the tissues—so that deep destruction is often greater than the visible damage on the surface. Quite apart from the obvious necessity of extinguishing burning clothing, delay in removing clothing saturated with hot liquids will maintain the local temperature and this can be of serious consequence on the thin skin of small infants where a superficial scald may rapidly become deeper. Accompanying the cellular damage there are vascular effects which are of considerable importance. Abnormal capillary permeability allows rapid loss of circulating fluid and this is accentuated by vasodilatation with increased rate of local blood flow Superficial loss of fluid causes blister formation or copious exudate from the surface where the superficial epithelium has been destroyed. Large quantities are also lost into the subcutaneous tissues as oedema (Fig. 37, 2A). The fluid loss is rapid at first and continues at a diminishing rate for as long as 48 hours after burning. After that time oedema fluid will rapidly reabsorb (Fig. 37, 2B).

DEPTH OF BURN

The initial diagnosis of depth is not easy. At the two extremes the erythema or thin blistering of the superficial scald and the scorched, coagulated surface of the deep flame burn may be readily distinguished. Partial-thickness burns may be accompanied by thick, opaque blisters, and where the superficial layers are absent the stippled appearance of exposed dermal papillae will be seen. Often however, there is a mottled, reddish appearance with absence of colour return on pressure which may be present in either partial-thickness or full-thickness burns. An added difficulty is due to a large proportion of these injuries being of mixed depth with areas of superficial and deep burning shading into each other.

In the *superficial* (1st degree) burn or scald with involvement of epidermis only there is erythema and thin transient blistering. Spontaneous healing should normally occur within five to seven days without any residual scarring. Very occasionally in

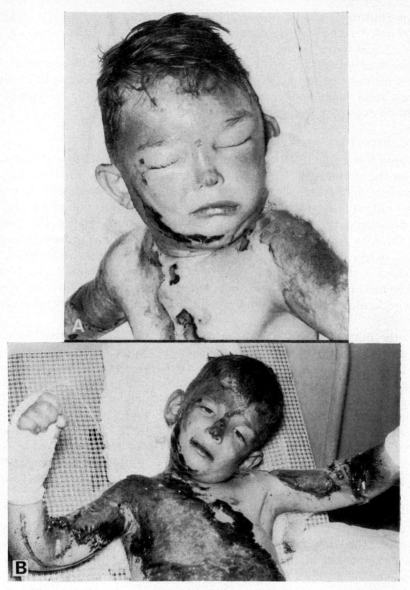

Fig. **37**, 2

(A) 5-year-old boy shortly after admission with 34 per cent. burn. (B) Facial oedema absorbed by fourth day.

young children slight pigmentation may remain for a month or two. In children of coloured race a patchy depigmentation may be seen but rarely persists beyond two or three weeks.

In the deeper *partial-thickness* (2nd degree) burn the dermis is involved to a variable depth and whether or not spontaneous healing will occur depends on the proportion of viable epithelial elements remaining. These are so scattered in the deep dermal burn that skin grafting is usually needed. Even in the less deep partial-thickness burns where trouble-free healing has occurred in rather less than two weeks, it is not uncommon to find hypertrophic scarring a few weeks later.

The *full-thickness* (3rd degree) burn has destroyed the whole depth of the dermis with possible damage to underlying deeper structures and healing can only occur in very small areas where epithelium can grow in from the periphery. Skin grafting will therefore be necessary in the great majority of these cases.

SYSTEMIC EFFECTS

The rapid loss of fluid from the damaged capillaries leads to a diminution in the volume of the circulation. This is at first countered by vasoconstriction and then by withdrawal of fluid from other areas of the body, leading to dehydration and thirst. The renal output falls with the drop in glomerular filtration rate and, if vasoconstriction is prolonged the kidney may suffer damage from anoxia. Continuing vasoconstriction may also affect the intestine so that absorption is prevented and vomiting may occur when the patient drinks. The amount of fluid lost and the degree of oligaemic shock is directly related to the extent of the burn. In small infants the surface area of the head is great in proportion to the rest of the body and the lax tissues of the face and neck allow considerable oedema formation so that shock is often very marked in these cases.

When the burn is extensive and deep there is some loss of red blood cells, not usually great in extent but sometimes sufficient to produce haemoglobinuria which is usually transient. At a later stage delayed haemolysis, the presence of extensive unhealed areas, blood loss at operations and nutritional problems may lead to a continuing anaemia which may hinder healing unless adequately treated.

Hypoproteinaemia will be encountered in the more extensive cases. The severe catabolic response occurring early after the injury is followed by continuing loss of protein in the exudate from the burn wound: if the patient is allowed to continue in negative nitrogen balance there will be rapid loss of weight accompanied by delayed healing and poor graft takes.

INFECTION

The susceptibility of the burn wound to infection is a major factor in influencing the survival of the burned child, and the wide variety of anti-bacterial agents and more sophisticated methods of combating cross-infection have had little effect in diminishing the size of the problem. Improved methods of treatment in the shock stage and a better understanding of metabolic requirements has led to the survival of the more extensively burned patients and the presence of these very large areas of skin destruction has increased the difficulties of limiting infection—which is now generally regarded as the most important single factor in mortality.

The haemolytic streptococcus does not present a common or serious problem nowadays, although minor outbreaks may occur in a burns unit, particularly at times when there is an increased carrier-rate in the general population. If it does become established on a burned surface it may cause delayed healing or graft failure.

Staphylococcus aureus will be present in the vast majority of cases although rarely giving rise to serious trouble. When large raw areas are extensively colonised there is the risk of invasive infection, and with the lowered defences in such cases septicaemia may occur. After death in an extensively burned child post-mortem examination may reveal the presence of multiple metastatic abscesses which have occurred in the terminal stages.

Gram-negative organisms include *Pseudomonas pyocyanea* and *Proteus vulgaris*, both of which tend to appear towards the end of the first week. They are more commonly encountered when closed dressings are used; and in those centres where exposure treatment is preferred they usually appear after the first grafting operation when the patient first goes into dressings. These organisms are difficult to eliminate and, as they give rise to large quantities of exudate, healing and graft takes may be seriously interfered with. Pseudomonas infection has presented an increasingly difficult problem in recent years and in certain centres a high incidence of septicaemia has been recorded. The outlook in these cases has been poor (Fig. **37**, 3) owing to the lack of an effective antibiotic, and many of the recent measures against burn wound sepsis which will be referred to later have been directed specifically against this organism.

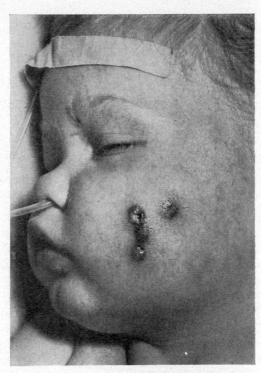

FIG. **37**, 3

Areas of skin gangrene which appeared shortly before death in a 2-year-old child who developed pseudomonas septicaemia.

E. coli is found as a contaminant of the burned surface more commonly in children than in adults but does not persist for long periods and does not usually present a serious problem. Care must be taken, however, to prevent urinary infection, particularly when an indwelling catheter has to be employed, and the the urine should be cultured at regular intervals.

TREATMENT

Immediately after admission any clothing or temporary dressings are removed and the extent of the burned area assessed. The child's weight should also be accurately determined at this point. In Roehampton intravenous replacement of circulating fluid is considered essential if the burn exceeds 12 per cent. of the body surface area in children (18 per cent. in adults). Infants with burns of lesser extent must be carefully watched and if adequate oral fluids cannot be given an intravenous drip must be considered. The variations in surface area of different parts of the body during growth must be taken into account in determining the extent of the burn and special charts should be referred to for this purpose (Table **37**, 1). Clinical appearance and blood pressure can be very misleading during the first few hours after burning, and if the burn exceeds 12 per cent. body surface area there must be no hesitation in setting up an intravenous drip.

Table **37**, 1

SURFACE AREA VALUES

Adults:—

Head and neck	9%
Trunk	34%
Upper limbs	19%
Lower limbs (including buttocks)	38%

Surface area modified for children

Age in years	1	2	3	4	5	6	7	8	9	10	11	12
Head and neck (%)	20	19	18	17	16	15	14	13	12	11	10	9
Trunk (%)	37	37	37	37	37	37	37	37	37	36	36	36
Upper limbs (%)	16	16	16	16	16	16	16	16	16	17	17	17
Lower limbs (%)	27	28	29	30	31	32	33	34	35	36	37	38

A suitable vein is chosen in the arm or leg, or the external jugular vein if the limbs are not available, and exposed by cutting down. Polythene tubing is preferred to any other type of cannula. In extensive burns there may be no alternative to cutting down on a vein through a burned area although, naturally, this is avoided wherever possible.

Restoration and maintenance of the blood volume throughout the period of continuing fluid loss must be achieved by the use of a colloid solution, and plasma is used for this purpose at most burns centres. The occasional case of hepatitis and questions concerning the availability and storage of plasma in conditions of mass disaster led to the introduction of dextran as a plasma substitute in treating burns. It has been used instead of plasma in our unit for 17 years and in some respects can be considered to be more efficient than plasma as the albumen content of the latter is more rapidly lost through the damaged capillaries than the larger dextran molecules. There have been no complications following the use of dextran, and the only practical difficulty is in blood grouping or cross-matching unless a blood sample is withdrawn before the administration of dextran is commenced. The recent introduction of dextran with a slightly lowered molecular weight (Dextran 110) with less tendency to rouleaux formation has led to fewer difficulties in cross-matching (Ricketts, 1966). The use of low-molecular dextran is not advised, although it has been recommended in some quarters for its possible beneficial effect on peripheral blood flow. However, it is lost very rapidly from the circulation and does not maintain the blood volume adequately for a sufficiently lengthy period.

In the extensive deep burn the early loss and the expected continuing destruction of red blood cells should be met by giving blood, and this may be given in quantities of up to one-quarter of the total colloid requirements during the first 48 hours. Apart from dextran (or plasma) and blood no other solutions are given and saline or other electrolyte solutions should not be considered necessary if restoration of the blood volume is efficiently carried out.

Metabolic requirements are met by giving oral fluids according to the child's age and weight. If this is not possible owing to vomiting or burns of the mouth or pharynx the appropriate amount of 5 per cent. glucose must then be given intravenously.

In assessing the amount of intravenous colloid required it must be remembered that fluid loss continues, although at a diminishing rate, for as long as 48 hours from the time of burning and the whole of this period must be covered. It is helpful, therefore, to have an initial estimate of the quantities which will probably be required and to vary them later according to the patient's clinical response and the effect on haemoconcentration. Many formulae have been devised for this purpose, taking into account the extent of the burn and the age and weight of the patient, The formula used at Roehampton has been used successfully for many years and is shown in Table **37**, 2.

Table **37**, 2

FLUID REPLACEMENT FORMULA IN CHILDREN

A. Burns less than 30% body surface area

	Birth–3 mths	*3–6 mths*	*6–9 mths*	*9–12 mths*	*1–2 yrs*	*2–3 yrs*	*3–4 yrs*	*4–5 yrs*	for each 1%
Dextran (ml)	15	21	24	27	30	42	48	54	

	5–6 yrs	*6–7 yrs*	*7–8 yrs*	*8–9 yrs*	*9–10 yrs*	*10–11 yrs*	*11–12 yrs*	for each 1%
Dextran (ml)	63	69	81	87	93	102	111	

The above figure multiplied by the % area of the burn gives the total quantity of dextran (or plasma if preferred) to be given during the 48 hours after burning as follows:—

$\frac{1}{3}$ in first 8 hours after burn
$\frac{1}{3}$ in next 16 hours
$\frac{1}{3}$ in final 24 hours.

B. Burns greater than 30% body surface area

Calculate 10% of body weight.
This gives the total quantity of dextran (or plasma) to be given during the 48 hours after burning as follows:—

$\frac{1}{2}$ in first 8 hours after burn
$\frac{1}{4}$ in next 16 hours
$\frac{1}{4}$ in final 24 hours.

Deep burns. Up to $\frac{1}{4}$ of total quantity may be given as whole blood in place of dextran.

For burns of less than 30 per cent. body surface area a quantity of dextran is given for each 1 per cent. of the burn and this varies according to the age of the child. For burns greater than 30 per cent. body surface area the amount given by this formula would exceed 10 per cent. of the body weight and we follow Wallace's recommendation (Kyle and Wallace, 1951) in limiting the total quantity at this level, at least for the initial estimate.

Haemoglobin levels and haematocrit readings are recorded every 2 hours during the first 10 to 12 hours and then 4-hourly until the end of the shock period. The rate at which the intravenous drip is being given may then be adjusted according to the rate at which haemoconcentration is being corrected. Fluid balance must be carefully recorded and this should be continued for several days beyond the shock period, an indwelling catheter being used for burns greater than 30 per cent. body surface area. The renal output will be low for the first 12 hours but will then gradually increase. Should the output remain persistently low (less than 8 to 10 ml/hour from birth to 4 years: 10 to 20 ml/hour from 4 to 12 years) any decision to increase the fluid dosage must only be made after considering other factors such as haemoconcentration and the general condition of the patient.

Care of the burned surface

Even with strict measures against cross-infection and the use of air-conditioned single cubicles it is difficult to prevent pathogenic organisms from gaining access to the burned surface. The use of occlusive dressings combined with topical antibiotics has met with limited success because of the warm, moist conditions under such dressings. As Wallace (1949) pointed out dryness, coolness and exposure to light are unfavourable to bacterial growth and if such conditions can be obtained on the burned surface then infection can be considerably reduced. Exposure treatment is regarded as the method of choice in Roehampton for burns of all degrees of severity and in patients of all ages. Its value in the treatment of children has been particularly apparent when contrasted with closed dressings which in burns of the lower part of the body in younger infants so often became contaminated with urine and faeces. The discomfort and irritation of such dressings and constant wriggling of the child added further trauma to the burned surface, and the unpleasant smell added to the problem of maintaining adequate nutrition.

Technique. After shock has been brought under control the burned areas are gently cleansed with warm cetrimide and chlorhexidine solution followed by isotonic saline. Blisters are opened, loose epithelium trimmed away with scissors and the whole area finally dried with gauze swabs. This cleansing process is performed in the patient's own bed either in the resuscitation room or cubicle, and general anaesthesia is not required. The child may be sedated with Nepenthe in the dose appropriate to the age.

In order to achieve adequate drying of the burned surface the child must be positioned so as to avoid any contact with the burn, either from bedding or some other part of the body. Where only one surface is involved this usually presents no great problem (Fig. **37**, 4) although a restless child may require splinting or some other form of restraint. A cradle carrying a sheet is then placed over the child as a protection from draughts but must be left open at both ends to allow drying. In extensive circumferential burns of the trunk the patient obviously has to lie on some part of the burned area which will therefore tend to become moist and liable to infection. Sectional mattresses and turning frames have been of limited value, and we have preferred to use for some years a special exposure frame (Evans, 1957 and 1966). This is surfaced with a plastic mesh on which are placed sheets of sterilised polyurethane foam and the patient is nursed directly in contact with the foam (Fig. **37**, 5). This allows evaporation from the burned surface through the foam and underlying mesh, and the drying process can be accelerated by placing a fan-heater

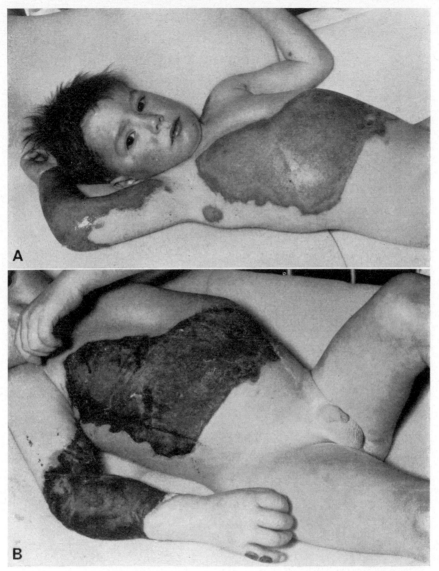

FIG. 37, 4
(A) Superficial scald in 2½-year-old boy. (B) Satisfactory coagulum six days later.

under the frame to maintain a current of slightly warmed dry air. Polyurethane foam is chemically inert and there is minimal adhesion to the damaged tissues. Adhesion can be further reduced by spraying the surface of the foam with silicone solution. The foam is sterilised by autoclaving and is changed daily, perhaps more frequently during the first few days when the exudate is greatest. Small frames which fit into the ordinary hospital cot are used for the smaller children (Fig. 37, 6).

As the burn dries a crust or coagulum forms which gradually deepens in colour to

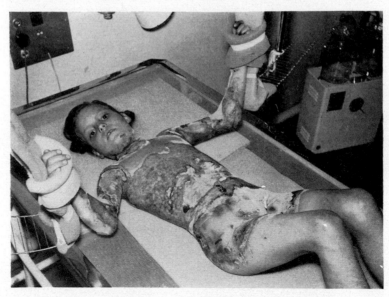

FIG. 37, 5
A 10-year-old girl with clothing burns of 31 per cent. body surface area nursed on polyurethane foam on frame.

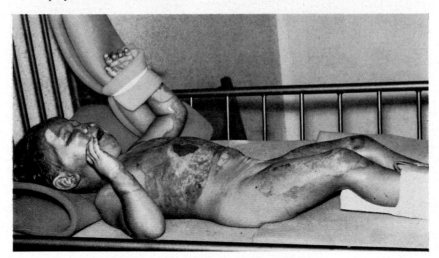

FIG. 37, 6
Small frame which fits into standard hospital cot.

a dark brown. In the superficial burn the crust is raised above the surface while in the deeper areas the coagulated tissue remains flat or even slightly contracted below the surface, a difference which becomes more apparent by the end of the first week and is a useful guide to the necessity for skin grafting. Some limitation of movement should be aimed at during the first few days to prevent the development of cracks in the coagulum. These are more likely to occur in the neighbourhood of joints and may be treated with an antibiotic powder (bacitracin and polymixin) or by inlaying strips of gauze impregnated with Furacin (nitrofurazone).

The face requires special attention, and lips and nostrils should be lightly coated with chlorhexidine cream. The eyes should be examined as early as possible before increasing oedema makes this more difficult, and if damage to the eye is suspected expert ophthalmological advice must be sought. The mouth and chin should be carefully cleaned of food debris and saliva after feeding and if it is found impossible to maintain a satisfactory coagulum a strip of Furacin gauze may be laid across the area. The neck creases in small babies will often remain moist and here again it may be necessary to use Furacin gauze.

Hands may be exposed in older children provided they are carefully elevated and positioned, and assuming there is expert nursing and physiotherapeutic supervision

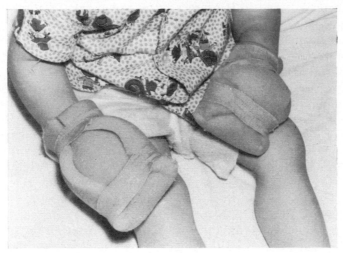

FIG. **37**, 7

In most burns centres closed dressings are preferred for all but older children, using tulle gras, gauze and cotton wool, with the hand bandaged as far as possible into the position of function. In younger children at Roehampton a compromise is achieved by enclosing the hand in a 'boxing glove' of polyurethane foam with foam wedges between the fingers, thus providing protection without too much maceration (Fig. **37**, 7).

Special consideration must be given to the deep encircling burn of the limb as this may produce a tourniquet effect and threaten the distal circulation. This is not due, as is sometimes supposed, to the formation of a coagulum by exposure but is the result of coagulation in depth at the time of burning. It is most likely to be seen at wrist or ankle, although sometimes extending to higher levels, and is usually marked by failure of oedema of hand or foot to subside in spite of elevation, and by continued pain. The constriction must be relieved by one or more vertical incisions through the eschar, no anaesthesia being required as the tissues are insensitive. As decompression occurs the incisions gape widely and there may be a short-lived venous ooze until the pressure subsides. A strip of Furacin gauze is then laid into the incision.

After a period of 12 to 14 days the coagulum of the less deep burn is ready to separate and may be cautiously removed with forceps and scissors. Earlier attempts at removal by the younger patient should be firmly discouraged and arm splints or the wearing of mittens may be advisable. Small adherent areas may be left for a few days further as it is usually clear at this stage that epithelialisation is going ahead satisfactorily.

Skin grafting

In the full-thickness and deeper partial-thickness burns surgical resurfacing will be necessary. With closed dressing techniques the necrotic tissue formed a moist slough and this was allowed to separate gradually, the process being aided by keeping the dressings moist or by the application of eusol compresses. The liability to infection was thereby increased, and in the larger burns some deterioration in the patient's general condition was inevitable. Chemical debridement by enzymes and other agents has also proved disappointing, largely because of failure to digest the tough collagen element of the slough.

Surgical removal of the necrotic areas is preferred in our unit and in most cases this is performed at about the fourteenth day after burning. The exposed areas can be kept reasonably dry in most patients up until this point, but from then onwards softening and infection of the slough is more likely to occur. The child's general condition has usually reached a satisfactory level at this time, but is likely to deteriorate if large necrotic areas are allowed to remain. In the more extensive cases it will be realised that the operation makes great demands on the patient and every effort must be made to ensure that he comes to the theatre in the best possible state. Haemoglobin levels will have been checked frequently, and if necessary a 'topping-up' blood transfusion will be given two or three days beforehand. Further quantities of blood are cross-matched and made available for the operation itself. If at all possible the diet will have been increased for two or three days to allow for diminished intake in the immediate post-operate period. Antibiotic cover is not given as a routine but the sensitivity of the organisms present should be known in case postoperative treatment becomes necessary. Pre-operative antibiotics may be given in certain special circumstances. If the haemolytic streptococcus is present penicillin should be commenced the day preceding operation, if indeed the patient is not already receiving it. In the case of the full-thickness burn involving more than 30 per cent. of the body surface area and which is growing a heavy culture of pseudomonas pyocyanea there is a real risk of invasive infection by this organism and a course of carbenicillin should be commenced as soon as the organism is identified.

Where skin donor sites are limited the necessary arrangements for obtaining homografts will have been made, either from suitable donors or from the skin bank where such facilities are available.

The operation is preferably divided into a 'dirty' and a 'clean' stage.

1. The burned surfaces are thoroughly cleansed with warm cetrimide-chlorhexidine solution followed by warm saline. Necrotic tissue is now removed starting with areas of raised coagulum which are carefully lifted off. The flat end of a Howarth's elevator slipped under the edge of the coagulum is particularly useful for this purpose. In deep

dermal burns a cleavage level is often found, and here blunt dissection aided by occasional snips of the scissors permits rapid stripping with very little bleeding. In younger infants forceful stripping must be avoided in this process as adherent co-agulum may readily tear away the soft and almost friable subcutaneous fat. The deeper areas of full-thickness destruction will require sharp dissection, scissors or scalpel being used for small areas. For extensive deep areas a widely-set Humby knife is much more rapid and efficient although several horizontal slices may have to be excised to ensure a uniformly viable surface. As each area is cleared of necrotic material warm saline packs are applied to stop bleeding. When the whole procedure is complete, further cleansing with fresh cetrimide-chlorhexidine solution is carried out and the whole area again covered with warm saline packs. Mackintoshes and towels are now removed and the patient placed on a clean mackintosh. All dirty materials, swabs, dressing bins, trolleys, bowls, etc., are removed from the theatre and the floor swabbed clean. Gowns and gloves are changed in readiness for the next stage.

2. Trolleys with grafting instruments and dressings are now brought into the theatre for the 'clean' phase. Skin preparation of donor sites is carried out and these areas towelled off. Thighs and calves are the preferred sites but in most extensive cases choice is limited to such undamaged areas of the trunk and limbs as are available. Thin split-skin grafts are necessary, firstly because the thinner grafts have a better chance of survival in adverse conditions, and secondly, because the donor sites heal rapidly and will permit further crops of skin to be cut after about $2\frac{1}{2}$ to 3 weeks. The Braithwaite knife with roller adjustable for variable depths and using disposable blades is used in most cases, but for the more extensive burns the Brown electric dermatome will cut very large areas with great speed and efficiency. When cutting grafts free-hand great care is needed in babies and small infants even when a guarded knife is used. The combination of a thin dermis with thick rolls of sub-cutaneous fat can be very treacherous, and accidental penetration of the dermis may allow the subcutaneous fat to bulge through almost as if under pressure. Careful suture is necessary should this occur but this may not prevent the formation of a hypertrophic linear scar. After the grafts are cut the donor sites are dressed with tulle gras, gauze, cotton wool and crepe bandage. If this is not immediately possible owing to the presence of adjacent burned areas warm saline packs are applied to limit bleeding until the whole area can be dressed. Grafts are spread on sheets of tulle gras for ease of handling and then cut into various shapes and sizes as required. Ideally large sheets should be used to secure complete coverage but this is only possible when the burned areas are not very extensive. Usually the larger sheets are applied to priority areas such as the face, front of neck, hands and the flexor surfaces of the large joints. The remaining areas are covered with strips or patches of skin placed 0·5 to 1 cm apart. The growing edges of a large number of discontinuous grafts will enable epithelialisation of large areas to go ahead quite rapidly and with the most economical use of limited quantities of autograft skin. The cosmetic result is somewhat inferior but has to be accepted particularly in resurfacing large 'silent' areas of the trunk or thighs. Patch grafts are also advisable when infected granulations have to be covered as this will permit the escape of exudate and limit the amount of possible graft loss.

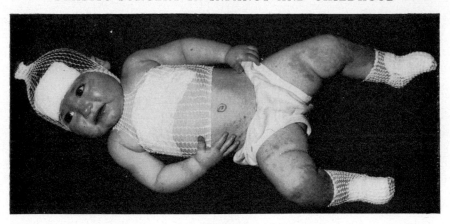

Fig. 37, 8

Large sheets are anchored with a few sutures but strips and patches are held in place with sheets of tulle gras.

Grafts do extremely well if they can be left exposed, but this is of limited value in children. Grafts on the face are routinely exposed, and in many cases grafts on the anterior surface of the trunk can also be left open although arms may have to be restrained to prevent interference. Dressings are usually necessary on the limbs, and when axillae or groins are involved plaster of Paris splints are applied over the dressings to limit movements in these areas where grafts are easily dislodged. On the trunk and limbs the macerating effect of a bulky dressing may often be avoided by covering the grafts with a layer of tulle gras and perhaps a single layer of gauze held in place by Netelast (Fig. 37, 8).

While in the majority of cases desloughing and skin grafting are performed at the same operation, in certain cases the application of grafts may be deferred to a second stage. This may be advisable if the patient's general condition has been so poor that in the anaesthetist's opinion the procedure should cease after the stage of excision, or if there are doubts concerning the degree of infection or the viability of the recipient sites. If this is decided upon, Furacin dressings are applied to the excised areas and the grafting operation performed a few days later.

Homografts. Skin grafts taken from another individual will take initially just as well as the patient's own skin but will be rejected after about $2\frac{1}{2}$ to 3 weeks. In a child with extensive raw areas the temporary cover obtained in this way can be of great value in limiting fluid and protein loss and in minimising infection. Where a moderate amount of autograft skin is available this can be used for priority sites and homografts used to cover other areas until the autograft donor sites are sufficiently stable for a second crop. Another method of diluting the autograft skin is to apply alternating strips of autografts and homografts as described by Jackson (1954). With this technique (Fig. 37, 9) the outgrowing epithelium from the autografts gradually replaces the homografts and the area eventually requiring regrafting is greatly reduced. Skin is often donated by a parent or other relative, but this can give rise to the unhappy situation where an extensively burned child fails to survive operation while the parent

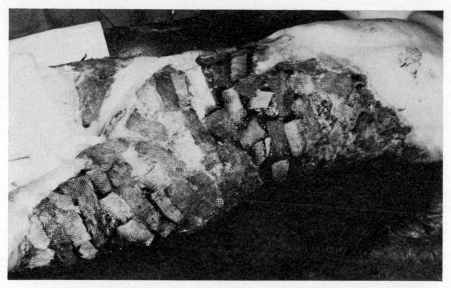

FIG. **37**, 9
Autografts (lighter colour) mixed with homografts.

has to remain in hospital until the donor site heals. At Roehampton we have preferred to use skin from our own skin-bank, and the necessary quantities can often be obtained from patients undergoing abdominal lipectomy or reduction mammaplasty. Skin obtained in this way is stored in a refrigerator at 4°C. Cadaver skin has been used on an increasing scale in recent years, both in the fresh state and after freeze-drying which permits prolonged storage but is rather less effective as the lyophilised graft can only provide dead cover. The increased availability of homograft skin from such sources has led to interesting developments in technique such as the application of homografts for short periods of up to a week followed by their removal and replacement by a fresh set. This not only helps to stabilise the patient's general con-dition but it is also claimed that the granulating surface is kept in the best possible state to receive the patient's own skin when this becomes available.

POSTOPERATIVE CARE

If a transfusion has been given it may be advisable to continue with intravenous glucose saline for 24 hours to cover any deficiencies of oral intake during this period. Any necessary antibiotics can be given in the drip, and before the cannula is removed the haemoglobin level should be checked in case further blood is needed.

Dressings are normally changed on the fourth or fifth postoperative day although the outer layers may need replacing before this if they become excessively moist or if there is contamination with urine or faeces. Hyperpyrexia is occasionally seen when extensive bulky dressings have been applied and these will then have to be removed completely or in part. The first postoperative dressing change is normally carried out under sedation but in the more extensive cases anaesthesia will be needed, particularly if only partial skin cover of large raw areas has been possible.

PS T

General treatment

A high-protein high-calorie diet is considered necessary because of the early catabolic response and the continuing loss of protein in the exudate from the burned areas. Failure to maintain adequate intake will be reflected in progressive loss of weight, increased susceptibility to infection, delayed healing and poor graft takes. The burned child is usually a poor eater, and care should be taken in finding out his normal likes and dislikes. When a child is proving to be particularly difficult in this respect it is often helpful if the mother can be present to assist in feeding. In many cases, however, reliance must be placed on supplementary liquid feeds in addition to such solid food as the child will take. Complan (Glaxo) has been found acceptable in most cases although it occasionally causes diarrhoea. The reduced activities of a child confined to bed lowers its energy requirements, and recent studies by Sutherland and Batchelor (1966) have supported earlier suggestions by other workers that the protein and calorie needs of the burned child are no greater than in normal health. It is vitally important, however, that these levels are maintained consistently and it is necessary to aim at an intake above normal to allow for anaesthetics and repeated dressing procedures. Accurate weight charts must be kept, and a bed-weighing machine may be found helpful, particularly with the larger children.

Haemoglobin levels should not be allowed to fall, and in children with extensive burns repeated blood transfusions will be needed, usually given at the time of further grafting operations or dressings under anaesthesia. To aid erythropoiesis colloidal iron is given daily. The diet is further supplemented by one of the vitamin-containing syrups and an additional 300 mg of ascorbic acid daily.

Prevention of infection

In the initial stages the child should be nursed in isolation in a separate cubicle at least until a dry coagulum is formed. Attending staff and visitors should be gowned and masked and the normal requirements of barrier nursing followed. Swabs for bacteriological culture will have been obtained on admission from nose, throat and rectum as well as from the burned surface. Further wound swabs should be taken at least twice weekly and the antibiotic sensitivity of contaminating organisms ascertained. Nose and throat swabs are obtained weekly from the staff, and in any centre where burns are regularly treated bacteriological monitoring of the environment is a necessary routine.

In recent years the problem of cross-infection in the treatment of burns has received increasing attention. In most new burns centres patients are nursed in specially designed cubicles supplied with filtered air under positive pressure and with control of temperature and humidity. The nursing of burned patients in ventilated plastic isolators (Haynes and Hench, 1966) goes a step further in providing protection against contamination, and although presenting certain nursing difficulties encouraging results have been obtained (Cason et al., 1966).

The application of moist compresses of 0·5 per cent. silver nitrate (Moyer et al., 1965) has been shown to have considerable prophylactic value against pseudomonas pyocyanea contamination (Cason et al., 1966). The treatment should be commenced from the day of admission as it has little effect on established infection, and serum electrolyte levels should be carefully watched as deaths in children have been reported from electrolyte disturbances.

Sulfamylon (p-aminomethylbenzene sulphonamide) applied in a thick cream to the entire burned surface has also been shown to be of value in reducing burn wound sepsis, and in particular the incidence of pseudomonas infection. (Lindberg *et al.*, 1965). The sulfamylon acetate now available is less painful when applied than the original sulfamylon hydrochloride which also had the disadvantage of producing hyperchloraemia. To be effective the cream must be washed off and reapplied at least once a day.

Antibiotics. Penicillin is given for the first five days after admission and broad spectrum antibiotics reserved for later use. Apart from early respiratory complications indications for such further treatment are not usually encountered until the end of the second week. Erythromycin, tetracycline or cloxacillin may then be considered according to the sensitivity of the organisms present. Serious infection with pseudomonas pyocyanea has been difficult to treat and has been associated with a high mortality. The position has recently improved following the introduction of two new antibiotics, carbenicillin and gentamicin. In the absence of a positive blood culture we prefer to give carbenicillin, and to reserve gentamicin, with its risk of vestibular nerve damage, for the patient with septicaemia.

Respiratory tract damage

Damage to the respiratory tract is relatively infrequent but response to treatment is often poor and the mortality is high. It is usually the result of inhalation of irritant fumes and products of combustion which may occur when a child is trapped in a burning room or building. Burns around the mouth and nose are often associated. When rescue has been delayed there may be rapid death from oxygen lack or the child may reach hospital unconscious and die shortly afterwards. Carbon monoxide poisoning may be present and in these circumstances hyperbaric oxygen treatment may present the only hope of survival.

In the presence of respiratory tract damage tracheostomy will be indicated if there are signs of respiratory distress, and will facilitate intermittent suction to remove secretions. Particular care is needed when suction is being carried out as the tip of the catheter may readily damage the hyperaemic mucosa. It has been suggested that tracheostomy should be performed when there is presumed respiratory tract damage and before actual distress supervenes, but the present tendency is towards a conservative approach in view of the real risk of introducing pathogenic organisms from the upper respiratory tract to the lower respiratory tree.

Oedema of face and neck without inhalational damage may present an alarming appearance but is unlikely to cause obstruction, and although these cases must be carefully watched we have rarely found tracheostomy to be necessary (Fig. **37**, 10). The deep circumferential burn of the trunk deserves special attention as movement of chest and upper abdomen may be severely restricted, and this has been regarded as an important indication for early excision (Jackson *et al.*, 1960). Bronchopneumonia may sometimes occur in younger children within the first few days after burning, and not infrequently there is a history of upper respiratory infection present at the

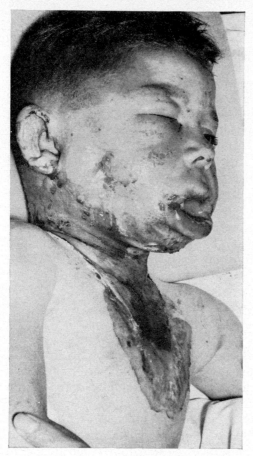

FIG. 37, 10

Deep burn of chin and neck with considerable oedema but not causing respiratory obstruction.

time of the accident. It usually responds satisfactorily to treatment unless the burn itself is very extensive.

Complicating factors

The common *infectious diseases* of childhood may introduce complicating factors, and unexpected swings of temperature, anorexia, vomiting or other symptoms may cause disquiet until the cause is established. A less usual example was provided by a child of 15 months admitted with scalds of 17 per cent. body surface area who developed a high fever two or three days later and whose general condition by the sixth day was causing concern. Investigations, including chest and abdominal X-rays, blood and stool cultures, were negative and although the staphylococcus was present on his burns invasive infection did not seem likely. He then developed multiple discrete, umbilicated vesicles on his face (Fig. 37, 11) and it was apparent that he was suffering from vaccinia; he had been vaccinated against smallpox a few days before his accident! He responded satisfactorily to intra-muscular postvaccinial gamma globulin and his burns subsequently healed following skin-grafting without any difficulty. There was no residual scarring from the vaccinial lesions.

Encephalopathy in burned children has been described by Emery and Reid (1962), and they reported deaths from raised intracranial pressure in patients with burns of moderate extent where overhydration could be excluded and electrolyte disturbances were not present. While the aetiology in these cases is obscure, cerebral oedema may also be encountered following anoxia as in the case of a 9-year-old boy who was rescued from a burning house and had sustained burns of 34 per cent. body surface area (Fig. 37, 12). His father, who repeatedly went into the house to rescue the boy and other children, died of carbon monoxide poisoning. By the fifth day the patient's blood pressure was 220/150 mm Hg, temperature 40°C (104°F), and he became semi-comatose with frequent convulsions. He was treated by hypothermia, his temperature being reduced to 31°C (88°F) by external ice packs for a period of 18 hours, general anaesthesia mainly with nitrous oxide and oxygen being maintained throughout that period (Jeffs *et al.*, 1966). On rewarming there were no further complications and skin-grafting and healing followed the normal course.

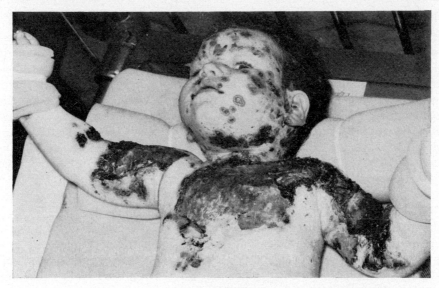

FIG. 37, 11
Vaccinial lesions which appeared seven days after burning.

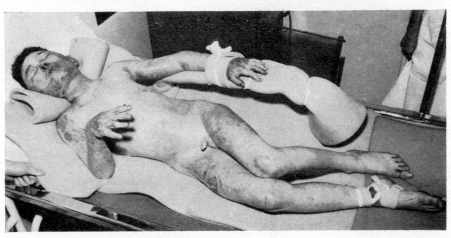

FIG. 37, 12
A 9-year-old boy who developed cerebral oedema which was successfully treated by hypothermia.

The *psychological effects* on a child of a burning accident and the necessary hospital treatment that follows may be great, and the high incidence of emotional problems in burned children admitted to the Birmingham Burns Unit was emphasised by Joan Woodward (1959). Children suffering from even minor burns will tend to regress to babyhood, and reversion to bed-wetting and thumb-sucking is common. Regular visiting by parents should be encouraged and considerable benefit can be achieved by enlisting the aid of the hospital social worker (Woodward and Jackson, 1961).

Mortality

Death from oligaemia or renal failure is rare when early and adequate treatment has been carried out. There were 19 deaths in a series of 714 burned children admitted to the Roehampton Unit from April 1959 to March 1968, and none of these died from oligaemia or renal failure. In six fatal cases respiratory complications were predominant, death occurring early, on average at 6·6 days, and in the younger children, average age being 1 year 10 months. The average extent of the burn was 30 per cent body surface area. Infection was responsible for 11 deaths, these occurring later, on average at 26·5 days, and in older children whose average age was 3 years 11 months. The burns were more severe, the average extent being 48·4 per cent body surface area.

Surgical Problems

Hypertrophic scarring

Healing of partial-thickness burns is often followed in children by hypertrophic scarring, and this may also be seen in deeper burns at the periphery of skin grafts, sometimes producing a checker-board pattern when patch grafts have been used. Over a period of several weeks after healing, the scarred area, at first flat and soft,

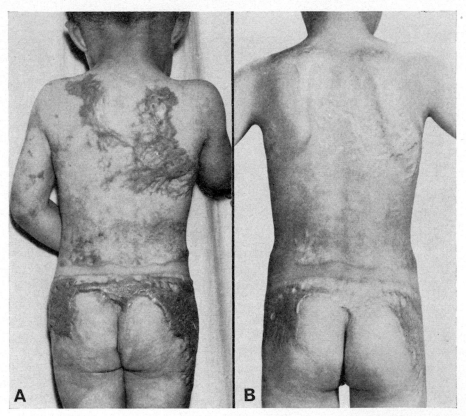

Fig. 37, 13
Gradual decrease in post-burn scarring.

becomes thickened and raised with a red, shiny surface (Fig. **37**, 13A). This is accompanied by intense irritation, usually worse when the child is warm in bed. It reaches its peak by about the third month and then over a further three to six months the irritation becomes less severe and gradually the scarring becomes paler and eventually flatter over a period of a year or more (Fig. **37**, 13B). Parents will need reassuring that this form of scarring commonly follows healing and that gradual resolution will certainly occur. Although plastic surgery may eventually be needed for the correction of residual defects it should be made clear that any form of surgery during the acute phase is contraindicated and may increase the severity of the scarring. Pruritis may be eased by the application of calamine lotion or Eurax lotion or cream. When the irritation is very intense sedatives may be necessary to enable the child, and the parents, to get some sleep.

Face

The upper half of the face is less commonly involved in children and then usually in scalding accidents when the damage is superficial and skin grafting rarely needed.

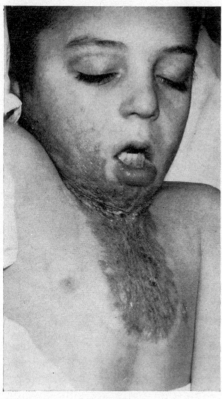

FIG. **37**, 14
Early neck contracture 2½ months after burning.

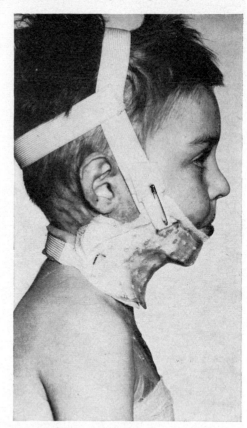

FIG **37**, 15
After release of neck contracture.

Deep flame burns are usually the result of clothing catching fire and tend to involve the lower half of the face and neck (Fig. **37**, 10). Eyelid burns are therefore less frequently encountered than in adults and skin cover to the lids is not often necessary. Should the lids be involved every care must be taken to prevent exposure of the cornea. If the coagulum prevents full lid closure the eye should be protected with chloramphenicol ointment until the coagulum separates. If there is full-thickness skin loss split-skin grafts will be applied initially to secure healing. These early grafts will contract and will have to be replaced within two or three weeks using the standard technique for correction of ectropion in which the grafts are applied, raw surface outwards, over stent moulds. The upper lids are resurfaced first with split-skin grafts and the lower lids repaired later preferably with post-auricular Wolfe grafts.

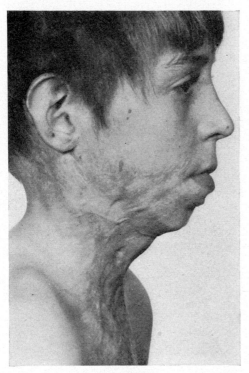

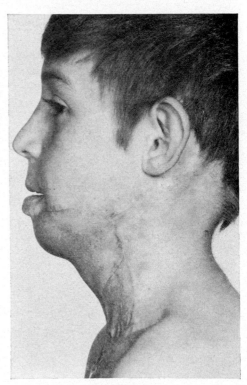

FIG. **37**, 16
After release of neck contracture.

FIG. **37**, 17
Later replacement of skin graft by a tube pedicle flap.

Neck

Burns of the front of the neck commonly lead to some degree of contracture and in some cases this may develop extremely rapidly. Even when early grafting has been followed by trouble-free healing it is sometimes difficult in children to control the position of the neck by splinting, particularly while the grafts are still unstable (Fig. **37**, 14). When stable healing has been achieved the contracture is released and medium-thickness skin grafts inserted. An accurately-fitting plastic splint is then worn for several months (Fig. **37**, 15 and **37**, 16). Although eventual repair by a skin flap may be considered desirable for appearance or function (Fig. **37**, 17) preliminary release by free grafts is necessary in children not only to gain time but to make future anaesthetics less difficult.

Hands

Burns of the dorsal surface of the hand may occur in association with clothing burns, but in general are seen less frequently than in adults. Burns of the flexor surface may occur in the same way but perhaps the most common variety is the deep contact burn, the most severe of these resulting from grasping the elements of an electric fire (Figs. **37**, 18 and **37**, 19).

While primary excision is sometimes advocated for deep burns of the hand or fingers it is often difficult at the outset to be certain of the depth of the injury and there

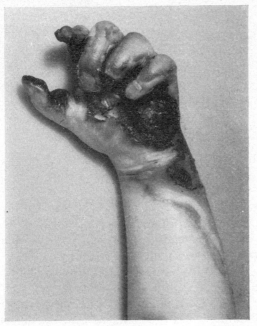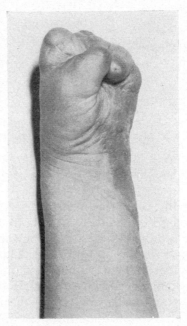

FIGS. **37**, 18 and **37**, 19
Severe electric fire burn with multiple loss of digits.

may be difficult decisions concerning tendon exposure. Primary skin flap closure is not a practical proposition in this type of case. By delaying surgery for 12 to 14 days healing will be well advanced in the less deep areas and the necrotic tissues of the full-thickness burn can be excised with confidence and skin grafts applied. When tendon or bone is exposed a conservative approach should be adopted and dressings continued as granulation tissue gradually reduces the area of the exposed structure. Grafts are applied to the encroaching granulations and dead bone and tendon removed as they are ready to separate. Splints should be applied after grafting and the fingers kept in extension for a period of six weeks. Forcible extension must be avoided, and

PS U

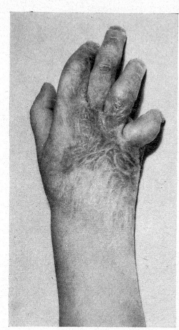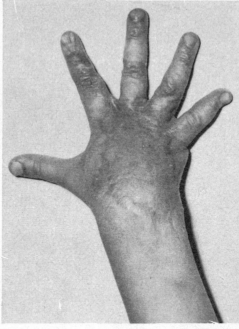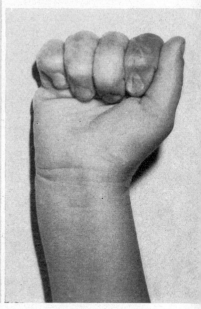

FIGS. **37**, 20 to **37**, 22
Contraction of extensor surface repaired with medium-thickness split-skin graft.

if splinting in full extension cannot be achieved this must be accepted as otherwise the skin may remain unstable and any further delay in healing may increase the deposition of deep scar tissue.

A period of at least six months should elapse before correction of scar contractures, particularly when there have been active hypertrophic changes. Contractures of the dorsum are relatively uncommon in children and do not present great problems in repair (Figs. **37**, 20 to **37**, 22). Under tourniquet the scar tissue is excised so as to allow maximal correction of the deformity and planned to avoid marginal scars in undesirable sites which might produce linear contractures. Web spaces may need release but lateral capsulotomy of the metacarpo-phalangeal joints is rarely necessary in children. A medium-thickness split-skin graft is then sutured into the defect with interdigitation of the edges where necessary.

The most severe flexion contractures follow electric fire burns involving the distal palm and extending on to the flexor surfaces of the fingers. Even when early and successful skin-grafting has been followed by careful splinting a large proportion of cases will require reparative surgery (Figs. **37**, 23 and **37**, 24). These injuries commonly occur at the age of 2 or 3 years at a period when there is rapid growth of the hand, and this tends to accentuate the deformity. Several operations may be needed to achieve full and stable correction and parents should be warned of this possibility during the period of initial treatment. As skin flap repair is rarely possible in these small children with multiple digital involvement careful dissection is needed to achieve maximal correction without exposure of flexor tendons. Because of this, only

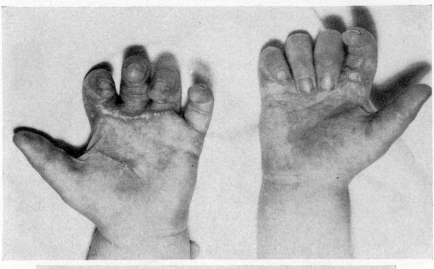

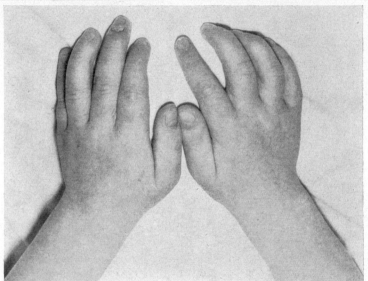

FIGS. 37, 23 and 37, 24

Bilateral flexion contractures which required several reparative operations before stable correction was achieved.

partial correction may at first be possible and further skin grafts will have to be added after an interval of six months to a year. Postoperative control of the position of these small digits is best obtained by the plastic 'sandwich' splint made in two halves from impressions taken of the flexor and extensor surfaces of the hand and held together by four screws (Figs. 37, 25 to 37, 27). This splint is worn continuously for six weeks and at night for a further four weeks. Parents are instructed in its application so that it may be removed for washing and powdering of the hand. Splinting may well be continued for longer periods than this but, although joint stiffness is not a

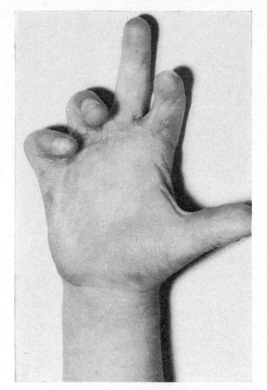

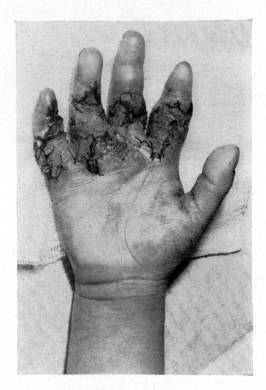

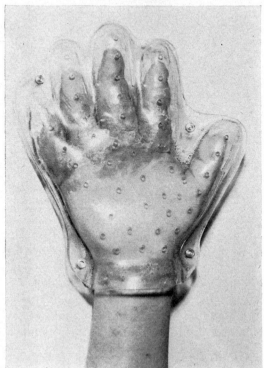

FIGS. **37**, 25 to **37**, 27
Release of flexion contracture followed by
application of plastic 'sandwich' splint.

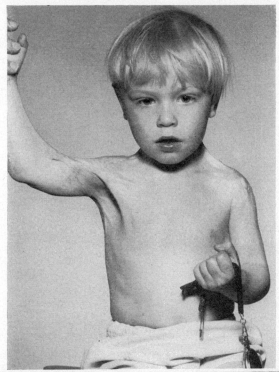

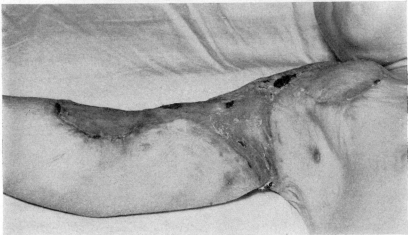

FIGS. 37, 28 and 37, 29
'Tri-radiate' contracture extending into axilla, cubital fossa and side of neck. Contracture bands released and split-skin graft let into the defect.

problem in children, use of the hand is necessary for full muscular development of the limb and nervous control of function. For this reason it is perhaps better to avoid very lengthy periods of immobilisation even at the expense of some degree of recurrence of contracture which may eventually need further release.

Scar contractures

Apart from the special situations described above these commonly occur over the front of the elbow, back of the knee, and in the axillae and groins. Release by Z-plasty alone is rarely adequate owing to the diffuse nature of the scarring and it is almost always necessary to add skin. In most cases free grafts will be suitable and they are inserted following division of scar bands and incision of the margins of the defect to

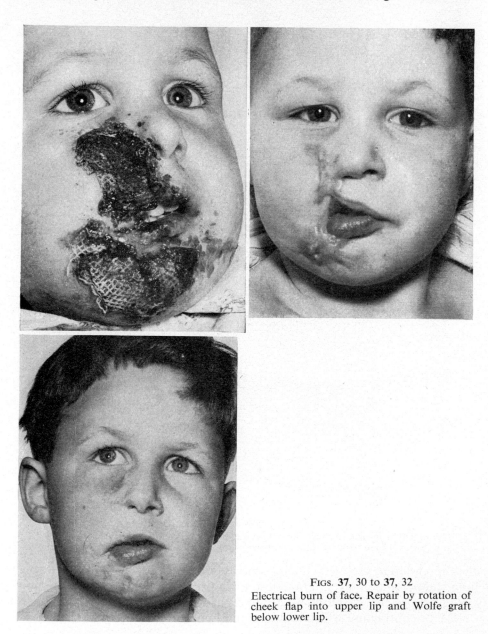

FIGS. **37**, 30 to **37**, 32
Electrical burn of face. Repair by rotation of cheek flap into upper lip and Wolfe graft below lower lip.

secure full correction (Figs. **37**, 28 and **37**, 29). Special attention must be paid to scarring of the anterior chest in female children, and they should be followed up into puberty to ensure that breast development is not interfered with. In most cases the overlying scar tissue softens and stretches with the growth of breast tissue, but there may be tightness extending from an axillary contracture or tethering of the lower pole by scar tissue, either or both of which will require release and insertion of additional skin.

ELECTRICAL BURNS

The passage of an electric current through the tissues may cause serious deep destruction, often involving bones, joints, tendons and nerves. Blood vessels, because of their conductivity, are readily damaged and thrombosis adds to the amount of necrosis and

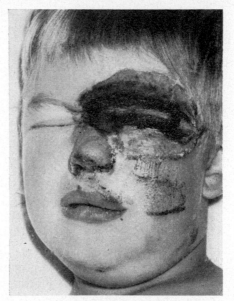

FIG. 37, 33
Live-rail electrical burn with destruction of left orbit.

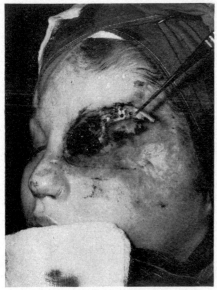

FIG. 37, 34
Forehead flap was brought down on twelfth day to cover nasal bones. Bony roof of orbit left to sequestrate while abdominal tube pedicle was prepared.

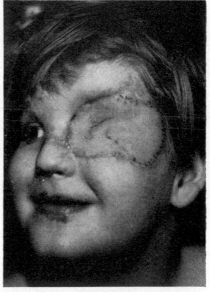

FIG. 37, 35
Cover of left orbit by tube pedicle flap. Later provided with prosthesis worn on spectacle frame.

predisposes to the slow healing which is characteristic of these injuries. Children are most likely to come into contact with the domestic electrical supply (220–250 V) and it is the hands which are most frequently affected. These injuries are treated in our unit on conservative lines, excision and grafting being performed at about 14 days. Amputation of digits, complete or partial, is sometimes necessary, particularly if digital vessels have been directly involved. The face is not often affected, but a small child may put the end of a live wire into the mouth causing intra-oral scarring and sometimes microstoma.

Outside the home more serious injuries may follow contact with higher voltage supplies, not infrequently the electric railway (660 V D.C.). In the case shown in Figure 37, 30, the result of contact with the live rail, advantage was taken of the scar alongside the nose (Fig. 37, 31) to rotate a cheek flap into the upper lip (Fig. 37, 32). In another live-rail accident a 7-year-old boy put his face down to the rail to listen for approaching trains and this resulted in complete destruction of the left orbit and its contents (Fig. 37, 33). After a short period of loss of consciousness he remained reasonably well until on the seventh day he developed meningitis which, however, responded satisfactorily to treatment. On the twelfth day the necrotic tissues were excised and a forehead flap brought down to cover the exposed but viable nasal bones and to make good the soft tissue loss which extended to the inner canthus of his remaining eye. It was decided to await sequestration of the bony roof of the orbit and during this period an abdominal tube pedicle flap was raised and then attached to his left wrist. Eventually, five months after the injury, the dead bone was removed and the flap inset to the defect (Figs. 37, 34 and 37, 35).

A. J. Evans

ACKNOWLEDGMENTS

My thanks for the photographic illustrations are due to Mr E. B. Ferrill, Department of Medical Illustration, Queen Mary's Hospital, Roehampton.

The following illustrations have appeared in previous publications and are reproduced here with permission. Figure 37, 2 from Rob and Smith, 1964, *Clinical Surgery*, London: Butterworth; Figure 37, 5 from Matthews, 1963, *Recent Advances in the Surgery of Trauma*, London: Churchill; Figure 37, 7 from Wallace and Wilkinson, 1966, *Research in Burns*, Edinburgh: Livingstone; Figure 37, 12 from Jeffs *et al.*, 1966, *British Journal of Plastic Surgery*, **19**, 361.

REFERENCES

Cason, J. S., Jackson, D. M., Lowbury, E. J. L. & Ricketts, C. R. (1966). *Br. med. J.* **2**, 1288.
Emery, J. L. & Reid, D. A. C. (1962). *Br. J. Surg.* **50**, 53.
Evans, A. J. (1957). *Br. med. J.* **1**, 547.
Evans, A. J. (1966). In *Research in Burns*. Ed. Wallace, A. B. & Wilkinson, A. W. Edinburgh: Livingstone.
Haynes, B. W. & Hench, M. E. (1966). In *Research in Burns*. Ed. Wallace, A. B. & Wilkinson, A. W. Edinburgh: Livingstone.
Jackson, D. M. (1954). *Br. J. plast. Surg.* **7**, 26.
Jackson, D. M., Topley, E., Cason, J. S. & Lowbury, E. J. L. (1960). *Ann. Surg.* **152**, 167.
Jeffs, J. V., Edwards, G. E. & Hoyle, J. R. (1966). *Br. J. plast. Surg.* **19**, 361.
Kyle, M. J. & Wallace, A. B. (1951). *Br. J. plast. Surg.* **3**, 144.
Lindberg, R. B., Moncrief, J. A., Switzer, W. E., Order, S. E. & Mills, W. (1965). *J. Trauma* **5**, 601.
Moyer, C. A., Brentano, L., Gravens, D. L., Margraf, H. W. & Monafo, W. W. (1965). *Archs Surg.* **90**, 812.
Ricketts, C. R. (1966). *Br. med. J.* **2**, 1423.
Sutherland, A. B. & Batchelor, A. D. R. (1966). In *Research in Burns*. Ed. Wallace, A. B. & Wilkinson, A. W. Edinburgh: Livingstone.
Wallace, A. B. (1949). *Br. J. plast. Surg.* **1**, 232.
Woodward, J. (1959). *Br. med. J.* **1**, 1009.
Woodward, J. & Jackson, D. M. (1961). *Br. J. plast. Surg.* **13**, 316.

CHAPTER XXXVIII

KELOIDS AND HYPERTROPHIC SCARS

A keloid (Greek: *Chele-oid*—like a crab's claw) is a tumour-like growth resulting from trauma to the skin, it is characterised by excessive fibroplasia extending outwith the confines of the original injury and showing little or no tendency to resolve. A hypertrophic scar on the other hand is confined to the area of injury and resolves very slowly. In clinical practice there is considerable merging from one to the other and the symptoms and degree of disfigurement may be similar.

Keloid is a more common entity in children than in adults (Garb and Stone, 1942). The causation is trauma, often thermal, surgical incisions, insect bites and vaccinations. Extensive keloids have been seen in Japanese children sustaining post atomic bomb burns but there is no definite proof to incriminate radiation in other circumstances. Dark-skinned races are more prone to keloid development than those with fair complexions. In the adult there is a predilection for the presternal and deltoid areas and also the ear lobes but no such well-marked distribution is seen in the child, the fore-arm and lower limb being frequently involved. The lesions may be multiple, but the fact that a keloid has developed once does not of necessity mean that this will always be the case. Nevertheless, the entity of the 'keloid former' does exist and should be borne in mind when faced with an operation on a child who has previously formed a keloid.

The appearance is that of a red, raised, hairless mass, having a sharp cut off at its junction with normal skin. The overlying epithelium is atrophic, being thin and shiny, the underlying vascular fibrous tissue has a vaguely translucent quality. Often there is evidence of superficial traumatisation due to scratching. On close examination telangectasia may be seen. The older lesion may be somewhat paler and flatter. On the presternal area the shape assumed is commonly that of a dumb-bell or butterfly.

Many keloids are asymptomatic especially in adults; children however are more troubled occasionally by pain, but much more frequently by itching. This is particularly so when they are warm in bed and may cause sleeplessness; pain on the other hand is associated with a cold environment.

The pathology of a keloid is related to the normal healing phase of a wound. In the latter fibroplasia is followed by resolution whereas in keloid the fibroplasia proceeds in an uncontrolled fashion showing little tendency to resolve.

Microscopically thick homogeneously eosinophilic bands of collagen are seen, mixed with thinner collagen fibres and large active fibroblasts. Sweat glands, sebaceous glands and arrectores pylorum muscles are atrophic or replaced by scar.

In 1966 Ohmori showed that dermatone grafts cut at 12 thousandths of an inch never caused keloids, while at 15 thousandths of an inch scattered keloids resulted and at 20 thousandths of an inch they invariably occurred. His explanation for this was that the dermis contains fine and coarse collagen: at 12 thousandths of an inch only the fine fibres are cut through whereas at 15 thousandths of an inch the coarse fibres are partly cut into and at 20 thousandths there are only coarse collagen fibres present. In addition the more superficial wounds healed in less than three weeks compared with those of 20 thousandths of an inch which took four to five weeks.

TREATMENT

The treatment of keloid and resistant hypertrophic scarring is the same, the latter of course will resolve eventually but often one wishes to speed up the process of resolution, sometimes for symptomatic and sometimes for cosmetic reasons.

In the early stages when the exact diagnosis is often uncertain, symptomatic measures alone are called for, particularly when the child is being kept awake at night or is becoming a social embarrassment due to continuous scratching. The most effective conservative treatment is the application of the steroid containing 0·025 per cent. fluocinolone acetonide cream (Synalar, I.C.I.), this is gently massaged into the affected areas three times daily and a mild sedative is given at night as required. This is usually all that is necessary in, for example, post-burn hypertrophic scarring; when true keloid is established or when the hypertrophic scarring affects the face and shows little sign of resolution, then other measures are usually necessary.

Excision alone, with or without a graft may sometimes succeed, but the change of recurrence, especially in the accepted 'danger areas' is so great that this is not recommended.

If excision is the chosen method certain precautions must be observed. The lesion should be completely excised both laterally and in depth; when direct closure is possible without any undue tension a 5/0 continuous intradermal nylon suture is inserted to buttress the wound against transverse stresses and to allow early removal of interrupted sutures. The wound edges are carefully approximated with 6/0 interrupted silk which can be removed in four or five days, the intra dermal suture being left *in situ* for three weeks. On removal of the interrupted sutures 0·1 per cent. triamcinolone Acetonide cream (Adcortyl—U.K., Kenalog, U.S.A.—Squibb) is applied to the suture line three times per day for a minimum period of three months after which time fresh keloid is unlikely to occur.

Several other methods have been advocated but there are objections to most of them.

Triamcinolone acetonide solution 1 to 3 ml may be instilled at the time of excision followed by an injection of this material into the wound at three-weekly intervals (Griffith, 1966). This runs the risk of subdermal atrophy which will be discussed later.

Excision within the confines of the lesion with primary closure or skin graft followed by oral administration of steroids, Dexamethazone 75 mg four times daily for a three-week period together with application of triamcinolone cream (Conway *et al.*, 1960) has the objection of giving oral steroids to children. Similarly excision and suture or graft followed by superficial radiation 800 to 1400 R, has been advocated, sometimes with oral steroid administration.

Fischer and Strock (1957) advised the use of irradiation therapy alone, especially where the lesion is of less than six months duration. In children the recommended course of treatment is X-rays 100 R weekly for four weeks and if necessary after two months two further treatments may be given (Paletta, 1957). Certainly, in adults,

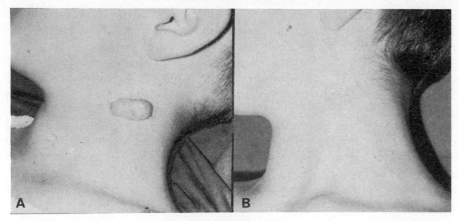

FIG. **38**, 1

This 8 year-old boy formed an area of keloid on the neck following a small burn with the tip of a glowing stick 1 year previously. It was treated with intralesional triamcinolone acetonide weekly injections for 4 weeks. (A) Pre-injection. (B) Post-injection (16 weeks).

this type of therapy may be effective in a proportion of cases. One is extremely reluctant, however, to use X-rays in children because of the hazard, albeit perhaps theoretical, to growing tissues, in particular the skeletal, haemopoetic and reticulo-endothelial systems.

In the writer's view the method of choice, especially for large keloids anywhere, or lesions of any size in 'danger areas' and certainly initially in facial lesions is the intralesional injection of steroid. Initially ACTH was used but now triamcinolone acetonide is preferred. This will accelerate resolution in the majority of scars with flattening and softening; symptoms are invariably relieved. These findings (Fig. **38**, 1) agree with other published reports (Murray, 1963; Griffiths, 1966).

Method

In the very young child under general anaesthesia, using a 23 or 25 gauge needle, as much triamcinolone acetonide aqueous suspension 10 mg/ml (Adcortyl—U.K., Kenalog—U.S.A.—Squibb) as possible, until the whole area is blanched, is injected into the lesion taking great care to stay within its confines both laterally and in depth. The initial injection is difficult because of the rigidity of the fibrous tissue but becomes progressively easier with subsequent injections. Considerable pain results from the injections and it is for this reason that a general anaesthetic is given. In older children it is possible to anaesthetise the area with Xylocaine and then inject a mixture of triamcinolone and local anaesthetic which has the effect of counteracting any post injection pain which may cause problems to the parents. A recent advance has been the use of the Dermojet (A. D. Krauth, Hamburg) which introduces monitored 0·1 ml doses to a depth of 0·5 mm below the epidermis. With this a mixture of tri-amcinolone and Xylocaine can be administered even to children of two or three years without any form of anaesthetic, the procedure being remarkably pain free although the child should be reassured about the noise of the trigger.

The lesion is injected weekly for one month and the course may be repeated a second, and if necessary a third time at six to eight week intervals. A word of caution must be introduced here. Should any triamcinolone be injected outwith the confines of the keloid then atrophy may result, the severity increasing directly with the depth of injection: this may also occur if a large dosage is delivered into a small area, regardless of depth. A concave scar is produced which extends beyond the boundaries of the keloid, the overlying epidermis is thinned and there may be hyperpigmentation. This phenomena has been described as a complication of intralesion steroid given for other conditions, e.g. psoriasis (Fisherman *et al.*, 1962; Schetman *et al.*, 1963). Fortunately as the months pass a gradual improvement occurs but the area will never completely revert to normal. Excision of scars resulting from this set of circumstances should not be approached lightly, all the precautions described earlier must be observed or keloid scarring may recur. Rarely small white nodules which are not 'milia' occur at the injection site but disappear in a few months.

The exact mechanism by which triamcinolone acts is not known but it has been suggested that it interferes in some way with protein syntheses thus interrupting collagen formation.

PROPHYLAXIS

This must be considered both before and after any skin injury occurs. Incisions in children should not, if possible, be made across natural crease lines; lesions in 'danger areas' should not be excised unless absolutely necessary although one should remember that unlike adults all areas are potentially dangerous in children. Where a child has formed a keloid previously any further skin incisions should be avoided.

If surgery is to be performed in 'danger areas' or in 'keloid formers' or where there is a burn or ulcer which does not heal within three weeks, or a donor site of over 15 thousandths of an inch thick prophylactic measures should be undertaken. Areas which do not heal within three weeks should be grafted, if they are too small or this is not possible for some other reason then they, like the other skin wounds described above, should have 1 per cent. triamcinolone acetonide cream applied three times daily for three months; this is commenced before or immediately after healing has occurred or sutures have been removed. In the lower limb a heavy elastic bandage of the Bisgaard type when the patient is out of bed may be of help, used for a period of two to three months.

Absorption of steroid applied to the skin for a long period may occur with a rise of 17 hydroxy corticosteroids in the plasma, a fall in the 17 ketosteroids in the urine and a fall in the circulating eosinophils; these changes are minimal, however, and no systemic upset has ever been recorded (Scroggins and Kliman, 1965).

I. T. JACKSON

REFERENCES

CONWAY, H., GILLETTE, R., SMITH, J. W. & FINDLEY, A. (1960). Differential diagnosis of keloids and hypertrophic scars by tissue culture technique with notes on therapy of keloids by surgical excision and Decadron. *Plastic reconstr. Surg.* **25**, 117.
FISCHER, E. & STROCK, H. (1957). Roentgen therapy of keloid. *Schweiz med. Wschr.* **87**, 1281.

FISHERMAN, E. W., FEINBERG, A. R., FEINBERG, S. M. (1962). Local subcutaneous atrophy. *J. Am. med. Ass.* **179**, 971.

GARB, J. & STONE, M. J. (1942). Keloids: review of literature and report of eighty cases. *Am. J. Surg.* **58**, 315.

GRIFFITH, B. H. (1966). The treatment of keloids with triacinolone acetonide. *Plastic reconstr. Surg.* **38**, 202.

MURRAY, R. D. (1963). Kenalog and the treatment of hypertrophied scars and keloids in negroes and whites. *Plastic reconstr. Surg.* **31**, 275.

OHMORI, S. (1966). The problem of keloid formation in burns in Japan. In *Transactions of the Second International Congress on Research in Burns*, p. 205. Ed. Wallace, A. B. & Wilkinson, A. W. Edinburgh: Livingstone.

PALETTA, F. X. (1967). *Pediatric Plastic Surgery*, Vol. 1, p. 228. St. Louis: Mosby.

SCHETMAN, D., HAMBRICK, G. W. & WILSON, C. E. (1963). Cutaneous changes following local injection of Triamcinolone. *Archs Derm.* **88**, 820.

SCROGGINS, R. B. & KLIMAN, B. (1965). Percutaneous absorption of corticosteroids. *New Engl. J. Med.* **273**, 831.

CHAPTER XXXIX

SCLERODERMA

Scleroderma is a rare disease of connective tissue which apparently involves only those of the caucasian race. This disorder occurs most frequently in the female (3 to 1) and is usually first noted in the second decade of life.

Visceral manifestations such as cardiac failure, pulmonary fibrosis, liver or renal failure, result in death in approximately 50 per cent. of patients. Often the first evidence of systemic symptoms is related to atony of the gut with difficulty in swallowing. Authorities suggest auto-immunization may be the basic disease abnormality.

The skin is affected severely. Interstitial oedema is first noted in such areas as the presternal region or extensor surface of the fingers where little subcutaneous tissue is present. Protein metabolism of the ground substance is abnormal with fibroblasts forming increased collagen. Collagen fibrils show fibrinoid degeneration; dermal appendages atrophy; vessel support to the area diminishes with thrombosis and fibroblastic replacement (Fig. **39**, 1). Elastic tissue fibres disappear. This disorder frequently will follow segmental peripheral nerve distribution especially in the ulnar nerve and fifth cranial nerve regions. Underlying structures, i.e. muscle, fat and bone, atrophy because of overlying skin tightness and pressure necrosis. Calcinosis will often be seen in the chronically involved areas of severe skin change. Bone shows the degeneration typical of prolonged ischaemia with severe osteoporosis developing.

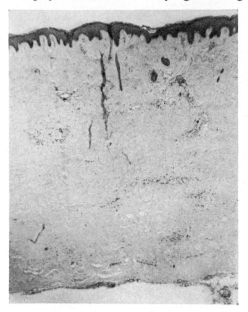

FIG. **39**, 1

A microphotograph of skin involved by scleroderma. Note the absence of dermal appendages, decreased blood vessels, and extensive fibroblastic infiltration. No calcification is present, but this is frequently seen in similar areas. Subcutaneous tissue in this specimen was completely absent.

Tongue function may become severely compromised by fibrosis of the lingual musculature. Malocclusion develops secondarily, and occasionally a marked thickening of the periodontal membrane, especially in the molar region, may occur. It becomes difficult to open the mouth because of facial skin tightening, secondary ankylosis of the temporomandibular joint, and tongue changes. Frequently the oral mucous membrane is atrophic and thickened.

Sjögren's syndrome with diminished secretion of the parotid and facial glands may result in dryness and atrophy of the conjunctiva, cornea, nasal and oral mucosa, and all other exocrine glands. Parotid swelling frequently occurs.

In many a rhematoid type of arthritis may be present.

There are three primary types of scleroderma: The *circumscribed* form frequently occurs as plaques, streaks or depressions, and is often initially surrounded by a violacous border (Fig. **39**, 2). These frequently occur on the face. Differentiation from Romberg's hemifacial atrophy may be impossible (Fig. **39**, 3). The streaks usually progress away from the centre, centrifugally. After an initial inflammatory phase, they fade to leave either a depression, atrophic and with little pigmentation, or a linear region of atrophy which often is accompanied by severe disabling contractures and associated fibrosis. This type is most frequently seen in children.

Acrosclerosis usually develops peripherally and progresses centrally. As the name implies a Raynaud's phenomena frequently is the first harbinger of scleroderma. Often arthritis will accompany progression. Skin changes develop as in the circumscribed form.

In the acrosclerotic, attempts to treat the intermittent spasms of the fingers with vasodilators, steroids, and chelating regi-

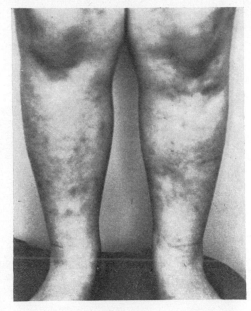

FIG. **39**, 2

The depressed scar-like streaks and plaques on this 22-year-old female remain as evidence of circumscribed scleroderma which first was noted at the age of 13 years. No other disorders have been seen.

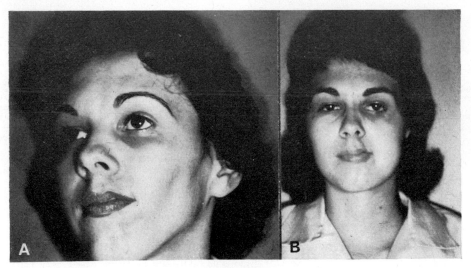

FIG. **39**, 3

(A) The left hemifacial atrophy which was first noted in this 23-year old X-ray technician at the age of 10 years, slowly progressed to this deformity by the age of 16. (B) Reconstruction of the lost subcutaneous tissue of the left cheek gave her some improvement with the implantation of three segments of silastic rubber. The deficiency of the left upper and lower lip and oral commissure persists.

mens have produced little permanent improvement. Frequently, these will be self-limiting problems. Sympathectomy has been of little value.

If the disorder is of the *severe systemic* type, scleroderma may involve the entire face and other areas and diffuse disease develops involving oesophagus, lung, myocardium, small bowel, kidney, and liver. This fulminating disease may result in death

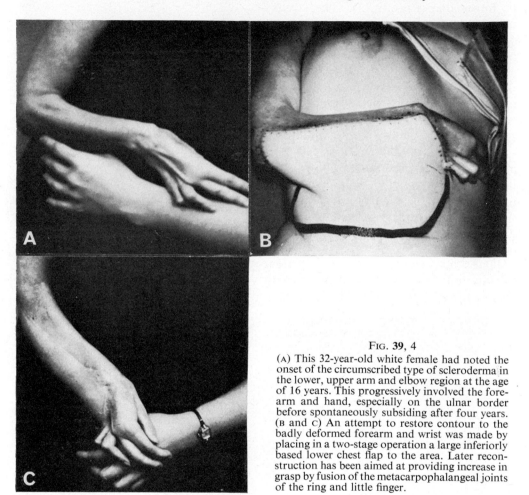

FIG. **39**, 4

(A) This 32-year-old white female had noted the onset of the circumscribed type of scleroderma in the lower, upper arm and elbow region at the age of 16 years. This progressively involved the forearm and hand, especially on the ulnar border before spontaneously subsiding after four years. (B and C) An attempt to restore contour to the badly deformed forearm and wrist was made by placing in a two-stage operation a large inferiorly based lower chest flap to the area. Later reconstruction has been aimed at providing increase in grasp by fusion of the metacarpophalangeal joints of the ring and little finger.

in a few months and 50 per cent of these patients do not survive more than three years. Death is usually caused by uremia, pulmonary fibrosis with pneumonia, congestive heart failure, or generalized cachexia related to gut immobility.

The earliest descriptions of scleroderma were reported in 1634 and 1752. Thirial in 1845 suggested the present name of scleroderma for the collection of symptoms which were noted.

The differential diagnosis of this disorder from such closely allied problems as dermatomyositis, erythematosus disseminata and pseudoscleromatis forms of cutaneous atrophy may be difficult. Dermatomyositis is usually the major alternative possibility with study of a skin biopsy often being inadequate for determining the diagnosis. The clinical course is important.

It is not the purpose of this review to discuss treatment of the systemic or visceral problems. Despite much research in this field, no major advances have been made.

The plastic surgeons' efforts for improvement are related to excision of skin and soft tissues contractures of the extremities and replacement with appropriate pedicle tissue to prevent as much as possible limitation of growth and development, breakdown and ulceration of severely damaged skin in areas of weight bearing and to improve circulation. Restoration of some function, especially in the hand, by excision of contractured diseased tissue, and fusion of bony parts to provide good position of remaining hand elements is attempted (Fig. **39**, 4). It is our feeling that the increased circulation brought into damaged areas by pedicle flap tissue inhibits the development of further contractures and enhances circulation of adjacent skin and subcutaneous structures.

In cases of hemifacial atrophy reconstruction using dermal pedicle flaps or synthetic implants has been successful (see Chap. XVIII). Subcutaneous injection of dimethyl polysiloxane fluids may prove valuable (see Chap. XVII). In those unfortunate patients with severe drying of the eyes, to prevent corneal scarring, parotid duct transfer may be indicated, but careful evaluation of parotid function should be made prior to such transfer. Fibrosis as seen in Mikulicz disease may involve the parotid.

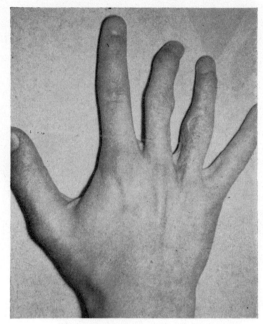

Fig. **39**, 5

The ring and middle fingers of the right hand of this 16-year-old school boy were involved by scleroderma at the age of 9. Because of progressive contracture on the ulnar side of the middle finger and radial side of the ring finger the contracting areas were excised and replaced with full thickness grafts at the age of 13. No progression of deformity has occurred. The full thickness grafts remained supple. There has been no evidence of systematic symptoms. The excision of the contracted, diseased tissue and replacement with full thickness grafts in this instance appeared to arrest the progressive course of the localized circumscribed form of scleroderma.

Multiple Z-plasties of a constricting band of the digits (ainhium) may be performed for small contractures, but for areas involving major portions of the extremity, wide excision and pedicle flap reconstruction is necessary. Full thickness grafts to the hand in which fibrotic syndactyly is beginning to develop have been successful in arresting the course of the disease in one instance with a six-year follow-up (Fig. **39**, 5).

Long-term evaluation of these patients is mandatory for the development of other manifestations of the disease, as well as treatment of further contractures that may occur with growth in children. Muscle balancing procedures with tendon transfers or

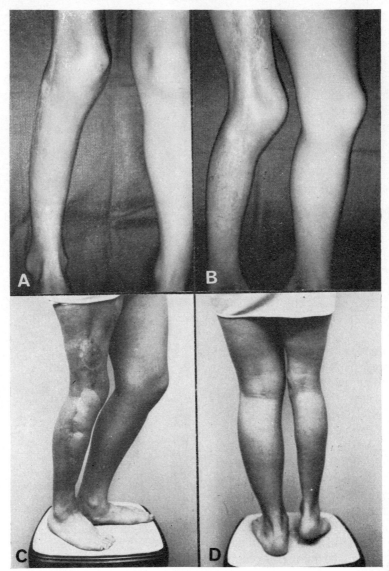

FIG. **39**, 6

(A and B) This 13-year-old girl developed scleroderma at the age of 6, involving the lower lateral thigh and calf. (C and D) The contracture progressed until a pedicle flap obtained from the abdomen was used to replace the diseased tissue. A marked decrease in growth and development of the extremity is demonstrated.

fusions in both the upper and lower extremities to provide appropriate function may be needed.

Until some definitive evidence is available as to the aetiology of this disorder we are limited to treating the results of the severe skin changes. It is our impression that early treatment of these manifestations seems to halt the progressive course (Fig. **39**, 6).

The rareness of the disorder has prevented any one group of plastic surgeons from obtaining a great personal experience to determine if this approach is the most valid one.

J. E. ADAMSON, C. E. HORTON AND R. A. MLADICK

REFERENCES

COBURN, R. F. & SCHMID, F. R. (1960). Progressive systemic sclerosis. *Q. Bull. N. West. Univ. med. Sch.* **34**, 49.

CRAMER, L. M. (1961). The management of the extravisceral manifestations of scleroderma. *Plastic reconstr. Surg.* **28**, 166–180.

LIPSCOMB, P. R., SIMONS, G. W. & WINKELMAN, R. K. (1969). Surgery for sclerodactylia of the hand. *J. Bone Jt Surg.* **51A**, 1112–1117.

LONGACRE, J. J. & WAGNER, E. A. (1952). The surgical management of disabling contractures due to linear scleroderma. *Plastic reconstr. Surg.* **9**, 369.

SCOPP, I. W. & SCHLAGEL, E. (196?) Scleroderma: its orofacial manifestations. *Oral Surg.* **15**, 1510–1514.

CHAPTER XL

UNRECOGNIZED TRAUMA IN INFANTS AND CHILDREN
(The Battered Baby Syndrome)

In 1957, Caffey published an article entitled 'Some traumatic lesions in growing bones other than fractures and dislocations', in which he stated this to be the least well known and the most abused subject in the entire field of paediatrics and radiology. In both Britain and America the problem is being recognized with increasing frequency and is now referred to as the 'battered baby syndrome'. The title is unfortunate in that it suggests injury produced by direct trauma in the form of blows or by striking the child against a static object. Such a mode of aggression will usually produce frank flat or long bone fractures and skin lesions, which are easily recognized. The common type of lesion is less easily recognized and may be missed.

The injury is produced by a severe shaking or twisting type of violence, causing metaphyseal fractures of long bones and slipping of the epiphyses. Either the upper or the lower limbs may be involved. The infant is brought to hospital because of

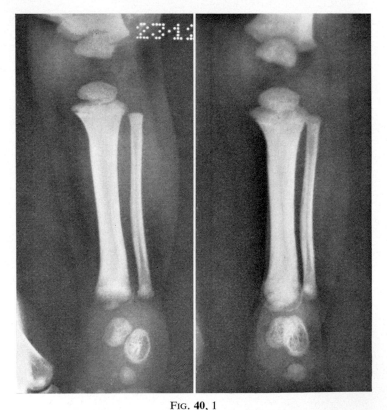

FIG. **40**, 1

(A) Minimal juxto-epiphyseal lesion of lower tibia when patient first seen.
(B) Radiographic appearances two weeks later. Increased calcification and subperiosteal new bone formation extending up shaft of tibia.

swelling of a limb, with a history of screaming when the limb is touched or because of failure to move the limb. A history of trauma is usually unobtainable. The syndrome may be seen at any age, but in general affected children are less than 3 years old. The general health is often poor, there is evidence of neglect—particularly poor skin hygiene—and there may be soft tissue injuries. I have never seen injuries of the facial bones nor lesions requiring the skilled services of a plastic surgeon. Examination may reveal evidence of old bruising suggestive of previous abuse of the child but the diagnosis is made by radiographic examination. The typical lesion is a small metaphyseal fracture which can be easily overlooked at an early stage unless the X-ray plate is carefully studied. The corroborative evidence is a small juxta-epiphyseal flake avulsed from the main body of the bone with the displaced epiphysis (Fig. **40**, 1A); within two weeks, subperiosteal new bone formation makes the diagnosis obvious (Fig. **40**, 1B). The lesions, though apparently minimal on X-ray, are by no means innocuous since if untreated, residual deformity may result.

Subdural haematoma with or without fracture of the skull is a frequent finding.

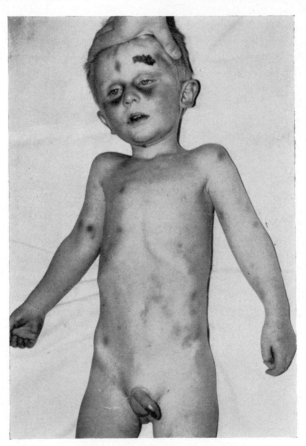

FIG. **40**, 2

Bruising of face, shoulder, arms, body and penis in abused infant.

Early recognition is of great importance since it may save the child from further injury or even death. Full radiographic examination of the child is desirable. Injury to internal organs can follow a blow on the chest or abdomen. Patients are sometimes admitted to a medical ward with a diagnosis of 'purpura' which is not reacting to vitamin supplements and the diagnosis is usually more obvious. The lesions are often linear and concentrated in clusters on the trunk, shoulders or buttocks (Fig. **40**, 2). Other lesions are due to tooth marks, cigarette burns and so-called ammoniacal dermatitis affecting the buttocks, thighs and calves. Like the bone lesions, the skin lesions may have been inflicted at different times and may be difficult to differentiate from lesions incurred by an accident or during play.

Immediate admission to hospital is important in any case of suspected 'battering', both to protect the child and to make a complete diagnosis. The family doctor who knows what to look for may be the first person to suspect the sort of family trouble which may lead to the types of injuries which have been described and sympathetic intervention may be all-important in saving the child from further injury.

While physical assaults by parents or guardians on helpless children are rightly regarded as criminal acts, it is not always wise to invoke the might of the law without knowledge of the underlying cause or causes of the assault. A long-term prison sentence may appease society's rage but it breaks up the family, imposes further social and economic problems and does little to reform the offender. The social service departments, the societies for prevention of cruelty to children, doctors and nurses all have their parts to play, but in many centres not enough use is made of the services of the department of child psychiatry.

It is important that the different manifestations of the syndrome should be recognized by both physicians and surgeons and all those whose work brings them into contact with children.

W. M. DENNISON

REFERENCES

British Medical Journal (1966). The Battered Baby, **1**, 601.
CAFFEY, J. (1946). *J. Pediat.* **29**, 541.
CAFFEY, J. (1957). *Br. J. Radiol.* **30**, 225.
SUSSMAN, S. J. (1968). *J. Pediat.* **72**, 99.

INDEX

A

Abbe flap, for lids, 228
  for lips, 21
Acrosclerosis of legs, 567
Acute osteomyelitis of maxilla, 131
Adamson, J. E., 322, 345, 443, 452, 566
Adeno-ameloblastoma, 143
Agenesis of vagina, 437
Alveolar mandibular protrusion, 56
Ameloblastic fibroma of jaw, 143
Ameloblastoma (adamantinoma) of jaw, 142
Angular dermoid, 231
Ankyloglossia (tongue tie), 121
Anlage-induced jaw deformities, 50
Annular grooves, of hands, 481
  of legs, 509
Anophthalmus, 232, 236
Apert's disease, 46, 73, 238, 254
Aplasia, vaginal, 438, 441
Arms, deformities of, 463
Arthrogryposis, 498
Athelia, female, 453
  male, 458
Atresia of nose, 261
Auricle, anatomy of, 274
  construction of, 276–291
  deformities of, 274–313
  loss of cartilage of, 305
  loss of skin of, 304
  traumatic deformities of, 304
Avulsion of teeth, 158
Axillary contracture, 502

B

Barsky, A. J., 463, 509
'Battered' baby syndrome, 572
Bell's phenomenon, 317
'Bent fingers' (clinodactyly), 499
Bifid nose, 268
Bifid tongue, 124
Bilateral cleft lip, 6, 14
Bilateral microtia, 291
'Bird-face' condition, 59
'Bird-face' deformity, 174
'Bird-face' profile, 193
Birth injuries, 178
Bladder exstrophy, 427
Bladder neck correction in epispadias, 432
Bone grafts, of face, 192
  of palate, 4, 9, 26, 45
Bony dysplasias of face, 148
Brachydactyly, 479
Branchial arch syndrome, 35, 75, 291
Branchial cleft anomalies, 366
Branchial cyst, 365, 368
Branchial sinus and fistula, 365, 367

Branchiogenic anomalies, 364
Branchiogenic carcinoma, 121
Breast, female, 452
  absence of, 453
  hypoplasia of, 453
  trauma of, 456, 459
  tumours of, 453, 455
Breast, male, 458
  tumours of, 459
Buccal mucosa, 126
Burns, 531
  damage due to, 547
  electrical, 559
  fluid replacement of, 537
  hypertrophic scarring of, 550
  infection of, 534, 546
  mortality of, 550
  of face, 551
  of hands, 553
  of lips, 111
  of neck, 552
  psychological effects of, 549
  scar contractures of, 558
  systemic effects of, 534
Burston, W. R., 37

C

Calcifying epithelial tumour of jaw, 143
Camptodactyly, 499
Cancrum oris, 112, 128
Capillary haemangioma, 519, 523
Carcinoma. *See* Tumours
Cauliflower ear, 304
Cellulitis, around mandible, 130
  orbital, 176
Cerebral meningocele, 348
Cervical cystic thymus, 372
Cervicofacial lymphadenitis, 131
Cherubism, 150
Chordee, 401, 408, 422
  without hypospadias, 404
Choristoma, 372
Cleft lip, 1
  bilateral, 6, 14
  classification of, 2
  embryology of, 2
  median, 33
  orthodontics of, 5, 37
  primary closure of, 9
    using bone graft, 4, 9
  repair technique of, Le Mesurier, 9
    Millard, 10
    Stellmach, 11
    Tennison, 10
  secondary soft tissue correction of, 19
  unilateral, 6, 9

Cleft palate, 1, 8, 16
  bone grafting of (late), 26, 45
  classification of, 2
  embryology of, 2
  operations of, 8, 16
  orthodontics of, 5, 37
Clefts, of alveolus, 2
  of cranium, 238
  of face, 3, 33, 94
  of foot, 511
  of hand, 511
  of lower lip, 3
  of nose, 3, 268
  oro-orbital, 34, 94
  transverse, of face, 34
  vertical, of face, 34, 94
Clinodactyly ('bent fingers'), 499
Club hand (talipomanus), 500
Coloboma of eyelid, 94, 98, 225
Composite grafts of auricle, 193
Concha, construction of, 287
Condylar hyperplasia, 63
Converse, J. M., 178, 248, 274
Coup de sabre, 326
Cranial nerve paralysis, 314, 323
Craniofacial dysostosis, 254
Craniofacial osteotomy, 248
Craniofacial synostosis, 73
Craniostosis, 238
Cranium bifidum, 348
Crouzon's disease, 46, 73, 238, 254
Cryptocia, 300
Cup ears ('shell' ears), 300
Cystic dysplasia of thyroid, 528
Cystic hygroma, 129, 373, 526
Cystic lesions of jaw, 134
Cystosarcoma phyllodes, 454
Cysts, dental, 135
  dentigerous, 136
  developmental, of jaws, 136
  eruption of, 134
  mucous, 115, 129
  of jaws, 134
  of neck, 373
  primordial, 138

D

Dennison, W. M., 176, 381, 526, 572
Dental cyst, 135
Dental lesions, 130, 132
Dentigerous cysts, 136
Dento-alveolar abscess, 130
Dermal sinus, 451
Dermoid, angular, 231
Dermoid cyst, of neck, 377
  of nose, 263
  of tongue, 125
Developmental cysts of jaw, 136

Developmental disturbance of facial bones, 171, 178
Developmental malformations, of face, 189
  of jaw, 46–93
Distichiasis, 230
Dogbites, 110
Double eyelashes, 230
Down's syndrome, 176
Drooling, 124
Dysostosis, craniofacial, 254
  mandibulofacial, 74, 98
  otomandibular, 75
Dysplasia, 148
  white, of buccal mucosa, 145

E

Ears, 274–313
  See also Auricles
Ectodermal tumours of head and neck, 120
Ectopic ear tissue, 367
Ectrodactyly, of finger, 483
  of thumb, 491
Ectrosyndactyly, 425
Elbow, contractures of, 507
Electrical burns, of face, 559
  of lips, 111
Encephalocele, 348
Encephalopathy in burns, 548
Endosteal carcinoma, primary, of jaw, 143
Eosinophilic granuloma of jaw, 152
Epiblepharon, 214
Epicanthus, 207, 212
Epidermoid carcinoma of mouth, 119, 121
Epispadias, 427
  treatment of, 429
Epithelioma of Malherbe, 377
Epulides, 132
Epulis, congenital, 145
Eruption cyst of jaw, 134
Evans, A. J., 531
Exstrophy, of bladder, 427
Eye, 207–237
  congenital absence of, 232
  See also Orbital region
Eyelid, coloboma of, 98, 225

F

Face, burns of, 551
  fractures of bones of, 161, 180
  haemangioma of, 337
  hemi-atrophy of, 326, 332
  hemihypertrophy of, 337
  injuries of, 178–206
  lymphangioma of, 339
  paralysis of, 314
Facial bone, developmental disturbance of, 171
  fractures of, 161, 180
Facial clefts, 3, 94

Facial paralysis, 314, 322
Facial scars, reconstructive surgery of, 191
Familial white folded dysplasia, 145
Feet, deformities of, 509
Female hermaphroditism, 445
Female hypospadias, 404
Fibromatosis gingivae, 146
Fibro-osseous neoplasm of jaws, 146
Fibrosarcoma of face, 119
Fibrous epulis, 133
First branchial arch syndrome, 75
Flame burns of lips, 111
Floating thumb (pouce flottant), 492
Fogh-Andersen, P., 437
Foreshortened nose, 202
Fractures, le Fort type, 170, 185, 188
  of facial bones, 161, 180
  of maxilla, 185
  of nose, 185
  of orbital floor, 188
  of teeth, 154, 157
  of zygoma, 188
Francesconi, G., 261
Francheschetti syndrome, 74, 98
Frenulum of lip, 108

G

Giant cell epulis, 133
Giant cell granuloma of jaw, 147
Giant fibroadenoma of breast, 454
Giant hairy naevus, 514, 517
Giantism, of face, 339
  of limb, 519
Giantomastia, 453
Gibson, T., 514, 519
Glioma of nose, 251, 267
Globulomaxillary cysts, 136
Glossitis, 122
Glossoptosis, 121
Granular-cell myoblastoma of tongue, 126
Granuloma, eosinophilic, of jaw, 152
Granulomatous epulis, 132
Gum-boil, 132
Gums, tumour of, 146
Gynaecomastia, 458

H

Haemangioma, 519, 528
  capillary, 519
  cavernous, 522
  of face, 337
  of fingers, 519
  of jaw, 138
  of lip, 106, 117
  of nose, 264
  of tongue, 126
Haemangiopericytoma of face, 119
Haematogenous osteitis of maxilla, 176

Haematoma, peri-orbital, 176
Hallux varus, 511
Hamartoma of jaw, 138
Hands, burns of, 553
  cleft, 486
  club, 500
  deformities of, 463
  five-fingered, 494
Hand-Schüller-Christian's disease, 152
Hare lip, 1
  See also Cleft lip
Head, tumours of, 118
Hemi-absence of nose, 267, 270
Hemi-atrophy of face, 326, 332
Hemigiantism of face, 337
Hemihypertrophy, of face, 337
  of tongue, 122
Hereditary fibromatosis gingivae, 146
Hermaphroditism, 443
Histiocytosis, 'X' of jaws, 152
Hodgkin's disease, 120
Homografts in burns, 544
Horton, C. E., 322, 345, 396, 443, 452, 566
Hydrocephalus, 352, 383
Hymen, imperforate, 438
Hyperplasia, condylar, 63
Hypertelorism, 238, 248, 251
Hypertrophic scarring, 191, 550, 561
Hypertrophy, virginal, of breast, 453
Hypomastia, 453
Hypoplasia, of mandible, 121
  of nasomaxilla, 195
  of tongue, 121
Hypospadias, 396
  'cripples', 404
  embryology of, 400
  female, 404
  incidence and classification of, 399
  pathological anatomy of, 401
  repair techniques of, Browne, 408
    Byars, 410
    Cecil, 411
    Horton-Devine, 413
    Mustardé, 421

I

Imperforate hymen, 438
Incisive papilla cysts, 136
Infection, Ludwig's angina, 126
  meningococcal, 114
  of burns, 534
  of jaw, 130
  of lips, 112
Injuries. See Trauma
Intersex, 444
Intracranial tumours, 118
Intra-oral tumours, 119
Intra-osseous nasopalatine cysts, 136

J

Jackson, I. T., 561
Jaw deformities, acquired, 46, 78
    ankylosis-induced mandibular micrognathism,
      78
    following cleft lip and palate repair, 79
    following irradiation injuries, 79
    postoperative, 89
    post-traumatic, 79
  aetiology of, 46
  anlage-induced, 46, 50
    aetiology, 50
    alveolar mandibular protrusion, 56
    'bird-face' condition, 59
    combined anomalies, 72
    macroglossia, 72
    mandibular asymmetry, 61
    mandibular protrusion, 52, 71
    mandibular retrusion, 58
    maxillary protrusion, 66
    microgenia, 57
    micromaxillism, 69
    open-bite, 64
    orthodontics in, 50
    prognathism, 52
    retromaxillism, 69
    retrusion of maxilla, 71
  congenital, 46, 73
    craniofacial synostosis, 73
    first branchial arch syndrome, 75
    mandibulofacial dysostosis, 74
    otomandibular dysostosis, 75
    Pierre Robin syndrome, 73
    Treacher-Collins syndrome, 74
    trismus, 73
  considerations regarding treatment, 47
  indications for treatment, 47
  traumatic lesions of, 154–175, 185
  tumours, 130–153

K

Keloids, 561
Keratodermia, 112

L

Laceration of lip, 108, 109
Le Fort type fracture, 170, 185, 188
Legs, deformities of, 509
Letterer-Siwe disease, 152
Limbs, deformities of, lower, 509
    upper, 463
Lindsay, W. K., 102, 360
Lingual thyroid, 126
Lip(s), 102, 111
  burns of, 111
  carcinoma of, 118
  congenital reduplication of, 106
  congenital soft tissue tumours of, 106

Lip(s)—*contd.*
  cyst of, 115
  fissures of, 112
  frenuli of, 108
  haemangioma of, 117
  infections of, 112
  laceration of, 108, 109
  lymphangioma of, 117, 529
  macrocheilia, 104
  mandibular pits of, 109
  microstoma, 102
  naevi of, 115
  papillomata of, 115
  sarcoma of, 118
  tumours of, 106, 115, 117
  verrucae of, 115
  webs of, 108
Lipoma, 528
Lop ear, 292, 305
Ludwig's angina, 126
Lymphadenitis, cervicofacial, 131
Lymphangioma, 526
  of axilla, 529
  of cheeks, 138
  of face, 339, 529
  of lips, 106, 117, 529
  of mouth, 129, 138, 373
  of neck, 529
  of tongue, 126, 138, 529
  other sites of, 530
Lymphoma, 121
Lymphosarcoma of face and jaws, 119, 120, 146

M

Macrocheilia, 104, 526
Macrodactyly, 494, 511
Macroglossia, 72, 121, 526
Macrostoma, 34
Maffuci's syndrome, 519
Male hermaphroditism, 445
Malignant teratoma of mouth, 120, 121
Mandible, deformities of, 46–93
  postnatal growth of, 189
  See also Jaw
Mandibular asymmetry, 61
Mandibular lip pits, 109
Mandibular micrognathism, 78, 193
Mandibular protrusion, 52, 71
  alveolar, 56
  skeletal, 52
Mandibular retrusion, 58
Mandibulofacial dysostosis (Treacher-Collins syn-
    drome), 74
Matthews, D. N., 1
Maxilla, fractures of, 185
  osteitis of, 131, 176
  protrusion of, 66, 88
  retrusion of, 71, 88
  tumours of, 119, 146

Maxillary osteotomy in cleft palate, 31
Median cleft lip, 33
Median dysraphia of face, 268
Median mandibular cyst, 136
Meningocele, 348, 382, 386
Meningococcaemia, 114
Meningomyelocele, 353, 383, 387
Mesodermal lesions of lips and tongue, 117, 126
Metastatic neoplasms of jaws, 147
Microgenia, 57
Microglossia, 121
Micrognathia, 1, 19, 73, 122, 193
Micrognathism, ankylosis-induced, mandibular, 78
Macromaxillism, 69
Microphthalmos, 232
Microstoma, 102
Microtia, 275, 291
Millard, R. D., 10, 20, 26
Mladick, R. A., 322, 345, 443, 452, 566
Möbius syndrome, 315
Monodactyly, 492
Mouth, infection of, 127
    tuberculous lesions of, 134
    tumours of, 129
    ulcers of, 114
Mustardé, J. C., 37, 202, 207, 251, 306, 337, 386, 410, 421
Myelocele, 383, 389
Myelomeningocele. *See* Meningomyelocele

N

Naevi, pigmented, 514
Naevus flammeus, 519
Nasal encephalocele, 265
Nasal fractures, 185
Nasal glioma, 267
Nasal reduction, 31
Nasolabial cysts, 136
Nasomaxillary complex, hypoplasia of, 195
    postnatal growth of, 190
Naso-orbital fractures, 185
Naso-orbital osteotomy, 197
Nasopharyngeal sarcoma, 121
Neck, branchiogenic anomalies of, 364
    burns of, 552
    dermoid cyst of, 377
    fissure and sinus of, 363
    haemangioma of, 376
    lymphangioma of, 373
    tumours of, 118, 373
    webbed, 360
    wry (torticollis), 361
Neoplasms. *See* Tumours
Neuroblastoma of face and neck, 119
Neurofibroma, of face, 341
    of lip, 106
    of tongue, 126
Neurofibromatosis, 146, 341
Nipple, absence of, female, 453

Nipple—*contd.*
    male, 458
Nixon, H. H., 447
Noma, 112, 128
Nose, atresia of, 261
    bifid, 268
    deformities of, 22
    dermoid cyst of, 263
    foreshortening of, 202
    haemangioma of, 264
    hemi-absence of, 267, 270

O

Oblique facial clefts, 94
Obwegeser, H. L., 46
Odontogenic fibroma, 143
Odontogenic myxoma, 145
Odontomes, 140
Open-bite conditions, 64
Oral ulceration, 114
Orbital cellulitis, 176
Orbital floor fractures, 188
Orbital region, abnormalities of, 207–237
Orbitofacial fissures, 94
Oro-orbital clefts, 34, 94
Orthodontics, in cleft lip and palate, 5, 37
    in jaw deformities, 49, 50
Osteitis of maxilla, 131, 176
Osteomyelitis (osteitis) of maxilla, 131, 176
Otohaematoma, 304
Otomandibular dysostosis (first and second branchial arch syndrome), 35, 75, 291

P

Palsy of face. *See* Paralysis
Papillomata of face and mouth, 115, 129
Paralysis, of cranial nerves, 323
    of face, 314, 322
Parotid tumour, 120
Penile correction in epispadias, 430
Penis, anomalies of, 396, 427
Perichondritis of ear, 304
Periostitis of jaw, 133
Pharyngoplasty, 23
Phocomelia, 502
Pierre Robin syndrome, 1, 19, 73
    treatment of, 122, 193
Pigmented naevi, 514
Pigmented tumour of jaw, 145
Pitanguy, I., 332
Plasmacytoma of neck, 121
Polydactyly, 472, 509
Polymastia, female, 452
    male, 458
Postnatal pits, 451
Pouce flottant (floating thumb), 492
Premaxilla, displaced, 6, 45, 82
Primordial cysts of jaw, 138

Proboscis, lateral, of nose, 34, 267, 273
Prognathism (skeletal mandibular protrusion), 52
Prolabium lengthening, Matthews, 20
  Millard, 20
Prominent ears, 292, 306
Psaume syndrome, 108, 124
Pseudohermaphroditism, 441, 443
Pterygium colli, 360
Ptosis, 214
  operations for, 216
Purpura fulminans, 114
Pyogenic granuloma of lip, 112
Pyramidal naso-orbitomaxillary osteotomy, 197

R

Ranula, 126
Raynaud's phenomenon, 567
von Recklinghausen's disease (neurofibromatosis
    of face), 341
Rees, T. D., 326
Reticulum-cell sarcoma of mouth, 119
Retinoblastoma, 118
Retromaxillism, 69
Rhabdomyosarcoma of face and mouth, 119,
    146
Rhinoschisis, 269
Rickham, P. P., 348, 352
Ring constrictions, 481, 509
Rogers, B. O., 314
Rowe, L. N., 130, 154

S

Sacrococcygeal teratoma, 447
Sarcoma of lip, 117
Scalds, 513
  See also Burns
Scalp, congenital defects of, 345
Scar, contractures in burns, 558
  hypertrophic, 561
  keloid, 561
Scleroderma, 566
  differential diagnosis of, 568
Sexual definition, 443
'Shell' ears, 300
Sjögren's syndrome, 566
Skeletal mandibular protrusion (prognathism), 52
Skin graft, of burns, 542
  of ear lobe, 284
  of face, 192
Sling operations of face, 224
Spider naevus, 519
Spina bifida, 381, 386
  cystica, 382
  occulta, 381, 386
  surgical treatment of, 386
Sternocleidomastoid muscle in facial paralysis,
    322
Stomatitis, gangrenous, 112, 128

Strawberry naevus, 519, 523
Sturge-Weber syndrome, 519
Sub-oribriform intercraniofacial osteotomy, 246
Subluxation of teeth, 158
Switch flap, 21, 228
Syndactyly, 465, 509
Synostosis, craniofacial, 73
Syringomyelocele, 383

T

Talipomanus, 500
Teeth, avulsion of, 155, 158
  fractures of, 155, 157
  subluxation of, 158
  trauma of, 130, 132, 154
  treatment of, 164
Telecanthus, 207, 213, 239
Teratoma, malignant, of mouth, 120, 147
  of premaxilla, 111
  sacrococcygeal, 447
Tessier, P., 94, 238, 254, 532
Thermal injury, 532
Thumb, floating, 492
Thyroglossal duct cyst, 369
Thyroid carcinoma, 119
Toe, macrodactyly of, 511
Tongue, congenital defects of, 121
  injuries of, 125
  tumours of, 125
Tongue tie, 121
Torticollis, 361
Transverse clefts of face, 3, 34
Trauma, of birth, 178
  of breast, 456, 459
  of ear, 304
  of face, 178, 180, 191
  of facial bones, 161, 189
  of facial nerve, 189
  of jaw, 79, 131, 154
  of lips, 110
  of maxilla, 185
  of nose, 185
  of orbital floor, 188
  of soft tissues of face, 179
  of teeth, 130, 154
  unrecognised ('battered' baby syndrome), 572
Treacher-Collins syndrome (mandibulofacial dys-
    ostosis), 74, 98
Triphalangism of thumb, 474
Trismus, congenital, 73
Tuberculous lesions of mouth, 134
Tumours, of breast, female, 453, 455
    male, 459
  of head, 118
  of jaws, 130–153
  of lips, 106, 115, 117
  of mouth, 129
  of neck, 118, 373, 377
  of sacrum, 447

Tumours—*contd.*
  of thyroid, 119
  of tongue, 125

U

Ulcers, of lip, 112
  of mouth, 114
  of scalp, 345
Unilateral cleft lip, 6, 9
Unrecognised trauma ('battered' baby syndrome), 572
Urethra, congenital short, 404
  reconstruction of, 407

V

Vaginal agenesis, 437
Vaginal aplasia, 438
Vaginal septa, 438
Veau-Wardill operation, 8

Verrucae, 115
Vertical facial clefts, 3, 34, 94
Virginal hypertrophy of breast, 453

W

Waardenburg's syndrome, 213
Web, of axilla, 502
  of lips, 108
  of neck, 360
Williams, D. I., 427
Wilms' tumour, secondary, of jaw, 148
Winter, G. B., 130, 154
Wood-Smith, D., 274
Worster Drought syndrome, 124
Wrestler's syndrome, 122
Wry neck (torticollis), 361

Z

Zygoma, 188